Evidence-Based Guide to Difficult Airway Management

Manuel Ángel Gómez-Ríos • André van Zundert
Editors

Evidence-Based Guide to Difficult Airway Management

Springer

Editors
Manuel Ángel Gómez-Ríos
Department of Anesthesiology
and Perioperative Medicine
Complejo Hospitalario Universitario de A Coruña (CHUAC)
A Coruña, Spain

André van Zundert
Department of Anaesthesia and
Perioperative Medicine
Royal Brisbane and Women's Hospital and
The University of Queensland
Brisbane, QLD, Australia

ISBN 978-3-032-30768-2 ISBN 978-3-032-30769-9 (eBook)
https://doi.org/10.1007/978-3-032-30769-9

This Springer imprint is published by the registered company Springer Nature Switzerland AG
The registered company address is: Gewerbestrasse 11, 6330 Cham, Switzerland

Foreword

“Clickbait” rules supreme in the current world, and yes, there’s no lack of information and opinion about airway management available on social media. What’s often lacking in that arena, though, is valid peer review: a sober second opinion on what’s being claimed, no matter the face validity of the “expert” (or how many “likes” they have). Therein lies the value of formally peer-reviewed publications. In the case of a textbook, this responsibility falls largely to the editors, and in *Evidence-Based Guide on Difficult Airway Management*, the reader can rest assured that the editors are world class in their airway pedigrees. Dr. Van Zundert has an extensive track record of research and publication about airway devices—especially supraglottic airways. Editor-in-chief Dr. Gómez-Ríos has been heavily involved in developing airway management guidelines: how to put airway devices to good and safe use, if you will. Collectively, their expertise spans much of the realm of airway management.

I’m happy to report that I know many of the text’s chapter authors personally or by reputation, and I’m privileged to count some as friends as well as professional colleagues. These and other of the text’s authors are regular speakers at national, international, and indeed, world congresses on airway management and/or anesthesia. And with good reason: they’re knowledgeable, they’re well-spoken, and they can eloquently put pen to paper. Perhaps most importantly, though, they’re *enthusiastic* about airway management.

There are many other textbooks on airway management, and especially in the era of search engines and artificial intelligence, it must be asked what exactly a new text of airway management might have to offer. Well, reading this one, the answer is plenty. The reader of this text will be a clinician who recognizes how fast knowledge is evolving and equally how frequently new airway management devices are being introduced. The value of a textbook such as this is that both the foundations of airway management and recent developments can be presented in juxtaposition, thus offering value to early-career and experienced clinicians alike.

We now have good insight into what is causing us trouble in managing patients’ airways, informed by published closed legal claims related to airway management, as well as airway-related morbidity and mortality database studies. The Internet bears further testament to what can go wrong, offering up coroner’s reports of tragic cases, in the public domain. Unfortunately, the areas causing us grief have remained stubbornly persistent over the decades, so it's gratifying to see these themes being addressed in dedicated chapters and being *re-visited* in many other chapters. For example, anchored by an excellent chapter on the topic, video laryngoscopy is a pervasive theme in many (and indeed, most) other chapters throughout this text—emphasizing, for example, its role in increasing first-attempt and overall tracheal intubation success; predictors of difficulty with its use, role in helping avoid unrecognized oesophageal intubation, as well as need for advocacy for its universal use to facilitate all tracheal intubations.

We know that there are substantial "human factors" issues involved in most adverse airway outcomes, yet it's a difficult topic to address well. Talks I've heard on the subject are often entertaining, but I've sometimes struggled to identify take-home points that I can apply the next day to make my patient safer. It's an important subject, and I'm happy to report that it's masterfully handled in the chapter on the topic and that it includes plenty of practical advice.

Human factors are front and center during the often-chaotic management of a cardiac arrest, of course, but another challenge, at least for me, has been to remain current on the latest outcome-based research on how best to manage the airway of an arrested patient. The chapter on this topic is an excellent synthesis of the currently available evidence base.

Ultrasound now helps with almost everything, it seems. It certainly helps identify the location of the cricothyroid membrane before managing an anticipated difficult airway—otherwise often unsuccessful if relying on external palpation. The senior author of the chapter on ultrasound was an early adopter of using ultrasound for this purpose and has continued to write and speak on the technique around the world, often with elegant and practical accompanying instructions and illustrations—as with this chapter. Appropriately, other applications of ultrasound in airway management are also addressed in this and other chapters, as another contemporary theme running through the text.

The chapter on documentation is one of the most comprehensive and well-written pieces I've read on the topic. While perhaps a slightly dry topic in airway management, often relegated to the end of an airway guideline or textbook, given that we now know that one of the best predictors of a difficult airway is a history of previously documented difficulty, it's also one of the most important.

Not a dry topic is airway management of the critically ill patient: regardless of your practice environment, who hasn't had a sick patient who made your heart rate exceed theirs? And with good reason, given a published cardiac arrest rate of 3% or more during airway management in that population. The concept of the "physiologically difficult airway" is relatively new, but arguably, it's low hanging fruit if seeking to decrease airway-related morbidity and mortality. The chapter on airway management in the critically ill patient is very instructive on how to avoid bad outcomes in this population and is written by a master on the topic. Parenthetically, in addressing use of video laryngoscopy in the critically ill patient, this chapter contains my favorite sentence in the entire text, which advises making "purchasing decisions [that] reflect the needs of the most junior operators…rather than idiosyncratic individual preferences of influential senior members of the department." Good advice indeed, and on that note, this quite possibly idiosyncratic and definitely senior writer will sign off. I hope that you enjoy your time reading all the chapters of this very engaging text as much as I did.

Halifax, Canada J. Adam Law

Contents

Editors and Contributors

About the Editors

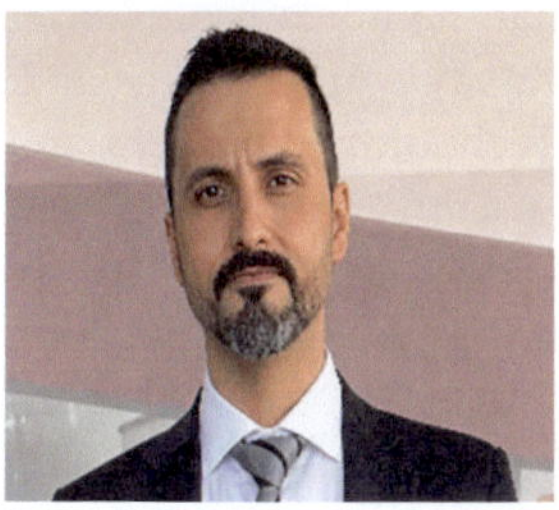

Manuel Ángel Gómez-Ríos, MD, PhD is a senior anesthesiologist, clinical researcher, and academic leader based in A Coruña, Spain. He is internationally recognized for his contributions to airway management, perioperative medicine, and patient safety, with a particular focus on videolaryngoscopy and the integration of human factors into clinical practice.

He works in the Department of Anesthesiology and Perioperative Medicine at the University Hospital Complex of A Coruña. He currently serves as Vice President of the Clinical Management Section of the Spanish Society of Anesthesiology, Resuscitation, and Pain Therapy (SEDAR) and is Co-founder of the Ibero-American Airway Society. He is also affiliated with the Cell Therapy and Regenerative Medicine Group at the University of A Coruña (UDC) and INIBIC and serves as Visiting Professor at Medical University of Łódź (Poland).

Dr. Gómez-Ríos has an extensive academic portfolio, with numerous peer-reviewed publications and active involvement in international collaborations and clinical guideline development. He holds editorial roles in journals such as *BMC Anesthesiology*, *Journal of Clinical Anesthesia*, and the *Spanish Journal of Anesthesiology and Resuscitation* and regularly reviews for high-impact journals.

His research focuses on airway management, perioperative risk assessment, and the application of artificial intelligence in healthcare. He has led and participated in clinical trials and innovative projects.

In addition to his research, he is actively engaged in postgraduate education and mentorship, supervising doctoral and master's students. His work integrates clinical excellence, scientific innovation, and leadership to advance safer, evidence-based anesthesiology worldwide.

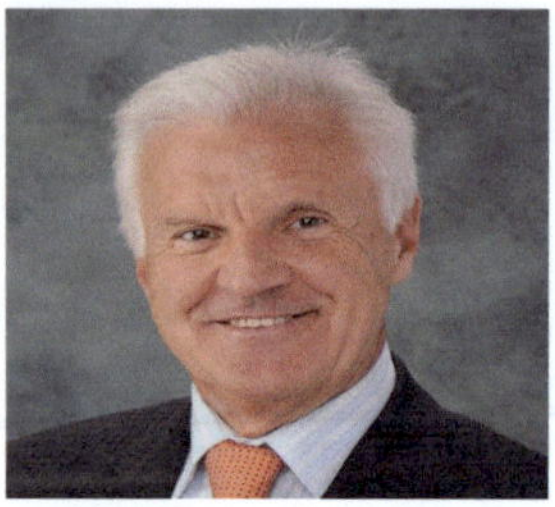

André van Zundert is a double-boarded anesthesiologist-intensivist who worked in Eindhoven, The Netherlands, for 30 years and relocated to Brisbane, QLD, Australia, in 2013, where he was asked to set up an academic department. Besides working at the Royal Brisbane and Women's Hospital, he holds professorial appointments at the University of Queensland, Queensland University of Technology, Queensland Brain Institute, and Udayana University (Denpasar, Indonesia). Recently, he was honored to lead the newly established "André van Zundert Research and Education Center" at the Shenzhen Institute of Advanced Technology and the Chinese Academy of Sciences.

Professor van Zundert's scholarly output includes some 150 airway-related scientific publications (out of a total of 550), including world guidelines on videolaryngoscopy. He is recognized as one of the "top ten world experts in airway management," contributing to the revolution in airway management. He is one of the foundational figures of videolaryngoscopy, moving the speciality "from mirrors to monitors." By championing the transition from "blind" clinical techniques to "vision-guided" precision, he achieved a monumental leap in patient safety. His clinical vision further led to the introduction of videolaryngeal mask airways into routine practice, providing clinicians with unprecedented control and positioning accuracy during difficult airway management.

In addition, Professor van Zundert pioneered safety in obstetric and regional anesthesia. The formula he proposed for safe and effective pain relief during childbirth is now a staple of clinical practice worldwide. He is one of the founders of the combined spinal-epidural regional anesthesia and introduced the segmental thoracic spinal anesthesia technique. Beyond clinical tools, Professor van Zundert is at the forefront of unravelling the molecular mechanisms of general anesthesia, including researching new reversal agents that counteract general anesthetics. His scientific work has been recognized by dozens of (inter)national awards. He supervised more than 50 PhD-Doctorates, which he considers his most important legacy.

Contributors

Carlos A. Artime Department of Anesthesiology, Critical Care, and Pain Medicine, McGovern Medical School at UTHealth Houston, Houston, TX, USA

Vassilis Athanassoglou Nuffield Department of Anaesthetics, Oxford University Hospitals, Oxford, UK

Lauren C. Berkow Division of Neuroanesthesia, University of Florida College of Medicine, Gainesville, FL, USA

Matthew Bigwood East Lancashire Hospitals, Lancashire, England, UK

Jon Blackshaw Liverpool Head and Neck Centre, Liverpool University Hospitals NHS Foundation Trust, Liverpool, UK

David J. Brewster School of Translational Medicine, Faculty of Medicine, Nursing and Health Science, Monash University, Melbourne, VIC, Australia

Intensive Care Unit, Cabrini Hospital, Melbourne, VIC, Australia

Christopher Choi Division of Critical Care Medicine, Department of Anesthesiology and Pain Management, University of Texas Southwestern Medical Center, Dallas, TX, USA

Stephen R. Collins Department of Anesthesiology, University of Virginia School of Medicine, Charlottesville, VA, USA

Rian Crandon Nuffield Department of Anaesthetics, Oxford University Hospitals, Oxford, UK

Vic Callanan Department of Anaesthetics, Townsville University Hospital, Douglas, QLD, Australia

Siddharth Dave Division of Critical Care Medicine, Department of Anesthesiology and Pain Management, University of Texas Southwestern Medical Center, Dallas, TX, USA

Neel Desai Guy's and St Thomas' NHS Foundation Trust, London, UK

Corinna von Deschwanden Institute of Anesthesiology and Perioperative Medicine, University Hospital Zurich, Zürich, Switzerland

Jeson Rajan Doctor Department of Anaesthesiology, Critical Care and Pain, Tata Memorial Hospital, Homi Bhabha National Institute, Mumbai, India

Daniel Edelman Alfred Hospital, Melbourne, VIC, Australia

Sandra Ellefsen Department of Anesthesia and Intensive Care Medicine, St. Olavs University Hospital, Trondheim, Norway

José M. Fandiño-Orgeira Emergency Department, University Hospital Complex of A Coruña, A Coruña, Galicia, Spain

Chris Frerk College of Life Sciences/Leicester Medical School, University of Leicester, Leicester, UK

University Hospitals of Northamptonshire, Northamptonshire, England, UK

Luis Gaitini Department of Anesthesiology, Bnai-Zion Medical Center, Haifa, Israel

Tony Garcia Division of Critical Care Medicine, Department of Anesthesiology and Pain Management, University of Texas Southwestern Medical Center, Dallas, TX, USA

Tomasz Gaszynski Medical University of Lodz, Lodz, Poland

Manuel A. Gómez-Ríos Department of Anesthesia and Perioperative Medicine, Complejo Hospitalario Universitario de A Coruña, A Coruña, Spain

Anesthesiology and Perioperative Medicine, University Hospital Complex of A Coruña, A Coruña, Galicia, Spain

Clinical Management Section of the Spanish Society of Anesthesiology, Resuscitation, and Pain Therapy (SEDAR), Madrid, Spain

Medical University of Lodz, Kosciuszki, Poland

Bastian Grande Institute of Anesthesiology and Perioperative Medicine, University Hospital Zurich, Zürich, Switzerland

Department of Health Sciences and Technology, ETH Zurich, Zürich, Switzerland

John F. Gray Department of Anesthesiology, Critical Care, and Pain Medicine, McGovern Medical School at UTHealth Houston, Houston, TX, USA

Peter Groom Liverpool Head and Neck Centre, Liverpool University Hospitals NHS Foundation Trust, Liverpool, UK

Haukur Týr Guðmundsson Anaesthesiology and Intensive Care Medicine, Oslo University Hospital, Oslo, Norway

Carin A. Hagberg Department of Anesthesiology & Perioperative Medicine, University of Texas MD Anderson Cancer Center, Houston, TX, USA

Jan Hansel Intensive Care Medicine, University of Manchester, Manchester, UK

Acute Intensive Care Unit, Wythenshawe Hospital, Manchester University NHS Foundation Trust, Manchester, UK

Neil Hauser Department of Anaesthesia and Pain Medicine, Perth Children's Hospital, Perth, WA, Australia

Perioperative Medicine Team, Perioperative Care Program, Kids Institute, Perth, WA, Australia

Division of Emergency Medicine, Anaesthesia and Pain Medicine, Medical School, The University of Western Australia, Perth, WA, Australia

Chloe Heath Department of Anaesthesia and Pain Medicine, Perth Children's Hospital, Perth, WA, Australia

Perioperative Medicine Team, Perioperative Care Program, Kids Institute, Perth, WA, Australia

Andy Higgs Intensive Care Medicine & Anaesthesia, Warrington Teaching Hospitals, Cheshire, UK

Kunal Karamchandani Division of Critical Care Medicine, Department of Anesthesiology and Pain Management, University of Texas Southwestern Medical Center, Dallas, TX, USA

El-Boghdadly Kariem Guy's and St Thomas' NHS Foundation Trust, London, UK

Hamelmal D. Kassahun Department of Anesthesiology, University of Virginia School of Medicine, Charlottesville, VA, USA

Michael Seltz Kristensen Copenhagen University Hospital, Copenhagen, Denmark

Robin Lohse Copenhagen University Hospital, Copenhagen, Denmark

Teresa López Department of Anesthesiology, Complejo Asistencial Universitario de Salamanca, Salamanca, Spain

Graham Trevor Lubinsky Department of Anesthesiology, Advocate Illinois Masonic Medical Center, Chicago, IL, USA

Kathleen Sheridan Lubinsky Department of Anesthesiology, Advocate Illinois Masonic Medical Center, Chicago, IL, USA

Alistair F. McNarry St John's Hospital, NHS Lothian, Livingston, UK

Western General Hospital NHS Lothian, Edinburgh, UK

Pavel Michalek General University Hospital, Prague, Czech Republic

First Medical Faculty, Charles University, Prague, Czech Republic

Basma Mohamed Department of Anesthesiology, Advocate Illinois Masonic Medical Center, Chicago, IL, USA

Sheila Nainan Myatra Department of Anaesthesiology, Critical Care and Pain, Tata Memorial Hospital, Homi Bhabha National Institute, Mumbai, India

Lauren M. Nakazawa Department of Anesthesiology, Critical Care, and Pain Medicine, McGovern Medical School at UTHealth Houston, Houston, TX, USA

Jaideep J. Pandit Nuffield Department of Anaesthetics, Oxford University Hospitals, Oxford, UK

Nuffield Department of Clinical Neuroscience, University of Oxford, Oxford, UK

Timthy Parr Liverpool Head and Neck Centre, Liverpool University Hospitals NHS Foundation Trust, Liverpool, UK

Anahi Perlas Toronto Western Hospital, University Health Network, Department of Anesthesiology and Pain Medicine, University of Toronto, Toronto, ON, Canada

Natalia C. Portela Mount Sinai Hospital, Department of Anesthesiology and Pain Medicine, University of Toronto, Toronto, ON, Canada

Jansie Prozesky Department of Anesthesiology, Penn State College of Medicine, Penn State Milton S. Hershey Medical Center, Hershey, PA, USA

Anuja Rathore Toronto Western Hospital, Department of Anesthesiology and Pain Medicine, University of Toronto, Toronto, ON, Canada

José Alfonso Sastre Department of Anesthesiology, Complejo Asistencial Universitario de Salamanca, Salamanca, Spain

Mostafa Somri Department of Anesthesiology, Bnai-Zion Medical Center, Haifa, Israel

Samuel Ern Hung Tsan Department of Anaesthesiology and Critical Care, Faculty of Medicine and Health Sciences, University of Malaysia Sarawak (UNIMAS), Kota Samarahan, Sarawak, Malaysia

Britta S. von Ungern-Sternberg Department of Anaesthesia and Pain Medicine, Perth Children's Hospital, Perth, WA, Australia

Perioperative Medicine Team, Perioperative Care Program, Kids Institute, Perth, WA, Australia

Division of Emergency Medicine, Anaesthesia and Pain Medicine, Medical School, The University of Western Australia, Perth, WA, Australia

Sonia Vaida Department of Anesthesiology, Penn State College of Medicine, Penn State Milton S. Hershey Medical Center, Hershey, PA, USA

Patrick A. Ward St John's Hospital, NHS Lothian, Livingston, UK

André van Zundert Department of Anaesthesia and Perioperative Medicine, Royal Brisbane and Women's Hospital and The University of Queensland, Brisbane, QLD, Australia

Tom C. R. V. Van Zundert Department of Emergency Medicine, Holy Heart Hospital, Mol, Belgium

Chapter 1
Facing the Difficult Airway: From Evidence to Action

Carin A. Hagberg and Manuel Ángel Gómez-Ríos

The greatest enemy of knowledge is not ignorance—it is the illusion of knowledge. (Stephen Hawking)

Highlights

- Difficult airway management (DAM) remains a major contributor to perioperative morbidity and mortality worldwide.
- National audit data continue to reveal significant challenges, including hypoxemia, failed intubation, and cognitive errors.
- Evidence-based medicine (EBM) provides a structured, dynamic framework to improve safety and clinical outcomes.
- Human factors, team performance, and cognitive aids are essential in minimizing preventable harm.
- The future of DAM will emphasize personalized care, immersive simulation, and interdisciplinary collaboration.

1.1 Introduction

Difficult airway management (DAM) remains one of the most critical and high-consequence responsibilities in modern clinical practice [1]. Despite decades of innovation and heightened awareness, airway-related complications continue to contribute disproportionately to perioperative morbidity and mortality. While

C. A. Hagberg
Department of Anesthesiology & Perioperative Medicine, University of Texas MD Anderson Cancer Center, Houston, TX, USA

M. Á. Gómez-Ríos (✉)
Anesthesiology and Perioperative Medicine, University Hospital Complex of A Coruña, A Coruña, Galicia, Spain

M. Á. Gómez-Ríos, A. van Zundert (eds.), *Evidence-based Guide to Difficult Airway Management*, https://doi.org/10.1007/978-3-032-30769-9_1

considerable progress has been made in areas such as videolaryngoscopy, supraglottic airway design, and reversal agents like sugammadex, the reality reflected in large-scale audits and incident reporting systems is sobering [2].

The past decade has ushered in not only rapid technological advances but also a shifting clinical landscape single space characterized by increasingly complex patients, an aging population, and rising obesity rates [3]. These evolving challenges require clinicians to adapt continuously, drawing upon both scientific evidence and experiential knowledge. The paradigm has expanded beyond technical proficiency to embrace the science of human factors, emphasizing communication, cognitive load management, and team dynamics as essential determinants of successful airway management [4].

Recent contributions, such as the Seventh National Audit Project (NAP7) [2] and updated consensus guidelines from the Difficult Airway Society [5], the American Society of Anesthesiologists [6] and the Spanish Society of Anesthesiology, Resuscitation, and Pain Therapy (SEDAR), the Spanish Society of Emergency Medicine (SEMES), and the Spanish Society of Otorhinolaryngology and Head and Neck Surgery (SEORL-CCC) [7, 8] have reinforced the urgent need for structured, evidence-informed approaches to airway care. These resources not only map the epidemiological terrain of airway-related harm but also offer practical, actionable frameworks designed to enhance safety and optimize decision-making under pressure.

This chapter provides a comprehensive introduction to the contemporary landscape of DAM. It draws upon the latest audit data, guideline statements, and systems-thinking approaches to set the foundation for understanding risk, reducing harm, and fostering excellence in airway care. By integrating technical, cognitive, and contextual considerations, the chapter aims to equip clinicians with the knowledge and tools necessary to navigate the complexities of the difficult airway in today's high-stakes environment.

1.2 Historical Background and Context

The evolution of DAM has been shaped by sentinel events and systematic reviews that exposed widespread deficiencies in clinical practice. A major turning point was the publication of the Fourth National Audit Project (NAP4), which analyzed over 1000 airway-related incidents across the United Kingdom [9, 10]. It found that the most serious outcomes resulted from a failure to plan for difficulty, poor decision-making, and misinterpretation of capnography, among other system-level issues. This catalyzed the implementation of several practice reforms, including the appointment of departmental airway leads, promotion of situational awareness, and adoption of the 'stop-and-think' approach during airway crises [5].

Airway management continues to evolve in response to demographic changes. The increasing prevalence of obesity, the aging surgical population, and the rise in comorbidities have created new challenges for clinicians [11]. These factors underscore the need for adaptable strategies that extend beyond the confines of controlled environments like operating rooms and into the prehospital, intensive care, and emergency medicine settings.

1.3 The Current Scope of the Problem

The recent publication of the Seventh National Audit Project (NAP7) has reaffirmed that airway-related complications remain a leading cause of perioperative morbidity and mortality [2]. Of the 24,721 anesthetic events analyzed, 421 involved airway complications, accounting for 22% of all serious perioperative incidents. These events ranged from laryngospasm (37%) and failed oxygenation (30%) to aspiration (6%). Many were preventable and associated with high rates of critical harm, including 113 cardiac arrests and 32 deaths, with hypoxemia being the predominant cause.

A recurring concern is the misinterpretation or neglect of capnographic data, [12] which continues to lead to unrecognized esophageal intubation and delayed rescue in CICO scenarios. These findings echo earlier patterns observed in NAP4 and illustrate that while awareness has improved, systemic vulnerabilities persist [13].

Certain patient populations remain disproportionately affected by DAM complications, including individuals with obesity, pediatric patients, and those undergoing procedures after-hours or in non-theatre environments [11, 14, 15]. These groups often present with anatomical or physiological challenges that require bespoke planning and increased vigilance.

1.4 Evidence-Based Medicine in Difficult Airway Management

EBM lies at the heart of modern airway management [16]. It offers a triad framework of best available evidence, clinical expertise, and patient preferences to guide decision-making—particularly vital in high-stakes, time-sensitive airway scenarios. This approach helps clinicians select the most appropriate tools—such as deciding between videolaryngoscopy and fiberoptic intubation—and informs the thresholds for escalating to surgical airway access in a CICO situation [1].

National audits like NAP7 provide real-world evidence by aggregating data from diverse practice settings and highlighting consistent themes, including common failure points and successful rescue techniques [17–19]. These data are augmented by systematic reviews and consensus statements, which synthesize large bodies of literature into actionable guidance [20].

By integrating evidence into every phase of airway management—from initial assessment to post-crisis debriefing—EBM fosters accountability, improves safety, and promotes reflective practice [7, 21]. This commitment to data-driven care is particularly important as new technologies and pharmacologic tools (e.g., sugammadex) continue to alter the clinical landscape.

1.5 Human Factors and Cognitive Aids: A Paradigm Shift

Human factors science has fundamentally reshaped our understanding of DAM [22, 23]. No longer viewed as purely a technical challenge, the difficult airway is now recognized as a complex, cognitive, and team-based endeavor [24]. Errors often stem not from a lack of equipment but from breakdowns in communication, failure to recognize evolving clinical cues, and lack of shared mental models [9, 10, 15].

The introduction of ergonomically designed algorithms and cognitive aids—such as the Vortex Approach [25] and the DAS [5] or SEDAR-SEMES-SEORL guidelines [7, 8]—has helped streamline decision-making and reduce cognitive overload during airway crises. These aids emphasize maintaining oxygenation at all times and recognize the importance of early transition to a definitive plan rather than repeating unsuccessful attempts.

Studies have consistently shown that the presence of checklists [26], clear role assignment, and shared situational awareness can dramatically improve the management of airway emergencies [27, 28]. Likewise, institutions that promote team-based simulation training and airway drills show improved performance and confidence during real events [29].

1.6 Planning and Multidisciplinary Decision-Making

Prevention is the cornerstone of successful airway management. A structured, team-based planning approach—incorporating both primary and fallback strategies—significantly improves outcomes [30]. Decision-making should begin preoperatively with robust airway assessment tools and include multidisciplinary input when necessary [7].

For anticipated difficult airways, awake tracheal intubation (ATI) is widely regarded as the safest approach [8, 31]. It allows for preservation of spontaneous ventilation and protective airway reflexes while providing a controlled setting for instrumenting the airway. Traditionally, flexible fiberoptic scopes were used, but videolaryngoscopy is now equally favored, especially when paired with effective topicalization and oxygenation techniques [8, 31, 32].

Effective planning also considers institutional capabilities and personnel experience. In facilities where advanced devices or ENT backup are unavailable, algorithms must be adapted to ensure safe and realistic options. Decision-making should be continuous and dynamic, with team members empowered to reassess the plan at any stage based on patient response or procedural progress [33].

1.7 The Airway Team: Roles, Communication, and Coordination

The concept of an "airway team" has emerged as a central pillar in modern DAM [34]. This team-centric approach ensures role clarity, anticipatory preparation, and seamless communication under pressure. Optimal outcomes depend not only on technical skill but on coordinated execution, particularly during airway emergencies.

Evidence from simulation studies and real-world clinical environments shows that interdisciplinary airway teams—comprising anesthesiologists, emergency physicians, ENT surgeons, and respiratory therapists—can reduce time to intervention and improve success rates in airway rescue [35]. The formal designation of airway leads within departments further enhances consistency in practice, facilitates equipment standardization, and promotes the implementation of guidelines [36–39].

Structured briefings, shared mental models, and closed-loop communication are now essential components of high-performing teams. Institutions are increasingly adopting in situ simulations and mock drills to foster team readiness and identify latent safety threats before they manifest during actual crises [28].

1.8 Legal and Ethical Implications

Ethical and legal challenges in DAM frequently arise during high-stakes, low-frequency events where clinicians must make urgent decisions under uncertainty. Core principles such as patient autonomy, informed consent, and non-maleficence intersect with the duty to act decisively and prevent harm [40].

Clear documentation of airway plans, communication of risk to patients or surrogates, and proactive contingency planning are all part of good clinical practice [7]. These steps not only fulfill ethical obligations but also serve as medicolegal safeguards. Debriefing and transparent disclosure after adverse events further strengthen trust in the patient-clinician relationship and support a culture of safety [41, 42].

From an institutional perspective, healthcare systems must ensure that airway practitioners have regular access to training, up-to-date equipment, and support for multidisciplinary collaboration [8]. Ethical concerns extend to ensuring equitable access to advanced airway care and simulation training, particularly in low-resource settings where the risk of poor outcomes is highest [43].

1.9 Future Directions

The future of DAM is being actively reshaped by an interplay of technological advancement, systems-level thinking, and an evolving understanding of human performance in high-stakes environments [44]. Central to this evolution is the move toward personalized airway strategies [45]. With the integration of advanced imaging modalities, machine learning algorithms, and refined risk stratification models, clinicians are increasingly able to tailor airway plans to the specific anatomical, physiological, and contextual characteristics of each patient [46]. This individualized approach moves beyond static predictors of difficulty and instead offers dynamic, data-informed decision-making that could significantly reduce unexpected complications.

Artificial intelligence (AI) is also beginning to play a transformative role in DAM [47]. Predictive analytics tools, fueled by large datasets and real-time monitoring, are being developed to identify potential airway challenges before they occur and to support clinician decision-making during critical phases of care [46]. For example, algorithms may assist in preoperative risk assessment or recommend context-appropriate strategies during airway crises. While these technologies are still in their early stages, the potential for AI to enhance situational awareness and mitigate cognitive overload is substantial [48], particularly in environments where rapid decisions must be made with incomplete information.

Education and training are likewise entering a new era. Immersive simulation—incorporating virtual reality (VR), augmented reality (AR), and haptic feedback—is emerging as a powerful modality to prepare providers for low-frequency, high-acuity airway emergencies [49]. Unlike traditional simulation, VR-based training allows for repetitive, lifelike rehearsal of technical maneuvers and team-based scenarios without the constraints of time, location, or patient safety [50]. These technologies also allow for the integration of cognitive stressors and team communication elements, supporting the development of both technical proficiency and non-technical skills such as leadership, resource management, and closed-loop communication [29].

At the global level, airway management is benefiting from increased collaboration across national boundaries and professional societies [51]. Harmonization of definitions, outcome measures, and educational standards is helping to create a shared vocabulary and benchmark for quality. Initiatives such as the International Airway Management Society and collaborative efforts among national airway groups are contributing to the creation of universal frameworks for training, research, and practice evaluation. These developments foster not only consistency in care but also the dissemination of best practices across diverse healthcare systems.

The future of DAM resides at the convergence of technological innovation, human factors science, and ethical professionalism. As new tools become available, clinicians must remain grounded in the fundamental principles of safety, patient-centered care, and clinical judgment. While automation and data science may enhance our capabilities, they must augment—not replace—the nuanced expertise of the airway clinician. It is within this balance of precision and compassion that the next generation of airway management will continue to evolve.

References

1. Yang IT, Tung A, Flores KS, Berenhaut KS, Choi JA, Bryan YF. Clinical decision-making and process complications during anticipated difficult airway management for elective surgery. Anesth Analg. 2025;140(2):295–305. https://doi.org/10.1213/ANE.0000000000007049.
2. Cook TM, Oglesby F, Kane AD, Armstrong RA, Kursumovic E, Soar J. Airway and respiratory complications during anaesthesia and associated with peri-operative cardiac arrest as reported to the 7th National Audit Project of the Royal College of Anaesthetists. Anaesthesia. 2024;79(4):368–79. https://doi.org/10.1111/anae.16187.
3. Naik H, Murray TM, Khan M, Daly-Grafstein D, Liu G, Kassen BO, et al. Population-based trends in complexity of hospital inpatients. JAMA Intern Med. 2024;184(2):183–92. https://doi.org/10.1001/jamainternmed.2023.7410.
4. Schnittker R, Marshall S, Horberry T, Young KL. Human factors enablers and barriers for successful airway management—an in-depth interview study. Anaesthesia. 2018;73(8):980–9. https://doi.org/10.1111/anae.14302.
5. Higgs A, McGrath BA, Goddard C, Rangasami J, Suntharalingam G, Gale R, et al. Guidelines for the management of tracheal intubation in critically ill adults. Br J Anaesth. 2018;120(2):323–52. https://doi.org/10.1016/j.bja.2017.10.021.
6. Apfelbaum JL, Hagberg CA, Connis RT, Abdelmalak BB, Agarkar M, Dutton RP, et al. 2022 American Society of Anesthesiologists practice guidelines for management of the difficult airway. Anesthesiology. 2022;136(1):31–81. https://doi.org/10.1097/ALN.0000000000004002.
7. Gómez-Ríos MA, Sastre JA, Onrubia-Fuertes X, López T, Abad-Gurumeta A, Casans-Francés R, et al. Spanish Society of Anesthesiology, reanimation and pain therapy (SEDAR), Spanish Society of Emergency and Emergency Medicine (SEMES) and Spanish Society of Otolaryngology, head and neck surgery (SEORL-CCC) guideline for difficult airway management. Part I. Rev Esp Anestesiol Reanim (Engl Ed). 2024;71(3):171–206. https://doi.org/10.1016/j.redare.2024.02.001.
8. Gómez-Ríos MA, Sastre JA, Onrubia-Fuertes X, López T, Abad-Gurumeta A, Casans-Francés R, et al. Spanish Society of Anesthesiology, reanimation and pain therapy (SEDAR), Spanish Society of Emergency and Emergency Medicine (SEMES) and Spanish Society of Otolaryngology, head and neck surgery (SEORL-CCC) guideline for difficult airway management. Part II. Rev Esp Anestesiol Reanim (Engl Ed). 2024;71(3):207–47. https://doi.org/10.1016/j.redare.2024.02.002.
9. Cook TM, Woodall N, Frerk C. Major complications of airway management in the UK: results of the fourth National Audit Project of the Royal College of Anaesthetists and the difficult airway society. Part 1: anaesthesia. Br J Anaesth. 2011;106(5):617–31. https://doi.org/10.1093/bja/aer058.
10. Cook TM, Woodall N, Harper J, Benger J. Major complications of airway management in the UK: results of the fourth National Audit Project of the Royal College of Anaesthetists and the difficult airway society. Part 2: intensive care and emergency departments. Br J Anaesth. 2011;106(5):632–42. https://doi.org/10.1093/bja/aer059.
11. McKechnie A, Iliff HA, Black R, Ahmad I, Chesworth A, Chesworth P, et al. Airway management in patients living with obesity: best practice recommendations from the Society for Obesity and Bariatric Anaesthesia: endorsed by the all Wales airway group, Scottish airway group and difficult airway society. Anaesthesia. 2025; https://doi.org/10.1111/anae.16647.

12. Chrimes N, Higgs A, Hagberg CA, Baker PA, Cooper RM, Greif R, et al. Preventing unrecognised oesophageal intubation: a consensus guideline from the project for universal management of airways and international airway societies. Anaesthesia. 2022; https://doi.org/10.1111/anae.15817.
13. Cook TM, Higgs A, Chrimes N. Time to replace 'No trace, wrong place' with 'Sustained exhaled carbon dioxide'. Comment on Br J Anaesth 2025; 134: 248-9. Br J Anaesth. 2025;134(4):1218–20. https://doi.org/10.1016/j.bja.2024.12.027.
14. Gibson J, Leckie T, Hayward J, Hodgson L, Chain SEAR. Non-theatre emergency airway management: a multicentre prospective observational study. Anaesthesia. 2023;78(11):1338–46. https://doi.org/10.1111/anae.16107.
15. Bordini M, Orsini L, Li SYW, Olsen J, Stein ML, Sarmiento Argüello LA, et al. Incidence of cognitive errors in difficult airway management: an inference human factors study from the pediatric difficult intubation registry. Br J Anaesth. 2025; https://doi.org/10.1016/j.bja.2025.04.033.
16. Gómez-Ríos MA, Van Zundert AAJ, Fernández-Vaquero MA. The relentless pursuit of excellence in airway management. Rev Esp Anestesiol Reanim (Engl Ed). 2025;72(4):501733. https://doi.org/10.1016/j.redare.2025.501733.
17. Cumberworth A, Lewith H, Sud A, Jefferson H, Athanassoglou V, Pandit JJ. Major complications of airway management: a prospective multicentre observational study. Anaesthesia. 2022;77(6):640–8. https://doi.org/10.1111/anae.15668.
18. Rosenstock C, Møller J, Hauberg A. Complaints related to respiratory events in anaesthesia and intensive care medicine from 1994 to 1998 in Denmark. Acta Anaesthesiol Scand. 2001;45(1):53–8. https://doi.org/10.1034/j.1399-6576.2001.450109.x.
19. Endlich Y, Davies EL, Kelly J. The nature of the response to airway management incident reports in high income countries: a scoping review. Anaesth Intensive Care. 2024;52(5):283–301. https://doi.org/10.1177/0310057X241227238.
20. Gómez-Ríos MA, Van Zundert AAJ, McNarry AF, Law JA, Higgs A, De Jong A, et al. Guidelines on strategies for the universal implementation of videolaryngoscopy. Eur J Anaesthesiol. 2025; https://doi.org/10.1097/EJA.0000000000002210.
21. Jarvis JL, Panchal AR, Lyng JW, Bosson N, Donofrio-Odmann JJ, Braude DA, et al. Evidence-based guideline for prehospital airway management. Prehosp Emerg Care. 2024;28(4):545–57. https://doi.org/10.1080/10903127.2023.2281363.
22. Heidegger T. Management of the difficult airway. N Engl J Med. 2021;384(19):1836–47. https://doi.org/10.1056/NEJMra1916801.
23. Kelly FE, Bailey CR, et al. Implementing human factors in anaesthesia: guidance for clinicians, departments and hospitals. Anaesthesia. 2023;78:458–78. https://doi.org/10.1111/anae.16003.
24. Kelly FE, Bailey CR, et al. Human factors in anaesthesia: a narrative review. Anaesthesia. 2023;78:479–90. https://doi.org/10.1111/anae.16004.
25. Chrimes N. The vortex: a universal 'high-acuity implementation tool' for emergency airway management. Br J Anaesth. 2016;117(Suppl 1):i20–i7. https://doi.org/10.1093/bja/aew175.
26. Marshall SD. Helping experts and expert teams perform under duress: an agenda for cognitive aid research. Anaesthesia. 2017;72(3):289–95. https://doi.org/10.1111/anae.13707.
27. Rall M, Gaba D, Howard S, Dieckmann P. Human performance and patient safety. Miller's anesthesia Philadelphia. Elsevier; 2005. p. 3027.
28. Kelly FE, Frerk C, Bailey CR, Cook TM, Ferguson K, Flin R, et al. Implementing human factors in anaesthesia: guidance for clinicians, departments and hospitals: guidelines from the difficult airway society and the Association of Anaesthetists: guidelines from the difficult airway society and the Association of Anaesthetists. Anaesthesia. 2023;78(4):458–78. https://doi.org/10.1111/anae.15941.
29. Nielsen RP, Nikolajsen L, Paltved C, Aagaard R. Effect of simulation-based team training in airway management: a systematic review. Anaesthesia. 2021;76(10):1404–15. https://doi.org/10.1111/anae.15375.

30. Law JA, Heidegger T. Structured planning of airway management. In: Cook T, Kristensen MS, editors. Core topics in airway management. 3rd ed. Cambridge: Cambridge University Press; 2020. p. 38–49.
31. Ahmad I, El-Boghdadly K, Bhagrath R, Hodzovic I, McNarry AF, Mir F, et al. Difficult airway society guidelines for awake tracheal intubation (ATI) in adults. Anaesthesia. 2020;75(4):509–28. https://doi.org/10.1111/anae.14904.
32. Alhomary M, Ramadan E, Curran E, Walsh SR. Videolaryngoscopy vs. fibreoptic bronchoscopy for awake tracheal intubation: a systematic review and meta-analysis. Anaesthesia. 2018;73(9):1151–61. https://doi.org/10.1111/anae.14299.
33. Law JA, Duggan LV. The airway assessment has come of age-or has it? Anaesthesia. 2019;74(7):834–8. https://doi.org/10.1111/anae.14658.
34. Tankard KA, Sharifpour M, Chang MG, Bittner EA. Design and implementation of airway response teams to improve the practice of emergency airway management. J Clin Med. 2022;11(21) https://doi.org/10.3390/jcm11216336.
35. Pandian V, Ghazi TU, He MQ, Isak E, Saleem A, Semler LR, et al. Multidisciplinary difficult airway team characteristics, airway securement success, and clinical outcomes: a systematic review. Ann Otol Rhinol Laryngol. 2022:34894221123124. https://doi.org/10.1177/00034894221123124.
36. McNarry AF, Cook T, Baker PA, O'Sullivan EP. The airway lead: opportunities to improve institutional and personal preparedness for airway management. Br J Anaesth. 2020;125(1):e22–e4. https://doi.org/10.1016/j.bja.2020.04.053.
37. Smith C, McNarry AF. Airway leads and airway response teams: improving delivery of safer airway management? Curr Anesthesiol Rep. 2020:1–8. https://doi.org/10.1007/s40140-020-00404-7.
38. Greenland KB. Introducing airway leads in Australia, vol. 2. Australian and New Zealand College of Anaesthetists; 2019.
39. Van Zundert AA, Endlich Y, Beckmann LA, Bradley WP, Chapman GA, Heard AM, et al. 2021 update on airway management from the Anaesthesia continuing education airway management special interest group. Anaesth Intensive Care. 2021;49(4):257–67. https://doi.org/10.1177/0310057X20984784.
40. McLeod ADM, Yentis SM. Legal and regulatory aspects of airway management. In: Calder I, Pearce A, editors. Core topics in airway management. 2nd ed. Cambridge: Cambridge University Press; 2010. p. 293–8.
41. Couper K, Salman B, Soar J, Finn J, Perkins GD. Debriefing to improve outcomes from critical illness: a systematic review and meta-analysis. Intensive Care Med. 2013;39(9):1513–23. https://doi.org/10.1007/s00134-013-2951-7.
42. Grande B, Kolbe M, Biro P. Difficult airway management and training: simulation, communication, and feedback. Curr Opin Anaesthesiol. 2017;30(6):743–7. https://doi.org/10.1097/ACO.0000000000000523.
43. Elendu C, Amaechi DC, Okatta AU, Amaechi EC, Elendu TC, Ezeh CP, et al. The impact of simulation-based training in medical education: a review. Medicine (Baltimore). 2024;103(27):e38813. https://doi.org/10.1097/MD.0000000000038813.
44. Gleeson S, Groom P, Mercer S. Human factors in complex airway management. BJA Education. 2016;16(6):191–7. https://doi.org/10.1093/bjaed/mkv045.
45. Natt BS, Malo J, Hypes CD, Sakles JC, Mosier JM. Strategies to improve first attempt success at intubation in critically ill patients. Br J Anaesth. 2016;117(Suppl 1):i60–i8. https://doi.org/10.1093/bja/aew061.
46. De Rosa S, Bignami E, Bellini V, Battaglini D. The future of artificial intelligence using images and clinical assessment for difficult airway management. Anesth Analg. 2025;140(2):317–25. https://doi.org/10.1213/ANE.0000000000006969.
47. Guo M, Hou Y, Liu Y, Yang B, Qiao C, Li J. From algorithms to airways: applying artificial intelligence to enhance airway assessment, management, and training. Trends Anaesth Crit Care. 2025;61:101548. https://doi.org/10.1016/j.tacc.2025.101548.

48. Choudhury A, Asan O. Human factors: bridging artificial intelligence and patient safety. Proc. Int. Symp. Hum. Factors Ergon. Health Care. 2020;9(1):211–5. https://doi.org/10.1177/2327857920091007.
49. Duffy CC, Bass GA, Yi W, Rouhi A, Kaplan LJ, O'Sullivan E. Teaching airway management using virtual reality: a scoping review. Anesth Analg. 2024;138(4):782–93. https://doi.org/10.1213/ANE.0000000000006611.
50. Battegazzorre E, Gino B, Strada F, Kapralos B, Dubrowski A, Lamberti F, et al. Enhancing difficult airway management training: the role of virtual reality and adaptive learning. Virtual Reality. 2025;29(1):22. https://doi.org/10.1007/s10055-025-01105-4.
51. Gómez-Ríos MA, Sastre J, Mayo-Yáñez M, Serrano-Moraza A. A new perspective on managing the difficult airway: the guidelines of the Spanish societies of anesthesiology, reanimation and pain therapy (SEDAR), emergency medicine (SEMES) and otorhinolaryngology and head and neck surgery (SEORL-CCC). Emergencias. 2024;36(4):303–8. https://doi.org/10.55633/s3me/039.2024.

Chapter 2
Airway Ultrasound

Robin Lohse, Sandra Ellefsen, and Michael Seltz Kristensen

Summary of Recommendations

- The cricothyroid membrane should be identified before initiating airway interventions (Grade D).
- If visual or palpation-based identification is uncertain, ultrasound should be used for identification and marking of the cricothyroid membrane (Grade A).
- The cricothyroid membrane should be identified with the neck fully extended, suitable for cricothyrotomy, as the marked position maintains its accuracy when the head is returned to this position (Grade C).
- For ultrasound identification of the cricothyroid membrane, the longitudinal technique, transverse technique, or a combination of both can be used (Grade B).
- Ultrasound should be used for tracheostomy procedures to identify tracheal rings, midline, depth, and location of any overlying vessels or pathology, particularly in cases of tracheal deviation (Grade C).
- Ultrasound can verify tracheal intubation as an adjunct to waveform capnography, confirming placement without requiring ventilation, and additionally aids in distinguishing between tracheal and endobronchial placement (Grade B).

R. Lohse (✉) · M. S. Kristensen
Copenhagen University Hospital, Copenhagen, Denmark
e-mail: robin.lohse@regionh.dk; Michael.Seltz.Kristensen@regionh.dk

S. Ellefsen
Department of Anesthesia and Intensive Care Medicine, St. Olavs University Hospital, Trondheim, Norway

M. Á. Gómez-Ríos, A. van Zundert (eds.), *Evidence-based Guide to Difficult Airway Management*, https://doi.org/10.1007/978-3-032-30769-9_2

2.1 Introduction

Airway management is essential in anesthesia and intensive care, but it remains a major cause of morbidity and mortality [1, 2]. Effective airway assessment is essential for preventing complications. Traditionally, assessments rely on bedside visual examinations and screening tests, but methods like endoscopy and imaging (e.g., CT and MRI) are often invasive, time-consuming, and impractical.

A commonly used bedside tool is the Simplified Airway Risk Index (SARI), which estimates the risk of difficult tracheal intubation based on seven assessment parameters: mouth opening, thyromental distance, Mallampati score, neck mobility, upper lip bite test, body weight, and previous tracheal intubation history. Clinical prediction like this is recommended as it will identify a significant fraction of the really difficult airways [3]. However, a Cochrane review by Roth D. et al. found these tests to have low sensitivity and high variability, making them unreliable as screening tools [4] (Grade B). Moreover, traditional bedside assessments may fail to detect hidden airway abnormalities, particularly as obesity and comorbidities become more prevalent. This is especially relevant for patients with head and neck pathology, who often require more precise airway evaluation techniques.

Ultrasound is a simple, portable, and noninvasive point-of-care tool that enhances airway assessment and planning. It provides a good overview and real-time visualization of upper airway anatomy and may improve the prediction of difficult laryngoscopy. Notably, ultrasound excels at easily and precisely identifying the cricothyroid membrane, a critical landmark for emergency airway access, which serves as the last resort in airway management. An inherent challenge in cricothyrotomy lies in accurately identifying the cricothyroid membrane [1, 5]. Studies show that palpation-only methods in emergency settings have a success rate of just 35% when performed by anesthesiologists [1], whereas ultrasound is significantly more accurate, especially in patients with abnormal anatomy [6, 7].

Additional applications of ultrasound in airway management include (1) confirming endotracheal tube placement, (2) planning and optimizing a tracheostomy, (3) selecting the correct endotracheal tube size, (4) assessing fasting status, and (5) enhancing airway evaluation in obstetric patients.

This chapter will explore the sonoanatomy of the upper airway, ultrasound-guided techniques for cricothyroid membrane identification, and methods for ruling out accidental esophageal intubation, ensuring accurate tracheal tube placement. Other applications of airway ultrasound will also be briefly discussed.

2.2 Sonoanatomy of the Upper Airway

Transcutaneous ultrasound allows the identification of anatomical features and hidden pathologies that are not detectable through direct inspection. This imaging modality facilitates precise real-time assessment of key airway components, including the thyroid cartilage, epiglottis, cricoid cartilage, cricothyroid membrane, tracheal rings, and esophagus, thereby enabling strategic planning of airway management. Ultrasound aids airway management by providing dimensional analysis and identification of potential obstruction, improving decision-making for selecting the optimal intervention.

2.2.1 Ultrasound Equipment and Image Formation

Most airway structures are superficial, located at a depth of 0.5–4 cm. A linear high-frequency transducer (3–15 MHz) is optimal for scanning these structures. However, a curvilinear transducer is preferred when a broader field of view is required, particularly in submandibular and supraglottic assessments [8] (Grade D).

Ultrasound imaging relies on acoustic impedance differences between tissues. When ultrasound waves encounter a transition between tissues with differing impedance, they are reflected, with greater impedance differences resulting in increased reflection. Homogeneous tissues, such as noncalcified cartilage and fluid within vessels, efficiently transmit ultrasound, exhibit minimal reflection, and thereby appear dark (hypoechoic) in ultrasound images, typically with bright borders. In contrast, heterogeneous tissues, such as fat or connective tissue, generate brighter (hyperechoic) signals, revealing structure within the tissue.

2.2.2 Air-Tissue Interface and Ultrasound Artifacts

In airway ultrasound, the transition to air is a key consideration. Like bone and calcified cartilage, air poorly transmits ultrasound waves, preventing visualization beyond the air-tissue interface. As a result, any structure appearing within an air-filled space is considered an ultrasound artifact. Nevertheless, the transition from tissue to air creates a significant impedance shift, producing a distinct bright white line at the air-tissue interface. This characteristic feature is crucial in airway ultrasound, aiding in the identification of important anatomical structures.

2.2.3 Regions of Interest for Airway Ultrasound

Submandibular Region: Placing a curvilinear transducer in the sagittal plane under the chin allows for optimal visualization of the floor of the mouth, extending from the mandibular symphysis to the hyoid bone, and of the tongue (Fig. 2.1). This is particularly useful for detecting base-of-tongue pathology.

Vocal Cords: Ultrasound can effectively visualize the vocal cords and detect associated pathologies, even when deeper structures beyond the air-tissue interface

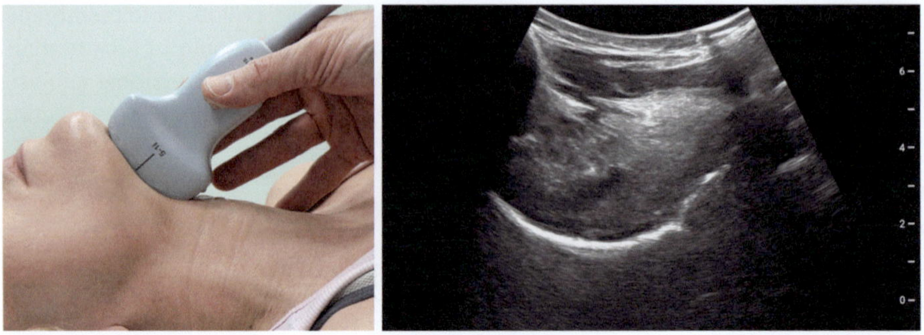

Fig. 2.1 Floor of mouth ultrasoundUltrasound imaging of the floor of the mouth. The shadows of the mandibular mentum (left side of the ultrasound image) and the hyoid bone (right side) are visible, with the tongue positioned between them. (Reproduced with permission from The Scandinavian Airway Management Course, www.airwaymanagement.dk)

remain obscured. This capability is particularly valuable for identifying tumors or abscesses affecting the anterior airway and aiding in airway management planning (Grade C).

Tracheal Mapping: Ultrasound is invaluable for tracing the course of the trachea, identifying the cricothyroid membrane, and locating overlying vessels. This information is essential for both emergency front-of-neck access and planned tracheostomy procedures.

Esophageal Identification: In the lower neck, ultrasound facilitates esophageal identification, assisting in the verification of correct endotracheal tube placement by ruling out esophageal intubation.

The following sections will explore specific ultrasound techniques for airway assessment and intervention.

2.3 Clinical Techniques for Locating the Cricothyroid Membrane

The success rate of cricothyrotomy, even among trained anesthesiologists, remains low. One of the main challenges is the inaccurate identification of the cricothyroid membrane, leading to frequent misplacements [1, 5]. This issue is particularly pronounced in obese patients and individuals with poorly defined neck landmarks, where palpation-based identification has a reported success rate ranging from 0% to 39% [6, 9–12].

2.3.1 Ultrasound-Guided Identification

Cricothyrotomy is typically a last-resort procedure in airway management. To enhance success rates, identifying and marking the cricothyroid membrane before airway interventions is recommended [13] (Grade D).

Ultrasound has proven valuable in cases where palpation or visual identification is unreliable. Studies demonstrate that ultrasound significantly increases accuracy in localization of the cricothyroid membrane [6, 7, 14–17] (Grade A) while also reducing procedural complications [18] (Grade B). Additionally, it provides precise measurements such as skin-to-membrane depth and precise detection of overlying vessels (Fig. 2.2).

2.3.2 Ultrasound Techniques for Identification

Two primary ultrasound techniques are used to locate the cricothyroid membrane [19]: (1) longitudinal approach—"string of pearls" technique (Fig. 2.3). It provides a clear view of the tracheal trajectory and is the most extensively studied technique. It is ideal when neck extension is possible. (2) Transverse approach—"TACA" technique (thyroid cartilage-airline-cricoid-airline) (Fig. 2.4): it is preferred in patients with short necks or limited neck extension, as positioning the transducer longitudinally can pose difficulties (Grade D).

Both techniques have demonstrated effectiveness when landmark palpation is challenging [20] (Grade B) and can be completed in less than 1 min [7] (Grade B).

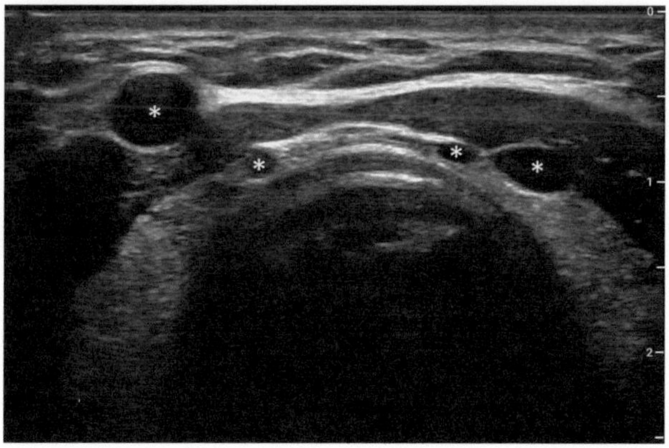

Fig. 2.2 Trachea and vesselsTransverse ultrasound image of the upper trachea. The anterior part of the trachea appears centrally as a round structure, while adjacent vessels are marked with asterisks. (Reproduced with permission from The Scandinavian Airway Management Course, www.airwaymanagement.dk)

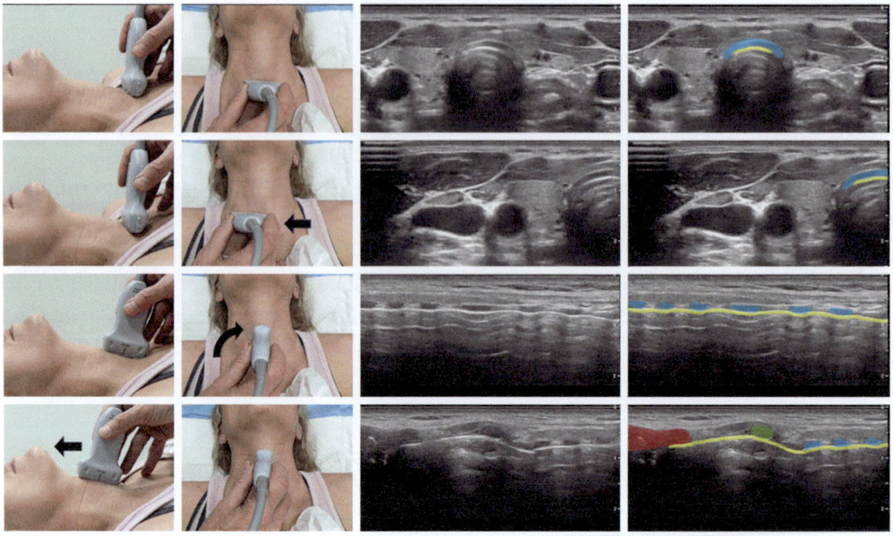

Fig. 2.3 String of pearls techniqueThe longitudinal "string of pearls" (SOP) technique for identifying the cricothyroid membrane and the interspaces between tracheal rings, as described in the text. Blue = anterior part of the tracheal ring; yellow = air-tissue border; green = anterior part of the cricoid cartilage; red = caudal end of the thyroid cartilage. (Reproduced with permission from The Scandinavian Airway Management Course, www.airwaymanagement.dk)

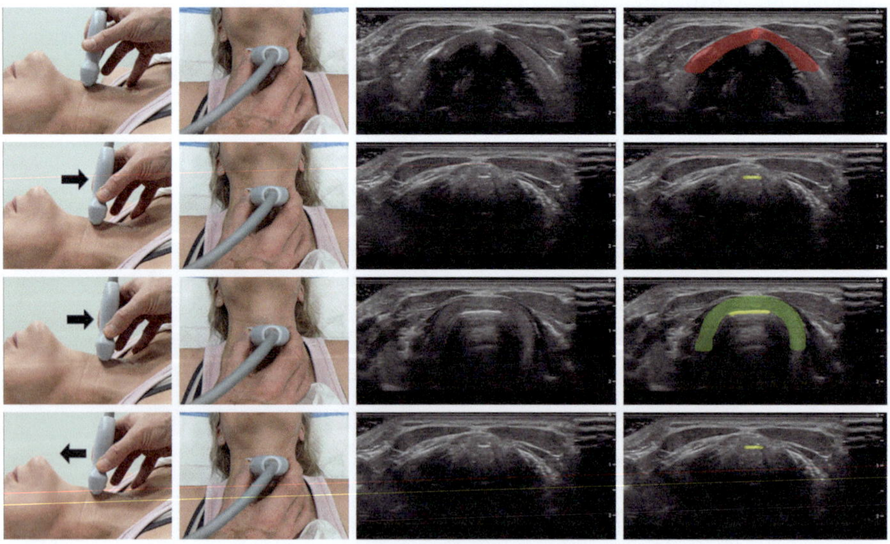

Fig. 2.4 TACA techniqueThe transverse "thyroid-airline-cricoid-airline" (TACA) technique for identifying the cricothyroid membrane, as described in the text. Red = thyroid cartilage, characterized by a distinct triangular shape; yellow = air-tissue border; green = anterior part of the cricoid cartilage, recognizable by its distinct horseshoe shape. (Reproduced with permission from The Scandinavian Airway Management course, www.airwaymanagement.dk)

When marking the cricothyroid membrane using either technique, the neck should be fully extended to a position suitable for cricothyrotomy (Grade C). After marking, the head can be repositioned as needed for the planned airway intervention. Studies indicate that even after repositioning, the marked location of the cricothyroid membrane remains accurate if the head is returned to the original marking position during a failed airway scenario [21] (Grade C).

Clinical Scenario

A 70-year-old man was admitted for a diagnostic biopsy. He had a BMI of 28 and a history of laryngeal cancer treated with radiotherapy, which had previously required a temporary tracheostomy. Airway assessment revealed normal mouth opening, neck extension, and lower jaw mobility, with a Mallampati class of 1. However, during nasoendoscopy, the surgeon encountered limited visualization of the vocal cords due to phlegm accumulation in the hypopharynx and significant swelling of the aryepiglottic fold. Additionally, post-radiation fibrosis made palpation of the trachea and cricothyroid membrane difficult. As a result, the medical team planned to perform tracheal intubation using an awake flexible bronchoscopic technique.

Ultrasound was used to locate and mark the cricothyroid membrane, after which an infrared light-guide was positioned on the skin. Tracheal intubation was attempted under light sedation and topical airway anesthesia using a 6.0 mm tracheal tube mounted on a disposable flexible bronchoscope. Guided by the infrared light through the skin, the bronchoscope was successfully advanced into the trachea after several attempts, navigating past a triangular tracheal stenosis caused by the previous tracheostomy. The tracheal tube was then placed without complications. Biopsy results later confirmed recurrent malignancy. Several weeks later, the patient underwent a laryngectomy using the same awake nasotracheal intubation technique [22].

2.3.3 Stepwise Approach to the "String of Pearls" Technique (Longitudinal Scan)

1. Positioning the Transducer

   Palpate the sternum, then place the ultrasound transducer transversely on the patient's neck, just above the suprasternal notch. This positioning provides a clear view of the trachea, which appears as a dark horseshoe-shaped structure with a distinct posterior white line (Fig. 2.3, first row).

2. Lateral Adjustment

   Slide the transducer toward the patient's right side until its right edge aligns with the tracheal midline. This adjustment divides the ultrasound image of the tracheal rings in half on the screen (Fig. 2.3, second row).

3. Rotating for a Longitudinal View

   Keeping the right end of the transducer along the tracheal midline, rotate the left end 90° into the sagittal plane. This maneuver generates a longitudinal scan, revealing a sequence of dark (hypoechoic) rings anterior to a prominent white hyperechoic line, marking the air-tissue interface. This pattern resembles a "string of pearls," where the dark hypoechoic "pearls" represent the anterior portions of the tracheal rings (Fig. 2.3, third row).

4. Identifying the Cricoid Cartilage

   Maintain the transducer in a longitudinal orientation and gently slide it cephalad until the cricoid cartilage is visualized. The cricoid cartilage appears as a larger, more elongated, and anteriorly positioned "pearl," distinct from the other tracheal rings. As scanning continues cephalad, the distal segment of the thyroid cartilage also becomes visible (Fig. 2.3, fourth row).

5. Needle Placement for Marking

   While stabilizing the ultrasound transducer with the dominant hand, use the non-dominant hand to carefully advance a needle (selected as a marker for its shadow-casting capability in the ultrasound image) between the transducer and the patient's skin. Position the needle at the cranial end of the transducer, ensuring that its tip remains away from the skin, and advance it until its shadow is positioned midway between the caudal edge of the thyroid cartilage and the cephalad edge of the cricoid cartilage.

6. Marking the Cricothyroid Membrane

   Withdraw the transducer, leaving the needle as a guide to pinpoint the center of the cricothyroid membrane in the transverse plane. Mark this location on the skin with a pen.
   Demonstration video: http://airwaymanagement.dk/pearls

2.3.4 *Stepwise Approach to the "TACA" Technique (Transverse Scan)*

1. Positioning the Transducer

   Place the transducer transversely on the front of the neck at the level of the thyroid cartilage. Slide it until the thyroid cartilage is clearly visualized as a hyperechoic triangular structure (Fig. 2.4, first row).

2. Identifying the Cricothyroid Membrane

   Slide the transducer caudally until the cricothyroid membrane is identified. It appears as a hyperechoic white line formed by the air-tissue interface of the mucosal lining, often accompanied by parallel white lines (reverberation artifacts) below (Fig. 2.4, second row).

3. Locating the Cricoid Cartilage

   Continue moving the transducer caudally until the cricoid cartilage is recognized. It resembles a horizontally oriented "C" with a distinct white lining (Fig. 2.4, third row).

4. Pinpointing the Cricothyroid Membrane

   Adjust the transducer slightly cephalad to precisely center the cricothyroid membrane (Fig. 2.4, fourth row).

5. Marking the Cricothyroid Membrane

   For accurate localization, mark the cricothyroid membrane on the skin in both transverse and sagittal planes using a pen. If the ultrasound machine includes a centerline function, utilize it for precise transverse plane marking. The upper and lower boundaries of the cricothyroid membrane can be identified by recognizing the characteristic shapes of the thyroid and cricoid cartilages.
   Demonstration video: http://airwaymanagement.dk/taca

2.4 Tracheostomy Planning with Ultrasound

Assessing the trachea and selecting the optimal tracheostomy site can be challenging, especially in patients with risk factors such as obesity, neck pathology, or a history of neck surgery or radiation therapy. These conditions may hinder palpation and lead to tracheal deviation. Ultrasound has proven to be a valuable tool in tracheostomy procedures, particularly for patients with tracheal deviation [23] (Grade C). It aids in determining the tracheal midline and depth, identifying overlying vessels, and visualizing tracheal rings, enhancing procedural accuracy and effectiveness (Grade C).

The ultrasound techniques used for cricothyroid membrane identification—longitudinal and transverse approaches—can also be applied to locate the ideal tracheostomy site. The longitudinal approach typically provides a superior view of the tracheal rings, while the transverse approach offers a clearer visualization of overlying vessels. Combining both techniques can optimize preparation and planning, ensuring a safer and more precise tracheostomy procedure (Grade C).

2.5 Confirmation of Tracheal Intubation

Ultrasound is a valuable tool for verifying tracheal intubation, particularly when combined with waveform capnography, demonstrating high accuracy [24] (Grade B). Additionally, it can detect mainstem bronchial intubation. Various ultrasound methods exist for confirming tracheal intubation, with one commonly used approach involving the identification of the esophagus and exclusion of esophageal intubation by directly scanning the anterior neck during or immediately after intubation [25, 26] (Grade B).

2.5.1 Ultrasound-Guided Esophageal Identification

Direct visualization of the esophagus via ultrasonographic scans of the anterior neck can be performed in three distinct areas: (1) transversely at the level of the cricothyroid membrane, (2) longitudinally along the visible length of the trachea, or (3) transversely in the midline, slightly cranial to the suprasternal notch [27]. The latter approach provides a clear distinction between the trachea and the esophagus, aided by characteristic ultrasound artifacts. To perform this method, place a linear, high-frequency transducer transversely in the midline, just cranial to the suprasternal notch, and slide it slightly toward the patient's left. The trachea will appear, while the esophagus, located posterolateral to the trachea, will present as a rounded or oval multi-layered structure with a lighter perimeter and a central dark area (Fig. 2.5).

Ultrasound of the esophagus is ideally performed in awake patients, allowing for the observation of dynamic expansion and contraction during swallowing (Grade B). Air movement within the esophageal lumen may generate ultrasound artifacts. A slight rightward flexion of the patient's head can improve esophageal visualization.

2.5.2 Detecting Esophageal Intubation

In cases of esophageal intubation, the esophagus may resemble the trachea, displaying a uniformly round shape and an air-tissue border that obscures posterior structures—commonly referred to as the "double trachea sign" [28]. This ultrasound technique allows for rapid confirmation of tracheal intubation without requiring ventilation (Grade B).

2.5.3 Alternative Confirmation via Lung Ultrasound

Another method for verifying endotracheal tube placement involves placing the ultrasound transducer in the midaxillary line on either side of the patient's chest to assess the pleural line. The presence of bilateral lung sliding confirms intra-airway

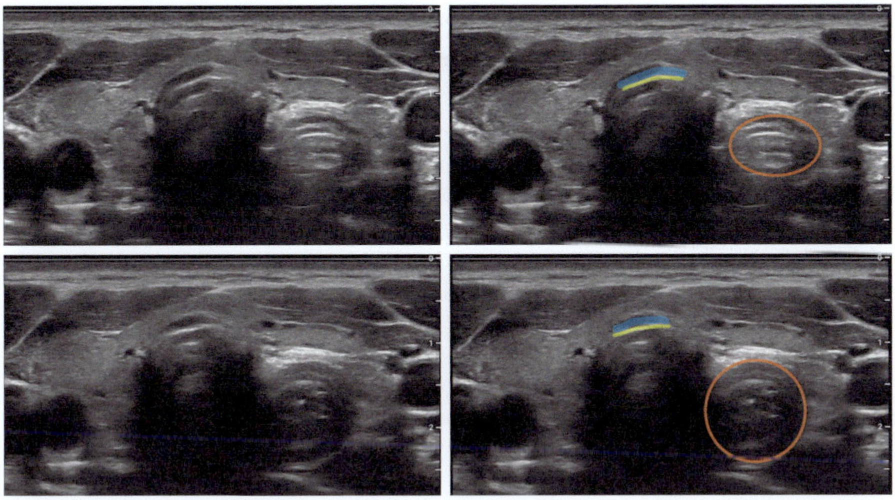

Fig. 2.5 Esophagus ultrasoundTransverse ultrasound scan just cranial to the suprasternal notch. Top row: the esophagus appears as a round structure positioned left of the trachea, lacking the hypoechoic and hyperechoic structures seen in the trachea. Bottom row: the esophagus during fluid swallowing, forming a round hypoechoic structure that resembles the appearance of esophageal intubation. However, unlike in esophageal intubation, the area posterior to the esophagus remains visible, and there is an absence of a distinct air-tissue border. Blue = anterior part of tracheal cartilage; yellow = air-tissue border; orange circle = esophagus. (Reproduced with permission from The Scandinavian Airway Management Course, www.airwaymanagement.dk)

tube placement. Lung sliding can also help detect right mainstem bronchial intubation, where sliding is present on the right lung but absent on the left, replaced by a lung pulse [29, 30] (Grade C). M-mode scanning further enhances lung sliding detection, aiding in differentiation between tracheal and mainstem bronchial intubation [31].

While ultrasound is highly sensitive for distinguishing between tracheal and esophageal intubation, its sensitivity for detecting mainstem bronchial intubation is comparatively lower [32].

2.5.4 Application in Double-Lumen Tube Placement

Thoracic ultrasound can assess double-lumen tracheal tube placement, offering sensitivity and specificity comparable to flexible bronchoscopy but with a shorter procedure time [33] (Grade C).

2.5.5 Key Advantages of Ultrasound in Intubation Confirmation

- Early detection of esophageal intubation before ventilation, irrespective of CO_2 monitoring, prevents gastric insufflation, which is particularly crucial in emergency scenarios where aspiration risk is high [34, 35] (Grade B).
- Effective in noisy environments, where auscultation may be unreliable.
- Essential for medical personnel to complement other tracheal intubation confirmation techniques to handle diverse clinical contexts.

2.5.6 Limitations of Ultrasound for Confirmation of Intubation

Despite its benefits, ultrasound has limitations:

- Subcutaneous emphysema can compromise the reliability of airway ultrasound.
- Neck tumors or trauma may hinder direct ultrasound examination.
- Pneumothorax, pneumonia, or malignancy can preclude the use of lung sliding to confirm tracheal intubation.

2.6 Additional Applications of Ultrasound in Airway Management

Ultrasound has several additional applications in airway management. Below, some key uses are outlined, though not in exhaustive detail.

2.6.1 Obstetric Airway Management

Obstetric patients present significant challenges in airway management, with failure-to-intubate rates up to eight times higher than in non-obstetric patients [36, 37]. Pregnancy induces notable changes in airway anatomy and physiology, including increased airway edema and an elevated aspiration risk [37].

Cricothyroid membrane identification in obstetric patients has shown low accuracy [38]. However, research indicates that ultrasound can improve this accuracy, albeit with a slightly extended identification time, typically within a 30-s range [39] (Grade C). Given the increased airway risks in this population, a prudent approach involves ultrasound-guided identification of the cricothyroid membrane before anesthesia induction, particularly when palpation is difficult (Grade C).

This is especially relevant in time-sensitive situations, such as emergency caesarean sections, where ultrasound can be used during preoxygenation, provided it is readily available, and resources allow for its utilization (Grade D).

2.6.2 Assessing Fasting Status

The NAP4 study identified aspiration as the leading cause of morbidity and mortality in patients undergoing general anesthesia [2]. Traditionally, aspiration risk assessment relies on fasting times. However, fasting guidelines do not apply universally, as certain patients experience delayed gastric emptying due to acute gastrointestinal conditions, acute pain, or comorbidities.

Notably, the use of GLP-1 receptor agonists has increased, and these medications have been shown to slow gastric emptying [40]. Given the importance of evaluating gastric content, ultrasound has emerged as a cost-effective, rapid, and noninvasive bedside tool that provides insights into gastric volume and composition [41]. Gastric ultrasound is covered in detail in a separate chapter in this book.

2.6.3 Tracheal Tube Size

Ultrasound is a reliable method for accurately measuring tracheal diameter, aiding in the optimal selection of endotracheal and tracheostomy tube sizes. It is superior to clinical assessment in both adult and pediatric patients [42, 43] (Grade B). This advantage is particularly evident in pediatric patients, where ultrasound outperforms age- and height-based estimations [43], and in double-lumen endotracheal tubes, where precise lumen sizing is crucial (Grade B).

Tracheal diameter measurement via ultrasound is typically performed using a transverse scan at the mid-tracheal level, *which is related* to thc outer diameter of the endotracheal tube.

2.6.4 Predicting Difficult Laryngoscopy

Currently, no single clinical predictor reliably forecasts difficult laryngoscopy or intubation, making unexpected difficult airways a persistent challenge in airway management. Ultrasound has been explored as a tool for predicting difficult laryngoscopy and intubation, offering several measurable parameters. Among them, the skin-to-epiglottis distance, skin-to-hyoid bone distance, and hyomental distance have demonstrated the highest accuracy in predicting airway difficulty. However, the clinical applicability and predictive accuracy of these ultrasound parameters remain uncertain [44, 45] (Grade C).

2.7 Frequently Encountered Problems and Solutions

Problem	Solution
Unable to identify the airway using ultrasound above the suprasternal notch	The trachea moves dorsally on its course caudally. Increase ultrasound depth or angle the transducer slightly cranially so the ultrasound beam is perpendicular to the trachea. Slide the transducer laterally to both sides to check for tracheal deviation
Difficulty obtaining the "string of pearls" view after rotating the transducer 90 degrees into the longitudinal view	Position the edge of the transducer over the tracheal midline and rotate around the transducers edge while looking down on the transducer. Adjust by sliding the transducer slightly to optimize the image
Inability to maintain the "string of pearls" view, because of inadvertent lateral movement	Hold the probe closer to the patient and rest your hand on the patient for stabilization
Difficulty identifying the thyroid cartilage/mistaking the cricoid cartilage for the thyroid cartilage in the "string of pearls" approach=	Slide the transducer cranially until both the thyroid and cricoid cartilages are visible. The air-tissue border will only be partially, if at all, visible underneath the thyroid cartilage because it is most often calcified. The cricoid cartilage is visible as a round or oval hypoechoic structure with the air-tissue border visible underneath
Challenges in scanning the neck and positioning the ultrasound probe	Keep the neck fully extended when identifying the cricothyroid membrane. In patients with a very short neck, the TACA approach may be preferable

References

1. Cook TM, Woodall N, Frerk C, Fourth National Audit Project. Major complications of airway management in the UK: results of the fourth National Audit Project of the Royal College of Anaesthetists and the difficult airway society. Part 1: anaesthesia. Br J Anaesth. 2011;106:617–31.
2. Cook TM, Woodall N, Harper J, Benger J, Fourth National Audit Project. Major complications of airway management in the UK: results of the fourth National Audit Project of the Royal College of Anaesthetists and the difficult airway society. Part 2: intensive care and emergency departments. Br J Anaesth. 2011;106:632–42.
3. Teoh WH, Kristensen MS. Prediction in airway management: what is worthwhile, what is a waste of time and what about the future? Br J Anaesth. 2016;117:1–3.
4. Roth D, Pace NL, Lee A, Hovhannisyan K, Warenits A-M, Arrich J, Herkner H. Airway physical examination tests for detection of difficult airway management in apparently normal adult patients. Cochrane Database Syst Rev. 2018;5:CD008874.
5. Zasso FB, Lait D, Siddiqui N, Perelman VS, Ye XY, You-Ten KE. Role of ultrasonography in an impalpable tissue larynx model during a simulated front-of-neck access scenario: a randomized simulation study. Can J Emerg Med. 2022;24:862–6.
6. Siddiqui N, Yu E, Boulis S, You-Ten KE. Ultrasound is superior to palpation in identifying the cricothyroid membrane in subjects with poorly defined neck landmarks: a randomized clinical trial. Anesthesiology. 2018;129:1132–9.
7. Lohse R, Wagner N, Kristensen MS. Palpation versus ultrasonography for identifying the cricothyroid membrane in models of laterally deviated larynx. Anesth Analg. 2024;139(1):195–200.

8. Kristensen MS. Ultrasonography in the management of the airway. Acta Anaesthesiol Scand. 2011;55:1155–73.
9. Lamb A, Zhang J, Hung O, Flemming B, Mullen T, Bissell MB, Arseneau I. Accuracy of identifying the cricothyroid membrane by anesthesia trainees and staff in a Canadian institution. Can J Anaesth. 2015;62:495–503.
10. Hiller KN, Karni RJ, Cai C, Holcomb JB, Hagberg CA. Comparing success rates of anesthesia providers versus trauma surgeons in their use of palpation to identify the cricothyroid membrane in female subjects: a prospective observational study. Can J Anesth/J Can Anesth. 2016;63.807–17.
11. Elliott DSJ, Baker PA, Scott MR, Birch CW, Thompson JMD. ORIGINAL ARTICLE: accuracy of surface landmark identification for cannula cricothyroidotomy. Anaesthesia. 2010;65:889–94.
12. Aslani A, Ng S-C, Hurley M, McCarthy KF, McNicholas M, McCaul CL. Accuracy of identification of the cricothyroid membrane in female subjects using palpation: an observational study. Anesth Analg. 2012;114:987.
13. Kristensen MS, Teoh WHL, Baker PA. Percutaneous emergency airway access; prevention, preparation, technique and training. Br J Anaesth. 2015;114:357–61.
14. You-Ten KE, Desai D, Postonogova T, Siddiqui N. Accuracy of conventional digital palpation and ultrasound of the cricothyroid membrane in obese women in labour. Anaesthesia. 2015;70:1230–4.
15. Kristensen MS, Teoh WH, Rudolph SS, Tvede MF, Hesselfeldt R, Børglum J, Lohse T, Hansen LN. Structured approach to ultrasound-guided identification of the cricothyroid membrane: a randomized comparison with the palpation method in the morbidly obese. Br J Anaesth. 2015;114:1003–4.
16. Hung K-C, Chen I-W, Lin C-M, Sun C-K. Comparison between ultrasound-guided and digital palpation techniques for identification of the cricothyroid membrane: a meta-analysis. Br J Anaesth. 2021;126:e9–e11.
17. Altun D, Ali A, Koltka K, Buget M, Çelik M, Doruk C, Çamcı AE. Role of ultrasonography in determining the cricothyroid membrane localization in the predicted difficult airway. Ulus Travma Acil Cerrahi Derg. 2019;25:355–60.
18. Siddiqui N, Arzola C, Friedman Z, Guerina L, You-Ten KE. Ultrasound improves cricothyrotomy success in cadavers with poorly defined neck anatomy: a randomized control trial. Anesthesiology. 2015;123:1033–41.
19. Kristensen MS, Teoh WH, Rudolph SS. Ultrasonographic identification of the cricothyroid membrane: best evidence, techniques, and clinical impact. Br J Anaesth. 2016;117(Suppl 1):i39–48.
20. Kristensen MS, Teoh WH, Rudolph SS, Hesselfeldt R, Børglum J, Tvede MF. A randomised cross-over comparison of the transverse and longitudinal techniques for ultrasound-guided identification of the cricothyroid membrane in morbidly obese subjects. Anaesthesia. 2016;71:675–83.
21. Bowness J, Teoh WH, Kristensen MS, Dalton A, Saint-Grant AL, Taylor A, Crawley S, Chisholm F, Varsou O, McGuire B. A marking of the cricothyroid membrane with extended neck returns to correct position after neck manipulation and repositioning. Acta Anaesthesiol Scand. 2020;64:1422–5.
22. Jauho KR, Johannsen ML, Hesselfeldt RT, Kristensen MS. Infrared flashing light through the cricothyroid membrane to guide flexible bronchoscopic tracheal intubation. Anaesth Rep. 2021;9:114–7.
23. Arora P, Arora R, Karim HMR, Neema PK, Panda CK. Transillumination and point-of-care ultrasonography to delineate tracheal deviation for challenging tracheostomy: a case report. Cureus. 15:e37164.
24. Gottlieb M, Holladay D, Peksa GD. Ultrasonography for the confirmation of endotracheal tube intubation: a systematic review and meta-analysis. Ann Emerg Med. 2018;72:627–36.

25. Chou EH, Dickman E, Tsou P-Y, Tessaro M, Tsai Y-M, Ma MH-M, Lee C-C, Marshall J. Ultrasonography for confirmation of endotracheal tube placement: a systematic review and meta-analysis. Resuscitation. 2015;90:97–103.
26. Das SK, Choupoo NS, Haldar R, Lahkar A. Transtracheal ultrasound for verification of endotracheal tube placement: a systematic review and meta-analysis. Can J Anaesth. 2015;62:413–23.
27. Rosenblatt WH, Popescu WM. Master techniques in upper and lower airway management. 1st ed. Lippincott Williams & Wilkins (LWW); 2015.
28. Teoh WH, Kristensen MS. Ultrasonography for airway management. In: Cook T, Kristensen MS, editors. Core topics in airway management. Cambridge University Press; 2020. p. 63–71.
29. Weaver B, Lyon M, Blaivas M. Confirmation of endotracheal tube placement after intubation using the ultrasound sliding lung sign. Acad Emerg Med. 2006;13:239–44.
30. Karacabey S, Sanrı E, Gencer EG, Guneysel O. Tracheal ultrasonography and ultrasonographic lung sliding for confirming endotracheal tube placement: speed and reliability. Am J Emerg Med. 2016;34:953–6.
31. Avila J, Smith B, Mead T, Jurma D, Dawson M, Mallin M, Dugan A. Does the addition of M-mode to B-mode ultrasound increase the accuracy of identification of lung sliding in traumatic Pneumothoraces? J Ultrasound Med. 2018;37:2681–7.
32. Kristensen MS, Teoh WH, Graumann O, Laursen CB. Ultrasonography for clinical decision-making and intervention in airway management: from the mouth to the lungs and pleurae. Insights Imaging. 2014;5:253–79.
33. Kanavitoon S, Raksamani K, Troy MP, Suphathamwit A, Thongcharoen P, Suksompong S, Oh SS. Lung ultrasound is non-inferior to bronchoscopy for confirmation of double-lumen endotracheal tube positioning: a randomized controlled noninferiority study. BMC Anesthesiol. 2022;22:168.
34. Abbasi S, Farsi D, Zare MA, Hajimohammadi M, Rezai M, Hafezimoghadam P. Direct ultrasound methods: a confirmatory technique for proper endotracheal intubation in the emergency department. Eur J Emerg Med. 2015;22:10–6.
35. Chou H-C, Tseng W-P, Wang C-H, et al. Tracheal rapid ultrasound exam (T.R.U.E.) for confirming endotracheal tube placement during emergency intubation. Resuscitation. 2011;82:1279–84.
36. Kinsella SM, Winton AL, Mushambi MC, Ramaswamy K, Swales H, Quinn AC, Popat M. Failed tracheal intubation during obstetric general anaesthesia: a literature review. Int J Obstet Anesth. 2015;24:356–74.
37. Quinn AC, Milne D, Columb M, Gorton H, Knight M. Failed tracheal intubation in obstetric anaesthesia: 2 yr national case-control study in the UK. Br J Anaesth. 2013;110:74–80.
38. Qasem F, Khalaf R, Sebbag I, Lavi R, Jones PM, Singh SI. Efficacy of surface landmark palpation for identification of the cricoid cartilage in obstetric patients: a prospective observational study. J Anaesthesiol Clin Pharmacol. 2019;35:335–9.
39. Lavelle A, Drew T, Fennessy P, McCaul C, Shannon J. Accuracy of cricothyroid membrane identification using ultrasound and palpation techniques in obese obstetric patients: an observational study. Int J Obstet Anesth. 2021;48:103205.
40. American Society of Anesthesiologists Consensus-Based Guidance on Preoperative Management of Patients (Adults and Children) on Glucagon-Like Peptide-1 (GLP-1) Receptor Agonists. https://www.asahq.org/about-asa/newsroom/news-releases/2023/06/american-society-of-anesthesiologists-consensus-based-guidance-on-preoperative. Accessed 3 Jan 2024
41. Van de Putte P, Perlas A. Ultrasound assessment of gastric content and volume. Br J Anaesth. 2014;113:12–22.
42. Lakhal K, Delplace X, Cottier J-P, Tranquart F, Sauvagnac X, Mercier C, Fusciardi J, Laffon M. The feasibility of ultrasound to assess subglottic diameter. Anesth Analg. 2007;104:611–4.
43. Shibasaki M, Nakajima Y, Ishii S, Shimizu F, Shime N, Sessler DI. Prediction of pediatric endotracheal tube size by ultrasonography. Anesthesiology. 2010;113:819–24.

44. Giordano G, Alessandri F, Zulian A, Bilotta F, Pugliese F. Pre-operative ultrasound prediction of difficult airway management in adult patients: a systematic review of clinical evidence. Eur J Anaesthesiol. 2023;40:313–25.
45. Carsetti A, Sorbello M, Adrario E, Donati A, Falcetta S. Airway ultrasound as predictor of difficult direct laryngoscopy: a systematic review and meta-analysis. Anesth Analg. 2022;134:740.

Chapter 3
Human Factors, Cognitive Aids, Checklists, and Airway Trolley

Peter Groom, Jon Blackshaw, and Timthy Parr

> **Highlights**
> - Human factors significantly impact airway management, with failures often linked to cognitive overload, poor communication, and stress-induced performance deterioration.
> - Cognitive aids, checklists, and decision-support tools improve adherence to airway management protocols, reducing errors in high-stakes situations.
> - The Vortex Approach provides a structured framework for managing airway emergencies by emphasizing rapid recognition of ventilation failure and progression through airway interventions.
> - Checklists enhance team coordination and safety, with the WHO Surgical Safety Checklist and the DAS 2017 critical care intubation checklist proving effective.
> - Difficult airway trolleys improve equipment accessibility, reduce cognitive overload, and support standardized airway management.
> - Education and simulation-based training strengthen non-technical skills (NTS), improving decision-making, communication, and teamwork in critical airway scenarios.
> - Recent DAS and AAGBI recommendations advocate for integrating human factors principles into anesthetic practice to improve both patient safety and clinician well-being.

P. Groom (✉) · J. Blackshaw · T. Parr
Liverpool Head and Neck Centre, Liverpool University Hospitals NHS Foundation Trust, Liverpool, UK
e-mail: jonblackshaw@doctors.net.uk; timothy.parr@liverpoolft.nhs.uk

M. Á. Gómez-Ríos, A. van Zundert (eds.), *Evidence-based Guide to Difficult Airway Management*, https://doi.org/10.1007/978-3-032-30769-9_3

3.1 Introduction

Human factors is a scientific discipline focused on preventing harm by understanding how humans interact with systems [1, 2]. Interventions in human factors aim to enhance performance and safety by acknowledging human fallibility, particularly in high-stress, time-sensitive scenarios, where decision-making can deteriorate [3].

To build safe systems, human factors integrates engineering, psychology, social and physical anthropology, and other disciplines to minimize reliance on faultless human performance [2, 3, 4]. This requires organizational commitment, including investment in system design to prevent errors, the establishment of robust barriers against error progression, and the implementation of effective mitigation strategies [2, 3, 4].

In safety-critical industries, such as aviation, nuclear energy, offshore oil, and healthcare, human factors principles are used to design working environments that make it easy to "do the right thing" and difficult or impossible to "do the wrong thing" [2, 3, 4]. Additionally, risk reporting systems, education, and training investments are crucial to enhancing safety.

3.2 Human Factors in Airway Management

Maintenance of oxygenation during airway management is a core anesthetic skill. Failure to anticipate, identify, and resolve airway issues quickly can lead to rapid deterioration, resulting in preventable patient harm [5]. The United Kingdom's Fourth National Audit Project (NAP4) examined major complications in airway management and found significant human factors failures in 40% of adverse outcomes [5]. Key recurring issues included poor team performance, task fixation, and loss of situational awareness [5]. High operator stress and associated deterioration of individual and team performance have contributed to high-profile airway-related deaths in the United Kingdom [5, 6]. Elaine Bromiley's death in 2005 was a landmark case that propelled the importance of human factors in airway management into sharp focus [4, 6]. Her husband, Martin Bromiley, a commercial airline pilot, advocated for integrating human factors training into medical education and healthcare management [4]. He highlighted the importance of non-technical skills (NTS) and checklists, which are cornerstones of safety in the airline industry.

3.2.1 The Importance of Non-technical Skills (NTS)

NTS are cognitive, social, and personal resource skills that support safe and efficient task performance [7, 8]. These include [7, 8]:

- Situational awareness.
- Decision-making.

- Teamwork and task management.
- Leadership and communication.
- Followership and delegation.
- Prioritization and coping with distractions.
- Managing stress.

Recognizing their value, the Anaesthetic Non-technical Skills Framework was introduced in 2003 [7, 8]. Given the crucial role of human factors in anesthesia and airway management, the Difficult Airway Society (DAS) and the Association of Anaesthetists of Great Britain and Ireland (AAGBI) published two key papers in 2023:

- A narrative review of human factors in anesthesia [9].
- Guidelines for Implementing human factors in anesthesia [10].

3.3 Conceptual Models in Human Factors Science

As human factors science has evolved, many attempts have been made to conceptualize the myriad factors that contribute to human failures and to propose strategies to prevent their recurrence. Three of these models are described below.

3.3.1 Reason's Three Bucket Model

The Three Bucket Model, proposed by James Reason, explains the likelihood of errors during airway management [11]. According to Reason, errors result from a dynamic interplay of contributory factors, grouped into three key categories ("buckets"), each containing potential risks ("bad stuff") that are constantly in flux.

The Clinician
Factors affecting individual performance:

- Fatigue, hunger, or illness.
- Emotional stress (anger, intimidation).
- Lack of knowledge, confidence, or experience.

The Task
Challenges related to the procedure itself:

- Production pressure and time constraints.
- Lack of support or poor communication.
- Unfamiliar environment.
- Defective, inadequate, or unavailable equipment.

The Context
Environmental and situational distractions:

- Unusual or unexpected circumstances.
- Routine, mundane tasks that may lead to complacency.
- External interruptions or competing demands.

3.3.1.1 Strategies for Error Prevention

To minimize errors, clinicians must remain self-aware of their own three "buckets" at all times. Reason emphasizes the following key principles:

- Accept that errors can and will occur, and plan accordingly.
- Assess the local "*bad stuff*" before embarking upon a task.
- Have contingencies ready to deal with anticipated problems.
- Be prepared to seek more qualified assistance.
- Avoid allowing professional courtesy to get in the way of checking your colleagues' knowledge and experience, particularly when they are strangers.
- Appreciate that the path to adverse incidents is paved with false assumptions.

3.3.1.2 Task Fixation and the CICO Emergency

One of the greatest risks in airway management is task fixation, where repeated, unsuccessful intubation attempts delay alternative oxygenation strategies (e.g. face mask ventilation, supraglottic airway, or cricothyroidotomy). This can lead to severe hypoxia, cardiac arrest, hypoxic encephalopathy, and ultimately, death [5].

The "can't intubate can't oxygenate" (CICO) scenario is a time-critical, high-pressure emergency that requires the multidisciplinary team to act decisively and efficiently under extreme stress [5]. Proper team coordination, cognitive aids, and adherence to predefined protocols are essential to ensure successful management and prevent catastrophic outcomes.

3.3.2 The Yerkes-Dobson Model

The Yerkes and Dobson model [1] complements Reason's framework by focusing on psychological and neurocognitive processes in stressful scenarios. This model illustrates how increasing perceived stress progressively impairs task performance.

First, a "*Zone of Frazzle*" is entered, with the individual feeling distressed due to the release of stress-response hormones. If the individual fails to recognize this state and seek assistance, stress levels will increase further until a "*Zone of Freeze*" is reached, where performance plummets as analytical thought is overwhelmed [12, 13].

3.3.2.1 Cognitive Overload and Stress Response

- Cognitive overload occurs when working memory—capable of holding only four pieces of information at a time—is overwhelmed, leading to failure in the "*Zone of Freeze*" [12].
- In this state, decision-making shifts from logical reasoning to the amygdala ("primitive brain"), triggering limbic hijacking and the "*fight-or-flight response*."
- Prioritization of gross motor skills over fine motor skills and the consequent reduction in manual dexterity and narrowing of the visual field contribute to loss of situational awareness [13].

3.3.2.2 Role of High-Fidelity Simulation

One of the key goals of high-fidelity simulation is to expose participants to the physiological effects of escalating stress. By experiencing and recognizing their "*buckets filling*" and entering the "*Zone of Frazzle*," clinicians can identify warning signs early and seek help before reaching the "Zone of Freeze."

3.3.3 Hierarchy of Controls Model

According to NAP4, a human factors approach to improving system safety should account for all contributory factors and their interactions. These factors are structured within a Hierarchy of Controls Model [14], which categorizes safety interventions based on their relative effectiveness [15] (Fig. 3.1).

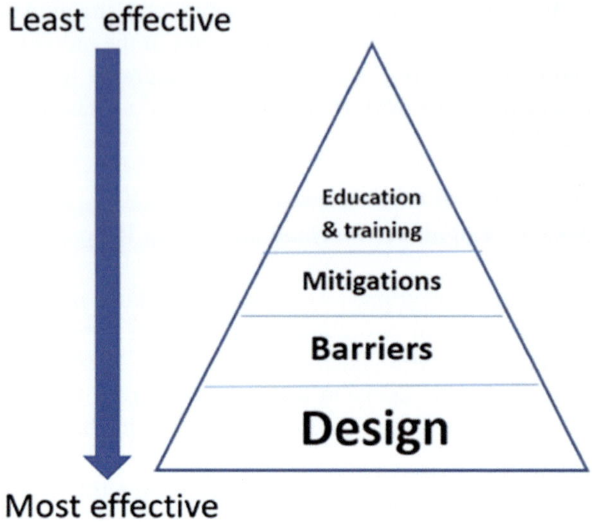

Fig. 3.1 Hierarchy of controls model. (Reproduced with permission from [9])

3.4 Design

Well-designed working environments are among the most effective human factors interventions for enhancing safety [1, 2, 16].

Examples of human factors-informed design in airway management include capnography as a minimum standard for all anesthetic machines and a well-stocked difficult airway trolley [5]. Further improvements in carbon dioxide monitoring could be achieved by standardizing the color and morphology of capnography and peak airway pressure traces as well as implementing smart alarms that integrate capnography with peripheral capillary oxygen saturation.

Another key aspect of workplace design is resource management. Ensuring adequately skilled personnel are available to handle anticipated difficult airways is an example.

3.5 Barriers

Robust barriers, the second stage of the hierarchy of controls, play a crucial role in trapping errors before they cause patient harm. These can be physical, administrative, or personal. Barriers can be physical, administrative, or personal.

Physical Barriers

Removing high-risk equipment associated with negative outcomes and replacing it with safer alternatives. A notable example is replacing Macintosh direct laryngoscopes with videolaryngoscopes, which has been supported by meta-analysis [17].

Administrative Barriers

- Standard operating procedures and protocols to reduce practice variation and promote safety.
- Particularly valuable in healthcare systems that rely on itinerant workforces.

Personal Barriers

Two person verification for:

- Videolaryngoscopy views.
- Capnography trace combined with the use of an assertiveness tool, such as CUS (concerned, uncomfortable, safety issue), to challenge authority when necessary [18].

3.6 Mitigations

Mitigations act as the last line of defense, aiming to limit the consequences of errors and prevent harm propagation. For mitigations to be effective, errors must be identified promptly. They serve to protect both patients and the healthcare professionals involved—the so-called second victims.

3.6.1 Cognitive Aids and Decision Support Tools

Examples of mitigations in airway management include guidance tools, specifically cognitive aids, algorithms, and guidelines. They aim to reduce cognitive overload and provide a standardized framework for appropriate decision-making [19], and improve patient outcomes [5].

3.6.2 Trauma Risk Management (TRiM)

TRiM is a trauma-focused peer support system designed to protect "second victims" —clinicians who experience traumatic or potentially traumatic events from post-traumatic stress disorder [20]. TRiM allows peers to understand likely reactions to traumatic incidents and to conduct structured risk assessments, aiming to identify colleagues who need early referral to qualified psychological support.

3.6.3 Incident Reporting and Systemic Learning

Difficult airway reporting, airway alert cards, and audits serve to highlight problems and guide improvements to the system. Traditional incident investigations in healthcare have disproportionately focused on individual scrutiny, often resulting in policy updates and staff training rather than meaningful system redesign [21]. Newer, system-focused methodologies, such as the Yorkshire Contributory Factors Framework [22], align with modern human factors principles and offer a more balanced approach to incident analysis.

3.7 Education and Training

Education and training, the fourth and final stage of the hierarchy of controls model, equip individuals and teams with essential knowledge to operate effectively within the system. Various DAS airway management guidelines serve as key educational resources [23, 24, 25, 26, 27]. Most difficult airway guidelines do not explicitly address the integration of human factors [28]. However, the DAS guidelines for unexpected difficult airway management [23], obstetric airway [25], critical care intubation [26], and awake tracheal intubation [27] incorporate human factors within their algorithms. The 2015/2018 DAS guidelines prompt teams to "call for help," "declare a failed intubation," "stop and think," and "invite ideas from the team" [23, 26]. Effective communication encourages teamwork—a skill that can deteriorate under stress [23].

3.7.1 National Educational Initiatives

3.7.1.1 "No Trace, Wrong Place" Campaign (2017)

A UK-wide educational initiative by The Royal College of Anaesthetists' (RCoA) aimed at reinforcing the principle that a flat capnography trace during cardiopulmonary resuscitation indicates esophageal intubation until proven otherwise [29]. Clinicians were encouraged to *voluntarily* watch an instructional YouTube video [29].

3.7.1.2 "Unrecognized Oesophageal Intubation Flashcard Simulation" (2021–2022)

Following further patient deaths due to unrecognized esophageal intubation, the RCoA launched a second national educational program [30]. This program required every UK hospital airway lead to conduct a 5-min, face-to-face flashcard simulation for all multidisciplinary operating theatre teams before starting their lists.

3.7.2 *Multidisciplinary Team Training and Adherence to Guidelines*

Training as a multidisciplinary team is essential for all members to learn and rehearse their roles in preventing patient harm during emergency airway management. Beyond improving communication and flattening hierarchical barriers, simulation training is crucial for practicing airway management guidelines, cognitive aids, and checklists in real time [31].

Education and training are critical. One study revealed that more than 50% of anesthetists had varying levels of understanding of an airway management guideline [32], while another found that 97% experienced difficulties recalling its content [33]. Even when an algorithm is retained, adherence is inconsistent [34]. Reported adherence to airway management tools ranges from 19% to 94% [35, 36], with clinicians who have greater clinical experience demonstrating higher adherence rates [37, 38].

Poor adherence may stem from challenges in interpreting algorithms or the lack of a universal algorithm [28]. Addressing these barriers through targeted education, hands-on training, and standardized airway management protocols is essential to improving patient safety.

3.8 Guidance Tools in Airway Management

Airway management guidelines generally consist of a flowchart outlining discrete management steps, with two or more alternative outcomes. The NAP4 report emphasized the importance of clinicians being aware of, understanding, and properly following a well-designed airway management guideline during emergencies [5].

NAP4 rated airway management as good in 16% of cases, mixed in 43% and poor in 35% [5]. Poor clinical judgment or a lack of education and training contributed to complications in 62% and 47% of cases, respectively [5]. These findings align with the American Society of Anaesthesiologists' (ASA) closed claims analysis, which revealed that anesthetist's airway management was substandard in nearly half of the cases, particularly due to repeated failed attempts at direct laryngoscopy [39]. After a comprehensive literature review, the ASA later stated that there is insufficient evidence to evaluate patient outcomes related to the use of visual aids, cognitive aids, or algorithms for unanticipated or emergency difficult airways [16]. Regardless, the ASA recommends that "When appropriate, refer to an algorithm and/or cognitive aid" and published their own revised algorithms and new infographics as part of their 2022 guideline document [16].

3.8.1 Airway Guidelines

3.8.1.1 Impact of Institutional Airway Guidelines

Several studies suggest that the routine adoption of institutional airway guidelines improves success rates and patient safety [40, 41, 42, 43].

- In a single-center study, intubation was successful in 95 out of 100 cases when staff adhered to an algorithmic approach for unanticipated difficult intubation [40].
- A prospective evaluation of various algorithmic approaches to difficult intubation reported a failure rate of just 0.05% (6 out of 13,248 cases) [41].
- A hospital implementing a difficult airway management algorithm achieved a 100% success rate across 12,225 patients, including 125 difficult airway cases, managed by 15 experienced anesthetists [42].
- Another study demonstrated that establishing an institutional difficult airway program led to a sustained reduction in the need for surgical airway rescue over 11 years, despite a rising number of cases [43].

National anesthesia and airway societies, including the UK's DAS, the ASA, and international airway groups such as the Project for Universal Management of Airways (PUMA), have reviewed the literature and applied evidence-based practices to develop clinical guidelines for airway management. These guidelines aim to limit the number of attempts using any single method to secure the airway [17, 23, 25, 26, 44]. They incorporate cognitive aids, infographics, algorithms, and checklists, all of which are strongly recommended tools for managing difficult airways [5, 45]. These terms are often used interchangeably, as reflected in the definitions provided by the American Psychological Association (APA) dictionary of psychology [46].

Cognitive Aid: Any guidance tool specifically designed for use *during* a task's performance. Cognitive aids support a mental process and prevent the user forgetting critical tasks. Formats include: checklist, algorithm, emergency manual, poster, visual aid or mnemonic.

Algorithm: A well-defined procedure or set of rules to solve a problem or accomplish a task or that is used for conducting a series of computations. Algorithms are often represented visually as flowcharts. The term is derived from the name of the ninth-century Arab mathematician al-Khwarizmi.

Checklist: A structured list of items that must to be observed, recorded, corrected, or considered to ensure compliance with a process.

Infographic [47]: A visual representation of information or data, such as charts or diagrams. Although the term is used by the American Society of Anaesthesiologists [16], it is not recognized by the APA.

3.8.1.2 Evidence and Limitations of Airway Guidelines

Despite widespread adoption, there is limited published evidence on whether airway management guidelines lead to changes in clinical practice and improved patient outcomes [17, 28]. Key concerns include:

- Lack of high-quality studies: There are insufficient large-scale, well-designed, multicenter trials evaluating the effectiveness of airway algorithms [53, 54].
- Reliance on observational data: Many recommendations, such as limiting SAD insertion attempts to three, stem from a single observational study of one anesthetist's practice [55].
- Short study follow-ups: Most available research consists of small sample sizes with brief follow-up periods [53].

Given the challenges of conducting randomized controlled studies on airway emergencies, most airway algorithms are based on expert consensus than robust evidence [54, 17]. This limits their reliability and longevity, requiring frequent updates as medical knowledge and technology evolve. Some experts suggest guidelines should be reviewed every 3–4 years to prevent obsolescence [56, 57].

3.8.1.3 Standardization of Airway Algorithms

In 2019, Edelman reviewed 38 published airway management algorithms, finding that 58% were published between 2014 and 2019 [28]. Since then, new guidelines have emerged, including:

- 2020 DAS thyroid hematoma guidelines [51]
- 2022 PUMA unrecognized esophageal intubation guidelines [52]
- 2022 ASA difficult airway guidelines [17]
- www.elsevier.es/redar

Most airway algorithms employ a four-step process, as represented by a flow chart, with progression from tracheal intubation, face mask ventilation, and supraglottic airway device use, to a rescue emergency surgical airway [28]. Although these guidelines are largely similar, inconsistencies in terminology and approach highlight the need for a single, universally recognized airway management algorithm applicable to all difficult airway management situations [28].

3.8.1.4 Towards a Unified Approach: PUMA Initiative

Recognizing the fragmentation in airway management, PUMA was established in 2016. Its mission is to [44]:

- Promote collaboration among international airway societies.
- Standardize terminology and best practices.
- Develop a unified, evidence-based airway management algorithm.

By consolidating research and expert consensus, PUMA aims to improve patient safety by harmonizing airway guidelines globally.

3.8.2 Designing Effective Guidance Tools

The design of a guidance tool—including its graphics, color, content, language, and information presentation—determines its suitability for either education and training (Planning Stage) or mitigation (Performance Stages) [48].

The term "*cognitive aid*" specifically refers to a guidance tool designed for use *during* task performance [28, 48]. Cognitive aids are especially valuable in time-critical emergency scenarios [80] and function as a mitigation strategy within the hierarchy of controls model (Fig. 3.1). Cognitive aids follow a standard iterative design process used in other medical and safety-critical devices. They incorporate human factors principles, intuitive graphic design, color-coded cues, and simple, low-content language [28, 48]. A cognitive aid should have four key attributes [31]:

- ***Content*** → based on best-practice guidelines.
- ***Design*** → Optimized for emergency use.
- ***Familiarity*** → Rehearsed format in practice and ***training***.
- ***Team alignment*** → Ensures cohesive and efficient teamwork.

Studies in aviation [49] and healthcare [50] suggest that cognitive aids lacking any of these four elements may promote wrong action sequences, potentially leading to patient harm. By highlighting critical steps in a task, cognitive aids [31, 51]:

- Reduce cognitive load, facilitating a structured approach.
- Minimize errors and enhance decision-making.
- Improve communication and task execution.
- Increase speed and precision of performance.

The Vortex Approach was the first custom-designed cognitive aid for airway management [48].

3.8.3 The Vortex Approach

The Vortex differs from other airway management guideline tools as it focuses on difficult ventilation by any route—face mask, supraglottic airway device (SAD), or endotracheal tube—rather than solely addressing failed intubation [28]. In contrast, most other airway guidance tools assume intubation as the primary objective [28]. This approach has been endorsed by DAS in its 2018 critical care intubation guidelines [26] and has influenced the design of both the 2019 DAS awake tracheal intubation guidelines [27] and the 2022 ASA practice guidelines for the management of the difficult airway [17].

3.8.4 *Checklists*

For over 70 years, checklists have been a cornerstone of aviation safety [58], standardizing procedures, minimizing human error, and improving efficiency. In aviation, checklists are categorized based on their purpose [59]:

- **Prevention Checklists**: Designed to prevent errors, mistakes, or mishaps in high-hazard work areas where mistakes could lead to serious harm or fatalities.
- **Preparation Checklists** ("shopping list"): used in multiple-step situations to ensure effective resource management and clear communication of planning.
- **Procedural Checklists** ("read-and-do"): Applied to complex or infrequent tasks, ensuring all steps are performed sequentially.
- **Problem-Solving Checklists**: Multiple-point, question-type checklists used for troubleshooting complex procedures or tasks to pinpoint what went wrong, areas of difficulty, or solutions to barriers blocking forward movement.

3.8.4.1 Checklist Implementation in Healthcare

Integrating checklists into clinical practice requires complex cultural and organizational adaptation, balancing both technical and socio-adaptive elements [60]. One of the most notable examples of checklist effectiveness in healthcare is the 2006 Michigan Keystone Project, which successfully reduced central venous catheter infections in over 100 intensive care units through standardized infection control checklists [61].

3.8.4.2 The WHO Surgical Safety Checklist

Introduced globally in 2009, the World Health Organization (WHO) Surgical Safety Checklist is one of the most recognized and widely used safety checklists in healthcare [62]. Studies have shown that it reduces post-operative complications and improves patient safety [62, 63]. Its three-stage process reinforces accepted safety practices and fosters better interdisciplinary communication [64]. In airway management, the WHO checklist prompts teams to [65]:

- Identify and discuss potential risks before intubation.
- Enhance communication and develop a shared mental model among team members.
- Flatten hierarchy barriers by encouraging team members to contribute, empowering all staff to raise concerns and challenge decisions if necessary.

3.8.4.3 Checklists in Anesthesia and Critical Care

Beyond surgical safety, checklists have proven benefits in anesthesia, particularly for handover processes and planning during emergencies and for specific procedures [66]. Checklists are also a key component of NHS England's National Safety Standards for Invasive Procedures (NatSSIPs), introduced in 2015 to standardize patient safety practices and reduce medical errors in invasive procedures across various clinical settings [67]. In response, the Intensive Care Society (ICS) developed six ICU-specific checklists, including those for percutaneous tracheostomy insertion, ITU intubation, and bronchoscopy [68]. Similar to the WHO checklist, these tools share a structured format that includes pre-procedural actions such as assigning roles, sourcing equipment, and identifying risks, a time-out phase for final safety verification before the procedure, and a sign-out process to confirm completion of all necessary actions, including proper handover and documentation.

3.8.4.4 The DAS 2017 Critical Care Intubation Checklist

The 2017 DAS guidelines for intubation in critically ill patients introduced a three-stage checklist designed for team-based execution [26]. The driver for this checklist was the recognition that human factors errors were prominent in NAP 4 [5] and deficits such as lack of patient preparation, insufficient equipment checks, or protocol deviation occur in up to 50% of ICU critical incidents [69]. The DAS 2017 checklist focuses on patient preparation, equipment checks, team communication, role allocation, and planning for potential airway difficulties.

The DAS critical care checklist serves as both a preparation checklist, ensuring readiness before induction, and a prevention checklist, reducing risks by standardizing best practices. It condenses key elements of the detailed guideline into a concise format for use before induction. The authors stress the importance of team familiarity with the guidelines and locally available equipment while encouraging practice and simulation-based training [26].

3.8.4.5 Checklists During the COVID-19 Pandemic

The COVID-19 pandemic introduced new challenges to airway management, including:

- Risk of operator infection.
- Unfamiliar environments and inexperienced staff.
- Barriers to communication (e.g. personal protective equipment).
- Tracheal intubation of profoundly hypoxic patients.

To address these challenges, a COVID-specific intubation checklist was developed [70], incorporating:

- A two-phase preparation process (inside vs. outside the patient's room), that includes an exhaustive checklist of required items.
- Detailed PPE verification and risk-reduction measures.
- Team discussion of airway plans before entering the room to optimize decision-making in controlled conditions.

3.8.5 Difficult Airway Trolley

The difficult airway trolley is a key advancement in integrating human factors principles into airway management. Over the past decade, the importance of standardized airway equipment has been recognized following studies linking human factors to airway complications [5, 48, 56, 71].

In 2010, just over 50% of UK ICUs had a dedicated difficult airway trolley [72]. Following the NAP4, this figure increased to over 90% [73], and by 2018, nearly all pediatric ICUs in the United Kingdom had access to a local airway trolley [74].

3.8.5.1 Key Principles for Airway Trolley

The availability, uniformity, and presentation of airway equipment on an airway trolley are key components of well-designed airway management [75]. Based on NAP4 recommendations [5], airway trolleys should adhere to the following principles:

- National standardization of airway trolleys across relevant areas.
- Local customization of advanced airway trolley contents.
- High-resource availability to manage unanticipated difficult airway scenarios.
- Immediate access to difficult airway trolleys in ICUs and emergency departments, standardized in content and layout to match those in theatre departments.
- Regular checking maintenance, and equipment replacement to ensure functionality.

3.8.5.2 Structured Layout: Aligning the Trolley with Airway Algorithms

For optimal usability, airway trolleys should be stocked and structured in alignment with local difficult airway management plans. The four-drawer organization commonly follows [19, 76]:

- **Plan A**—tracheal intubation.
- **Plan B**—supraglottic airway device (SAD).
- **Plan C**—face mask ventilation.
- **Plan D**—cricothyroidotomy.

Integrating a cognitive aid or algorithm into the structured layout of the trolley is an example of effective human factors design. This approach transforms the trolley into an extension of the corresponding airway algorithms [19, 76], guiding the team through each stage and reinforcing a shared mental model. As a result, it facilitates timely progression through each stage of the algorithm and ensures a swift transition to cricothyroidotomy rescue when all other attempts have failed.

3.8.5.3 Human Factors in Airway Trolley Design

To enhance usability and safety, airway trolleys should incorporate:

- Clear labeling for quick identification of equipment.
- Color coding and icons to aid cross-referencing with cognitive aids.
- Shadow board systems, where items are placed on designated templates during setup, ensuring proper equipment placement [77].
- Scenario-based simulation training, improving staff familiarity with trolley layout [78] and its integration into clinical workflows [19].

3.8.5.4 Standardization and Rationalization of Airway Equipment

Initially, airway trolleys lacked standardization, leading to variable layouts and excess equipment [19]. This hindered clinical performance during airway crises and prompted a more structured approach to equipment selection and presentation [79]. Devices that perform the same function should be eliminated and equipment that achieves a specific challenge should be prioritized [19]. Rationalizing in this way has the following benefits:

- Minimized Cognitive Overload → Reduced clutter and enhanced visibility facilitate access and streamline decision-making, preventing delays in airway management. This approach mitigates both choice overload—where an excess of options leads to indecision or inaction—and choice fatigue—where repeated decision-making under stress results in deteriorating judgment and an increased risk of error.
- Improved Efficiency → Clinicians become proficient with a limited yet effective range of equipment.
- Customizability → Trolleys can be tailored to local requirements, with contents that suit the users and the context. Dedicated adult or pediatric trolleys [80], for example, may stock a smaller range of sizes than those trolleys catering for all age ranges.

3.8.5.5 Guidelines on Difficult Airway Equipment

International airway management guidelines vary in their recommendations regarding difficult airway trolleys (Fig. 3.2).

Guideline	Year	Equipment/Airway Trolley Advice
American Society of Anaesthesiologists	2022	Recommends the use of a difficult airway trolley with specific recommendations on contents. Suggests customization to meet specific needs of the practitioner and healthcare facility.
Canadian Airway Focus Group	2021	No specific recommendations regarding content of a DAT. General advice regarding immediate availability of equipment for difficult airway management. Emphasis on the need for adequate equipment in obstetrical units.
All India Difficult Airway Association	2016	Specific suggestions for content of a difficult airway cart, including drawer organization. List of mandatory equipment and desirable equipment
All India Difficult Airway Association (Obstetric)	2016	Guidelines focused on unanticipated difficult tracheal intubation in obstetric patients. Brief recommendations regarding selection of equipment
Difficult Airway society (UK)	2015	Detailed recommendations regarding setup, organization, and implementation of a DAT. Advice about the design and contents of an ideal DAT. Emphasizes limiting the number of devices to improve decision-making
Difficult Airway Society OAA	2015	Guidelines concerning difficult/failed tracheal intubation in obstetrics. Standardization of airway equipment within the hospital is recommended. Limited recommendations regarding which equipment to include in a DAT
German Society of Anaesthesiology and Intensive Care	2015	List of minimum equipment for the anesthesiologists' workstation. Airway management equipment should be readily available also in the PACU and ICU. No comments regarding a DAT
Japanese Society of Anaesthesiologists	2014	Rescue airway devices should be accessible "within seconds from any operating room," e.g., in a DAT. Limited recommendations regarding specific equipment
Australia and New Zealand College of Anaesthetists	2012	List of essential (minimum) equipment. Additional items "may be added at the discretion of each individual department." List of supplementary equipment. Emphasizes careful selection of items.
Italian Scientific Society of Anaesthesiologists, Intensivists and Pain Therapists	2005	List of mandatory devices and devices which should be available upon request.
Swedish Society of Anaesthesia and Intensive Care Medicine	2005	Difficult airway trolleys with standardized equipment at all sites where anesthesia or intensive care is provided. Brief, general advice regarding equipment

Fig. 3.2 Difficult airway guidelines containing recommendations for difficult airway trolley

However, there is broad consensus that [81]:

- Difficult airway equipment should be available in all locations where anesthesia or intensive care is provided [82].
- Equipment standardization must be promoted to improve safety and efficiency [82].
- Guidelines provide varying levels of detail on device selection and trolley organization [23, 25].

3.9 Recommendations for Implementing Human Factors in Anesthesia

In 2023, DAS and the AAGBI published the first guidelines for integrating human factors in anesthesia to improve patient safety and staff well-being [10]. These 12 recommendations, based on the hierarchy of controls model [14] provide a structured approach for anesthetists, anesthetic departments, and hospitals to implement human factors principles across five key domains:

3.9.1 Design

1. Design of medical equipment should include input from human factors experts at an early stage. The medical equipment procurement process should include human factors assessments.
2. Design of drug ampoules and packaging should incorporate human factors principles to optimize readability and reduce the risk of mis-selection. Anesthetists, pharmacists and procurement departments should ensure that these principles are prioritized during the purchasing processes.
3. Design of safe working environments should incorporate human factors principles to enhance workflow and reduce errors. Regular reviews should be carried out to ensure that safety has not been compromised.

3.9.2 Barriers

4. Operating theatre list planning and scheduling should include additional time allocated for complex cases and high-turnover lists to reduce time pressure on staff and allow adequate preparation.
5. Cognitive aids, including algorithms and checklists, should be designed and tested using human factors principles to ensure usability and efficacy.
6. Non-technical skills should be practiced daily to strengthen decision-making, communication, and teamwork abilities among staff.

3.9.3 Mitigations

7. Investigation of critical incidents and adverse events should involve teams trained in human factors and use human factors investigative tools. Lessons learned should be shared systematically across teams to improve future practice.
8. Morbidity and mortality meetings should be a routine part of anesthetic practice, including cases with positive outcomes to encourage learning from success. Hospitals should allocate time within job plans to ensure staff can prepare for and attend these meetings.

3.9.4 Education and Training

9. Human factors education and training should be provided at an appropriate level for all anesthetists and theatre teams. It should include the role of good design in healthcare, an appreciation of a systems perspective, the importance of non-technical skills, and strategies to improve these.
10. Non-technical skills training and interprofessional simulation training: Teams that work together should train together. Non-technical skills should be integrated during classroom learning, in-theatre teaching, anesthetic workshops and courses, and regular interprofessional simulation training. Time and resources should be allocated to support these training initiatives.

3.9.5 Well-Being

11. Staff well-being should be optimized by hospitals and anesthetic departments by implementing organizational strategies.

3.9.6 Strategy

12. Each anesthetic department should appoint a human factors lead with appropriate training. Every hospital should have a patient safety leads with formal human factors qualifications, as recommended by Health Education England.

References

1. https://iea.cc/what-is-ergonomics/. Accessed 22/10/22.
2. https://ergonomics.org.uk/resource/human-factors-in-health-and-social-care.html. Accessed 22/10/22.

3. Shorrock S, Williams C. Human factors and ergonomics in practice: improving system performance and human wellbeing in the real world. CRC Press, 2017.
4. https://www.health.org.uk/funding-and-partnerships/programmes/clinical-human-factors-group?gclid=EAIaIQobChMI7q-O6eOR-AIVjJftCh0J1AzxEAAYASAAEgLRDfD_BwE. Accessed 22/10/22.
5. Cook TM, Woodall N, Frerk C. Major complications of airway management in the UK: results of the fourth National Audit Project of the Royal College of Anaesthetists and the difficult airway society. Part 1: anaesthesia. Br J Anaesth. 2011;106:617–31.
6. Bromiley M. Have you ever made a mistake? R Coll Anaesth Bull. 2008;48:2442–5. https://studylib.net/doc/18282697/have-you-ever-made-a-mistake%3F. Accessed 22/10/22
7. Flin R, O'Connor P, Crichton M. Safety at the sharp end: a guide to non-technical skills. Farnham: Ashgate; 2008.
8. Flin R, Patey R, Glavin R, Maran N. Br J Anaesth. 2010;105:38–44.
9. Kelly FE, Frerk C, Bailey CR, et al. Human factors in anaesthesia: a narrative review. Anaesthesia 2023; https://doi.org/10.1111/anae.15941
10. Kelly FE, Frerk C, Bailey CR, et al. Implementing human factors in anaesthesia: guidance for clinicians, departments and hospitals. Anaesthesia. 2023; https://doi.org/10.1111/anae.15941.
11. Reason J. Beyond the organisational accident: the need for "error wisdom" on the front line. BMJ Quality & Safety. 2004;13:ii28–33.
12. Wickens CD. Multiple resources and performance prediction. Theor Issues Ergon Sci. 2002;3:159–77.
13. Hearns S. Peak performance under pressure. Somerset: Class Professional Publishing, 2019.
14. Manuele FA. Achieving risk reduction, effectively. Human factors Management. 2006;84:184–90.
15. Cook TM, MacDougall-Davis SR. Complications and failure of airway management. Br J Anaesth. 2012;109(Suppl 1):i68–85.
16. Dul J, Bruder R, Buckle P, et al. A strategy for human factors/ergonomics: developing the discipline and profession. Ergonomics. 2012;55:377–95.
17. Apfelbaum JL, Hagberg CA, Connis RT, et al. 2022 American Society of Anesthesiologists Practice Guidelines for Management of the Difficult Airway. Anesthesiology. 2022;136:31–81.
18. Eppich W. "Speaking up" for patient safety in the pediatric emergency department. Clin Pediatr Emerg Med. 2015;16:83–9.
19. Chrimes N, Bradley WPL, Gatward JJ, Weatherall AD. Human factors and the 'next generation' airway trolley. Anaesthesia. 2019;74:427–33.
20. Kelly FE, Osborn M, Stacey MS. Improving resilience in anaesthesia and intensive care medicine—learning lessons from the military. Anaesthesia. 2020;75:720–3.
21. Microsoft Word—Imperial College Report for NHS London—Never Events Analysis—final (imperial-anaesthesia.org.uk). Accessed 12/9/22.
22. Lawton R, McEachan RRC, Giles SJ, et al. Development of an evidence-based framework of factors contributing to patient safety incidents in hospital settings: a systematic review. BMJ Qual Saf. 2012;21:369–80.
23. Frerk C, Mitchell VS, McNarry AF, et al. Difficult airway society 2015 guidelines for management of unanticipated difficult intubation in adults. Br J Anaesth. 2015;115:827–48.
24. Popat M, Mitchell V, Dravid R, et al. Difficult airway society guidelines for the management of tracheal extubation. Anaesthesia. 2012;67:318–40.
25. Mushambi MC, Kinsella SM, Popat M, et al. Anaesthesia. 2015;70:1286–306.
26. Higgs A, McGrath BA, Goddard C, et al. Guidelines for the management of tracheal intubation in critically ill adults. Br J Anaesth. 2018;120:323–52.
27. Ahmad I, El-Boghdadly K, Bhagrath R, et al. Difficult airway society guidelines for awake tracheal intubation (ATI) in adults. Anaesthesia. 2020;75:509–28.
28. Edelman DA, Perkins EJ, Brewster DJ. Difficult airway management algorithims: a directed review. Anaesthesia. 2019;74:1175–85.
29. https://www.youtube.com/watch?v=t97G65bignQ. Accessed 3/10/2022.

30. https://www.rcoa.ac.uk/sites/default/files/documents/2021-11/Unrecognised-Oesphageal-Intubation-Flash-Cards.pdf. Accessed 3/10/2022
31. Marshall S. The use of cognitive aids during emergencies in anesthesia: a review of the literature. Anesth Analg. 2013;117:1162–71.
32. Knudsen K, Poder U, Nilsson U, et al. How anaesthesiologists understand difficult airway guidelines-an interview study. Ups J Med Sci. 2017;122:243–8.
33. Rosenstock C, Ostergaard D, Kristensen MS, et al. Residents lack knowledge and practical skills in handling the difficult airway. Acta Anaesthesiol Scand. 2004;48:1014–8.
34. Borges BCR, Boet S, Siu LW, et al. Incomplete adherence to the ASA difficult airway algorithm is unchanged after a high-fidelity simulation session. Can J Anesth. 2010;57:644–9.
35. Borg PAJ, Stuart C, Dercksen B, et al. Anaesthetic management of the airway in The Netherlands: a postal survey. Eur J Anaesthesiol. 2001;18:730–8.
36. Ezri T, Konichezky S, Geva D, et al. Difficult airway management patterns among attending anaesthetists practising in Israel. Eur J Anaesthesiol. 2003;20:619–23.
37. Kristensen MS, Moller J. Airway management behaviour, experience and knowledge among Danish anaesthesiologists—room for improvement. Acta Anaesthesiol Scand. 2001;45:1181–5.
38. Rochlen LR, Housey M, Gannon I, et al. Assessing anesthesiology residents' out-of-the-operating-room [OOOR] emergent airway management. BMC Anesthesiol. 2017;17:96.
39. Peterson GN, Domino KB, Caplan RA, Posner KL, Lee LA, Cheney FW. Management of the difficult airway. A closed claims analysis. Anesthesiology. 2005;103:33–9.
40. Combes X, Le Roux B, Suen P, et al. Unanticipated difficult airway in anesthetized patients. Prospective validation of a management algorithm. Anesthesiology. 2004;100:1146–50.
41. Heidegger T, Gerig HJ, Ulrich B, et al. Validation of a simple algorithm for tracheal intubation: daily practice is the key to success in emergencies—an analysis of 13,248 intubations. Anesth Analg. 2001;92:517–22.
42. Amathieu R, Combes X, Abdi W, et al. An algorithm for difficult airway management, modified for modern optical devices (Airtraq laryngoscope; LMA CTrach™). Anesthesiology. 2011;114:25–33.
43. Berkow LC, Greenberg RS, Kan KH, et al. Need for emergency surgical airway reduced by a comprehensive difficult airway program. Anesth Analg. 2009;109:1860–9.
44. Project for Universal Management of Airways. 2019. https://www.universalairway.org. Accessed 3/10/2022.
45. Crosby ET, Cooper RM, Douglas MJ, et al. The unanticipated difficult airway with recommendations for management. Can J Anesth. 1998;45:757–76.
46. https://dictionary.apa.org. Accessed 3/10/2022.
47. https://www.google.co.uk/search?q=infographic+definition&ei=edFnY-roCIeV8gLyhpjoAw&ved=0ahUKEwiqibug7pn7AhWHilwKHXIDBj0Q4dUDCA4&uact=5&oq=infographic+definition&gs_lcp=Cgxnd3Mtd2l6LXNlcnAQAzIFCAAQgAQyBQgAEIAEMgUIAB-CABDIGCAAQFhAeMgYIABAWEB4yBggAEBYQHjIGCAAQFhAeMgYIABAWEB4y-BggAEBYQHjIICAAQFhAeEA86CggAEEcQ1gQQsAM6BwgAELADEEM6DQgAEOQ-CENYEELADGAE6EgguEMcBENEDEMgDELADEEMYAjoVCC4QxwEQ0QMQ1AI-QyAMQsAMQQxgCOgcIABCxAxBDOgQIABBDOgUIABCGA0oECE0YAUoECEEY-AEoECEYYAVDOC1jDGmDCHmgBcAF4AIABpgGIAbsHkgEDOS4ymAEAoAEByAES wAEB2gEGCAEQARgJ2gEGCAIQARgI&sclient=gws-wiz-serp. Accessed 3/10/2022.
48. Chrimes N. The vortex: a universal 'high-acuity implementation tool' for emergency airway management. Br J Anaesth. 2016;117:i20–7.
49. Mosier KL, Palmer EA, Degani A. Electronic checklists: implications for decision making. Proceedings of the human factors society 36th annual meeting. 1992 Atlanta, GA (Human factors and ergonomics society) (Degani A, Wiener EL). Cockpit checklists: concepts, design and use. Hum Factors. 1993;35:345–59.
50. Carthey J, Clarke J The 'how to guide' for implementing human factors in healthcare patient safety first, UK. 2009. Available at: http://www.patientsafetyfirst.nhs.uk/ashx/Asset.

ashx?path=/Intervention-support/Human%20Factors%20How-to%20Guide%20v1.2.pdf. Accessed 3/10/2022 .
51. Iliff HA, El-Boghdadly k, Ahmad I, et al. Anaesthesia. 2022;77:82–95.
52. https://www.universalairway.org/puoi (accessed 3/10/2022).
53. Ahmad I, Onwochei DN, Muldoon S, et al. Airway management research: a systematic review. Anaesthesia. 2019;74:225.
54. Ahmad I, El-Boghdadly K. From evidence based on practice to evidence-based practice: time for a difficult airway management research strategy. Anaesthesia. 2019;74:135.
55. Cook TM, Gibbison B. Analysis of 1000 consecutive uses of the ProSeal laryngeal mask airway by one anaesthetist at a district general hospital. Br J Anaesth. 2007;99:436–9.
56. Cook TM. Strategies for the prevention of airway complications—a narrative review. Anaesthesia. 2018;73:93–111.
57. Shekelle PG, Ortiz E, Rhodes S, et al. Validity of the agency for healthcare research and quality clinical practice guidelines. How quickly do guidelines become outdated? JAMA J Am Med Assoc. 2001;286:1461–7.
58. Webster CS. Checklists, cognitive aids, and the future of patient safety. Br J Anaesth. 2017;119(2):178–81.
59. Higgins WY, Boorman DJ. An analysis of the effectiveness of checklists when combined with other processes, methods and tools to reduce risk in high Hazard activities. Boeing Tech J. 55(11):1217–30.
60. Flin R, Fioratou E, Frerk C, et al. Human factors in the development of complications of airway management: preliminary evaluation of an interview tool. Anaesthesia. 2013;68:817–25.
61. Pronovost P, Needham D, Berenholtz S, et al. An intervention to decrease catheter-related bloodstream infections in the ICU. N Engl JMed. 2006;355:2725–32.
62. Haynes AB, Weiser TG, Berry WR, et al. A surgical safety checklist to reduce morbidity and mortality in a global population. N Engl J Med. 2009;360:491–9.
63. Haugen AS, Sevdalis N, Søfteland E. Impact of the World Health Organization surgical safety checklist on patient safety. Anesthesiology. 2019;131:420–5.
64. Safety, WHO Patient, and World Health Organization. Implementation manual WHO surgical safety checklist 2009: safe surgery saves lives. World Health Organization; 2009.
65. Pattni N, Arzola C, Malavade A, et al. Challenging authority and speaking up in the operating room environment: a narrative synthesis. Br J Anaesth. 2019;122:223–44.
66. Saxena S, Krombach JW, Nahrwold DA, Pirracchio R. Anaesthesia-specific checklists: a systematic review of impact. Anaesth Crit Care Pain Med. 2020;39(1):65–73.
67. https://www.england.nhs.uk/wp-content/uploads/2015/09/natssips-safety-standards.pdf. Accessed 1/11/2022.
68. https://www.ficm.ac.uk/standardssafetyguidelinessafety/safety-checklists-for-invasive-procedures. Accessed 1/11/2022.
69. Chopra V, Shojania KG. Recipes for checklists and bundles: one part active ingredient, two parts measurement. BMJ Qual Saf. 2013;22:93–6.
70. Cook TM, El-Boghdadly K, McGuire B, et al. Consensus guidelines for managing the airway in patients with COVID-19: guidelines from the difficult airway society, the Association of Anaesthetists the Intensive Care Society, the Faculty of Intensive Care Medicine and the Royal College of Anaesthetists. Anaesthesia. 2020;75:785–99.
71. Watterson L, Rehak A, Heard A, et al. Transition from supraglottic to infraglottic rescue in the "can't intubate can't oxygenate" (CICO) scenario. Report from the ANZCA Airway Management Working Group; 2014. Available from http://www.anzca.edu.au/Documents/Report-from-the-ANZCA-Airway-Management-Working-Gr.pdf. Accessed 1/11/2022
72. Jeanrenaud P, Girotra V, Wharton T, et al. Difficult airway trolleys for the critical care unit. J Intensive Care Soc. 2010;7:23–5.
73. Cook TM, Woodall N, Frerk C. A national survey of the impact of NAP4 on airway management practice in United Kingdom hospitals: closing the safety gap in anaesthesia, intensive care and the emergency department. Br J Anaesth. 2016;117:182–90.

74. Foy KE, Mew E, Cook TM, et al. Paediatric intensive care and neonatal intensive care airway management in the United Kingdom: the PIC-NIC survey. Anaesthesia. 2018;73:1337–44.
75. Schnittker R, Marshall S, Horberry T, et al. Human factors enablers and barriers for successful airway management—an in-depth interview study. Anaesthesia. 2018;73:980–9.
76. Chishti K. Setting up a Difficult Airway Trolley (DAT). https://www.das.uk.com/content/difficult_airway_trolley. Accessed 1/11/22.
77. Leigh A, Salih T, Same M, et al. Airway trolley shadow board incorporating intubation checklist for critically ill adults. Br J Anaesth. 2019;123(3):E451.
78. Sathananthan C, Hulme A. Raising the standard: difficult airway trolleys on the intensive care unit. Trends Anaesth Crit Care. 2017;12:44.
79. Baker PA, Flanagan BT, Greenland KB, et al. Equipment to manage a difficult airway during anaesthesia. Anaesth Intensive Care. 2011;39:16–34.
80. Weatherall AD. The airway trolley—something old? Something new? 2018; https://songsorstories.com/2018/04/09/the-airway-trolley-something-old-something-new/. Accessed 1/11/2022
81. Bjurstrom MF, Bodelsson M, Sturesson LW. The difficult airway trolley: a narrative review and practical guide. Anesthesiol Res Pract. 2019; https://doi.org/10.1155/2019/6780254. Accessed 1/11/22
82. ANZCA. Professional document PG 56 (a): guidelines on equipment to manage difficult airways. West End: ANZCA; 2021. https://www.anzca.edu.au/getattachment/02fe1a4c-14f0-4ad1-8337-c281d26bfa17/PS56-Guideline-on-equipment-to-manage-difficult-airways

Chapter 4
Airway Leads

Patrick A. Ward and Alistair F. McNarry

Highlights

- The position of Airway Lead was formally established in 2012 as a response to the findings of the UK Fourth National Audit Project into complications relating to airway management.
- The Airway Lead role has evolved over time, but remains central to *local* delivery of airway training, airway guideline dissemination and implementation, airway equipment provision and standardisation, and surveillance and audit of airway management practices and outcomes at individual hospitals.
- Appointment of a local airway representative enables national directives to be delivered most effectively by applying awareness and knowledge of local organisational structures and resources.
- The Airway Leads project has played a crucial role in the development of important nationally implemented airway safety interventions, including the "No trace=wrong place" campaign and institutional preparedness for the Coronavirus 2019 pandemic.

P. A. Ward
St John's Hospital, NHS Lothian, Livingston, UK

A. F. McNarry (✉)
St John's Hospital, NHS Lothian, Livingston, UK

Western General Hospital NHS Lothian, Edinburgh, UK

M. Á. Gómez-Ríos, A. van Zundert (eds.), *Evidence-based Guide to Difficult Airway Management*, https://doi.org/10.1007/978-3-032-30769-9_4

4.1 Introduction

A chapter on the evidence supporting the existence of an Airway Lead, their function, and the requirement to have one appointed in every hospital could be very short indeed, as randomised controlled trial data or meta-analyses in this area simply do not exist. Despite this, recently published airway management guidelines consistently advocate the presence of an Airway Lead in every department [1], and their existence is presumed in others [2]. (Evidence Level: Grade D).

4.1.1 Evolution of Airway Management

Airway management has evolved radically over the past 40 years since the advent of the Laryngeal Mask Airway in 1983 [3], with the introduction of second-generation supraglottic airways, videolaryngoscopes, and apnoeic oxygenation techniques [4–6], among other technological advances. Airway guidelines to direct airway management behaviours have been produced since the early 1990s [7], and are now available in several languages [8, 9] and are even in their second and third iterations [1, 2, 10, 11].

All of these airway equipment innovations were designed to facilitate a higher success rate with tracheal intubation, provide effective airway management, and improve patient oxygenation when the primary airway plan is unsuccessful. Multiple systematic reviews and meta-analyses have been published describing the potential [12–16] benefit of these devices in a variety of settings and/or patient groups. New pharmacological agents have also become available (e.g. rocuronium and sugammadex) that, when used appropriately, should also facilitate easier primary airway management [17–20] and secondary rescue oxygenation techniques.

4.1.2 Persistent Airway-Related Morbidity and Mortality

Unfortunately, over the same time period, evidence of airway-related morbidity and mortality has continued to accumulate, where patients' airways were not managed optimally/effectively (irrespective of the underlying cause). The American Society of Anesthesiologists' (ASA) closed claims analysis (1990) found that adverse respiratory events represented the single largest group of claims (34%), and that death or brain damage were common events. Airway management issues were also highlighted in the Australian Incident Monitoring Study (AIMS) [21]. The AIMS report also recognised "human failure" and (ineffective) "crisis management" to be contributory factors. The publication of the ASA Practice guidelines for management of the difficult airway in 1993 made a positive impact in reducing the number of difficult airway events occurring at induction of anaesthesia [22], but unfortunately, adverse events relating to airway management did not disappear. Similarly, the UK fourth National Audit Report (NAP4) undertaken by the Royal College of Anaesthetists (RCoA) and Difficult Airway Society (DAS) recorded 188 cases of death, brain damage, unanticipated intensive care unit (ICU) admission or the need for the creation of an emergency front of neck airway [23]—for which data collection started 4 years *after* the publication of the first unanticipated difficult tracheal intubation guidelines [24].

4.1.3 Establishing the Airway Lead Role

The NAP4 report explicitly called for the creation of the Airway Lead role within hospitals, stating that, "the anaesthetic department should have an anaesthetist responsible for difficult airway management. The responsible person along with departmental colleagues should develop or adopt protocols for dealing with difficult airways in all areas of the organisation, ensure the purchase of suitable equipment to manage difficult airways and that regular multidisciplinary training for difficult airway management takes place."

However, this was not the first time that a recommendation had been made that an individual should be appointed with the specific responsibility of coordinating airway training within every anaesthetic department (a so-called airway representative). Indeed, Adrian Pearce, the founder of DAS in the United Kingdom, had proposed precisely such a role in 2002 (A. Pearce, personal communication). However, at that particular time, there was concern that centralising training decisions to just one individual might decrease department-wide involvement in airway training.

The subsequent recommendation in the NAP4 report was received more positively, however, resulting in the call to create the Airway Lead role, issued by the Council of the RCoA in 2012 [25]. By 2020, there was an Airway Lead in over 97% of UK hospitals [26], with similar networks established in New Zealand and Australia [27, 28].

A recent editorial described the role of the Airway Lead as being, "to ensure supply, quality and storage of airway equipment, promote the use of current practice guidelines as well as the organisation of training and audits [29]." This rather succinctly summarises the role specifications that were originally outlined by the RCoA (Box 4.1). Initially, the role was centred upon four distinct domains of activity, but it now encompasses other relevant areas. It is desirable that the roles of the Airway Lead are not restricted to the RCoA-DAS definition, and it is encouraged that the Airway Lead responsibilities may extend into other relevant areas, with a degree of flexibility expected within the role, adapted according to local requirements, logistics, personnel, and organisational structures. For example, the Airway Lead may also play a pivotal role in: airway device procurement, audit of guideline adherence, audit of complications, promotion of best practice, establishment of regular morbidity and mortality review, implementation of systems for surveillance of high-risk airways, participation in relevant national surveys and national audits, promotion of consistency in airway assessment and planning, and provision of support to staff following an adverse airway management event.

Box 4.1: The Four Domains of Activity Initially Identified by the RCoA and DAS That Defined the Role and Functions of the Airway Lead

1. Overseeing local airway training for anaesthetists and assisting in airway training more widely.
2. Ensuring local policies exist and are disseminated for predictable airway emergencies.
3. Ensuring that difficult airway equipment is appropriate to the local guidelines and standardised within the organisation.
4. Liaising specifically with the ICU and emergency department to ensure consistency.

4.2 Nationally Engaged, Locally Focussed

Whilst many aspects of an Airway Lead's role require engagement with national bodies and organisations, the crucial delivery element of their role is provided *locally,* which is best illustrated with examples:

(i) When the updated DAS guidelines for management of unanticipated difficult intubation were launched in 2015, they were presented many times at relevant meetings throughout the United Kingdom and around the world; however, whilst these presentations disseminated the message of the updated guidelines, they did not deliver the necessary change in equipment availability that was necessitated. This was particularly apparent in relation to "Plan D" (cricothyroidotomy), for which the revised guidance recommended a change from the existing cannula/low-frequency manual jetting technique (for which training and equipment had been provided in most hospitals) to a "scalpel-bougie-tube" technique.

Such a change did not simply mean that the Manujet device in the "Plan D" drawer of the airway trolley could merely be replaced by a scalpel, bougie, and a tube. Rather, the decision to follow the updated guideline involved the individual Airway Lead at each hospital arranging the sourcing of the equipment, ensuring that all staff who might be involved in an airway emergency received the necessary teaching, and an opportunity to practice the scalpel-bougie-tube technique. The final and crucial safety step in this process was the designation of an appropriate changeover day when all of the necessary training had been undertaken and the new equipment had been procured.

It is recognised that the education and training sessions for adoption of the new "Plan D" will have been delivered differently in different hospitals, ranging from lectures to workshops, or a combination of both [30], but it is precisely this ability to adapt to the local circumstances that is a fundamental benefit of the Airway Lead's Project. Indeed, a local clinician empowered to make decisions about how to implement national directives at a local level is likely to have far more success than an edict from a national body—by enabling local clinicians to choose the best time to run education sessions, how best to reach the anaesthetic support staff etc., since these decisions will be best made with the knowledge of how each individual department functions.

(ii) The evidence on the benefits of videolaryngoscopy in airway management is increasing [31, 32], and calls for its routine use have been made in academic journals on more than one occasion [33–36]. Examples of how universal videolaryngoscopy can be adopted in hospitals have been presented at a previous Airway Leads Day (annual meeting of Airway Leads at the RCoA) [37], but alternate strategies have also been described [38, 39]. Crucially, the decisions regarding which specific model of videolaryngoscope to choose require consideration of a variety of *local* factors (Fig. 4.1).

At the core of the duties/role of an Airway Lead is the ability to coordinate strategy across a hospital/hospital group (organisation). For example, there is the potential for different models of videolaryngoscopes to be acquired in different clinical areas within the same hospital, e.g. in operating theatres, on labour ward, and in ICU (with inevitable deleterious consequences), unless an individual or a team of individuals assumes the responsibility of coordinating the procurement process.

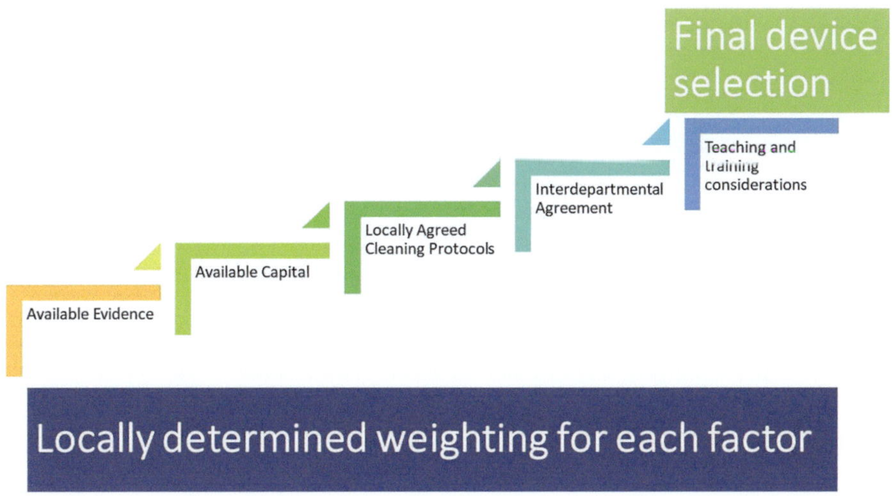

Fig. 4.1 Elements of a videolaryngoscope selection process that must be determined locally, not nationally

4.3 Best Practice

The Airway Leads Day (discussed later) and the Airway Leads network have served to encourage sharing of ideas and promote best clinical practice, so that strategies that have been implemented successfully at a local level by individual Airway Leads might be replicated in other hospitals throughout the United Kingdom. Sharing local success stories enables good practice ideas and behaviours to thrive in other hospitals and regions, by allowing adaptation to individual hospitals' specific requirements and capabilities.

Examples of best practice that have been promoted through the Airway Leads network are described in the following three "case studies" (Boxes 4.2, 4.3, and 4.4):

Box 4.2: Case Study: "Trachy Tracey" [40]
Case study 1: "Trachy Tracey"

Educational aims:

- Deliver essential training on the management of tracheostomy emergencies to a multidisciplinary audience. Significant morbidity and mortality have been associated with dislodged/blocked tracheostomies.

Educational challenges:

- Delivering airway training to a multidisciplinary audience.
- Delivering airway training without incurring significant costs or organisational burden.
- Delivering airway training that requires minimal teaching faculty.
- Delivering airway training that does not require the learner to have significant time away from clinical work.

Educational solution:

- "Trachy Tracey" was an educational tool designed first in *NHS Lothian*. It involved modification of a commercially available doll's head to include a tracheostomy stoma and tube, permitting widespread *bedside* training in the management of tracheostomy emergencies (blocked or dislodged tracheostomy tubes) to be successfully delivered across the region.

Educational success:

- Within 3 months of its introduction within *NHS Lothian*, 70% of ICU staff had been trained, with a demonstrable improvement in familiarity with the steps described in the tracheostomy emergencies management algorithm.
- Such a low cost, simple, and portable education tool that does not necessitate the learner to leave their workplace and requires minimal teaching faculty is precisely the type of intervention that can be (and has been) put into practice relatively easily by other Airway Leads at other hospitals.

Box 4.3: Case Study: Bath "Tea Trolley Training" [41, 42]
Case study 2: "Tea Trolley Training".

Educational aims:

- Deliver essential airway management training on a range of different topics to a multidisciplinary audience.

Educational challenges:

- Delivering airway training to a multidisciplinary audience.
- Delivering airway training without incurring high costs or organisational burden.
- Delivering airway training that requires minimal teaching faculty.
- Delivering airway training that does not require the learner to have significant time away from clinical work.
- Delivering airway training in manageable quantities to facilitate knowledge and skill retention.
- Encourage engagement with airway training by delivering training in a practical, fun, and effective way.

Educational solution:

- "Tea Trolley Training" was a novel educational modality first utilised at the *NHS Royal United Hospitals, Bath*. It consists of a small teaching faculty (one or two people) wheeling a modified surgical equipment trolley directly to staff during their normal working day. The mobile teaching materials and equipment are transported to the operating theatre, post-anaesthesia care unit or ICU, where short, targeted "bite-sized" teaching sessions can be conducted to a multidisciplinary audience—with the subsequent reward of tea and cake.

Educational success:

- This project has been successfully implemented across numerous hospitals nationally (reported at subsequent DAS annual conferences as abstracts/posters), and has been used to deliver training on emergency front-of-neck airways, rescue intubation through a supraglottic airway using an Aintree Intubating Catheter and flexible bronchoscope, and failed intubation drills, to name a few.

Box 4.4: Case Study: Regional Airway Networks

Case study 3: Regional Airway Networks

Organisational/management aims:

- Promote regional harmonisation and collaboration, rationalisation and standardisation of equipment across multiple hospital sites. Whilst the Airway Leads project was designed to be delivered by an individual representative at single organisations (hospital or hospitals within the same Trust/health board), it is recognised and encouraged that Airway Leads work together with other Airway Leads by sharing ideas, learning, resources, and structures, and establish regional networks that facilitate this process.

Organisational/management challenges:

- Inconsistency in airway management equipment and training across different hospitals within the same region, through which anaesthetic trainees rotate.
- Different equipment procurement teams, priorities, policies, and funding within different hospitals within the same region.

Organisational/management solution:

- Establishment of regional Airway Leads networks. This process has been undertaken successfully in a number of different regions throughout the UK, including in *NHS Cheshire and Merseyside hospitals.*

Organisational/management success:

- In this particular region, Consultants from 11 out of 13 departments collaborated on airway management equipment decisions, leading to the standardisation of equipment (paediatric airway equipment and cricothyroidotomy sets) across multiple organisations. Specifically, there was a successful rationalisation of cricothyroidotomy equipment from nine different sets to just two agreed pieces of equipment.
- This example demonstrates the power of the Airway Leads network in enabling consistency in equipment procurement and provision, particularly relevant to trainees rotating throughout the region on training attachments.
- Clearly, this type of local cooperation has potential benefits in maintaining patient safety, ensuring both consistent training and delivery of techniques, and can be replicated in other regions throughout the UK, aided by communication through the Airway Leads network.

4.4 Airway Leads Day

Since the inception of the Airway Lead role, there has been an annual meeting held at the RCoA in London (the first held in 2013), convened by the RCoA-DAS national Airway Lead Coordinator, open to all Airway Leads from across the United Kingdom. This annual meeting was designed to act as a forum for the sharing of best practices, facilitate learning from other Airway Leads, and promote collaboration between individuals and regions, building connections and strengthening the Airway Leads network. The scientific programme is also designed to promote discussion to address specific current/upcoming challenges facing Airway Leads, for example, delivery of airway training aligned to a new anaesthesia curriculum (2021), delivery and assessment of competence in advanced airway management techniques, incorporating human factors simulation training into airway management etc.

The Airway Leads Day has also served to enable recruitment of Airway Lead volunteers for working groups to address national projects, e.g. participating in the establishment of a framework for national procurement of airway management devices.

The meeting has also provided the platform for several critically important airway management interventions:

(i) The origins of the "No trace = wrong place" campaign [43] can be mapped to the 2015 annual meeting. This national campaign, coordinated through the RCoA, was introduced to highlight the correct use of capnography to prevent undetected oesophageal intubation. The campaign focussed upon the technical skill of reading the capnograph, but also extended into non-technical skills, empowering all members of the team to speak up if a flat capnograph is seen and encouraging multidisciplinary team simulation training. Ultimately, this campaign has been superseded by the Preventing unrecognised oesophageal intubation: a consensus guideline, which has been devised by an international collaboration of international airway societies [11].

(ii) More recently, the 2020 event (held in March, a few weeks before the United Kingdom entered "lockdown" as the spread of the Coronavirus 2019 accelerated) permitted crucial information to be presented to the right audience at the right time—facilitating the dissemination of learning into local hospitals (with Airway Leads organising and coordinating the delivery of training), rapid sharing of knowledge, and swift development and implementation of adapted airway management guidelines (personal and institutional preparedness) [44, 45]. (Evidence Level: Grade D).

4.5 Role Recognition and Support

For the Airway Lead role to be successfully established, maintained, and maximally effective, formal recognition by relevant national bodies and associations—namely, the RCoA and DAS, was necessary. Formal endorsement by the RCoA was fundamental in assisting individuals in gaining the support of their local department and facilitated essential discussions around the allocation of appropriate time to deliver the role.

To improve airway management locally, Airway Leads also need the support and authorisation of their local hospital's management team. For an individual Airway Lead to implement new or updated national guidelines, deliver airway management education, purchase airway training equipment, purchase new devices, establish robust audit and reporting systems, and organise regular review of practices and outcomes, the significance of their role must be recognised by staff and management alike. Secondly, as local training is such a core component, staff must have sufficient time allocated to effectively engage with the teaching away from their clinical duties.

Any Airway Lead can seek assistance from the Airway Leads network, gain support from other Airway Leads at local hospitals within their region (through establishing regional networks), and may also apply for financial investment (in the form of funding grants) for larger projects directly through both the RCoA and DAS.

4.6 Airway Leads National Advisor

This post was created as a joint role, representing a collaboration between the RCoA and DAS. The post-holder was appointed specifically to establish and progress the role and functions of the Airway Lead, promote and facilitate the activities of Airway Leads at a local level, as well as set priorities and coordinate projects at a national level. The National Advisor was also established as a single point of contact for any ideas or questions generated by individual Airway Leads, as well as having the responsibility of collating the findings of completed NAP4 Recommendations audits (submitted by Airway Leads) and gathering examples of best practice. Additionally, the National Advisor convenes the annual Airway Leads Day at the RCoA, liaising with individual Airway Leads to set a relevant meeting agenda that identifies the priorities for action (new guidelines, current challenges, etc.).

4.7 Difficult Airway Response Teams

Where the Airway Leads initiative has been described as a quality improvement project on a national scale [46], Difficult Airway Response Teams represent a quality improvement programme at a hospital-based level. Difficult Airway Response Teams were first created by a multidisciplinary team at the Johns Hopkins Hospital in Baltimore, USA [47]. Just as Airway Leads arose from the recognition that the problems identified in NAP4 needed to be addressed in a coordinated fashion, DART teams were instituted in response to a 3-year time span between 2005 and 2008, during which it was discovered that all adverse airway events at Johns Hopkins Hospital occurred outside the operating room.

Anesthesiologists, otolaryngologists, trauma surgeons, and emergency physicians worked together with hospital risk managers to create a highly skilled multidisciplinary team to attend and manage patients who were found to have or who were known to have difficult airways requiring emergency management. The original DART programme comprised three core components—an operational component, a safety component, and an educational component. The scheme shares many similarities with the ambitions of the Airway Leads programme, with the provision of standardised DART equipment carts at strategic positions across the hospital, similar to the calls to standardise airway trolleys across hospitals in the United Kingdom.

4.7.1 DART Review, Simulation, and Education

Mirroring the Airway Lead call for coordinated airway-specific Morbidity and Mortality meetings, all DART activations are reviewed in real time with a quarterly multidisciplinary DART case review conference. In situ simulations are held to address deficiencies in the process, and the specific education component of the DART programme focuses on enhancing individual knowledge, but targets all members of the multidisciplinary team.

4.7.2 Expanding the DART Model

In his editorial, Joffe acknowledged that generalising the DART Program to other institutions may not be straight forward [48], but that every institution should aim to have "Some Kind of Multidisciplinary Airway Response Team" (Evidence Level: Grade D). Such a team-centred approach, that is dictated by local resources, is remarkably similar to the Airway Leads approach, whereby individuals with local knowledge of a hospital's skills set, presenting pathologies and readily available resources, are best placed to coordinate airway training and education.

Chmielewska et al. [49] encouraged hospitals that could not support a fully-fledged DART programme to develop contingency plans so that their rapid response systems could deal with emergency airway management at a local level.

DART teams were established with a specific remit in a specific institution and so have been able to demonstrate a reduction to zero of airway-related deaths, sentinel events, or malpractice claims in adult patients—clear evidence of their success (Evidence Level: Grade C) [50].

4.7.3 DART Model Adaptations

Long et al. describe the single institution success of a hospital-wide "Alpha-Team [51]." They stated that difficult airway management required application of the R3P3 principle—"Right People, Right Parts and Right Place." Again, education was a common core to their programme.

Whilst the cause and incidence of difficult airways in the paediatric population differs to the adult population [52], a Pediatric Difficult Airway Response Team [53] and similar services [54] have been described. As with all DARTs, the rationale of the pDART is to "rapidly mobilise specialised airway equipment as well as personnel with advanced airway expertise to the bedside during airway emergencies." This was coupled, unsurprisingly, with a rigorous training programme so that clinicians had both competence and confidence to use the available airway equipment.

4.7.4 DART and Airway Leads: Complementary Models

Airway Leads and Difficult Airway Response Teams tackle the same problem—improving airway management across a hospital. They are not mutually exclusive—a hospital can have a DART team *and* an Airway Lead. For example, a hospital with an Airway Lead may institute a DART team to manage airway emergencies outside the operating theatre complex. The roles of Airway Leads and DARTs share common themes—education, equipment provision, audit and feedback on airway-related events, among others.

A recent editorial co-authored by the President of the US-based Society of Airway Management outlined the benefits and potential opportunities that having an Airway Lead can bring [29] (Evidence Level: Grade D). Figure 4.2 illustrates the ideal relationship between local stakeholders—which vary depending on the clinical specialities in an individual hospital and their direct link through an Airway Lead to national bodies and organisations.

Most importantly, this represents a three-way relationship, with information being relayed from national organisations to local hospitals (and vice-versa), as well as allowing for the transfer of locally implemented strategies (that have proved effective) from one hospital to another, through the Airway Leads network—adapted to suit as necessary.

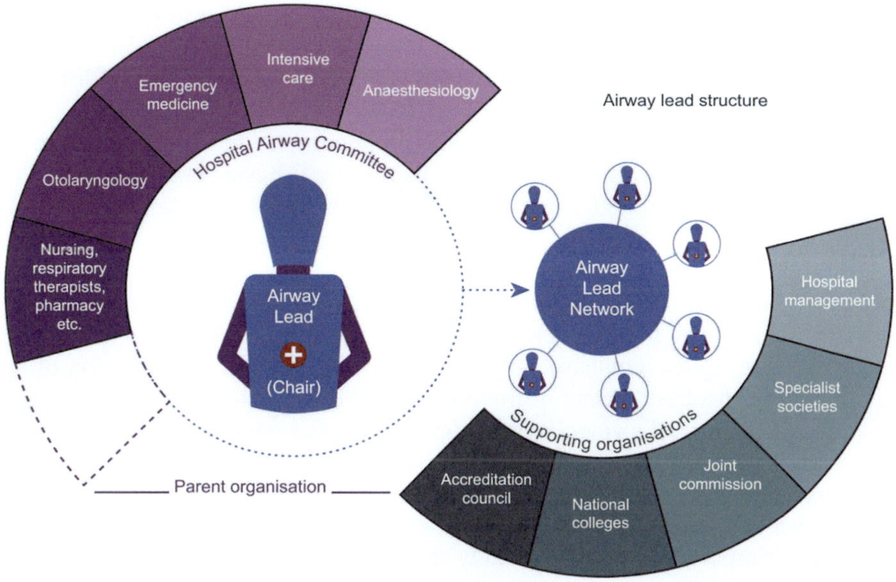

Fig. 4.2 Interactions and coordinating role of an Airway Lead [29] (courtesy of the BJA)

4.8 Evidence of Success/Progress

It is difficult to directly measure the relative success or impact of the Airway Lead/Airway Leads Project, as it is not an intervention that lends itself easily to objective investigation through randomised controlled trials or meta-analyses. It is equally impossible to collate the findings and assess the positive effect of the many hundreds of local airway management quality improvement projects led or coordinated by Airway Leads. Therefore, the relative success and/or progress that has resulted from the creation and evolution of the Airway Lead role must be assessed by other, less tangible metrics.

Following the creation and formal recognition of the role in 2012, the network expanded rapidly. The number of Airway Leads across the United Kingdom was recorded as 197 in 2015. Since then, the proportion of UK hospitals with an appointed Airway Lead has been maintained successfully at over 97% year on year.

In 2013–2014, a year after the Airway Lead network was formed, a survey of Airway Leads identified major changes in airway practices throughout the United Kingdom [55]. As a result, 98% of hospitals had made changes in practice, including closing the safety gap (the gap between ideal practice and actual practice based on NAP4 recommendations) of approximately 40% in anaesthesia, 50% in ED, and 60% in ICU. (Evidence Level: Grade D).

Accurately measuring the positive effect of an Airway Lead is challenging, as the data gathered may be potentially misleading. For example, we speculate that during the early phase of introduction of an Airway Lead or DART programme at an institution, the incidence of 'adverse airway events' may appear to *increase*—as a core element of these roles is the identification and reporting of adverse events, allowing them to be investigated and then to provide the appropriate local learning and training.

Perhaps the greatest endorsement of the programme comes from the desire to replicate the Airway Leads model, with similar networks having been established in Ireland, New Zealand, and Australia, with interest in the programme in North America as well.

The benefits of targeted interventions in certain areas of airway management have also been clearly demonstrated (Evidence Level: Grade C). Pedersen et al. instigated a bundle of five interventions: the immediate administration of neuromuscular blocking agents; emphasis on proper preoxygenation; implementation of an airway safety checklist; a clear instruction to hand over intubation after the second attempt; and the use of a videolaryngoscope. These interventions reduced the number of cases with airway-related events from 566/3668 to 433/3786 (RR 0.74) [56]. This exemplifies the use of a locally directed package that made targeted changes following a baseline assessment. It is not clear whether such a package would have a universal impact, but it is very likely that locally conducted assessments with locally defined interventions are likely to be of benefit—which is precisely the remit of the Airway Lead.

4.9 Conclusion

The need for a person to coordinate and standardise core elements of airway care and behaviour within an institution is recommended by many national bodies around the world. Similarly, the benefits of limiting choice and standardising equipment are being recognised [57, 58]. Shared learning between groups of such individuals in a network is an obvious next step, so that knowledge and methods of improving outcomes are not contained within a single institution.

Airway Leads are also vital to ensure the smooth, effective, and safe introduction of nationally agreed guidelines within a local setting. Their role must also include reviewing complex airway cases to ensure that any potential learning points for the institution, the airway team, or individual airway managers are identified, and appropriate education delivered.

Difficult Airway Response Teams have also shown a benefit in managing airways outside the operating theatre environment, and hospitals should consider how their local resources can best be coordinated to manage these high-risk episodes.

Recommendations

- All hospitals should identify an individual to coordinate and optimise airway care throughout the entire hospital, wherever an airway might be managed.
- Duties of an Airway Lead depend upon the needs of the institution in which they are based, but should include national guideline adoption, equipment standardisation, complex airway case review, and education and training for the entire airway team.
- Airway Leads should not work in isolation, but should feed into a network of Airway Leads at local, regional, and national levels. This allows shared learning, shared strategy planning, and the possibility of information sharing between local hospitals and national bodies, between national bodies and local institutions, *and* between individual hospitals that are otherwise geographically separated (three-way communication, via the network).
- Targeted interventions within an institution's airway management strategy can improve safety, and should be considered after conducting an analysis of local airway events.
- All hospitals should have an operational strategy for dealing with complex airway situations outside the operating theatre environment.
- The possibility of collating adverse event reporting or research projects across an Airway Leads network is recognised and should be investigated by national bodies.

References

1. Law JA, Duggan LV, Asselin M, et al. Canadian airway focus group updated consensus-based recommendations for management of the difficult airway: part 1. Difficult airway management encountered in an unconscious patient. Can J Anaesth. 2021;68:1373.
2. Frerk C, Mitchell VS, McNarry AFF, Mendonca C, Bhagrath R, Patel A, O'Sullivan EPP, Woodall NM, Ahmad I. Difficult airway society 2015 guidelines for management of unanticipated difficult intubation in adults. Br J Anaesth. 2015;115:827–48.
3. BRAIN AIJ. The laryngeal mask- a new concept in airway management. Br J Anaesth. 1983;55:801–6.
4. Cook TM, Lee G, Nolan JP. The ProSeal laryngeal mask airway: a review of the literature. Can J Anaesth. 2005;52:739–60.
5. Cooper RM, Pacey JA, Bishop MJ, McCluskey SA. Early clinical experience with a new videolaryngoscope (GlideScope) in 728 patients. Can J Anaesth. 2005;52:191–8.
6. Patel A, Nouraei SAR. Transnasal humidified rapid-insufflation Ventilatory exchange (THRIVE): a physiological method of increasing apnoea time in patients with difficult airways. Anaesthesia. 2015;70:323–9.
7. Practice guidelines for management of the difficult airway. A report by the American Society of Anesthesiologists Task Force on Management of the Difficult Airway. Anesthesiology 78:597–602; 1993.
8. Langeron O, Bourgain J-L, Francon D, et al. Difficult intubation and extubation in adult anaesthesia. Anaesth Crit Care Pain Med. 2018;37:639–51.

9. Piepho T, Cavus E, Noppens R, Byhahn C, Dörges V, Zwissler B, Timmermann A. S1 guidelines on airway management: guideline of the German society of anesthesiology and intensive care medicine. Anaesthesist. 2015;64(Suppl 1):27–40.
10. Kriege M, Noppens RR. Evaluation of the McGrath MACTM and Macintosh laryngoscope for tracheal intubation. Br J Anaesth. 2020;125:e209.
11. Chrimes N, Higgs A, Hagberg CA, et al. Preventing unrecognised oesophageal intubation: a consensus guideline from the project for universal Management of Airways and international airway societies*. Anaesthesia. 2022;77:1395–415.
12. Abdelgadir IS, Phillips RS, Singh D, Moncreiff MP, Lumsden JL. Videolaryngoscopy versus direct laryngoscopy for tracheal intubation in children (excluding neonates). Cochrane Database Syst Rev. 2017; https://doi.org/10.1002/14651858.CD011413.pub2.
13. Hansel J, Rogers AM, Lewis SR, Cook TM, Smith AF. Videolaryngoscopy versus direct laryngoscopy for adults undergoing tracheal intubation. Cochrane Database Syst Rev. 2022; https://doi.org/10.1002/14651858.CD011136.PUB3.
14. Nicholson A, Cook TM, Smith AF, Lewis SR, Reed SS. Supraglottic airway devices versus tracheal intubation for airway management during general anaesthesia in obese patients. Cochrane Database Syst Rev. 2013;(9):CD010105.
15. Qamarul Hoda M, Samad K, Ullah H. ProSeal versus classic laryngeal mask airway (LMA) for positive pressure ventilation in adults undergoing elective surgery. Cochrane Database Syst Rev. 2017; https://doi.org/10.1002/14651858.CD009026.pub2.
16. Qureshi MJ, Kumar M. Laryngeal mask airway versus bag-mask ventilation or endotracheal intubation for neonatal resuscitation. Cochrane Database Syst Rev. 2018; https://doi.org/10.1002/14651858.CD003314.pub3.
17. Caldwell JE, Miller RD. Clinical implications of sugammadex. Anaesthesia. 2009;64(Suppl 1):66–72.
18. Mirakhur RK. Sugammadex in clinical practice. Anaesthesia. 2009;64:45–54.
19. Popat M, Mitchell V, Dravid R, Patel A, Swampillai C, Higgs A. Difficult airway society guidelines for the management of tracheal extubation. Anaesthesia. 2012;67:318–40.
20. Ahmad I, El-Boghdadly K, Bhagrath R, Hodzovic I, McNarry AF, Mir F, O'Sullivan EP, Patel A, Stacey M, Vaughan D. Difficult airway society guidelines for awake tracheal intubation (ATI) in adults. Anaesthesia. 2019;75:509–28.
21. Webb RK, Currie M, Morgan CA, Williamson JA, Mackay P, Russell WJ, Runciman WB. The Australian incident monitoring study: an analysis of 2000 incident reports. Anaesth Intensive Care. 1993;21:520–8.
22. Peterson GN, Domino KB, Caplan RA, Posner KL, Lee LA, Cheney FW. Management of the difficult Airway: a closed claims analysis. J Am Soc Anesthesiol. 2005;103:33–9.
23. Cook T, Woodall N, Frerk C. 4th National Audit Project of the Royal College of Anaesthetists and the difficult airway society (NAP4) major complications of airway management in the United Kingdom. London: Report and findings.
24. Henderson JJ, Popat MT, Latto IP, Pearce AC. Difficult airway society guidelines for management of the unanticipated difficult intubation. Anaesthesia. 2004;59:675–94.
25. Cook TM, Woodall N, Frerk C, O'Sullivan E, McNarry A, Drake SGM. The college department airway lead and NAP4 follow-up surveys: an announcement. Bull R Coll Anaesth. 2012;76:37–8.
26. Smith C, McNarry AF. Airway leads and airway response teams: improving delivery of safer airway management? Curr Anesthesiol Rep. 2020;10:370–7.
27. Baker PA. New Zealand Society of Anaesthetists: establishing a New Zealand airway leads network. 2019.; Available from www.anaesthesiasociety.org.nz/about/networks/airway-leads-network
28. Greenland KB. Introducing airway leads in Australia. ANZCA Bull. 2019:22–5.
29. Baker PA, Behringer EC, Feinleib J, Foley LJ, Mosier J, Roth P, Wali A, O'Sullivan EP. Formation of an airway Lead network: an essential patient safety initiative. Br J Anaesth. 2022;128:225–9.

30. Warnakulasuriya SR, Harvey R, McNarry AF. Translation of national guidelines into local practice. Clin Teach. 2019;16:604–9.
31. Lewis SR, Butler AR, Parker J, Cook TM, Schofield-Robinson OJ, Smith AF. Videolaryngoscopy versus direct laryngoscopy for adult patients requiring tracheal intubation: a Cochrane systematic review†. BJA Br J Anaesth. 2017;119:369–83.
32. Hansel J, Rogers AM, Lewis SR, Cook TM, Smith AF. Videolaryngoscopy versus direct laryngoscopy for adults undergoing tracheal intubation: a Cochrane systematic review and meta-analysis update. Br J Anaesth. 2022;129:612–23.
33. Zaouter C, Calderon J, Hemmerling TM. Videolaryngoscopy as a new standard of care. Br J Anacsth. 2015;114:181–3.
34. Hemmerling TM, Zaouter C. Videolaryngoscopy: is there a path to becoming a standard of Care for Intubation? Anesth Analg. 2020;131:1313–6.
35. De Jong A, Pardo E, Rolle A, Bodin-Lario S, Pouzeratte Y, Jaber S. Airway management for COVID-19: a move towards universal videolaryngoscope? Lancet Respir Med. 2020;8:555.
36. Cook TM, Aziz MF. Has the time really come for universal videolaryngoscopy? Br J Anaesth. 2022;129:474–7.
37. Cook TM, Boniface NJ, Seller C, Hughes J, Damen C, MacDonald L, Kelly FE. Universal videolaryngoscopy: a structured approach to conversion to videolaryngoscopy for all intubations in an anaesthetic and intensive care department. Br J Anaesth. 2018;120:173–80.
38. De Jong A, Sfara T, Pouzeratte Y, Pensier J, Rolle A, Chanques G, Jaber S. Videolaryngoscopy as a first-intention technique for tracheal intubation in unselected surgical patients: a before and after observational study. Br J Anaesth. 2022;129:624–34.
39. De Jong A, Pouzeratte Y, Laplace A, et al. Macintosh Videolaryngoscope for intubation in the operating room: a comparative quality improvement project. Anesth Analg. 2021;132:524–35.
40. Riley E, Payne S, Jones J, Cook TM, Kelly FE, Robinson O, Baruah R. 'Trachy Tracey'—an education tool for tracheostomy training. Anaesthesia. 2018;73:1044–5.
41. Corbett L, Davies A, McDonald M, Kelly F, Jordan L. Bath tea trolley' training; part 1. Bull R Coll Anaesth. 2020;119:28–30.
42. O'Farrell G, McDonald M, Kelly FE. 'Tea trolley' difficult airway training. Anaesthesia. 2015;70:104.
43. Cook TM, Harrop-Griffiths AWW, Whitaker DKDK, McNarry AF, Patel A, McGuire B. The 'no trace=wrong place' campaign. Br J Anaesth. 2019;122:e68–9.
44. Cook TM, El-Boghdadly K, McGuire B, McNarry AF, Patel A, Higgs A. Consensus guidelines for managing the airway in patients with COVID-19: guidelines from the difficult airway society, the Association of Anaesthetists the Intensive Care Society, the Faculty of Intensive Care Medicine and the Royal College of Anaesthetists. Anaesthesia. 2020;75:785–99.
45. Lockie C, Ward P. A timely airway (leads) intervention. Bull R Coll Anaesth. 2021;125:59.
46. McNarry AF, Cook TM, Baker PA, O'Sullivan EP. The airway Lead: opportunities to improve institutional and personal preparedness for airway management. Br J Anaesth. 2020;125:e22–4.
47. Mark LJ, Herzer KR, Cover R, et al. Difficult airway response team. Anesth Analg. 2015;121:127–39.
48. Joffe AM. Use your SMARTs (some kind of multidisciplinary airway response team) for emergent airway management outside the operating room. Anesth Analg. 2015;121:11–3.
49. Chmielewska M, Winters BD, Pandian V, Hillel AT. Integration of a difficult airway response team into a hospital emergency response system. Anesthesiol Clin. 2015;33:369–79.
50. Mark L, Lester L, Cover R, Herzer K. A decade of difficult airway response team: lessons learned from a hospital-wide difficult airway response team program. Crit Care Clin. 2018;34:239–51.
51. Long L, Vanderhoff B, Smyke N, Shaffer LET, Solomon J, Steuer JD. Management of difficult airways using a hospital-wide "alpha team" approach. Am J Med Qual. 2010;25:297–304.
52. Burjek N. The difficult pediatric airway: predictors, incidence, and complications. In: Jagannathan N, Fiadjoe J, editors. Management of the Difficult Pediatric Airway. Cambridge: Cambridge University Press; 2019. p. 8–19.

53. Kelly GS, Deanehan JK, Dalesio NM. Pediatric difficult airway response team utilization in the emergency department: a case series. Pediatr Emerg Care. 2021;37:E1462–7.
54. Sterrett EC, Myer CM, Oehler J, Das B, Kerrey BT. Critical airway team: a retrospective study of an airway response system in a pediatric hospital. Otolaryngol—Head Neck Surg (United States). 2017;157:1060–7.
55. Cook TM, Woodall N, Frerk C. A national survey of the impact of NAP4 on airway management practice in United Kingdom hospitals: closing the safety gap in anaesthesia, intensive care and the emergency department. Br J Anaesth. 2016;117:182–90.
56. Pedersen TH, Ueltschi F, Hornshaw T, Greif R, Theiler L, Huber M, Kleine-Brueggeney M. Optimisation of airway management strategies: a prospective before-and-after study on events related to airway management. Br J Anaesth. 2021;127:798–806.
57. Gibbins M, Kelly FE, Cook TM. Airway management equipment and practice: time to optimise institutional, team, and personal preparedness. Br J Anaesth. 2020;125:221–4.
58. McNarry AF, Patel A. The evolution of airway management-new concepts and conflicts with traditional practice. Br J Anaesth. 2017; https://doi.org/10.1093/bja/aex385.

Chapter 5
Pre-procedure Assessment and Planning

Lauren M. Nakazawa, John F. Gray, and Carlos A. Artime

Highlights

- A structured pre-procedure airway assessment is critical to identifying risk factors for difficult airway management and ensuring optimal preparation.
- A thorough review of the patient's medical, surgical, and anesthetic history—especially prior airway management challenges—provides key predictive information.
- Obesity, congenital disorders, musculoskeletal diseases, and obstructive sleep apnea (OSA) are significant risk factors for difficult mask ventilation (DMV), supraglottic airway (SGA) failure, and difficult intubation (DI).
- Bedside airway examination tools, such as Mallampati classification, thyromental distance, sternomental distance, and upper lip bite test, assist in predicting difficult airway scenarios but should be used in combination rather than individually.
- Advanced airway assessment techniques, including preoperative endoscopic airway evaluation, ultrasonography, and imaging studies, can further refine risk assessment and guide airway management plans.

(continued)

L. M. Nakazawa · J. F. Gray · C. A. Artime (✉)
Department of Anesthesiology, Critical Care, and Pain Medicine, McGovern Medical School at UTHealth Houston, Houston, TX, USA
e-mail: Lauren.M.Nakazawa@uth.tmc.edu; John.F.Gray@uth.tmc.edu; carlos.artime@uth.tmc.edu

M. Á. Gómez-Ríos, A. van Zundert (eds.), *Evidence-based Guide to Difficult Airway Management*, https://doi.org/10.1007/978-3-032-30769-9_5

- The American Society of Anesthesiologists (ASA) and the Canadian Airway Focus Group (CAFG) strongly recommend structured airway evaluations before initiating airway management or extubation.
- Pre-procedure planning should incorporate equipment availability, personnel coordination, communication strategies, and backup airway plans to enhance patient safety.

5.1 Introduction

After induction of anesthesia and ablation of spontaneous respiration, the anesthesia clinician has only a few minutes to secure an airway before the development of hypoxia. Difficulty in securing the airway can lead to adverse outcomes, including airway trauma, cardiac arrest, anoxic brain injury, and death. To ensure success and prevent patient harm, the airway manager should proactively identify risk factors for difficult airway management and make adequate preparations.

An evaluation of the patient's medical history and a targeted physical exam including an airway assessment should be performed prior to airway management to predict whether the patient has a potentially difficult airway or is at increased risk of aspiration. The 2022 American Society of Anesthesiologists (ASA) Practice Guidelines for the Management of the Difficult Airway, authored by an international task force of anesthesiologists, strongly recommends conducting a structured airway physical examination and risk assessment [1]. Similarly, the Canadian Airway Focus Group (CAFG) advises airway evaluation before both airway management initiation and tracheal extubation or discontinuation of airway support [2].

The Fourth National Audit Project (NAP4) of the United Kingdom, one of the largest studies on airway-related major complications, concluded that the lack of an airway evaluation and a planned airway strategy was predictive of adverse outcomes, including increased patient morbidity and mortality [3]. A comprehensive review of a patient's medical and surgical history, along with a physical examination to assess facial features and airway anatomical measurements and landmarks, can provide valuable information for risk stratification. This assessment helps predict difficult mask ventilation (DMV), difficult supraglottic airway (SGA) ventilation, and/or difficult intubation (DI)—all critical considerations in developing a tailored airway management plan and ensuring optimal preparation.

5.2 Patient History

During a preoperative or pre-airway evaluation, the presence of certain clinical conditions or history may suggest difficulty with airway management. The clinician should review the patient's past medical, surgical, and anesthetic history, paying careful attention to predisposing factors and underlying diseases. Prior medical and anesthetic records should be reviewed, with special attention to intubation notes and documentation of previous airway management. The Canadian Airway Focus Group notes that a history of difficulty with airway management may be more predictive of a difficult airway than a bedside physical examination [2].

5.2.1 *Congenital Disorders*

Certain congenital disorders resulting in craniofacial abnormalities can indicate airway difficulty.

- Pierre Robin sequence: Micrognathia and glossoptosis (incorrect placement of the tongue leading to obstruction).
- Treacher Collins syndrome: Malar and mandibular hypoplasia.
- Klippel-Feil syndrome: Cervical abnormalities—two or more cervical vertebrae are fused, resulting in decreased neck mobility.
- Goldenhar syndrome: Facial asymmetry, macrostomia, and mandibular hypoplasia [4].
- Beckwith-Wiedemann syndrome: Generalized overgrowth, including macroglossia [5].

Mucopolysaccharidoses are an array of diseases resulting from genetic enzymatic defects leading to the accumulation of glycosaminoglycans in tissue that vary in severity and presentation. Macroglossia is a clinical feature of mucopolysaccharidosis. Additionally, airway obstruction may worsen due to deposits in the soft tissues of the airway. In a multiyear view at one pediatric institution, 8 of 16 patients with mucopolysaccharidosis had a difficult airway [6].

Trisomy 21 (Down syndrome) has many anesthetic implications, including multiple airway challenges:

- Predisposition to upper airway obstruction due to macroglossia, large tonsils, and adenoids.
- Laryngomalacia and a short palate.
- Subglottic stenosis and a smaller trachea, which may necessitate the use of a smaller endotracheal tube.
- Atlantooccipital (AO) instability [7, 8]. Upright cervical radiographs are a useful tool for evaluating AO instability.

5.2.2 *Obesity/Obstructive Sleep Apnea*

With increasing rates of obesity worldwide, its effect on airway difficulty has been extensively studied. In one investigation, morbid obesity (BMI > 40 kg/m^2) was found to be associated with DMV; however, morbid obesity did not increase the likelihood of DI [9]. In another study, obese patients had a higher incidence of a difficult airway compared to lean patients. However, the only independent identifiable risk factor was a Mallampati score of III or IV [10].

Clinical features of obesity, such as large neck circumference and a large tongue, may more specifically predict difficulty with intubation and mask ventilation (MV). One study showed that a neck circumference of 40 cm demonstrated a 5% probability of DI, while a 60 cm neck circumference increased the probability of DI to 35% [11]. Large, immobile neck and pharyngeal adipose tissue deposits in obesity predispose patients to airway obstruction, which can complicate airway management and MV. Decreased functional residual capacity in obese individuals leads to reduced apnea time and a shorter time to desaturation, which are key considerations when managing an airway.

Obstructive sleep apnea (OSA) is a syndrome characterized by disordered breathing through apneas and hypopneas. Daytime tiredness and somnolence, heavy snoring, frequent accidents, and memory impairment are suggestive of OSA. The gold standard for diagnosis is polysomnography. OSA is significantly underdiagnosed in the surgical population. The STOP-BANG questionnaire is an OSA screening tool that demonstrates high sensitivity and high positive predictive value and has been validated in a surgical population [12]. It is a key clinical tool in recognizing undiagnosed OSA prior to anesthesia. OSA itself is a risk factor for DMV [13, 14]. Additionally, OSA is associated with an increased risk of postoperative complications, ICU admission, and a greater length of hospital stay.

5.2.3 Musculoskeletal Disease (RA, Ankylosing Spondylitis, TMJ Dysfunction, Diabetes Mellitus)

Several medical comorbidities can affect the musculoskeletal system, leading to rigidity and decreased mobility of joints throughout the body. If these joints are in the head and neck, decreased mobility and stiffness may contribute to difficult airway management due to a decreased range of motion and immobility.

Rheumatoid arthritis (RA) is an autoimmune disorder with various bony and systemic side effects. Cricoarytenoid arthritis is a common manifestation of RA, which can complicate intubation or reveal itself after extubation with a sore throat, hoarseness, and even stridor. Special care should be taken during airway management to avoid airway trauma. Patients with RA also warrant an assessment of cardiovascular or pulmonary disease involvement [15]. Cervical spine disease may be present, and anesthesiologists should be aware of possible asymptomatic cervical instability. The patient history elicited from those with RA should include the duration of disease, steroid use, cervical symptomatology, and any other disease-modifying drugs. No specific guidelines exist for preoperative cervical radiographs in RA patients; however, if performed, they should include flexion-extension views [16].

Another rheumatologic disease, *ankylosing spondylitis*, leads to body rigidity and joint fusion. Cervical spine involvement is associated with DI. Neurologic injury may occur with excessive neck extension during laryngoscopy [17].

RA and ankylosing spondylitis may also involve the *temporomandibular joint (TMJ)*; other conditions or prior trauma may contribute to TMJ dysfunction, leading to pain, TMJ clicking and popping, diminished mouth opening, and/or jaw locking. The examination should include an assessment of mouth opening, range of motion, hypermobility, facial asymmetry, and TMJ joint palpation. In patients with severely restricted mouth opening and TMJ dysfunction, laryngoscopy is likely to be unsuccessful [18].

Diabetes mellitus is a metabolic disorder that causes hyperglycemia from defects in insulin secretion or action. It is commonly comorbid with obesity, which, as discussed previously, presents its own airway challenges. Diabetes also affects the musculoskeletal system through glycosylation of proteins, microvascular changes, and collagen accumulation. The non-enzymatic glycosylation of collagen most commonly affects the small joints but can also affect the spine. The prayer sign and palm print test can indicate joint immobility and collagen deposition, which may hint at possible AO or laryngeal joint involvement, increasing the risk of DI [19].

5.2.4 Head and Neck Tumors/Abscess

Head and neck tumors are often not visible during a cursory physical examination but have significant implications for airway management. Masses of the larynx and pharynx may lead to airway obstruction and distortion of normal airway anatomy. External airway assessment parameters may fail to detect internal airway obstruction. Patients with head and neck cancer may have received radiation as part of their treatment. Radiation-induced changes to the neck were found to be the most significant predictor of impossible mask ventilation (IMV) [14].

Infections of the mouth, tonsils, retropharyngeal space, submandibular space, and neck—including epiglottitis and Ludwig's angina—can distort the airway. Patients should be assessed for dysphonia, trismus, and dysphagia, as well as respiratory compromise and stridor, as these are clinical signs of airway obstruction. Progression of infection, along with expanding abscess formation and edema, can lead to complete obstruction and airway collapse.

Clinicians should prepare for airway management by reviewing computed tomography (CT), ultrasound, and magnetic resonance imaging (MRI) of the head and neck to assess the degree of anatomic distortion. Endoscopic airway evaluation using a flexible nasal endoscope may be beneficial in patients with head and neck tumors or infection.

5.2.5 *Acromegaly*

Acromegaly is a disorder caused by the oversecretion of growth hormone by the pituitary gland, causing bony and soft tissue overgrowth. Patients with acromegaly have DI rates four to five times higher than those of the general population [20]. Schmitt and colleagues found that patients with acromegaly had an increased incidence of Cormack and Lehane grade 3 view on first-attempt laryngoscopy (25%) compared to the previously reported population rate of 6%. Features of acromegaly that contribute to difficult airway management include macroglossia, prognathism, laryngeal and pharyngeal soft tissue overgrowth, and enlarged epiglottis [21].

5.2.6 *Pregnancy*

Pregnancy is a known risk factor for an unanticipated difficult airway. The obstetric airway is discussed further in the chapter "Obstetric Airway Management."

5.3 Bedside Airway Examination

5.3.1 *Mallampati Classification*

"Can you open your mouth and stick out your tongue?" is a ubiquitous phrase used by anesthesiologists when performing an airway exam. This allows for the grading of the patient's Mallampati classification while also assessing oral aperture and any limitations in mouth opening. The Mallampati system (originally with three classifications) was updated in 1987 to the modified Mallampati system (four classifications) and is widely used as a tool to assess and predict difficult airways [22]. The modified Mallampati classification system (classes I–IV) relates tongue size to mouth opening and provides a general approximation of the space available for laryngoscopy (Fig. 5.1 [23]). As tongue size increases, it obstructs oropharyngeal structures. As the Mallampati score increases, structures of the soft palate are gradually obstructed.

Classification:

I: Soft palate, uvula, and tonsillar pillars visible.
II: Soft palate and uvula visible.
III: Soft palate and base of the uvula visible.
IV: Soft palate not visible; only the hard palate is seen.

For optimal assessment of the modified Mallampati class, the patient would be in the sitting position without phonation, with the observer positioned in front of the

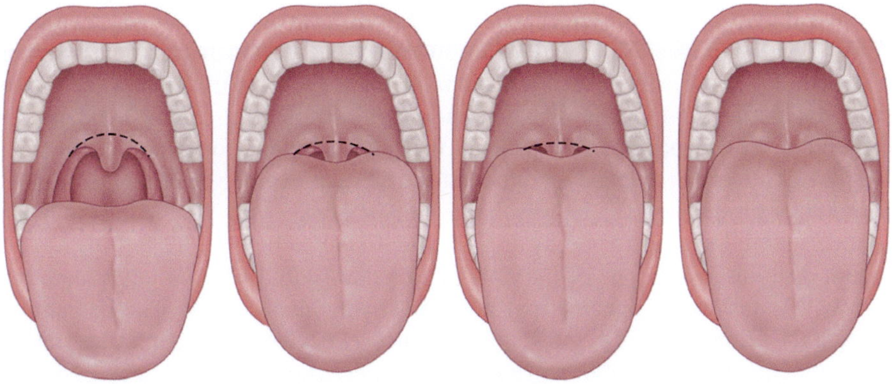

Fig. 5.1 Mallampati classification [23]

patient, looking straight forward. Supine positioning may elevate the Mallampati score; however, a study by Tham and colleagues found this elevation to be small and not statistically significant, concluding that supine Mallampati scores could be interpreted similarly to sitting scores [24]. Another study by Bindra and colleagues found that Mallampati assessment in the supine position was a more accurate predictor of airway difficulty than sitting assessment [25]. Phonation raises the soft palate, which may lower the Mallampati score; this was confirmed in the study by Tham and colleagues [24]. Clinicians should be mindful that patients may unintentionally phonate on examination, even when asked to remain silent.

The modified Mallampati score is widely used to predict difficult laryngoscopy and DMV. Throughout multiple studies, Mallampati scores of III and IV are consistently associated with difficult laryngoscopy and MV [9, 10, 13, 14, 26, 27]. However, a multivariate analysis by Lundstrom found that the Mallampati classification alone is an insufficient standalone test, with only 35% of DIs identified as Mallampati class III or IV. They emphasized that the Mallampati score should be considered as one of many factors in predicting a difficult airway [28].

5.3.2 Mouth Opening/Oral Aperture

Mouth opening is best measured as the distance between the upper and lower incisors, known as the interincisor distance (IID). An IID of less than 3 cm is considered limited. Fingerbreadths are often used to approximate the IID, with two adult fingers being roughly equivalent to less than 3 cm. Mouth opening helps estimate the available space for airway device placement. TMJ dysfunction and other disorders affecting the TMJ joint and masseter muscle, such as burns, scarring, contractures, and prior temporal craniotomy, can decrease mouth opening. Mouth opening is largely controlled by a hinge-like movement of the mandible onto the maxilla.

The use of mouth opening as a predictor of difficult airways is advantageous because it has high interobserver reliability among both anesthesiologists and residents [29]. A multicenter study by Yildiz and colleagues found that a mouth opening of less than 4 cm was the most sensitive predictor of DI (43%), even more sensitive than Mallampati III–IV (35%). They found a significant increase in the incidence of difficult airway management in patients with limited mouth opening, Mallampati III–IV classification, reduced thyromental and sternomental distances, or decreased mandibular protrusion [27]. However, in a meta-analysis by Shiga, the sensitivity of limited mouth opening for predicting DI was found to be only 22% [30]. Again, mouth opening is only one of multiple factors that should be used to evaluate the airway. A small mouth opening may alter the airway management plan, potentially leading the clinician to select an alternative airway device that occupies less space in the mouth, such as flexible scope intubation.

5.3.3 *Thyromental Distance*

Thyromental distance (TMD) is measured with the neck extended as the distance between the superior thyroid notch and the tip of the chin (mentum). TMD reflects the mandibular space and can help assess the ease of tongue displacement during laryngoscopy [30]. An inadequate thyromental distance is considered to be less than 6 cm. Just as fingerbreadths can be used as a rough approximation for mouth opening, they are also used to approximate thyromental distance, with approximately three fingerbreadths corresponding to 6 cm. However, this measurement can vary widely. In a study by Baker and colleagues, the range of three fingerbreadths among anesthesiologists and trainees varied from 4.9 to 7.0 cm, with an average of 5.9 cm. They also found that using a ruler to measure TMD increased the sensitivity of predicting DI from 16% to 48% [31].

To further refine TMD, the ratio of height to thyromental distance (RHTMD) has been studied. RHTMD modifies the original TMD measurement by adjusting for patient size. Schmitt and colleagues determined that an RHTMD of 25 (height in centimeters divided by TMD in centimeters) was the optimal threshold for predicting DL. While sensitivity for both TMD and RHTMD was 81%, RHTMD increased specificity from 73% (for TMD alone) to 91% [32]. Shah and colleagues used an RHTMD cutoff of 23.5 and found RHTMD to again be superior to TMD at predicting difficult laryngoscopy [33].

5.3.4 *Sternomental Distance*

The sternomental distance (SMD) is measured as the straight-line distance from the upper border of the manubrium to the bony tip of the mentum, with the neck extended and mouth closed. SMD provides a more accurate measurement of head extension compared to more subjective assessments and is predictive of DI if it is less than 12.5 cm [34]. In a study by Savva, SMD, as a screening test for DI, had higher sensitivity and specificity (82.4% and 88.6%, respectively) than TMD (64.7% and 81.4%), the modified Mallampati score (64.7% and 66.1%), and mandibular protrusion (29.4% and 85%) [34].

5.3.5 *Neck Range of Motion*

Neck flexion and extension should be examined for any limitations and should be assessed while the patient is in the seated position. Neck flexion can be assessed by having the patient bring their chin down to their chest. Neck extension can be assessed by having the patient look upwards, tilting their head back as far as possible. Mobility of the head and neck is important for proper patient positioning and optimizing laryngeal views during direct laryngoscopy. The sniffing position is considered to provide the optimal view of the glottis. Neck flexion aligns the pharyngeal and laryngeal axes, while head extension at the AO joint brings the oral axis in alignment with the other two axes [35].

Patients with cervical spine limitations are more likely to experience a difficult airway throughout the continuum of airway management. Mashour and colleagues demonstrated that in patients less than 60 years old, cervical spine limitations increased difficulty with MV, laryngoscopy, and intubation. In patients aged 60 years and older, cervical spine limitations increased the difficulty with laryngoscopy and intubation [36]. In this cohort, age $\geq$ 48 years, TMD < 6 cm, and a Mallampati score of III or IV were independent risk factors for DI in patients with limited cervical spine mobility.

Calder and colleagues demonstrated an increased incidence of difficult laryngoscopy, defined as Cormack and Lehane grades 3 and 4, in patients with cervical spine disease, particularly those with AO disease [37]. See Fig. 5.2 for an illustration of the Cormack and Lehane classification system [23]. In these patients, AO disease was associated with poor mandibular protrusion, which is important in direct laryngoscopy. Additionally, loss of joint space between the first and second cervical vertebrae on lateral radiographs was the most successful predictive variable for difficult laryngoscopy. Despite these findings, the authors did not recommend routinely

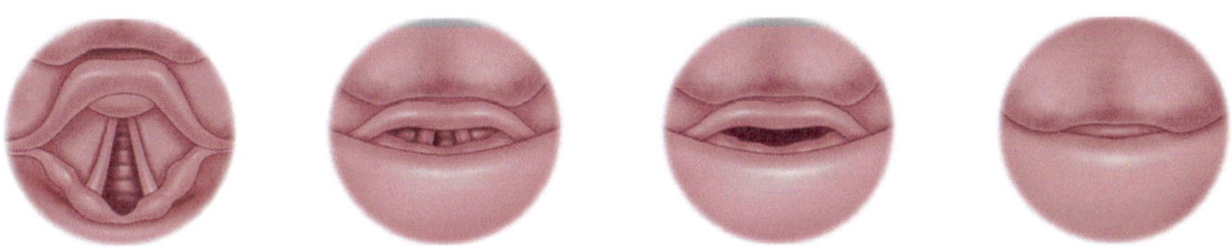

Fig. 5.2 Cormack-Lehane classification. Grade 1: full view of the vocal cords; grade 2: partial view of the vocal cords or arytenoid cartilage; grade 3: only the epiglottis is visible; grade 4: no visualization of the epiglottis or glottis

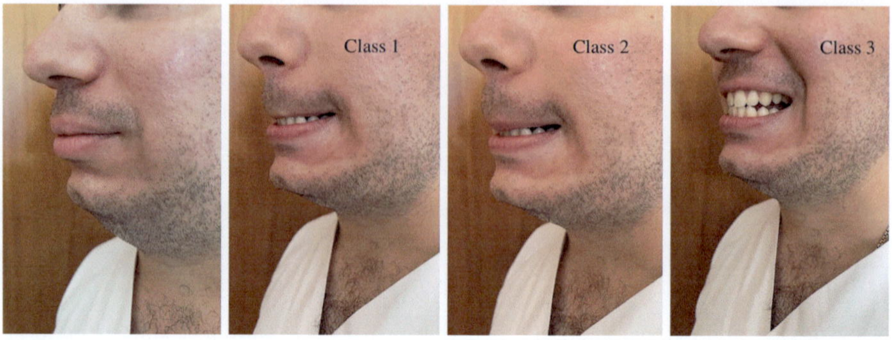

Fig. 5.3 Upper lip bite test. [38]

obtaining lateral cervical radiographs solely to examine cervical joint spaces. Instead, they recommend using physical examination as the primary basis for clinical decision-making.

5.3.6 Mandibular Protrusion

Mandibular protrusion is assessed by having the patient protrude their lower jaw so that the lower incisors are in front of the upper incisors. Mandibular protrusion depends on proper TMJ function and serves as an indicator of mandibular subluxation during laryngoscopy. A more objective test is the upper lip bite test (ULBT), which evaluates the patient's ability to bite the upper lip with their lower incisors. Patients are classified based on the following criteria (Fig. 5.3 [39]):

Class I: Lower incisors can bite the upper lip above the vermilion line.
Class II: Lower incisors can bite the upper lip below the vermilion line.
Class III: Lower incisors cannot bite the upper lip.

In edentulous patients, the ULBT can be replaced with the upper lip catch test (ULCT), which is performed by asking the patient to raise their lower lip above the vermillion border of the upper lip [40] (Fig. 5.4 [41, 42]). The authors demonstrated that the ULCT had a sensitivity, specificity, and accuracy of 75.0%, 89.4%, and 89.3%, respectively—higher than the sensitivity, specificity, and accuracy of the Mallampati test. The ULCT also had a high negative predictive value of 99.4% [40]. Therefore, the authors concluded that the ULCT is a useful predictor for difficult laryngoscopy in edentulous patients.

Khan and colleagues studied 380 adult patients and found a 5% prevalence of difficult laryngoscopy, defined as Cormack-Lehane grade 3 or 4. This study demonstrated that the sensitivity, specificity, and accuracy of the ULBT were 78.95%, 91.96%, and 91.05%, respectively [43]. In comparison to other tests such as TMD,

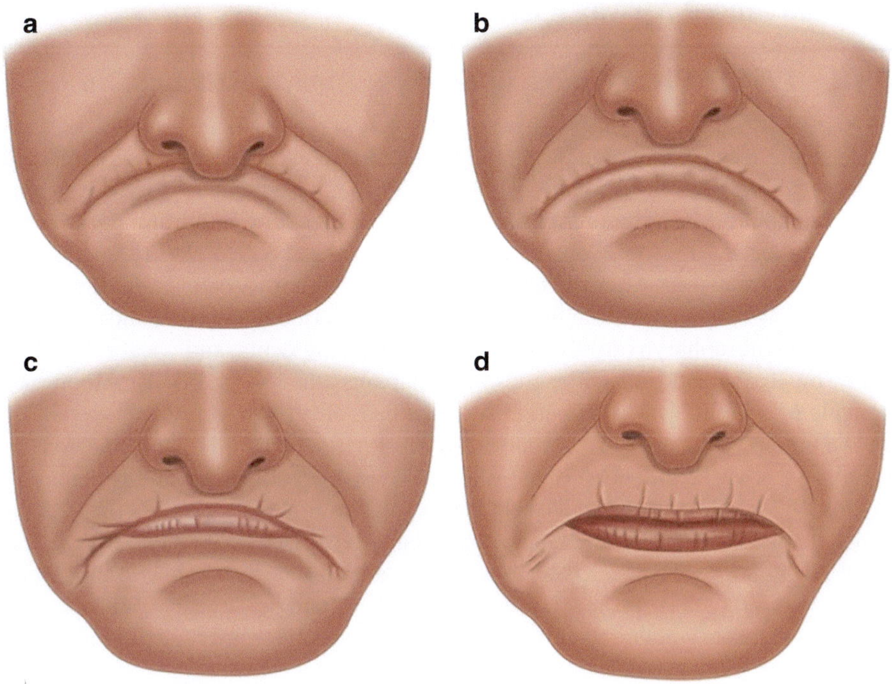

Fig. 5.4 Upper lip catch test. (**a**) Class 0: the lower lip can advance to the rhinion or any point above the midpoint of the vermilion line to the rhinion; (**b**) class I: the lower lip can advance between 2 mm above the vermilion line and the midpoint of the vermilion line to the rhinion; (**c**) class II: the lower lip can advance to the vermilion line or within 2 mm above it; (**d**) class III: the lower incisors cannot advance to the vermilion line. [41]

SMD, and IID, the ULBT had significantly increased specificity (82.27%, 70.64%, and 82.27%, respectively) and accuracy (71.32%, 81.84%, and 76.58%, respectively). Combining the ULBT with SMD improved sensitivity compared to the ULBT alone. In contrast, combining the ULBT with the other tests did not improve the specificity or positive/negative predictive values.

The ULBT demonstrated greater specificity and accuracy compared to the Mallampati score (specificity of 88.7% vs. 66.8%), but sensitivity and positive and negative predictive values between the tests were similar [44].

These findings contrast with the work of Myneni and colleagues, who evaluated the ULBT in 6882 adult patients for predicting difficult laryngoscopy [45]. They found a sensitivity of 8.1% and a positive predictive value of 8.2%, concluding that the ULBT is a poor predictor of difficult laryngoscopy and should not be used as a sole bedside screening test.

5.4 Advanced Airway Assessment

5.4.1 PEAE (Preoperative Endoscopic Airway Examination)

Endoscopic airway examination is a tool commonly used by otolaryngologists to inspect the nasopharynx, larynx, and glottis. It can be used to assess airway tumors and evaluate vocal cord mobility. PEAE can provide additional information about the upper airway that may not be apparent from the medical history or external physical examination. After the nares are prepared with a vasoconstrictor and topical anesthetic, a small flexible fiberoptic scope is inserted into a naris and advanced through the nasopharynx to visualize the epiglottis, vallecula, and vocal cords. In a study by Rosenblatt and colleagues, 138 patients underwent PEAE. Among 44 patients for whom awake intubation was planned, only 16 were thought to require awake intubation after PEAE. Conversely, in 94 patients initially planned to secure the airway after the induction of anesthesia, the plan was changed in 8 patients following PEAE, who instead underwent awake intubation. In total, 26% of the patients had a change in their airway management plan after PEAE [46]. While routine use of PEAE is not recommended for elective surgery, it can be a valuable tool when airway pathology is suspected. Findings from PEAE can guide airway management decisions, such as whether to perform awake intubation versus a standard induction.

5.4.2 Airway Imaging

5.4.2.1 Radiographs, Computed Tomography, Magnetic Resonance Imaging

Given the limited predictive power of bedside screening tests for DI, there has been growing interest in using diagnostic imaging—including radiographs (X-ray), computed tomography (CT), and magnetic resonance imaging (MRI)—as alternative tools. Parameters on lateral neck radiography, including reduced AO space and maxillopharyngeal angle, along with decreased angle between the lines from the hyoid bone to the thyroid cartilage, are predictive of DI [47, 48]. In a meta-analysis of 17 studies involving 8779 patients, the modified Mallampati score had a pooled sensitivity, specificity, and positive likelihood ratio of 0.61, 0.63, and 2.11, respectively. These values were significantly lower than those of CT, X-ray, and ultrasonography (USG) [48]. The authors concluded that the diagnostic value of predicting DI was similar between USG, CT, and X-ray. Given the significant limitations of CT and X-ray, including radiation exposure, cost, and lack of portability, the authors recommended ultrasound as the preferred diagnostic modality. While diagnostic imaging is not recommended as a routine screening tool for difficult airways, it can be useful in patients with known or suspected airway pathology. For example, CT and MRI can provide critical information about the location and size of a goiter, airway tumors that may compress the airway or cause tracheal deviation, or extrinsic masses such as abscesses that can distort airway anatomy. Information gleaned from a review of airway imaging can be helpful in developing an airway management plan.

5.4.2.2 Airway Ultrasonography

USG is a portable and non-invasive tool that can be used for airway visualization, from the mouth to the lungs. It offers several advantages over other imaging modalities—it is safe (no radiation exposure), quick, dynamic, can be performed at the bedside, and is widely available. USG is comparable to MRI and CT in measuring subglottic airway diameter and, in both adult and pediatric populations, is superior to clinical assessment in predicting the appropriate size of single- and double-lumen endotracheal tubes [49]. USG guidance can accurately localize the cricothyroid membrane, and cadaveric studies show that its use improves the success rate of cricothyrotomy [50]. The cricothyroid membrane is a key landmark for percutaneous airway access, but can be challenging to localize in obese patients. Prior to the management of patients with suspected or known difficult airways, using USG guidance to identify and mark the cricothyroid membrane can be a useful safety measure. Additionally, USG can be used to obtain various airway measurements, including skin to hyomental distance, tongue volume, and the distance from the skin to the epiglottis.

Studies examining USG as a tool to predict a difficult airway have yielded conflicting results. Kundra and colleagues found that pretracheal soft tissue thickness at the level of the vocal cords was a good predictor of difficult laryngoscopy in the obese population [51]. Conversely, Komatsu and colleagues concluded that the thickness of the pretracheal soft tissue at the level of the vocal cords was not a predictor of difficult laryngoscopy in obese patients [52]. Another study evaluating the pre-glottic space thickness found that an increased distance from the skin to the epiglottis was predictive of worsening Cormack-Lehane grades and difficulty with laryngoscopy and intubation [53]. However, this study did not find a significant correlation between USG measurements at the level of the vocal cords and difficult laryngoscopy.

5.5 Predictors of Difficult Mask Ventilation, SGA Ventilation, and Tracheal Intubation

While the goal of reviewing a patient's history and conducting an anesthesia-focused physical exam is to predict the risk of difficulty with ventilation and intubation, most difficult airways are unexpected. In a review of 188,064 patients from the Danish Anesthesia Database, the accuracy of anesthesiologists' predictions of DI was low. Among 3391 DIs, 93% were unanticipated [54]. Conversely, out of 929 patients where difficulty was anticipated, only 25% were difficult. Similarly, 94% of cases of DMV were unanticipated. When DMV was anticipated, it only occurred in 22% of cases. These findings highlight the challenges in airway prediction and the critical importance of maintaining constant preparedness for unexpected difficulties.

5.5.1 Performance of Airway Screening Tests

Numerous studies have examined whether bedside airway assessment tools can reliably predict difficulty with airway management. A meta-analysis of bedside screening tests found that screening tests had low to moderate sensitivity (20–62%) and moderate to fair specificity (82–97%) [30]. Shiga and colleagues concluded that a combination of tests adds incremental value compared to using a single test alone. The most useful test combination was the Mallampati score and TMD, which had a positive likelihood ratio of 9.9 for predicting DI [30]. A Cochrane review analyzed 133 studies with 844,204 patients to assess airway physical examination tests for predicting difficult airway management in apparently normal adult patients [55]. For difficult laryngoscopy, sensitivity ranged from 0.22 (mouth opening test) to 0.67 (ULBT), and specificity ranged from 0.80 (modified Mallampati test) to 0.95 (Wilson risk score). The ULBT had the highest sensitivity to predict difficult laryngoscopy, and the modified Mallampati test had the highest sensitivity for predicting difficult tracheal intubation. While single tests have limited predictive value, bedside airway examination can alert clinicians to potential difficulties with MV, SGA ventilation, and tracheal intubation. These assessments also provide valuable insight for developing an airway management plan.

5.5.2 Difficult Mask Ventilation (DMV)

MV is a critical aspect of airway management, particularly for patients with difficult airways. In a review of 22,000 anesthetics, 1.4% of patients experienced DMV, and 0.16% were deemed impossible to mask ventilate (IMV) [13]. In this study, DMV was defined as MV that was inadequate to maintain oxygenation, unstable MV, or MV requiring two providers, while IMV was defined as absent end-tidal carbon dioxide measurement and lack of chest wall movement. A later study of over 53,000 anesthetics reported an IMV incidence of 0.15% [14]. In this study, DMV was defined as inadequate ventilation despite multiple adjuvants and providers, while IMV was defined as the inability to exchange air during BMV attempts, despite multiple providers, airway adjuvants, or neuromuscular blockade. Of the 77 patients

Table 5.1 Predictors of difficult mask ventilation [2, 9, 14, 56–60]

Obesity
Older age
Male sex
Mallampati classification III or IV
Large neck circumference
Short thyromental distance (<6 cm)
History of neck radiation
Limited mandibular protrusion
Edentulous
Obstructive sleep apnea (OSA)
Snoring
Presence of a beard or facial hair
Avoidance of neuromuscular blocking agents (NMBA)

who were impossible to mask ventilate in the study, 25% also experienced difficulty with intubation. Langeron and colleagues reported an incidence of DMV at 5%, defined as the inability of an unassisted anesthesiologist to maintain oxygen saturations above 92% or failure to prevent/reverse signs of inadequate ventilation during positive pressure MV under general anesthesia [56]. In these studies, the definitions of DMV and/or IMV vary, and the lack of a standardized definition may explain the variability in incidences.

Risk factors have been identified for DMV and are presented in Table 5.1. The greater the number of risk factors present, the higher the risk of DMV or IMV.

5.5.3 Difficult Supraglottic Airway (SGA) Ventilation

Since the laryngeal mask airway (LMA) was introduced into clinical practice in the 1980s, it has become increasingly popular for patients undergoing general anesthesia. SGAs, including the LMA, play a key role in the management of the difficult airway and are integral to difficult airway algorithms, including the ASA Practice Guidelines for Management of the Difficult Airway [1]. In a study of over 15,000 adult patients, LMA failure occurred in 1.1% of patients. LMA failure was defined as an airway event requiring LMA removal and tracheal intubation. Among patients with LMA failure, 5.6% also experienced DMV [61]. The LMA failure rate was consistent with previous studies showing LMA failure to range from 0.19% to 4.7% [62, 63]. Proper SGA size selection is critical for successful placement. While a wide variety of brands and styles exist, most manufacturers recommend weight-based size selection [57].

Risk factors for difficult SGA ventilation are presented in Table 5.2.

Table 5.2 Predictors of difficult supraglottic airway ventilation [2, 58, 61, 64, 65]

Obesity
Male sex
Mallampati classification III or IV
Large neck circumference (>44 cm)
Decreased cervical spine motion
Neck radiation
Glottic, subglottic, or hypopharyngeal pathology
Poor dentition/edentulous
Limited mouth opening (limited interincisor distance)
Avoidance of neuromuscular blocking agents (NMBA)

5.5.4 *Difficult Tracheal Intubation*

Adverse respiratory events, including difficult tracheal intubation, are associated with patient morbidity and mortality and can result in hypoxemia, brain injury, and death. The ASA Closed Claims Project is a database of anesthesia-related adverse outcomes collected from professional liability insurance claims. Adverse respiratory events were identified as the most common cause of anesthesia malpractice claims, with brain damage and death most frequently attributed to respiratory system events, including inadequate ventilation, esophageal intubation, and difficult tracheal intubation [66]. It is important, therefore, to understand the incidence and risk factors for difficult tracheal intubation to ensure adequate preparation and reduce adverse patient outcomes. A meta-analysis of 35 studies involving 50,760 patients demonstrated a DI incidence of 5.8%, defined as Cormack-Lehane grade 3 or greater [30]. Another study of over 100,000 patients found that the rate of difficult laryngoscopy was 4.9%, defined as Cormack-Lehane 3 or 4 [67].

Table 5.3 presents risk factors for DI, with the most predictive being a history of prior DI, limited cervical spine mobility, and short TMD. The likelihood of DI increases with the number of risk factors present [58].

5.5.5 *Role of Videolaryngoscopy in Difficult Airway*

Videolaryngoscopy is a useful tool for managing difficult airways. It has been shown to improve Cormack-Lehane laryngeal views and increase the likelihood of successful intubation compared to direct laryngoscopy [71]. Therefore, videolaryngoscopy is a valuable rescue technique if direct laryngoscopy fails. Because videolaryngoscopy follows a different approach than direct laryngoscopy, the risk factors also differ.

Risk factors for difficult videolaryngoscopy are listed in Table 5.4.

Table 5.3 Predictors of difficult tracheal intubation using direct laryngoscopy [2, 9, 39, 55, 58, 67–70]

History of difficult intubation
+/− increased BMI (conflicting evidence)
Age >46 years
Male sex
Mallampati classification III or IV
Limited mouth opening (interincisor distance <4 cm)
Large neck circumference (>40 cm)
Short thyromental distance (<6 cm)
Short sternomental distance (<12.5 cm)
Decreased cervical spine motion
History of neck radiation
History of head and neck surgery, cardiac surgery, or oral/maxillofacial surgery
Limited mandibular protrusion or high score on the upper lip bite test (ULBT)
Prominent dentition
Obstructive sleep apnea (OSA)
Avoidance of neuromuscular blocking agents (NMBA)

Table 5.4 Predictors of difficult tracheal intubation using videolaryngoscopy [2, 58, 72–74]

High Cormack-Lehane grade on previous direct laryngoscopy
Limited mouth opening
Large tongue
Short sternothyroid distance
Decreased cervical spine motion
Abnormal neck anatomy (e.g., neck radiation, head, and neck masses)
History of head and neck surgery or cardiac surgery
Limited mandibular protrusion (high ULBT score)

5.6 Pre-procedure Planning

Once the patient's medical history is reviewed, an airway-focused physical exam is performed to assess risk, and relevant diagnostic studies are considered, an anesthetic and airway management plan can be formulated. This strategy must account for not only the clinical assessment and context, but also the risks and benefits of different options.

Since the majority of DIs are unanticipated and any strategy can unexpectedly fail, it is imperative to consider backup plans and ensure adequate training to manage the difficult airway. The ASA Difficult Airway Algorithm is a tool for planning the approach for a patient with a potentially difficult airway and addressing unexpected problems that can arise during airway management [1]. The 2022 ASA Practice Guidelines for the Management of the Difficult Airway recommends considering awake tracheal intubation if difficult intubation is suspected, especially if at least one of the following conditions is present: difficult ventilation, increased aspiration risk, inability to tolerate brief periods of apnea, and/or predicted difficulty with emergency invasive airway access [1]. It is important to consider the patient's age and ability to cooperate before planning an awake tracheal intubation, as this technique poses greater challenges in pediatric and uncooperative patients.

Once an airway plan is formulated, the next step is to ensure adequate preparation, including [1]:

- Availability of necessary equipment and trained personnel.
- Comprehensive patient preparation, incorporating the discussion of anticipated challenges.
- Communication of the airway management plan.
- Preoxygenation.
- Proper patient positioning.
- Local anesthetic administration (if awake, intubation is planned).

For further details, see the chapter "Previous Preparation for Airway Management."

References

1. Apfelbaum JL, Hagberg CA, Connis RT, Abdelmalak BB, Agarkar M, Dutton RP, et al. 2022 American Society of Anesthesiologists practice guidelines for management of the difficult airway. Anesthesiology. 2022;136(1):31–81.
2. Law JA, Duggan LV, Asselin M, Baker P, Crosby E, Downey A, et al. Canadian Airway Focus Group updated consensus-based recommendations for management of the difficult airway: part 2. Planning and implementing safe management of the patient with an anticipated difficult airway. Can J Anaesth. 2021;68(9):1405–36.
3. Cook TM, Woodall N, Frerk C, Fourth National Audit Project. Major complications of airway management in the UK: results of the Fourth National Audit Project of the Royal College of Anaesthetists and the Difficult Airway Society. Part 1: anaesthesia. Br J Anaesth. 2011;106(5):617–31.
4. Brambrink AM, Braun U. Airway management in infants and children. Best Pract Res Clin Anaesthesiol. 2005;19(4):675–97.
5. Sequera-Ramos L, Duffy KA, Fiadjoe JE, Garcia-Marcinkiewicz AG, Zhang B, Perate A, et al. The prevalence of difficult airway in children with Beckwith-Wiedemann syndrome: a retrospective cohort study. Anesth Analg. 2021;133(6):1559–67.
6. Baines D, Keneally J. Anaesthetic implications of the mucopolysaccharidoses: a fifteen-year experience in a children's hospital. Anaesth Intensive Care. 1983;11(3):198–202.
7. Hamilton J, Yaneza MM, Clement WA, Kubba H. The prevalence of airway problems in children with Down's syndrome. Int J Pediatr Otorhinolaryngol. 2016;81:1–4.
8. Watts R, Vyas H. An overview of respiratory problems in children with Down's syndrome. Arch Dis Child. 2013;98(10):812–7.
9. Moon TS, Fox PE, Somasundaram A, Minhajuddin A, Gonzales MX, Pak TJ, et al. The influence of morbid obesity on difficult intubation and difficult mask ventilation. J Anesth. 2019;33(1):96–102.
10. Juvin P, Lavaut E, Dupont H, Lefevre P, Demetriou M, Dumoulin JL, et al. Difficult tracheal intubation is more common in obese than in lean patients. Anesth Analg. 2003;97(2):595–600.
11. Brodsky JB, Lemmens HJ, Brock-Utne JG, Vierra M, Saidman LJ. Morbid obesity and tracheal intubation. Anesth Analg. 2002;94(3):732–6, table of contents.
12. Chung F, Yegneswaran B, Liao P, Chung SA, Vairavanathan S, Islam S, et al. STOP questionnaire: a tool to screen patients for obstructive sleep apnea. Anesthesiology. 2008;108(5):812–21.

13. Kheterpal S, Han R, Tremper KK, Shanks A, Tait AR, O'Reilly M, et al. Incidence and predictors of difficult and impossible mask ventilation. Anesthesiology. 2006;105(5):885–91.
14. Kheterpal S, Martin L, Shanks AM, Tremper KK. Prediction and outcomes of impossible mask ventilation: a review of 50,000 anesthetics. Anesthesiology. 2009;110(4):891–7.
15. Alotaibi M, Albazli K, Bissar L, Almoallim H. Perioperative management of patients with rheumatic diseases. In: Almoallim H, Cheikh M, editors. Skills in rheumatology. Singapore: Springer; 2021. p. 407–17.
16. Krause ML, Matteson EL. Perioperative management of the patient with rheumatoid arthritis. World J Orthop. 2014;5(3):283–91.
17. Woodward LJ, Kam PC. Ankylosing spondylitis: recent developments and anaesthetic implications. Anaesthesia. 2009;64(5):540–8.
18. Aiello G, Metcalf I. Anaesthetic implications of temporomandibular joint disease. Can J Anaesth. 1992;39(6):610–6.
19. Stevanovic K, Sabljak V, Toskovic A, Kukic B, Stekovic J, Antonijevic V, et al. Anaesthesia and the patient with diabetes. Diabetes Metab Syndr. 2015;9(3):177–9.
20. Ali Z, Bithal PK, Prabhakar H, Rath GP, Dash HH. An assessment of the predictors of difficult intubation in patients with acromegaly. J Clin Neurosci. 2009;16(8):1043–5.
21. Schmitt H, Buchfelder M, Radespiel-Troger M, Fahlbusch R. Difficult intubation in acromegalic patients: incidence and predictability. Anesthesiology. 2000;93(1):110–4.
22. Samsoon GL, Young JR. Difficult tracheal intubation: a retrospective study. Anaesthesia. 1987;42(5):487–90.
23. Fernandez MW, Beattie LK. Assessment of the difficult airway. In: Ganti L, editor. Atlas of emergency medicine procedures. New York: Springer; 2022. p. 89–92. https://doi.org/10.1007/978-3-030-85047-0_12.
24. Tham EJ, Gildersleve CD, Sanders LD, Mapleson WW, Vaughan RS. Effects of posture, phonation and observer on Mallampati classification. Br J Anaesth. 1992;68(1):32–8.
25. Bindra A, Prabhakar H, Singh GP, Ali Z, Singhal V. Is the modified Mallampati test performed in supine position a reliable predictor of difficult tracheal intubation? J Anesth. 2010;24(3):482–5.
26. Krobbuaban B, Diregpoke S, Kumkeaw S, Tanomsat M. The predictive value of the height ratio and thyromental distance: four predictive tests for difficult laryngoscopy. Anesth Analg. 2005;101(5):1542–5.
27. Yildiz TS, Korkmaz F, Solak M, Toker K, Erciyes N, Bayrak F, et al. Prediction of difficult tracheal intubation in Turkish patients: a multi-center methodological study. Eur J Anaesthesiol. 2007;24(12):1034–40.
28. Lundstrom LH, Vester-Andersen M, Moller AM, Charuluxananan S, L'Hermite J, Wetterslev J, et al. Poor prognostic value of the modified Mallampati score: a meta-analysis involving 177 088 patients. Br J Anaesth. 2011;107(5):659–67.
29. Rosenstock C, Gillesberg I, Gätke MR, Levin D, Kristensen MS, Rasmussen LS. Inter-observer agreement of tests used for prediction of difficult laryngoscopy/tracheal intubation. Acta Anaesthesiol Scand. 2005;49(8):1057–62.
30. Shiga T, Wajima Z, Inoue T, Sakamoto A. Predicting difficult intubation in apparently normal patients: a meta-analysis of bedside screening test performance. Anesthesiology. 2005;103(2):429–37.
31. Baker PA, Depuydt A, Thompson JM. Thyromental distance measurement—fingers don't rule. Anaesthesia. 2009;64(8):878–82.
32. Schmitt HJ, Kirmse M, Radespiel-Troger M. Ratio of patient's height to thyromental distance improves prediction of difficult laryngoscopy. Anaesth Intensive Care. 2002;30(6):763–5.
33. Shah PJ, Dubey KP, Yadav JP. Predictive value of upper lip bite test and ratio of height to thyromental distance compared to other multivariate airway assessment tests for difficult laryngoscopy in apparently normal patients. J Anaesthesiol Clin Pharmacol. 2013;29(2):191–5.
34. Savva D. Prediction of difficult tracheal intubation. Br J Anaesth. 1994;73(2):149–53.
35. Bannister FB, Macbeth RG. Direct laryngoscopy and tracheal intubation. Lancet. 1944;2:651–4.

36. Mashour GA, Stallmer ML, Kheterpal S, Shanks A. Predictors of difficult intubation in patients with cervical spine limitations. J Neurosurg Anesthesiol. 2008;20(2):110–5.
37. Calder I, Calder J, Crockard HA. Difficult direct laryngoscopy in patients with cervical spine disease. Anaesthesia. 1995;50(9):756–63.
38. Gogakos AS, Rallis T, Barbetakis N. Upper airways the Maxilar-Jaw effect. In: Esquinas AM, De Vito A, Barbetakis N, editors. Upper airway disorders and noninvasive mechanical ventilation. Cham: Springer; 2023.
39. Detsky ME, Jivraj N, Adhikari NK, Friedrich JO, Pinto R, Simel DL, et al. Will this patient be difficult to intubate?: the rational clinical examination systematic review. JAMA. 2019;321(5):493–503.
40. Khan ZH, Arbabi S, Yekaninejad MS, Khan RH. Application of the upper lip catch test for airway evaluation in edentulous patients: an observational study. Saudi J Anaesth. 2014;8(1):73–7.
41. Khan ZH, Khan RH. A new airway assessment classification for edentulous patients and its potential role in neurocritical care. In: Khan Z, editor. Challenging topics in neuroanesthesia and neurocritical care. Cham: Springer; 2017. p. 123–7. https://doi.org/10.1007/978-3-319-41445-4_9.
42. Khan ZH, Kashfi A. Evaluating a patient's airway. Anesth Analg. 2003;97(3):915–6.
43. Khan ZH, Mohammadi M, Rasouli MR, Farrokhnia F, Khan RH. The diagnostic value of the upper lip bite test combined with sternomental distance, thyromental distance, and interincisor distance for prediction of easy laryngoscopy and intubation: a prospective study. Anesth Analg. 2009;109(3):822–4.
44. Khan ZH, Kashfi A, Ebrahimkhani E. A comparison of the upper lip bite test (a simple new technique) with modified Mallampati classification in predicting difficulty in endotracheal intubation: a prospective blinded study. Anesth Analg. 2003;96(2):595–9, table of contents.
45. Myneni N, O'Leary AM, Sandison M, Roberts K. Evaluation of the upper lip bite test in predicting difficult laryngoscopy. J Clin Anesth. 2010;22(3):174–8.
46. Rosenblatt W, Ianus AI, Sukhupragarn W, Fickenscher A, Sasaki C. Preoperative endoscopic airway examination (PEAE) provides superior airway information and may reduce the use of unnecessary awake intubation. Anesth Analg. 2011;112(3):602–7.
47. Kamalipour H, Bagheri M, Kamali K, Taleie A, Yarmohammadi H. Lateral neck radiography for prediction of difficult orotracheal intubation. Eur J Anaesthesiol. 2005;22(9):689–93.
48. Ji C, Ni Q, Chen W. Diagnostic accuracy of radiology (CT, X-ray, US) for predicting difficult intubation in adults: a meta-analysis. J Clin Anesth. 2018;45:79–87.
49. You-Ten KE, Siddiqui N, Teoh WH, Kristensen MS. Point-of-care ultrasound (POCUS) of the upper airway. Can J Anaesth. 2018;65(4):473–84.
50. Siddiqui N, Arzola C, Friedman Z, Guerina L, You-Ten KE. Ultrasound improves cricothyrotomy success in cadavers with poorly defined neck anatomy: a randomized control trial. Anesthesiology. 2015;123(5):1033–41.
51. Kundra P, Mishra SK, Ramesh A. Ultrasound of the airway. Indian J Anaesth. 2011;55(5):456–62.
52. Komatsu R, Sengupta P, Wadhwa A, Akca O, Sessler DI, Ezri T, et al. Ultrasound quantification of anterior soft tissue thickness fails to predict difficult laryngoscopy in obese patients. Anaesth Intensive Care. 2007;35(1):32–7.
53. Falcetta S, Cavallo S, Gabbanelli V, Pelaia P, Sorbello M, Zdravkovic I, et al. Evaluation of two neck ultrasound measurements as predictors of difficult direct laryngoscopy: a prospective observational study. Eur J Anaesthesiol. 2018;35(8):605–12.
54. Norskov AK, Rosenstock CV, Wetterslev J, Astrup G, Afshari A, Lundstrom LH. Diagnostic accuracy of anaesthesiologists' prediction of difficult airway management in daily clinical practice: a cohort study of 188 064 patients registered in the Danish Anaesthesia Database. Anaesthesia. 2015;70(3):272–81.
55. Roth D, Pace NL, Lee A, Hovhannisyan K, Warenits AM, Arrich J, et al. Bedside tests for predicting difficult airways: an abridged Cochrane diagnostic test accuracy systematic review. Anaesthesia. 2019;74(7):915–28.

56. Langeron O, Masso E, Huraux C, Guggiari M, Bianchi A, Coriat P, et al. Prediction of difficult mask ventilation. Anesthesiology. 2000;92(5):1229–36.
57. Cattano D, Katsiampoura A, Corso RM, Killoran PV, Cai C, Hagberg CA. Predictive factors for difficult mask ventilation in the obese surgical population. F1000Res. 2014;3:239.
58. Rosenblatt WH, Artime C. Management of the difficult airway for general anesthesia in adults. In: Hagberg CA, editor. Waltham: UpToDate; 2022.
59. Leoni A, Arlati S, Ghisi D, Verwej M, Lugani D, Ghisi P, et al. Difficult mask ventilation in obese patients: analysis of predictive factors. Minerva Anestesiol. 2014;80(2):149–57.
60. Gautam P, Gaul TK, Luthra N. Prediction of difficult mask ventilation. Eur J Anaesthesiol. 2005;22(8):638–40.
61. Ramachandran SK, Mathis MR, Tremper KK, Shanks AM, Kheterpal S. Predictors and clinical outcomes from failed Laryngeal Mask Airway Unique: a study of 15,795 patients. Anesthesiology. 2012;116(6):1217–26.
62. Verghese C, Brimacombe JR. Survey of laryngeal mask airway usage in 11,910 patients: safety and efficacy for conventional and nonconventional usage. Anesth Analg. 1996;82(1):129–33.
63. Rose DK, Cohen MM. The airway: problems and predictions in 18,500 patients. Can J Anaesth. 1994;41(5 Pt 1):372–83.
64. Katsiampoura AD, Killoran PV, Corso RM, Cai C, Hagberg CA, Cattano D. Laryngeal mask placement in a teaching institution: analysis of difficult placements. F1000Res. 2015;4:102.
65. Di Filippo A, Adembri C, Paparella L, Esposito C, Tofani L, Perez Y, et al. Risk factors for difficult Laryngeal Mask Airway LMA-Supreme (LMAS) placement in adults: a multicentric prospective observational study in an Italian population. Minerva Anestesiol. 2021;87(5):533–40.
66. Cheney FW. The American Society of Anesthesiologists Closed Claims Project: what have we learned, how has it affected practice, and how will it affect practice in the future. Anesthesiology. 1999;91(2):552–6.
67. Heinrich S, Birkholz T, Irouschek A, Ackermann A, Schmidt J. Incidences and predictors of difficult laryngoscopy in adult patients undergoing general anesthesia: a single-center analysis of 102,305 cases. J Anesth. 2013;27(6):815–21.
68. Seet E, Chung F, Wang CY, Tam S, Kumar CM, Ubeynarayana CU, et al. Association of obstructive sleep apnea with difficult intubation: prospective multicenter observational cohort study. Anesth Analg. 2021;133(1):196–204.
69. Sheff SR, May MC, Carlisle SE, Kallies KJ, Mathiason MA, Kothari SN. Predictors of a difficult intubation in the bariatric patient: does preoperative body mass index matter? Surg Obes Relat Dis. 2013;9(3):344–9.
70. Joffe AM, Aziz MF, Posner KL, Duggan LV, Mincer SL, Domino KB. Management of difficult tracheal intubation: a closed claims analysis. Anesthesiology. 2019;131(4):818–29.
71. Aziz MF, Dillman D, Fu R, Brambrink AM. Comparative effectiveness of the C-MAC video laryngoscope versus direct laryngoscopy in the setting of the predicted difficult airway. Anesthesiology. 2012;116(3):629–36.
72. Aziz MF, Bayman EO, Van Tienderen MM, Todd MM, St AGEIG, Brambrink AM. Predictors of difficult videolaryngoscopy with GlideScope(R) or C-MAC(R) with D-blade: secondary analysis from a large comparative videolaryngoscopy trial. Br J Anaesth. 2016;117(1):118–23.
73. Aziz MF, Healy D, Kheterpal S, Fu RF, Dillman D, Brambrink AM. Routine clinical practice effectiveness of the Glidescope in difficult airway management: an analysis of 2,004 Glidescope intubations, complications, and failures from two institutions. Anesthesiology. 2011;114(1):34–41.
74. Tremblay MH, Williams S, Robitaille A, Drolet P. Poor visualization during direct laryngoscopy and high upper lip bite test score are predictors of difficult intubation with the GlideScope videolaryngoscope. Anesth Analg. 2008;106(5):1495–500, table of contents.

Chapter 6
Ultrasound Assessment of Gastric Content and Aspiration Risk

Natalia C. Portela, Anuja Rathore, and Anahi Perlas

Highlights

- Point-of-care gastric ultrasound (POCUS) is a non-invasive and reliable tool for assessing the composition and volume of gastric content.
- Multiple studies confirm its validity and applicability across diverse patient populations, including pregnant, obese, and pediatric patients.
- Particularly useful when aspiration risk is unclear, gastric ultrasound enables individualized risk assessment and guides anesthetic management to prevent pulmonary aspiration.
- A grade 0 or 1 antrum (or < 1.5 mL/kg of clear fluid) is consistent with fasting and low aspiration risk. In contrast, a grade 2 antrum (or > 1.5 mL/kg of clear fluid) or the presence of any solid content indicates a full stomach and a higher-than-baseline risk of aspiration.
- When the stomach contains clear fluid only, a mathematical model can accurately estimate gastric volume up to 500 mL.

N. C. Portela
Mount Sinai Hospital, Department of Anesthesiology and Pain Medicine, University of Toronto, Toronto, ON, Canada

A. Rathore
Toronto Western Hospital, Department of Anesthesiology and Pain Medicine, University of Toronto, Toronto, ON, Canada
e-mail: Anuja.Rathore@uhn.ca

A. Perlas (✉)
Toronto Western Hospital, University Health Network, Department of Anesthesiology and Pain Medicine, University of Toronto, Toronto, ON, Canada
e-mail: anahi.perlas@uhn.ca

M. Á. Gómez-Ríos, A. van Zundert (eds.), *Evidence-based Guide to Difficult Airway Management*, https://doi.org/10.1007/978-3-032-30769-9_6

6.1 Clinical Example

A 55-year-old female presents for diagnostic laparoscopy due to multiple abdominal collections suggestive of pelvic inflammatory disease. The procedure is urgent but not immediately life-threatening. The patient has fasted for more than 8 h and has a medical history of hypertension, dyslipidemia, and type II diabetes. She weighs 80 kg, and her airway evaluation shows no predictors of difficult tracheal intubation. She is hemodynamically stable, with an unremarkable electrocardiogram (ECG) and normal routine blood test. However, as the on-call anesthesiologist, you are concerned about the possibility of a full stomach despite adequate fasting, given her diabetes and acute intra-abdominal pathology.

6.1.1 Application of Gastric Ultrasound

You perform a point-of-care ultrasound (POCUS) assessment of her gastric content. The scan reveals a distended gastric antrum with hyperechoic mixed content, blurring the posterior antral wall—findings consistent with solid gastric content, indicating a "full stomach."

6.1.2 Management Decision

You prescribe aspiration prophylaxis with famotidine 20 mg, metoclopramide 10 mg, and sodium citrate. You decide to proceed with a rapid sequence induction (RSI) and endotracheal intubation. A nasogastric tube is not indicated, as it is unlikely to evacuate solid, particulate content before induction.

6.2 Introduction

Pulmonary aspiration of gastric contents is a serious anesthetic complication associated with aspiration pneumonia, prolonged mechanical ventilation, and increased mortality [1–6]. The incidence of aspiration ranges from 0.025% to 1% [1, 5, 7], with mortality rates from aspiration pneumonia reaching up to 5% [6].

Anesthesia predisposes patients to this complication by reducing esophageal sphincter tone and depressing airway protective reflexes. Up to 9% of all anesthesia-related deaths are linked to pulmonary aspiration [8, 9]. A key risk factor is the presence of gastric content at the time of anesthetic induction or sedation. The solid nature of the aspirate, a low pH (<2.5), and a high volume (>0.8 mL/kg) are strongly associated with increased morbidity and mortality following aspiration.

6.2.1 Factors Affecting Aspiration Risk

Even in healthy patients who adhere to standard preoperative fasting guidelines, residual gastric volumes up to 1.5 mL/kg (composed of clear gastric secretions) are not associated with significant aspiration risk [10, 11]. However, several conditions can increase the risk of regurgitation and aspiration, including inadequate preoperative fasting, pregnancy, altered consciousness or sedation, gastroesophageal reflux disease (GERD), diabetes mellitus, severe renal or hepatic dysfunction, intestinal obstruction, or any other cause of gastroparesis. Additionally, anxiety and prolonged fasting may increase gastric acid production and lower gastric pH, paradoxically raising the risk of aspiration pneumonitis.

6.2.2 Challenges in Aspiration Risk Assessment

Even for experienced anesthesiologists, assessing perioperative aspiration risk remains challenging. Several factors can complicate risk evaluation, including unreliable clinical history, limited patient communication (e.g., language barriers, altered consciousness), and medical comorbidities or physiologic conditions affecting gastric emptying. These limitations can lead to inaccurate risk assessment, one of the primary contributors to aspiration events [7].

6.2.3 Role of Point-of-Care Gastric Ultrasound

Given the importance of recognizing a full stomach in surgical settings, point-of-care gastric ultrasound (POCUS) has emerged in the past decade as a non-invasive, reliable tool for evaluating gastric content and volume [12–15]. Gastric ultrasound is particularly useful in scenarios where fasting status and aspiration risk are unclear. In these cases—when the pre-test probability of a "full stomach" approaches 50%—POCUS can provide critical information to guide anesthetic management [16, 17].

6.3 Technique

When performing a gastric ultrasound to assess gastric content and volume, the most reliable anatomical section to evaluate is the gastric antrum. The gastric body often contains significant air, which can interfere with the exam, while the gastric fundus is difficult to visualize via ultrasound [22, 25].

Several studies suggest that the antrum is best evaluated in a semi-sitting or right lateral decubitus (RLD) position, as gastric contents naturally shift toward dependent areas of the stomach [13, 15, 18–23]. Scanning should first be performed in the supine position, followed by RLD. If the patient cannot be positioned in RLD, an alternative is the semi-recumbent position (head elevated 45°).

In adults, a curved-array, low-frequency abdominal probe (2–5 MHz) is preferred due to its adequate penetration for visualizing anatomical landmarks [18]. In pediatric patients, a linear high-frequency transducer is often used [24].

The stomach is imaged in a sagittal plane, scanning the epigastric area, immediately inferior to the xiphoid and superior to the umbilicus. The examiner should swipe the transducer from left to right along the subcostal margin to obtain a transverse view of the antrum. Techniques such as sliding, rotating, and tilting the probe help optimize the image. However, excessive probe rotation may create oblique views, overestimating antral size.

6.4 Anatomic Characteristics and Landmarks

The gastric antrum is typically located superficially in the epigastric area, using a soft tissue acoustic window provided by the left lobe of the liver [14, 15, 22]. Studies confirm that assessing the antrum provides accurate information about gastric content in the entire organ [14, 15, 22].

6.4.1 Sonographic Landmarks

- The antrum appears as a superficial hollow viscus structure with a thick, multilayered wall, positioned between the left lobe of the liver (anteriorly) and the body of the pancreas (posteriorly) (Fig. 6.1) [15].
- The inferior vena cava (IVC) and aorta lie posterior to the antrum.
- Additional vascular landmarks include the superior mesenteric artery and vein.

6.4.2 Gastric Wall Structure (Adults)

The gastric wall is approximately 4–6 mm thick and comprises five distinct sonographic layers (from the inner to the outer surface): (1) mucosal-air interface, (2) muscularis mucosa, (3) submucosa, (4) muscularis propria, and (5) serosa (Figs. 6.2 and 6.3) [15]. With low-frequency transducers, only the muscularis propria is consistently visible. The thicker muscularis layer and distinct antral location help differentiate the stomach from other parts of the gastrointestinal tract, which have thinner, less prominent smooth muscle layers.

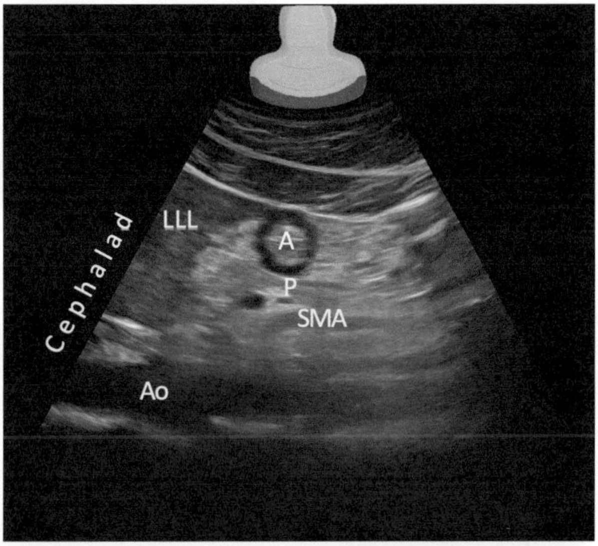

Fig. 6.1 Sagittal ultrasound scan of the gastric antrum. *A* gastric antrum, *LLL* left lobe of liver, *P* pancreas, *SMA* superior mesenteric artery, *Ao* aorta. (Permission obtained from Dr. Perlas Fontana Medicine Professional Corporation)

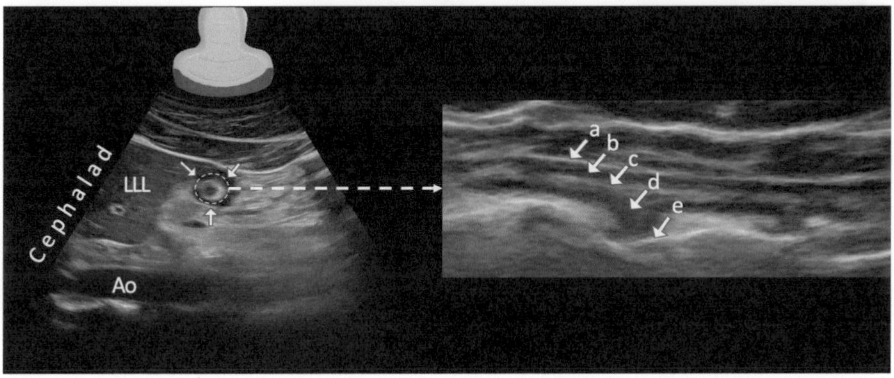

Fig. 6.2 Ultrasound depiction of gastric wall layers. (**a**) serosa, (**b**) muscularis propria, (**c**) submucosa, (**d**) muscularis mucosa, (**e**) mucosal-air interface. (Permission obtained from Dr. Perlas Fontana Medicine Professional Corporation)

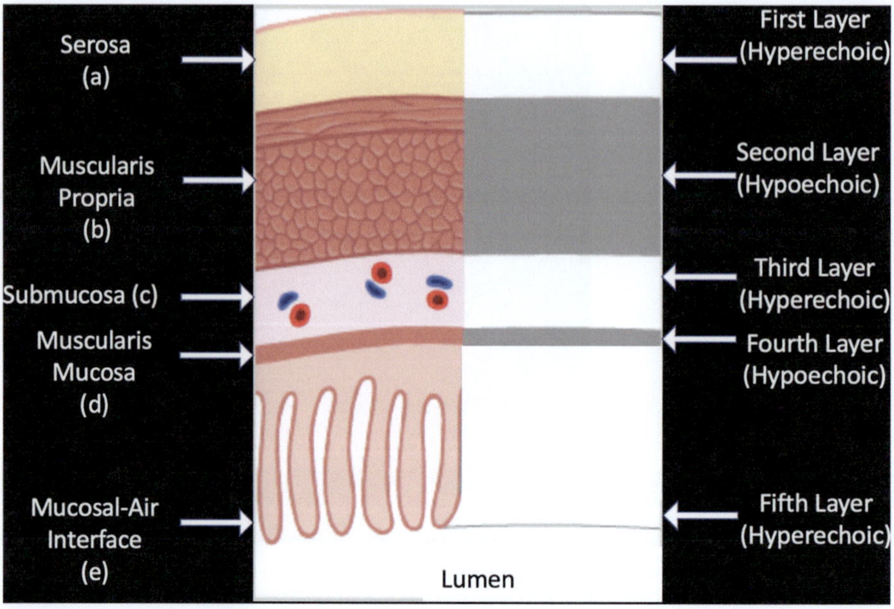

Fig. 6.3 Detailed view of gastric wall layers on ultrasound. (**a**) serosa, (**b**) muscularis propria, (**c**) submucosa, (**d**) muscularis mucosa, (**e**) mucosal-air interface. (Permission obtained from Dr. Perlas Fontana Medicine Professional Corporation)

6.5 Sonographic Evaluation and Interpretation

Once the gastric antrum is located, the initial assessment involves a qualitative evaluation of gastric content, categorized as empty, clear fluid, or thick fluid/solid.

6.5.1 Sonographic Patterns

- Empty stomach → The antrum appears flat or round with juxtaposed anterior and posterior walls, resembling a "bull's eye" or "target" pattern (Fig. 6.4) [15, 22].
- Clear fluid → Content appears hypoechoic or anechoic. As fluid volume increases, the antrum becomes round and distended with thin walls (Fig. 6.5).
- Thick fluid → Hyperechoic and usually homogenous.
- Solid food → During chewing, air mixes with the food bolus and tends to accumulate along the anterior wall of the antrum. Initially, this trapped air creates

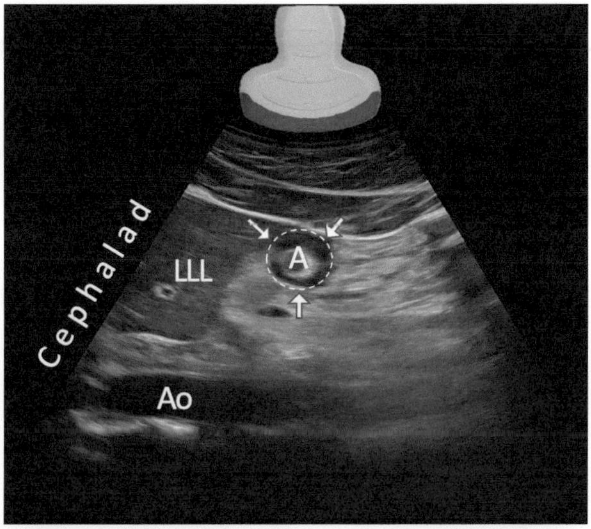

Fig. 6.4 Gastric antrum with an EMPTY stomach. The antrum appears small and empty with a characteristic "bull's eye" appearance. *LLL* left lobe of liver, *A* antrum, *Ao* aorta. (Permission obtained from Dr. Perlas Fontana Medicine Professional Corporation)

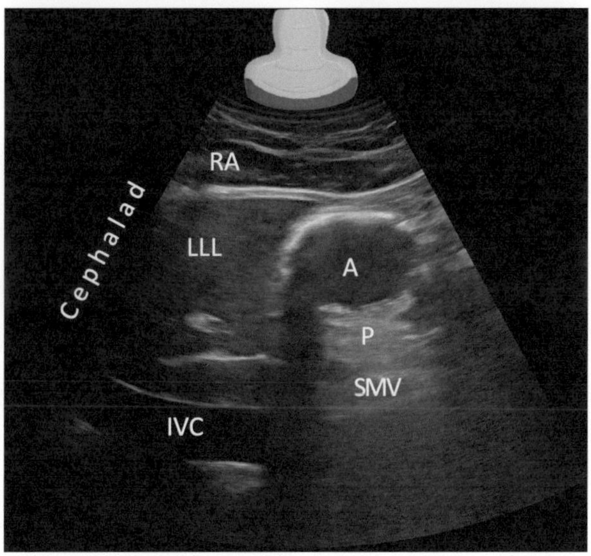

Fig. 6.5 Gastric antrum after ingestion of CLEAR FLUID. The antrum appears distended with hypoechoic or anechoic content. With increasing volume, it becomes round with thin walls. *RA* rectus abdominis, *LLL* left lobe of liver, *A* antrum, *IVC* inferior vena cava, *P* pancreas, *SMV* superior mesenteric vein. (Permission obtained from Dr. Perlas Fontana Medicine Professional Corporation)

anterior wall artifacts, blurring the posterior antral wall, pancreas, and aorta—a phenomenon known as the "frosted glass" pattern (Fig. 6.6) [15]. As digestion begins, air is displaced, causing the antrum to distend and revealing particulate content, which typically exhibits mixed echogenicity (Fig. 6.7).

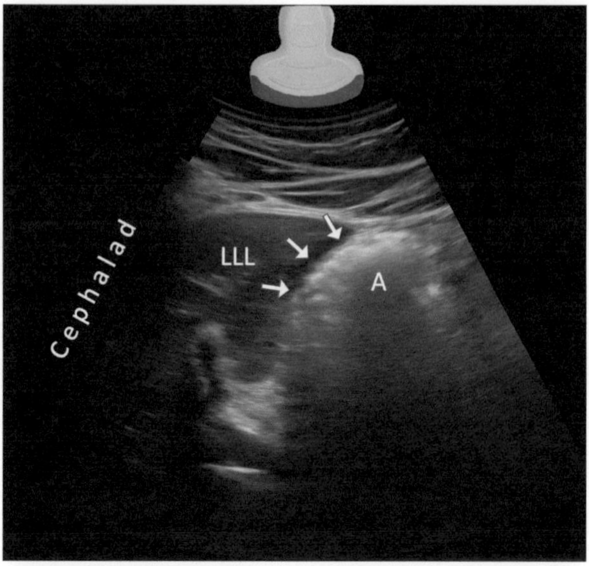

Fig. 6.6 EARLY SOLID content in the gastric antrum. The image resembles a "frosted glass" pattern (arrow). *LLL* left lobe of liver, *A* antrum. (Permission obtained from Dr. Perlas Fontana Medicine Professional Corporation)

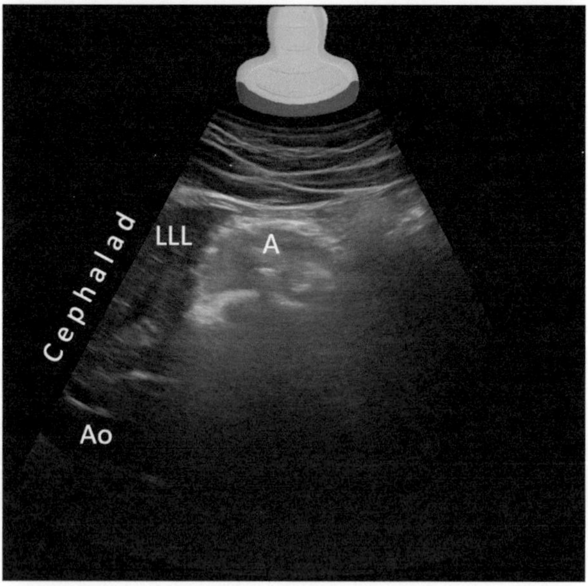

Fig. 6.7 Gastric antrum with mixed echogenicity, representing SOLID content. *LLL* left lobe of liver, *A* antrum, *Ao* Aorta. (Permission obtained from Dr. Perlas Fontana Medicine Professional Corporation)

6.5.2 *Clinical Implications*

- A completely empty antrum or one containing solid food has obvious clinical implications (empty vs. full stomach).
- Clear fluid in the antrum necessitates volume assessment to distinguish:
  - Low volume → baseline gastric secretions.
    High volume → suggestive of a "full stomach".

  Approximately 50% of healthy fasting patients have some amount of baseline secretions in the antrum with negligible aspiration risk [13]. While no universal threshold exists for a "safe" gastric volume, studies suggest that volumes ≤1.5 mL/kg are common in fasted, healthy individuals.

6.5.3 *Gastric Antrum Grading System [13, 14, 16]*

Grade 0: Antrum empty, no content in supine or RLD positions.
Grade 1: Small volume of baseline secretions, usually only visible in RLD (≤1.5 mL/kg).
Grade 2: Clear fluid in both supine and RLD positions; it correlates with higher volumes, suggesting a full stomach.

Table 6.1 summarizes the classification of the gastric antrum in grades 0, 1, and 2 [13].

6.6 Volume Assessment

When the stomach contains clear fluid, quantitative analysis complements qualitative assessment, differentiating between negligible baseline secretions and clinically significant volumes [13, 14, 16].

Table 6.1 Gastric antrum grading system based on fluid content assessment

Grade	Fluid in supine?	Fluid in RLD?	Estimated gastric volume	Aspiration risk
Grade 0	No	No	Near 0	Baseline
Grade 1	No	Yes	Usually <1.5 mL/kg	Baseline
Grade 2	Yes	Yes	Usually >1.5 mL/kg	Higher than baseline

Permission obtained from Dr. Perlas Fontana Medicine Professional Corporation
RLD Right lateral decubitus

6.6.1 *Gastric Volume Estimation Using Antral Cross-Sectional Area (CSA)*

Studies confirm a strong correlation between antral CSA and total gastric volume, particularly in the RLD position [22, 26–30]. Multiple mathematical models describe this relationship [14, 22, 23, 27, 31–34]. One validated formula, based on endoscopic suctioning in non-pregnant adults across a wide age and weight range, predicts gastric volume up to 500 mL: [14].

Gastric Volume (mL) = 27.0 + (14.6 x RLD CSA)—(1.28 x Age).

6.6.2 *Best Practices for Antral Measurement*

- Obtain antral CSA at the level of the aorta.
- Measure when the antrum is at rest (i.e., between peristaltic contractions).
- Use a free-tracing tool to follow the serosal (outer) surface of the antrum.

6.7 Applicability

Gastric ultrasound is particularly valuable in situations where aspiration risk is uncertain, allowing for individualized risk assessment.

- If imaging suggests an "empty stomach" (grade 0 or 1, or < 1.5 mL/kg) and no additional risk factors are present, it is likely safe to proceed with elective surgery and standard airway management (Fig. 6.8).
- Conversely, if the image is consistent with solid content or a high volume of clear fluid (grade 2 or > 1.5 mL/kg), it indicates an elevated aspiration risk (Fig. 6.8).

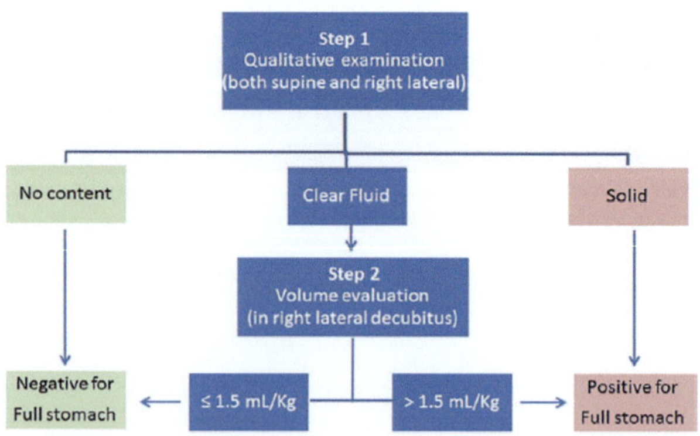

Fig. 6.8 Suggested algorithm for interpretation of gastric ultrasound findings

6.7.1 Clinical Management Considerations

Clinical management depends on several factors.

- Elective procedures: Postponement may be prudent in cases of high aspiration risk.
- Urgent/emergency procedures: Surgery may proceed, but airway protection with endotracheal intubation is recommended, either via awake tracheal intubation (ATI) or rapid sequence induction (RSI).
- High-volume clear fluid: Nasogastric decompression before anesthesia induction may be considered.

6.8 Special Populations

6.8.1 Patients with Obesity

Patients with obesity are traditionally considered at higher aspiration risk. While increased abdominal wall thickness and visceral adiposity can pose technical challenges, gastric ultrasound remains feasible in 95% of severely obese individuals [35, 36].

- Despite a slight overestimation, the mathematical model previously presented for gastric volume assessment remains accurate, even in severely obese patients (BMI > 40 kg/m^2) [36].
- Studies show that obese patients have a larger baseline antral CSA and total gastric volume compared to non-obese individuals [35, 36].

6.8.2 Pediatric Patients

- For children under 40 kg, a linear high-frequency transducer is recommended, while a curved transducer provides better imaging in larger pediatric patients [24].
- Spencer et al. [28] described a strong linear correlation between antral CSA and gastric volume, particularly in the RLD position.
- Gastric ultrasound has been successfully used for:
  - Management of hypertrophic pyloric stenosis [37].
    Detection and monitoring of ingested foreign bodies (e.g., batteries, hair clips, coins) [38–40].

6.8.3 Pregnant Patients

- In healthy, non-laboring pregnant women, gastric emptying is comparable to that of non-pregnant individuals. However, once labor begins, gastric emptying slows significantly and remains impaired for several hours postpartum [19, 41].
- Gastric ultrasound may be useful in obstetric anesthesia to provide a real-time assessment of gastric content when prandial status is uncertain.
- Identifying the gastric antrum in pregnant patients can be challenging due to:
  - Cephalad and rightward displacement of the stomach by the gravid uterus. Increased respiratory rate and hyperdynamic circulation, which may affect image acquisition [29, 30].
- Arzola et al. [42] proposed a gastric volume estimation model for third-trimester pregnant women, similar to the one described by Perlas et al.

Summary and Recommendations

1. Point-of-care gastric ultrasound may be considered at the bedside to assess gastric content and aspiration risk and guide airway management prior to anesthetic induction whenever prandial status or gastric content is uncertain based on clinical information alone—grade B evidence.
2. Gastric ultrasound has been mostly studied in adult patients in whom it has been validated as an accurate and reliable tool providing both qualitative and quantitative information on gastric content—grade A evidence.
3. In pediatric patients, a semi-quantitative grading system is likely more accurate than a volume assessment—grade B evidence.

References

1. Sakai T, Planinsic RM, Quinlan JJ, Handley LJ, Kim TY, Hilmi IA. The incidence and outcome of perioperative pulmonary aspiration in a university hospital: a 4-year retrospective analysis. Anesth Analg. 2006;103:941–7.
2. Neilipovitz DT, Crosby ET. No evidence for decreased incidence of aspiration after rapid sequence induction. Can J Anaesth. 2007;54:748–64.
3. Lockey DJ, Coats T, Parr MJ. Aspiration in severe trauma: a prospective study. Anaesthesia. 1999;54:1097–8.
4. Kluger MT, Short TG. Aspiration during anesthesia: review of 133 cases from the Australian anesthetic incidence monitoring study (AIMS). Anesthesia. 1999;54:19–26.
5. Kozlow J, Berenholtz S, Garrett E, Dorman T, Pronovost P. Epidemiology and impact of aspiration pneumonia in patients undergoing surgery in Maryland, 1999–2000. Crit Care Med. 2003;31:1930–7.
6. Warner MA, Warner ME, Weber JG. Clinical significance of pulmonary aspiration during the perioperative period. Anesthesiology. 1993;78:56–62.
7. Cook TM, Woodall N, Frerk C, Fourth National Audit Project. Major complications of airway management in the UK: results of the fourth National Audit Project of the Royal

College of Anaesthetists and the difficult airway society. Part 1: anaesthesia. Br J Anaesth. 2011;106:617–31.
8. Shime N, Ono A, Chihara E, Tanaka Y. Current status of pulmonary aspiration associated with general anesthesia: a nationwide survey in Japan. Masui. 2005;54:1177–85.
9. Lienhart A, Auroy Y, Pequignot F, et al. Survey of anesthesia related mortality in France. Anesthesiology. 2006;105:1087–97.
10. Agarwal A, Chari P, Singh H. Fluid deprivation before operation: the effect of a small drink. Anesthesia. 1989;44:632–4.
11. Read MS, Vaughan RS. Allowing pre operative patients to drink: effects on patients' safety and comfort of unlimited oral water until 2 hours before anaesthesia. Acta Anaesthesiol Scand. 1991;35:591–5.
12. Chan VW, Lupu CM, Mitsakakis N, Hanbidge A. Ultrasound assessment of gastric content and volume. Anesthesiology. 2009;111:82–9.
13. Perlas A, Davis L, Khan M, Mitsakakis N, Chan VW. Gastric sonography in the fasted surgical patient: a prospective descriptive study. Anesth Analg. 2011;113:93–7.
14. Perlas A, Mitsakakis N, Liu L, et al. Validation of a mathematical model for ultrasound assessment of gastric volume by gastroscopic examination. Anesth Analg. 2013;116:357–63.
15. Cubillos J, Tse C, Chan VW, et al. Bedside ultrasound assessment of gastric content: an observational study. Can J Anaesth. 2012;59:416–23.
16. Van de Putte P, Vernieuwe L, Jerjir A, Verschueren L, Tacken M, Perlas A. When fasted is not empty: a retrospective cohort study of gastric content in fasted surgical patients. Br J Anaesth. 2017;118:363–71.
17. Bouvet L, Desgranges FP, Aubergy C, et al. Prevalence and factors predictive of full stomach in elective and emergency surgical patients: a prospective cohort study. Br J Anaesth. 2017;118:372–9.
18. Sijbrandij LS, Op den Orth JO. Transabdominal ultrasound of the stomach: a pictorial essay. Eur J Radiol. 1991;13:81–7.
19. Carp H, Jayaram A, Stoll M. Ultrasound examination of the stomach contents of parturients. Anesth Analg. 1992;74:683–7.
20. Jayaram A, Bowen MP, Deshpande S, Carp HM. Ultrasound examination of the stomach contents of women in the postpartum period. Anesth Analg. 1997;84:522–6.
21. Jacoby J, Smith G, Eberhardt M, Heller M. Bedside ultrasound to determine prandial status. Am J Emerg Med. 2003;21:216–9.
22. Perlas A, Chan VW, Lupu CM, Mitsakakis N, Hanbidge A. Ultrasound assessment of gastric content and volume. Anesthesiology. 2009;111:82–9.
23. Fujigaki T, Fukusaki M, Nakamura H, Shibata O, Sumikawa K. Quantitative evaluation of gastric contents using ultrasound. J Clin Anesth. 1993;5:451–5.
24. Spencer AO, Walker AM. Antral sonography in the paediatric patient: can transducer choice affect the view? Br J Anaesth. 2015;114:1002–3.
25. Van de Putte P, Perlas A. Ultrasound assessment of gastric content and volume. Br J Anaesth. 2014;113:12–22.
26. Tomomasa T, Tabata M, Nako Y, Kaneko H, Morikawa A. Ultrasonographic assessment of intragastric volume in neonates: factors affecting the relationship between intragastric volume and antral cross-sectional area. Pediatr Radiol. 1996;26:815–20.
27. Schmitz A, Schmidt AR, Buehler PK, et al. Gastric ultrasound as a preoperative bedside test for residual gastric contents volume in children. Paediat Anaesth. 2016;26:1157–64.
28. Spencer AO, Walker AM, Yeung AK, et al. Ultrasound assessment of gastric volume in the fasted pediatric patient undergoing upper gastrointestinal endoscopy: development of a predictive model using endoscopically suctioned volumes. Paediat Anaesth. 2015;25:301–8.
29. Arzola C, Cubillos J, Perlas A, Downey K, Carvalho JC. Interrater reliability of qualitative ultrasound assessment of gastric content in the third trimester of pregnancy. Br J Anaesth. 2014;113:1018–23.

30. Arzola C, Perlas A, Siddiqui NT, Carvalho JC. Bedside gastric ultrasonography in term pregnant women before elective cesarean delivery: a prospective cohort study. Anesth Analg. 2015;121:752–8.
31. Ricci R, Bontempo I, Corazziari E, La Bella A, Torsoli A. Real time ultrasonography of the gastric antrum. Gut. 1993;34:173–6.
32. Hveem K, Hausken T, Berstad A. Ultrasonographic assessment of fasting liquid content in the human stomach. Scand J Gastroenterol. 1994;29:786–9.
33. Bouvet L, Miquel A, Chassard D, Boselli E, Allaouiche B, Benhamou D. Could a single standardized ultrasonographic measurement of antral area be of interest for assessing gastric contents? A preliminary report. Eur J Anaesthesiol. 2009;26:1015–9.
34. Bouvet L, Mazoit JX, Chassard D, Allaouchiche B, Boselli E, Benhamou D. Clinical assessment of the ultrasonographic measurement of antral area for estimating preoperative gastric content and volume. Anesthesiology. 2011;114:1086–92.
35. Van de Putte P, Perlas A. Gastric sonography in the severely obese surgical patient: a feasibility study. Anesth Analg. 2014;119:1105–10.
36. Kruisselbrink R, Arzola C, Jackson T, Okrainec A, Chan V, Perlas A. Ultrasound assessment of gastric volume in severely obese individuals: a validation study. Br J Anaesth. 2017;118:77–82.
37. Gagey AC, de Queiroz Siqueira M, Desgranges FP, et al. Ultrasound assessment of the gastric contents for the guidance of the anaesthetic strategy in infants with hypertrophic pyloric stenosis: a prospective cohort study. Br J Anaesth. 2016;116:649–54.
38. Salmon M, Doniger SJ. Ingested foreign bodies: a case series demonstrating a novel application of point-of-care ultrasonography in children. Pediatr Emerg Care. 2013;29:870–3.
39. Jeckovic M, Anupindi SA, Barbir SB, Lovrenski J. Is ultrasound useful in detection and follow-up of gastric foreign bodies in children? Clin Imaging. 2013;37:1043–7.
40. Horowitz R, Cico SJ, Bailitz J. Point-of-care ultrasound: a new tool for the identification of gastric foreign bodies in children? J Emerg Med. 2016;50:99–103.
41. O'Sullivan G. Gastric emptying during pregnancy and the puerperium. Int J Obstet Anesth. 1993;2:216–24.
42. Arzola C, Perlas A, Siddiqui NT, Downey K, Ye XY, Carvalho JC. Gastric ultrasound in the third trimester of pregnancy: a randomised controlled trial to develop a predictive model of volume assessment. Anaesthesia. 2018;73:295–303.

Chapter 7
Preparation Before Airway Management

Samuel Ern Hung Tsan

Highlights

- Proper planning and preparation before airway management significantly impact success and reduce emergencies.
- Effective teamwork, clear communication, and role assignment enhance efficiency in critical situations.
- Backup strategies and familiarity with rescue devices are essential to manage unexpected difficulties.
- Regular training and simulation improve decision-making and confidence in airway management.
- Structured decision-making enhance performance in high-pressure scenarios.

7.1 Introduction

Benjamin Franklin once said, "*By failing to prepare, you are preparing to fail.*" This wisdom holds true in all high-acuity scenarios, particularly in airway management. Optimal preparation is key to successful airway management, ensuring effective oxygenation of the patient without adverse effects. This becomes even more critical when a difficult airway is anticipated.

S. E. H. Tsan (✉)
Department of Anaesthesiology and Critical Care, Faculty of Medicine and Health Sciences, University of Malaysia Sarawak (UNIMAS), Kota Samarahan, Sarawak, Malaysia
e-mail: tehsamuel@unimas.my

M. Á. Gómez-Ríos, A. van Zundert (eds.), *Evidence-based Guide to Difficult Airway Management*, https://doi.org/10.1007/978-3-032-30769-9_7

7.2 Use of a Checklist

One key aspect of preparation before embarking on the management of the difficult airway is the use of a checklist. The 4th National Audit Project (NAP4) of the Royal College of Anaesthetists recommends using an intubation checklist in critically ill patients. This checklist ensures proper preparation of the patient, drugs, equipment, team roles, and backup plans [1]. This recommendation has been adopted by the "2018 Guidelines for the management of tracheal intubation in critically ill adults," published by the Difficult Airway Society (DAS), the Intensive Care Society, the Faculty of Intensive Care Medicine, and the Royal College of Anaesthetists.

Several single-centre observational studies have shown that preintubation checklists provide clear benefits. In a prospective study involving 141 Emergency Department patients, Smith et al. [2] found that the use of a preintubation checklist reduced intubation complications, shortened intubation time, and improved safety measures. Two additional studies that evaluated preintubation checklists as part of an intubation bundle-of-care also reported increased patient safety during intubation in the Emergency Department [3, 4]. Conversely, a randomized controlled trial by Janz et al. [5] found no significant differences in oxygen saturation, blood pressure, laryngoscopy attempts, or complications when comparing preintubation checklists to standard care in critically ill patients. However, this study was criticized for methodological limitations, and the lack of a comprehensive checklist [6, 7]. A recent systematic review and meta-analysis found that using a checklist reduced the incidence of hypoxia during tracheal intubation. However, no significant differences were observed in rates of oesophageal intubation, hypotension, or first-pass intubation success, possibly due to underpowered subgroup analyses [8].

Managing the airway in critically ill patients is also known as managing the physiologically difficult airway. It is a high-stress scenario with a high risk of cognitive overload. Based on evidence and recommendations from critically ill patient management, preintubation checklists are a valuable tool in difficult airway situations. In fact, the 2022 American Society of Anesthesiologists (ASA) Practice Guidelines for Management of the Difficult Airway recommended the first step in their airway management algorithm as reviewing the airway strategy. This functions as a mental checklist, ensuring the patient's airway and physiological status are assessed, equipment and monitoring devices are checked, team roles are assigned, and backup plans are in place [9]. Thus, the use of a preintubation checklist adds an extra layer of safety to a complex procedure, enhancing error prevention. Table 7.1 summarizes essential items that should be included in a preintubation checklist.

Table 7.1 Preintubation checklist: essential items (non-exhaustive list)

Preparation of the patient	Consent and explanation Positioning Preoxygenation (*discussed in another chapter*)
Preparation of equipment and drugs	Monitoring equipment Airway equipment and adjuncts Drugs
Preparation of the team	Role allocations Human factors (discussed in another chapter)
Preparation of backup plans	Airway strategy in the event of failure (*discussed in another chapter*) Management of anticipated complications

7.3 Preparation of the Patient

7.3.1 Consent and Explanation

Management of the difficult airway carries multiple risks for patients, including, but not limited to, death, brain injury, cardiopulmonary arrest, airway trauma, and dental damage. Therefore, patients or their responsible caregivers have the right to be informed of these risks, in accordance with the ethical principle of autonomy. The latest 2022 ASA Practice Guidelines for Management of the Difficult Airway recommended that patients undergoing tracheal intubation be informed of the specific risks and procedures involved. If the patient is underage or incapacitated, the responsible person of the patient should be informed. Among 174 expert consultants surveyed on this statement, 74% strongly agreed, 21% agreed, 3% were neutral, and 2% either strongly disagreed or disagreed [9].

7.3.2 Positioning

For most of the last 100 years, the widely accepted head position for laryngoscopy and tracheal intubation has been the supine sniffing position, achieved by flexion of the lower cervical spine and extension of the head at the atlanto-occipital joint from the horizontal plane. This technique is credited to Sir Ivan Magill, who first described it in 1936 as "a man standing in the normal erect position when he scents the air" [10]. The DAS 2015 Guidelines for Management of Unanticipated Difficult Intubation in Adults recommended this position for most patients, except for obese patients, who should be placed in the ramped position [11]. However, recent evidence suggests that the head-elevated position should be the standard for all tracheal intubations, not just for obese patients. This position can be achieved using pillows, blankets, or specialized devices. One of the simplest methods for head elevation is the bed-up-head-elevated (BUHE) position, which uses the bed control to elevate the head of the bed until the patient's sternal angle aligns with the external auditory meatus (by adjusting the bed at the hip level) (Fig. 7.1).

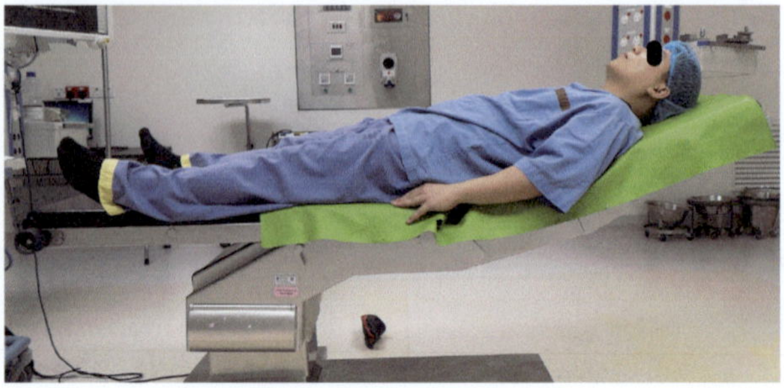

Fig. 7.1 Bed-up-head-elevated position

7.3.2.1 Improved Glottic Views with the Head-Elevated Position

The head-elevated position has been shown to improve glottic views during laryngoscopy. Lee et al. [12], in a randomized controlled trial (RCT), showed that this position improves the glottic view by nearly 25% compared to the supine position. Another RCT found that the head-elevated position significantly increases the rate of Cormack-Lehane grade 1 or 2 views, reducing the occurrence of grades 3 or 4 views [13]. A more recent RCT demonstrated that laryngoscopy in the head-elevated position was non-inferior to videolaryngoscopy in terms of glottic view [mean difference −6.3%, 98% confidence interval (CI) −13.2% to 0.6%, non-inferiority limit −15% at the lower 98% CI limit]. Additionally, the glottic view improved by up to 25.8% in the head-elevated position compared to the supine sniffing position [14]. These findings were confirmed by a systematic review and meta-analysis, which found that in patients undergoing tracheal intubation in the operating theatre, there was a significantly higher likelihood of achieving a Cormack-Lehane grade 1/2 view in the head-elevated position compared to the sniffing position (odds ratio 2.05, 95% CI 1.26–3.32, $p = 0.004$, $I^2 = 0\%$) [15]. The improved laryngeal view in the head-elevated position may be attributed to:

- Increased airway dimensions due to gravitational effects on laryngeal structures and the upper thorax.
- A change in biomechanics, where the force applied during laryngoscopy lifts the laryngoscope blade further forward rather than upward, optimizing the laryngeal view [12].

7.3.2.2 Impact on Intubation Success and Safety

Beyond improving glottic visualization, the head-elevated position also enhances tracheal intubation success rates. Lee et al. [13] in an RCT involving patients with anticipated difficult tracheal intubation, found that this position increased the success rate by 21% (defined as successful intubation within the first or second attempt) compared to the supine sniffing position. Observational studies have further shown this position is associated with fewer peri-intubation complications and reduced need for airway manoeuvres [16, 17].

7.3.2.3 Effect on Preoxygenation

Another major advantage of the head-elevated position is enhanced preoxygenation effectiveness. Multiple RCTs have shown that, compared to the supine position, this position prolongs the safe apnoea period, defined as the time taken for oxygen saturation to drop to a specified level during the peri-intubation apnoea period [18–20]. A recently published systematic review and meta-analysis by Tsan et al. [21] found that preoxygenation in the head-elevated position significantly extends the safe apnoea period by up to 61.99 s (95% CI 42.93 s to 81.05 s, $p < 0.00001$, $I^2 = 30\%$), with the authors grading the certainty of evidence as high based on the GRADE criteria. The physiological rationale behind this improvement includes:

- Increased functional residual capacity, as the raised torso position reduces diaphragmatic pressure from abdominal contents.
- Decreased weight of chest wall tissues on the lungs, allowing better oxygen reserve.

When managing patients with an anticipated difficult airway, special attention must be given to optimizing patient positioning to improve success rates and minimize complications. Recent evidence strongly supports the head-elevated position as the optimal choice for intubation due to its multiple benefits, lack of proven complications, and ease of implementation. Hence, it should be the standard position for tracheal intubation.

7.4 Preparation of Equipment

It is widely accepted that immediate access to difficult airway management equipment is essential during the procedure. However, there is a lack of direct clinical evidence evaluating the impact of having such equipment readily available. Despite this, expert opinions from airway management guidelines strongly recommend that essential airway equipment be both available and easily accessible during intubation [9, 22]. In addition, specialized equipment for difficult airway (though only required in specific situations) should be immediately accessible in a portable storage unit [9]. A summary of standard and specialized airway equipment that should be available is provided in Table 7.2.

7.4.1 Stylet

The stylet has been used as an intubation aid for decades due to its ability to preshape the endotracheal tube. A recent multicentre pragmatic RCT investigated the success of intubation using an endotracheal tube with a stylet versus an endotracheal tube alone. The study included 999 patients undergoing intubation in

Table 7.2 Airway equipment

Standard airway equipment for all intubations	Specialized airway equipment for difficult airway management[a]
Self-inflating bag-valve-mask Various sizes of face masks Various sizes of oropharyngeal and nasopharyngeal airways Various sizes of laryngoscope blades and handles Various sizes of endotracheal tubes Various sizes of supraglottic airways Yankauer suction tubes, suction catheters, suction tubing Tracheal tube stylets (malleable and rigid) Tracheal tube introducers (bougie) Equipment for emergency invasive airway management Magill forceps Water-soluble medical lubricant Nasal cannula Oxygen face masks Video laryngoscope with appropriate stylet Standard AAGBI monitoring equipment [23] Anaesthetic induction, maintenance, and rescue medications	Alternative intubation equipment Various sizes of tracheal tubes (including microlaryngeal tubes) Different designs and sizes of laryngoscope blades Specialized tracheal tube guides (semirigid stylets, lighted stylets) Intubating supraglottic airway Videolaryngoscope with appropriate stylet Optical laryngoscope Intubating video stylet Flexible intubating bronchoscope with bite block, topical anaesthetic, and equipment Aintree catheter Alternative/rescue ventilation equipment Various sizes of oropharyngeal and nasopharyngeal airways Various types (at least 2) and sizes of supraglottic airways High-flow nasal cannula Emergency airway equipment Equipment for emergency invasive airway management Jet ventilation equipment Miscellaneous Various sizes of airway exchange catheters Multiple exhaled carbon dioxide detectors Laminated version of difficult airway algorithm/cognitive aid/checklist Defogger

[a]Available and accessible in a portable storage unit
Abbreviation: *AAGBI* Association of Anaesthetists of Great Britain and Ireland

intensive care units, with the first-pass intubation success rate as the main outcome. The results showed a first-attempt intubation success rate of 78.2% in the stylet group, compared to 71.5% in the endotracheal tube alone group (relative risk 1.10, 95% CI 1.02–1.18, $p = 0.01$). The number needed to treat (NNT) to prevent an intubation failure was 14.8. Importantly, no significant differences were reported between groups regarding intubation-related complications or serious peri-intubation adverse events [24]. Given the evidence supporting its effectiveness as an adjunct, the stylet should be readily available during tracheal intubation, if not used as the primary approach.

7.4.2 Bougie

The tracheal tube introducer, commonly known as the gum elastic bougie, has proven to be an effective rescue device in unanticipated difficult tracheal intubations [25]. Evidence suggests that using a bougie may improve first-pass intubation success in patients with difficult laryngoscopy or intubation features. A large RCT by Driver et al. [26], involving 757 patients undergoing emergency intubation in the emergency department, compared bougie-assisted intubation versus endotracheal tube with stylet for first-pass intubation success. First-attempt intubation success was significantly higher in the bougie group (98%) compared to the endotracheal tube and stylet group (87%) (absolute difference 11%, 95% CI 7–14%). Among 380 patients with at least one difficult airway feature (defined as obscured laryngeal view, airway oedema or obstruction, obesity, short neck, large tongue, small mandible, facial trauma or cervical spine immobility), the bougie group had a higher first-attempt intubation success rate (96% vs. 82%, absolute difference 14%, 95% CI 8–20%, $p < 0.001$). First-attempt intubation success without hypoxemia was also higher in the bougie group (82% vs. 69%, absolute difference 12%, 95% CI 3–21%, $p = 0.006$). In recent times, a new class of tracheal tube introducers, widely known as dynamic introducers, has emerged. Dynamic bougies consist of articulated bougies and may include a fibreoptic bronchoscope when used as an introducer during direct or indirect laryngoscopy. A recent meta-analysis showed that the usage of dynamic bougies in patients with difficult airways reduced the time required for intubation and had a higher rate of first-attempt intubation success [27]. All these findings reinforce that the bougie is a valuable tool in the airway management armamentarium, particularly when a difficult airway is anticipated.

7.4.3 Continuous Capnography

Unrecognized oesophageal intubation can lead to hypoxaemia, cerebral injury, and even death. According to NAP4, the incidence of unrecognized oesophageal intubation leading to severe harm is estimated to be 1:1,000,000 for tracheal intubations during anaesthesia, 1:15,000 in the intensive care unit, and 1:10,000 in the emergency department [1]. Commonly used clinical tests to confirm tracheal intubation include the presence of misting, lung auscultation, and five-point auscultation. A systematic review and meta-analysis evaluated the accuracy of these clinical tests. They found that misting or auscultation has false positive rates that are too high to be considered safe. There was also insufficient evidence to conclude on the use of bougie "hang-up" or chest rise to confirm tracheal placement [28]. To prevent oesophageal intubation and confirm tracheal tube placement, multiple expert guidelines have recommended the use of continuous capnography as the "gold standard" to confirm successful endotracheal intubation [9, 11, 22, 29]. The 2022 consensus guideline from the Project for Universal Management of Airways for preventing unrecognized oesophageal intubation states that exhaled carbon dioxide monitoring should be used for all airway management procedures [29]. Several observational studies have demonstrated the effectiveness of continuous capnography to determine correct tube placement, with a 100% detection rate for oesophageal intubation [30–33]. Furthermore, continuous capnography has been shown to have 100% sensitivity and specificity even in low perfusion states, such as in patients experiencing cardiac arrest [34]. Taken together, the evidence strongly supports the use of continuous capnography during tracheal intubation to ensure correct endotracheal tube placement.

7.5 Preparation of the Team

7.5.1 Role Allocations

The airway, particularly a difficult airway, should be managed by appropriately trained operators. Role allocation should be procedure- and expertise-specific, rather than based on seniority. For instance, an anaesthetist with more airway management experience is designated as the team leader, while an otorhinolaryngology (ENT) surgeon may be on standby for emergency front-of-neck access.

Role allocations should be determined during the preparation phase, ideally as part of the team briefing. Establishing clear roles beforehand can help minimize confusion and cognitive overload in crisis scenarios. When each team member understands their designated responsibilities, decision-making becomes more efficient, and patient safety improves.

The 2022 ASA Guidelines for difficult airway management included a survey of 174 airway expert consultants, in which 94% strongly agreed, and 5% agreed that a skilled individual should be present or immediately available when managing a known or suspected difficult airway [9].

Effective leadership and communication are essential in crisis management. The team leader should ensure clear communication, facilitate real-time role adjustments if needed, and maintain situational awareness to optimize patient outcomes.

7.6 Prepare for Failure

7.6.1 Airway Strategy

One of the clinical themes identified in the NAP4 regarding complications in airway management was poor planning. When managing a known or suspected difficult airway, the NAP4 authors emphasized that an airway strategy, rather than a simple airway plan, should be developed. An airway plan typically refers to a single technique for securing the airway. An airway strategy, in contrast, consists of a coordinated series of contingency plans aimed at ensuring adequate oxygenation and minimizing complications [1]. A crucial element of an airway strategy is the incorporation of fail-safe measures for failure to intubate or failure to oxygenate. This was another clinical theme highlighted in the NAP4, where lack of backup plans often led to an uncoordinated response and ultimately poor patient outcomes [1]. Given these risks, multiple airway management guidelines strongly recommend developing structured backup plans before airway intervention. Preparation should include:

- Team coordination, ensuring clear role assignments in case of failure scenarios.
- Availability of alternative airway devices, such as supraglottic airways, video laryngoscopy, bougies, and front-of-neck access equipment.
- Predefined escalation pathways, ensuring rapid transition to emergency airway interventions if needed.

More detailed strategies for managing difficult airways will be discussed in later chapters.

Recommendations

- A preintubation checklist should be considered before managing an anticipated difficult airway to improve the success of endotracheal intubation (Table 7.1) (grade C).
- The patient or their responsible caregiver should be informed of the risks and procedures involved in managing a difficult airway (grade D).
- Patients undergoing tracheal intubation should be placed in the head-elevated position due to its multiple benefits and absence of complications (grade A).
- Standard airway management equipment should be immediately available during the intubation process. Specialized airway equipment should be available in a portable storage unit nearby in the event of a difficult airway scenario (grade D).
- The stylet should be immediately available during the endotracheal intubation procedure (grade A).
- The tracheal tube introducer (bougie) should be immediately available during the endotracheal intubation procedure (grade A).
- Continuous capnography should be used during tracheal intubation to confirm correct tracheal tube placement (grade B).
- Appropriately skilled personnel should be present or immediately available during the management of a known or suspected difficult airway (grade D).
- When managing a known or suspected difficult airway, an airway strategy should be devised during the preparation phase. The strategy must include plans for failure to intubate or oxygenate (grade D).

References

1. The Royal College of Anaesthetists and the Difficult Airway Society. Major complications of airway management in the United Kingdom: report and findings. Cook T, Woodall N, Frerk C, editors. The Royal College of Anaesthetists; 2011.
2. Smith KA, High K, Collins SP, Self WH. A preprocedural checklist improves the safety of emergency department intubation of trauma patients. Acad Emerg Med. 2015;22:989–92.
3. Fogg T, Alkhouri H, Vassiliadis J. The Royal North Shore Hospital Emergency Department airway registry: closing the audit loop. Emerg Med Australas. 2016;28:27–33.
4. Long E, Cincotta DR, Grindlay J, Sabato S, Fauteux-Lamarre E, Beckerman D, et al. A quality improvement initiative to increase the safety of pediatric emergency airway management. Pediatr Anesth. 2017;27:1271–7.
5. Janz DR, Semler MW, Joffe AM, Casey JD, Lentz RJ, deBoisblanc BP, et al. A multicenter randomized trial of a checklist for endotracheal intubation of critically ill adults. Chest. 2018;153:816–24.
6. Choudhary A, Angurana SK. Pre-intubation checklist: need of the hour. Chest. 2018;153:1075–6.
7. De Jong A, Jaber S. Do not throw the intubation checklist out with the bath water! Chest. 2018;153:771–3.
8. Turner JS, Bucca AW, Propst SL, Ellender TJ, Sarmiento EJ, Menard LM, et al. Association of checklist use in endotracheal intubation with clinically important outcomes: a systematic review and meta-analysis. JAMA Netw Open. 2020;3:e209278.
9. Apfelbaum JL, Hagberg CA, Connis RT, Abdelmalak BB, Agarkar M, Dutton RP, et al. 2022 American Society of Anesthesiologists practice guidelines for management of the difficult airway. Anesthesiology. 2022;136:31–81.
10. Magill IW. Endotracheal anesthesia. Am J Surg. 1936;34:450–5.
11. Frerk C, Mitchell VS, McNarry AF, Mendonca C, Bhagrath R, Patel A, et al. Difficult Airway Society 2015 guidelines for management of unanticipated difficult intubation in adults. Br J Anaesth. 2015;115:827–48.
12. Lee BJ, Kang JM, Kim DO. Laryngeal exposure during laryngoscopy is better in the 25 back-up position than in the supine position. Br J Anaesth. 2007;99:581–6.
13. Lee J-H, Jung H-C, Shim J-H, Lee C. Comparison of the rate of successful endotracheal intubation between the "sniffing" and "ramped" positions in patients with an expected difficult intubation: a prospective randomized study. Korean J Anesthesiol. 2015;68:116.
14. Tsan SEH, Lim SM, Abidin MFZ, Ganesh S, Wang CY. Comparison of Macintosh laryngoscopy in bed-up-head–elevated position with GlideScope laryngoscopy: a randomized, controlled, noninferiority trial. Anesth Analg. 2020;131:210–9.
15. Tsan SEH, Ng KT, Lau J, Viknaswaran NL, Wang CY. A comparison of ramping position and sniffing position during endotracheal intubation: a systematic review and meta-analysis. Rev Bras Anestesiol. 2021;70:667–77.
16. Khandelwal N, Khorsand S, Mitchell SH, Joffe AM. Head-elevated patient positioning decreases complications of emergent tracheal intubation in the ward and intensive care unit. Anesth Analg. 2016;122:1101–7.
17. Reddy RM, Adke M, Patil P, Kosheleva I, Ridley S. Comparison of glottic views and intubation times in the supine and 25 degree back-up positions. BMC Anesthesiol. 2016;16:113.
18. Altermatt FR, Munoz HR, Delfino AE, Cortinez LI. Pre-oxygenation in the obese patient: effects of position on tolerance to apnoea. Br J Anaesth. 2005;95:706–9.
19. Dixon BJ, Dixon JB, Carden JR, Burn AJ, Schachter LM, Playfair JM, et al. Preoxygenation is more effective in the 25° head-up position than in the supine position in severely obese patients: a randomized controlled study. Anesthesiology. 2005;102:1110–5.
20. Lane S, Saunders D, Schofield A, Padmanabhan R, Hildreth A, Laws D. A prospective, randomised controlled trial comparing the efficacy of pre-oxygenation in the 20° head-up vs supine position. Anaesthesia. 2005;60:1064–7.

21. Tsan SEH, Viknaswaran NL, Lau J, Cheong CC, Wang CY. Effectiveness of preoxygenation during endotracheal intubation in a head-elevated position: a systematic review and meta-analysis of randomized controlled trials. Anaesthesiol Intensive Ther. 2022;54:413–24.
22. Higgs A, McGrath BA, Goddard C, Rangasami J, Suntharalingam G, Gale R, et al. Guidelines for the management of tracheal intubation in critically ill adults. Br J Anaesth. 2018;120:323–52.
23. Checketts MR, Alladi R, Ferguson K, Gemmell L, Handy JM, Klein AA, et al. Recommendations for standards of monitoring during anaesthesia and recovery 2015: Association of Anaesthetists of Great Britain and Ireland. Anaesthesia. 2016;71:85–93.
24. Jaber S, Rollé A, Godet T, Terzi N, Riu B, Asfar P, et al. Effect of the use of an endotracheal tube and stylet versus an endotracheal tube alone on first-attempt intubation success: a multicentre, randomised clinical trial in 999 patients. Intensive Care Med. 2021;47:653–64.
25. Combes X, Le Roux B, Suen P, Dumerat M, Motamed C, Sauvat S, et al. Unanticipated difficult airway in anesthetized patients: prospective validation of a management algorithm. Anesthesiology. 2004;100:1146–50.
26. Driver BE, Prekker ME, Klein LR, Reardon RF, Miner JR, Fagerstrom ET, et al. Effect of use of a bougie vs endotracheal tube and stylet on first-attempt intubation success among patients with difficult airways undergoing emergency intubation: a randomized clinical trial. JAMA. 2018;319:2179–89.
27. Sastre JA, Gómez-Ríos MA, López T, Gutiérrez-Couto U, Casans-Francés R. Dynamic versus standard bougies for tracheal intubation with direct or indirect laryngoscopy in simulated or real scenarios: a systematic review and meta-analysis. Expert Rev Med Devices. 2024;21:427–38.
28. Hansel J, Law JA, Chrimes N, Higgs A, Cook TM. Clinical tests for confirming tracheal intubation or excluding oesophageal intubation: a diagnostic test accuracy systematic review and meta-analysis. Anaesthesia. 2023;78:1020–30.
29. Chrimes N, Higgs A, Hagberg CA, Baker PA, Cooper RM, Greif R, et al. Preventing unrecognised oesophageal intubation: a consensus guideline from the Project for Universal Management of Airways and international airway societies. Anaesthesia. 2022;77:1395–415.
30. Grmec Š. Comparison of three different methods to confirm tracheal tube placement in emergency intubation. Intensive Care Med. 2002;28:701–4.
31. Knapp S, Kofler J, Stoiser B, Thalhammer F, Burgmann H, Posch M, et al. The assessment of four different methods to verify tracheal tube placement in the critical care setting. Anesth Analg. 1999;88:766–70.
32. Silvestri S, Ralls GA, Krauss B, Thundiyil J, Rothrock SG, Senn A, et al. The effectiveness of out-of-hospital use of continuous end-tidal carbon dioxide monitoring on the rate of unrecognized misplaced intubation within a regional emergency medical services system. Ann Emerg Med. 2005;45:497–503.
33. Takeda T, Tanigawa K, Tanaka H, Hayashi Y, Goto E, Tanaka K. The assessment of three methods to verify tracheal tube placement in the emergency setting. Resuscitation. 2003;56:153–7.
34. Silvestri S, Ladde JG, Brown JF, Roa JV, Hunter C, Ralls GA, et al. Endotracheal tube placement confirmation: 100% sensitivity and specificity with sustained four-phase capnographic waveforms in a cadaveric experimental model. Resuscitation. 2017;115:192–8.

Chapter 8
Preoxygenation

Manuel Á. Gómez-Ríos and José M. Fandiño-Orgeira

Highlights

- *Preoxygenation is a core, physiology-based intervention* whose effectiveness depends on functional residual capacity, alveolar denitrogenation, oxygen consumption, and gas-exchange integrity, rather than time alone.
- *The lung is the dominant oxygen reservoir during apnea.* Expansion and stabilization of functional residual capacity before induction are the primary determinants of safe apnea time.
- *Pulse oximetry is an unreliable marker of preoxygenation quality.* End-tidal oxygen concentration ($EtO_2 > 90\%$) best reflects effective alveolar denitrogenation.
- *Failure of preoxygenation is physiologically predictable*, most commonly resulting from intrapulmonary shunt, reduced or unstable FRC, increased oxygen consumption, or loss of upper airway patency.
- *Patients with obesity, pregnancy, hypoxemia, or critical illness* have markedly reduced apnea tolerance, making conventional preoxygenation techniques frequently inadequate.

(continued)

M. Á. Gómez-Ríos (✉)
Anesthesiology and Perioperative Medicine, University Hospital Complex of A Coruña, A Coruña, Galicia, Spain

Clinical Management Section of the Spanish Society of Anesthesiology, Resuscitation, and Pain Therapy (SEDAR), Madrid, Spain

Medical University of Lodz, Lodz, Poland

J. M. Fandiño-Orgeira
Emergency Department, University Hospital Complex of A Coruña, A Coruña, Galicia, Spain

M. Á. Gómez-Ríos, A. van Zundert (eds.), *Evidence-based Guide to Difficult Airway Management*, https://doi.org/10.1007/978-3-032-30769-9_8

- *Patient positioning is a key modifiable factor.* Head-up and ramped positions increase FRC, improve airway patency, and enhance oxygen reserve before apnea.
- *Positive airway pressure strategies improve preoxygenation efficacy* by preventing alveolar collapse, increasing lung volume, and optimizing ventilation–perfusion matching.
- *Noninvasive ventilation is the most effective noninvasive strategy* for preoxygenation in shunt-dominant and critically ill patients, consistently reducing peri-intubation hypoxemia.
- *High-flow nasal oxygen provides continuous oxygen delivery* and effective apneic oxygenation, prolonging safe apnea time, though it is less effective than noninvasive ventilation (NIV) in severe shunt physiology.
- *Apneic oxygenation complements but does not replace preoxygenation*, and its success depends on prior maximization of alveolar oxygen content.
- *Safe airway management relies on aligning preoxygenation strategy with patient physiology*, rather than on any single device or technique.

8.1 Introduction

Preoxygenation is one of the most powerful, low-risk, and universally applicable interventions in airway management (Grade A) [1–3]. Its purpose is deceptively simple—to maximize the body's oxygen reserves before apnea [4]. Yet beneath this simplicity lies a rich interplay of respiratory physiology, patient-specific vulnerabilities, and technical execution [5] that determines whether an airway intervention proceeds safely or spirals into hypoxemia, hemodynamic collapse, or cardiac arrest [6, 7].

No other maneuver in airway management provides such a profound extension of the "oxygenation time budget" [8]. In ideal circumstances, effective preoxygenation can transform seconds into minutes of safe apnea [5]. In compromised physiology—obesity, pregnancy, shunt-dominant disease, or critical illness—the available window shrinks dramatically, and preoxygenation becomes not just important but essential [9]. In many of these patients, expertly optimized preoxygenation is the only barrier preventing catastrophic desaturation during induction [7].

Historically, preoxygenation was viewed as a brief prelude to anesthesia: 3 min of tidal breathing with a tight-fitting mask delivering FiO_2 1.0 [10]. Modern evidence has radically expanded this view [8]. Today, preoxygenation is a physiology-driven, dynamic, and customizable process whose success depends on much more than time alone. Modern airway management increasingly conceptualizes oxygen delivery as a continuous process, *peroxygenation*, encompassing both preoxygenation before apnea and oxygenation during the apneic phase. Positioning, positive pressure strategies, device selection, dual oxygenation, monitoring, and an understanding of individual physiological limitations all play decisive roles [1]. In this chapter, the term "peroxygenation" is used to describe an integrated strategy of oxygen delivery before, during, and immediately after airway management. The clinician's mastery of these elements directly influences patient safety, especially in high-risk populations.

This chapter presents an integrated framework for preoxygenation that unites foundational physiology with cutting-edge clinical practice, distilling decades of research into a coherent, practical strategy applicable across operating rooms, intensive care units, emergency departments, and austere environments, with the aim of translating physiology and evidence into actionable approaches that improve patient safety during airway management.

8.2 Physiology of Oxygen Reserve and Apnea

Preoxygenation prolongs the duration for which apnea can be safely tolerated by increasing oxygen reserves, thereby preventing—or at least attenuating—the onset and severity of hypoxemia during laryngoscopy and tracheal intubation. Consequently, its primary objective is to extend the safe apnea interval. Apnea time is defined as the period from the cessation of spontaneous or assisted ventilation to a decline in arterial oxyhemoglobin saturation to ≤90% [11]. Understanding preoxygenation requires first understanding the physiological landscape in which apnea unfolds. Every airway intervention is a race between oxygen consumption and oxygen reserve, and this race is won or lost long before the airway device touches the patient. Preoxygenation does not alter metabolic demand but profoundly alters the initial conditions of apnea. To master airway safety is to master this physiology [12, 13].

The following sections outline the core physiological principles underlying peroxygenation and apnea tolerance.

8.2.1 The Oxygen Reservoir: Distribution Across Lungs, Blood, and Tissues

At the onset of apnea, oxygen is drawn from three physiological compartments [12]. The lungs, specifically the functional residual capacity (FRC), constitute the dominant reservoir and the only one that can be directly modified before induction; both its volume and alveolar oxygen fraction determine apnea tolerance. The blood provides oxygen bound to hemoglobin, which is substantial in absolute terms but offers little buffering once alveolar oxygen declines, although severe anemia shortens tolerance by reducing total oxygen content despite preserved saturation. Tissues contain dissolved oxygen that is released only as partial pressures fall; their contribution is limited and cannot compensate for alveolar depletion.

These reservoirs interact dynamically, but only the alveolar reservoir can be expanded immediately before airway manipulation—hence the foundational role of preoxygenation. Effective preoxygenation therefore acts almost exclusively by expanding this compartment, which overwhelmingly determines apnea tolerance compared with all other body oxygen stores. Under room air conditions, total body oxygen stores are limited to approximately 1500 mL, of which only ~450 mL reside in the FRC. With effective preoxygenation, total oxygen stores can increase to over 4000 mL, with the FRC alone contributing up to 3000 mL—explaining why denitrogenation of the lungs dwarfs all other reservoirs in determining apnea tolerance [14, 15]. Conceptually, preoxygenation efficacy reflects the ability to achieve alveolar denitrogenation, whereas preoxygenation efficiency determines how long these oxygen reserves can sustain adequate arterial oxygenation during apnea, integrating functional residual capacity, oxygen consumption, and gas exchange [7].

8.2.2 *Functional Residual Capacity: The Central Determinant of Safe Apnea Time*

FRC is the lung volume at the end of passive exhalation. It represents the principal and most accessible oxygen store during apnea. Its size is influenced by body habitus, pregnancy, patient positioning, and lung and chest wall compliance [16, 17]. Obesity reduces FRC through chest wall loading and basal airway closure; pregnancy elevates the diaphragm; supine and Trendelenburg positions reduce lung volume; and conditions such as ARDS, pulmonary edema, abdominal hypertension, and thoracic rigidity further compromise FRC.

A low FRC compresses the safe apnea window, sometimes catastrophically. Mastery of airway physiology begins with understanding who is at risk and why.

8.2.3 *Alveolar Gas Dynamics: Oxygen Wash-In and Nitrogen Washout*

Room air comprises 78% nitrogen. During preoxygenation, nitrogen is replaced through:

- Oxygen wash-in (raising alveolar PO_2 as FiO_2 approaches 1.0).
- Nitrogen washout (expelling nitrogen from the FRC during exhalation).

The effectiveness of nitrogen washout is determined by the inspired oxygen fraction, the quality of the mask seal, fresh gas flow, duration of breathing, and number of lung units available for gas exchange.

With ideal conditions, alveolar oxygen fractions exceed 85–90%, enabling prolonged oxygen storage. However, nitrogen depletion increases susceptibility to absorption atelectasis [18, 19], particularly in dependent or poorly aerated regions. This phenomenon motivates many optimization strategies discussed later.

8.2.4 Oxygen Consumption and CO_2 Behavior During Apnea

At rest, adults consume approximately 200–300 mL of oxygen per minute, a rate that remains unchanged during apnea [10]. In contrast, CO_2 kinetics differ markedly: during early apnea, only ~10% of metabolically produced CO_2 reaches the alveoli, as most CO_2 remains buffered within blood and tissues owing to its high solubility [20]. Consequently, oxygen uptake substantially exceeds CO_2 delivery to the alveolar space.

As a result, while oxygen uptake remains near 230 mL/min, only ~20 mL/min of CO_2 enters the alveoli, producing a net alveolar gas loss of approximately 200 mL/min. This imbalance leads to a progressive reduction in alveolar volume and the generation of a subatmospheric intrapulmonary pressure gradient [21]. This negative pressure passively draws gas from the upper airway into the alveoli even in the absence of diaphragmatic movement, forming the physiological basis upon which apneic oxygenation strategies operate [22].

Although oxygenation can be prolonged through this mechanism, carbon dioxide inevitably accumulates—typically at a rate of 3–6 mmHg per minute—thereby defining the physiological limit of apnea duration even when hypoxemia is prevented [20].

8.2.5 Determinants of Safe Apnea Time

After optimal preoxygenation:

- *Healthy adults* may maintain $SpO_2 \geq 90\%$ for 6–8 min.
- *Pregnant patients* typically desaturate within 2–3 min.
- *Obese individuals* may reach desaturation in 90–150 s.
- *Critically ill or hypoxemic patients* may tolerate <60–120 s.
- *Infants* desaturate within 20–60 s due to very high oxygen consumption per kilogram and low FRC.

These differences arise from three physiological axes:

1. Size of the oxygen reservoir (FRC): A low FRC results in a small oxygen reservoir and rapid desaturation.
2. Oxygen consumption: High metabolic demand accelerates alveolar depletion.
3. Alveolar-to-arterial oxygen transfer: Shunt, V/Q mismatch, and lung injury impede oxygen uptake regardless of FiO_2.

   Understanding which axis dominates in an individual patient is the key to selecting the appropriate preoxygenation strategy.

8.2.6 Physiology of Apneic Oxygenation

Building on the gas exchange mechanisms described above, apneic oxygenation exploits the persistent negative intrathoracic pressure generated during apnea, which passively draws oxygen from the pharynx into the lungs when a source is available [12]. Its effectiveness depends on the maintenance of open alveolar units, upper airway patency, and a continuous supply of oxygen to the oropharynx or nasopharynx.

Apneic oxygenation does not remove carbon dioxide [20], cannot overcome shunt physiology, and is most effective only after alveolar oxygen content has been maximized by proper preoxygenation. It is therefore an adjunct—not a replacement—for preoxygenation.

8.2.7 Physiological Determinants of Preoxygenation Failure

Even optimal preoxygenation and airway technique are constrained by underlying respiratory and metabolic physiology. Failure of preoxygenation and safe apnea extension arises when one or more of the following dominant physiological mechanisms prevail:

1. *Shunt-dominant gas exchange impairment:* Alveolar units that are perfused but nonventilated contribute to intrapulmonary shunt, rendering increases in FiO_2 ineffective within these regions and limiting arterial oxygenation despite adequate preoxygenation.
2. *Reduced or unstable functional residual capacity:* A diminished or readily collapsible FRC reduces the size and stability of the alveolar oxygen reservoir, accelerating alveolar depletion during apnea. This is characteristic of obesity, pregnancy, supine positioning, and anesthesia-induced loss of lung volume.
3. *Elevated oxygen consumption:* Increased metabolic demand shortens apnea tolerance by accelerating oxygen extraction from the alveolar reservoir, as seen in fever, sepsis, trauma, agitation, and pediatric physiology.
4. *Loss of upper airway patency:* Obstruction of the upper airway interrupts both ventilation and apneic oxygen mass flow, abolishing the physiological mechanisms required to sustain oxygenation during apnea.

These constraints define the physiological boundaries within which airway management strategies must operate.

8.3 Indications for Preoxygenation

Preoxygenation is indicated whenever ventilation may be interrupted, impaired, or intentionally suspended [23]. Because apnea is inherent to airway management and hypoxemia remains a leading cause of periprocedural morbidity and mortality [24,

25], preoxygenation should be universal [1, 9]. Across operating rooms, emergency departments, and intensive care units, preoxygenation serves as a universal physiological safeguard, extending safe apnea time and reducing the risk of catastrophic deterioration during airway manipulation. Critically ill patients are increasingly recognized as having a "physiologically difficult airway," in which limited oxygen reserves and impaired gas exchange—rather than anatomical complexity—are the primary determinants of peri-intubation risk [26].

Preoxygenation before airway management is a standard of care and should be routinely performed in all patients (Grade A), with particular importance in those with an anticipated difficult airway, rapid desaturation risk, or when manual ventilation is undesirable or contraindicated [27, 28]. Indeed, it represents a fundamental element of rapid sequence induction (RSI) (Grade A) [10]. When properly performed, it converts physiological variability into predictable safety margins and transforms a time-limited process into a controlled, reproducible intervention.

The principal clinical indications for preoxygenation, together with their underlying physiological rationale and corresponding clinical requirements, are summarized in Table 8.1.

Table 8.1 Indications for preoxygenation and clinical implications

Clinical context	Physiological rationale	Clinical requirement
Routine induction of general anesthesia	Loss of spontaneous ventilation and upper airway tone during induction	Standard of care for all patients
Rapid sequence induction (RSI)	Immediate and uninterrupted apnea with limited rescue ventilation and frequent hemodynamic instability	Maximal, optimized preoxygenation is essential
Emergency and critical care airway management	Severe gas exchange impairment and limited cardiopulmonary reserve, with a high risk of cardiac arrest and intubation hypoxic injury	Mandatory; often requires advanced techniques
Procedural sedation and nonoperating room anesthesia	Risk of sudden apnea, hypoventilation, or airway obstruction	Recommended before moderate to deep sedation
Patients with limited apnea tolerance[a]	Reduced oxygen reserves and/or increased oxygen consumption	Essential; enhanced strategies are frequently required
Physiological states limiting standard preoxygenation	Shunt-dominant disease, low FRC, acidosis, fixed obstruction	Preoxygenation plus adjunctive strategies are required

[a]These populations include patients with obesity, which is associated with reduced functional residual capacity, early airway closure, increased oxygen consumption, and atelectasis. Pregnancy further decreases functional residual capacity while increasing metabolic demand and airway edema. Pediatric patients exhibit high oxygen consumption on a per-kilogram basis and possess very limited oxygen reserves. Critically ill or hypoxemic patients—including those with ARDS, pneumonia, cardiogenic pulmonary edema, COPD exacerbations, or systemic inflammation—often have severely impaired alveolar oxygen transfer. Agitated or dyspneic patients may also be unable to tolerate conventional mask-based preoxygenation without modified strategies

8.4 Devices for Delivering Oxygen

The choice of oxygen-delivery device is a key determinant of preoxygenation effectiveness. Although the physiological goals of preoxygenation are constant—maximizing alveolar oxygen content and minimizing nitrogen—devices differ markedly in their ability to deliver high FiO_2, maintain airway patency, preserve lung volume, and ensure patient comfort [12]. These differences are especially relevant in patients with limited physiological reserve or during time-critical airway interventions. Non-rebreather masks and low-flow nasal cannulae should not be used as sole preoxygenation strategies in high-risk patients due to unreliable FiO_2 delivery (*Grade B*).

Table 8.2 summarizes the main devices used for preoxygenation, including their mechanisms, strengths, limitations, and optimal clinical contexts. Anesthesia circuits provide the most reliable FiO_2 delivery but are largely confined to the operating room. Outside this setting, bag-valve-mask systems are widely used but remain highly dependent on mask seal and operator technique. Simpler devices offer greater tolerance but less consistent FiO_2 delivery, whereas advanced modalities such as high-flow nasal cannulae and noninvasive ventilation provide improved oxygenation and, in selected cases, alveolar recruitment.

Table 8.2 Devices for delivering oxygen for preoxygenation

Device	Mechanism	Strengths	Limitations	Optimal clinical context
Anesthesia circuits	Circle breathing system allowing precise control of FiO_2 (≈ 1.0), fresh gas flow, PEEP/CPAP, and continuous monitoring (EtO_2, $EtCO_2$)	Most reliable method to achieve $FiO_2 \approx 1.0$; minimal room-air entrainment; positive pressure integration; gold-standard EtO_2 confirmation	Limited to operating rooms; requires trained personnel; bulky and non-portable	Highest-performance preoxygenation when available; operating room standard
Bag-valve-mask (BVM)	Facemask attached to self- or flow-inflating bag; with reservoir and ≥ 15 L/min O_2 can approach $FiO_2 \approx 1.0$	Portable; allows manual ventilation; PEEP via valve; effective in emergency and prehospital settings	Seal-dependent; variable FiO_2; operator fatigue; gastric insufflation risk	Workhorse device outside the operating room
Non-rebreather mask (NRB)	One-way valve and reservoir bag reduce room-air entrainment.	Simple; lightweight; higher FiO_2 than simple masks	Highly variable FiO_2; no PEEP; inadequate for high-risk patients	Low-risk, spontaneously breathing patients

(continued)

Table 8.2 (continued)

Device	Mechanism	Strengths	Limitations	Optimal clinical context
Low-flow nasal cannula	Oxygen at 1–15 L/min via nasal prongs, providing a modest increase in FiO_2	Excellent tolerance; essential adjunct for dual oxygenation and apneic oxygenation	Inadequate alone; no PEEP; variable FiO_2	Adjunct device only; not suitable as a standalone preoxygenation strategy
High-flow nasal oxygen (HFNO)	Heated, humidified oxygen up to 60–70 L/min, providing high FiO_2 and flow-dependent low-level PEEP	Excellent tolerance; continuous oxygenation during laryngoscopy; improves mild-to-moderate hypoxemia	Less effective than CPAP/NIV in severe shunt physiology; PEEP variable and modest; provides no ventilatory support	Mild-to-moderate physiologic impairment
CPAP/NIV	Continuous positive airway pressure ± inspiratory support, promoting alveolar recruitment, ↑FRC, improved V/Q matching, and reduced work of breathing	Most effective noninvasive option for shunt physiology; provides oxygenation and ventilatory support; ideal for ARDS, cardiogenic pulmonary edema, and COPD exacerbations	Mask intolerance; gastric distention and aspiration risk; limited availability	Critically ill patients before intubation
Supraglottic airway devices (second generation)	Oropharyngeal seal allowing oxygenation and ventilation without requiring a face mask	Useful when mask seal is impossible (facial trauma, unusual anatomy, lack of cooperation); provides a stable airway	Requires tolerance or sedation; aspiration risk	Rescue preoxygenation; not a first-line device in routine scenarios

8.4.1 Choosing the Right Device: A Performance Framework

No single oxygen-delivery device is suitable for all patients or clinical scenarios. Effective device selection requires matching the device to the patient's physiological limitations, clinical environment, and urgency of airway management. Oxygen-delivery systems can therefore be viewed through a performance-based framework encompassing four domains: FiO_2 delivery capability, ability to increase functional

Table 8.3 Conceptual framework for oxygen delivery device selection

Performance domain	Relative device performance/examples
FiO_2 delivery capability	*Highest*: anesthesia circuit; BVM with reservoir *Moderate*: non-rebreather mask (NRB) *Variable*: nasal cannula systems
Ability to increase FRC or recruit alveoli	*NIV* > *CPAP* > *HFNC* ≫ simple face masks
Tolerance and comfort	*HFNC* > *NRB* > nasal cannula > mask-seal devices > *NIV/CPAP*
Applicability across clinical settings	*Operating room*: anesthesia circuit *Emergency department/ICU*: BVM, NIV, HFNC *Prehospital*: BVM ± NRB *Uncooperative patients*: HFNC *Difficult mask seal*: supraglottic airway devices (SGA)

residual capacity or recruit alveoli, patient tolerance and comfort, and applicability across clinical settings.

Table 8.3 integrates these domains to support rational, individualized device selection and to optimize oxygen reserves during airway management.

8.5 Core Techniques of Preoxygenation

A tight-fitting facemask delivering $FiO_2 \approx 1.0$ remains an effective preoxygenation technique in patients with preserved lung mechanics (Grade A). The most common approach to preoxygenation involves spontaneous breathing through a well-fitting face mask with 100% oxygen until adequate alveolar denitrogenation is achieved, typically defined by an end-tidal oxygen (EtO_2) concentration > 90% and an end-tidal nitrogen (EtN_2) fraction <5% prior to anesthetic induction [10]. Pulse oximetry is an unreliable surrogate of preoxygenation adequacy, as SpO_2 may reach 100% long before alveolar denitrogenation is complete; end-tidal oxygen and nitrogen concentrations remain the preferred physiological endpoints. Recent comparative analyses emphasize that end-tidal oxygen concentration reflects the efficacy of preoxygenation, whereas safe apnea time better captures its clinical effectiveness, integrating both oxygen loading and ongoing oxygen consumption during airway management [8].

Widely used preoxygenation strategies include 3 min of tidal volume breathing or a series of eight deep vital-capacity breaths [29, 30]. The effectiveness of these techniques has been extensively evaluated by analyzing the rate of arterial oxygen desaturation during apnea following induction and neuromuscular blockade, with "time to desaturation" (commonly to 95% or 90% SaO_2) serving as the primary outcome in many studies.

Inadequate mask seal and rebreathing of expired gases significantly reduce preoxygenation efficiency by preventing delivery of a true inspired oxygen fraction (FiO_2) of 1.0 [9]. Optimal mask sealing is best achieved through the use of a two-handed mask-holding technique whenever feasible, careful selection of an appropriately sized mask, and mandibular lift (jaw thrust) to enhance airway patency without applying excessive pressure [1, 3]. Inadequate mask seal represents a leading cause of failed preoxygenation and is a key determinant of the effectiveness of all mask-based techniques [31]. Proper system performance is suggested by appropriate reservoir bag movement, a normal capnographic waveform, and clearly identifiable inspired and end-tidal CO_2 ($EtCO_2$) values [10]. To minimize rebreathing, sufficient oxygen flow rates are required: approximately 5 $L{\cdot}min^{-1}$ for 3–5 min during tidal volume breathing, and 10 $L{\cdot}min^{-1}$ for 1 min when using the eight deep-breath technique [30]. The relative advantages, limitations, and clinical applicability of standard tidal breathing and accelerated vital-capacity techniques are summarized in Table 8.4.

Table 8.4 Comparison of standard and accelerated preoxygenation breathing techniques

Feature	Standard tidal breathing	Eight vital capacity breaths (60-s technique)
Core principle	Prolonged exposure to 100% FiO_2 allowing gradual oxygen wash-in and nitrogen wash-out	Rapid alveolar gas replacement using repeated maximal inspirations
Typical duration	3 min (≈30–60 tidal breaths)	~60 s (8 deep breaths)
Alveolar oxygen achieved	High (alveolar O_2 fraction >85–90%)	Near-equivalent in healthy, cooperative adults
Reliance on patient cooperation	Low	High
Physiological stress	Minimal	Moderate (increased work of breathing)
Performance consistency	High and predictable	Variable; highly patient-dependent
Speed of preoxygenation	Slow but reliable	Rapid
Effectiveness in normal physiology	Excellent	Good to excellent
Effectiveness in obesity, pregnancy, lung disease	Generally preserved, though may be reduced	Significantly reduced due to limited inspiratory capacity
Effectiveness in hypoxemia or dyspnea	Limited but more reliable	Poor
Mask tolerance required	Moderate	High
Primary advantages	Simplicity, reproducibility, minimal patient effort	Time-efficient when rapid airway control is required
Key limitations	Time-consuming; less effective in severe shunt physiology	Requires cooperation; unreliable in critically ill patients
Preferred clinical context	Elective airways; cooperative patients with stable cardiopulmonary function	Time-critical situations—such as emergent airway intervention or rapid deterioration—in healthy, cooperative patients
Role in practice	Reference and foundational technique	Selective alternative when time is limited

8.6 Optimization Strategies

Even when optimally applied, standard preoxygenation techniques have inherent limitations. Their effectiveness depends on patient cooperation and is reduced in uncooperative, dyspneic, or agitated patients. They cannot overcome significant intrapulmonary shunt, do not increase functional residual capacity, and are insufficient in the presence of markedly elevated oxygen consumption, leading to rapid depletion of oxygen reserves. Three minutes of tidal breathing or eight vital-capacity breaths are acceptable techniques in cooperative patients with normal physiology (Grade A), but are frequently inadequate in critically ill or hypoxemic patients (Grade B). The benefits of conventional preoxygenation are attenuated in patients at high risk of hypoxemia, in whom optimization strategies—such as head-up positioning, positive end-expiratory pressure (PEEP), apneic oxygenation, and, increasingly, noninvasive ventilation (NIV)—are required to maximize alveolar oxygen content and prolong safe apnea time [32]. These strategies target modifiable physiological variables—lung volume, airway patency, gas flow, and oxygen continuity—allowing each technique to operate at its full physiological potential.

Several optimization strategies, supported by different levels of evidence, can be applied to enhance preoxygenation efficacy and prolong safe apnea time.

Patient Positioning
Head-up (20–30°) and ramped positioning improve preoxygenation and prolong safe apnea time compared with the supine position (Grade A). On physiological grounds, these positions increase FRC, improve oxygen reserve and airway patency, and are therefore commonly recommended unless contraindicated (Grade D).

Positive Airway Pressure
The application of positive end-expiratory pressure (PEEP) or continuous positive airway pressure (CPAP) during preoxygenation improves alveolar recruitment and oxygenation and should be considered in patients with reduced functional residual capacity (Grade B).

Noninvasive Ventilation
Noninvasive ventilation improves preoxygenation efficacy and reduces peri-intubation hypoxemia in patients with hypoxemic respiratory failure or shunt-dominant physiology (Grade A).

High-flow Nasal Oxygen
High-flow nasal oxygen prolongs safe apnea time and provides apneic oxygenation during laryngoscopy (Grade A), but is less effective than noninvasive ventilation in patients with severe shunt physiology (Grade A).

Apneic Oxygenation
Apneic oxygenation should be used as an adjunct to preoxygenation to prolong safe apnea time, but it does not replace adequate preoxygenation (Grade D).

The mechanisms, physiological effects, and clinical applications of these optimization strategies are summarized in Table 8.5.

Table 8.5 Preoxygenation optimization strategies: mechanisms, benefits, and clinical use

Adjunct		Mechanism/ physiological effect	Key benefits	Optimal clinical context	Limitations/ considerations
Patient positioning	Head-up position (20–30°)	Reduces diaphragmatic compression; increases FRC; improves dependent alveolar aeration	Increases oxygen reservoir; reduces airway collapse; improves comfort and breathing mechanics	Default position for most patients unless contraindicated	May be limited by spinal precautions or hemodynamic instability
	Ramped position	Aligns external auditory meatus with sternal notch; improves upper airway patency and chest wall mechanics	Improves mask seal and comfort; enhances laryngoscopic view; increases FRC beyond simple head-up positioning	Obesity; pregnancy; reduced chest wall compliance; limited neck mobility	Requires preparation and positioning aids
Positive pressure	PEEP during spontaneous breathing (5–10 cmH_2O)	Prevents end-expiratory alveolar collapse; increases FRC; enhances denitrogenation	Improves oxygenation without pressure support; augments preoxygenation effectiveness	Low baseline FRC with preserved airway patency	Limited by mask seal quality and patient tolerance
	Continuous positive airway pressure (CPAP)	Provides continuous distending pressure; stabilizes small airways	Improves V/Q matching; reduces atelectasis; enhances oxygenation	Obesity; pregnancy; pulmonary edema; moderate hypoxemia	Requires tolerance of tight-fitting mask; aspiration risk
	Noninvasive ventilation (NIV)	Adds inspiratory pressure support; increases tidal volume and alveolar recruitment	Most effective noninvasive method for improving oxygenation; reduces work of breathing; improves shunt physiology	Hypoxemic respiratory failure; severe shunt-dominant conditions	Mask intolerance; aspiration risk; requires close monitoring
	Lung recruitment maneuvers (selective use)	Brief application of high airway pressures (e.g., 30–40 cmH_2O for 10–15 s) to reopen collapsed alveoli	Increases aerated lung volume; improves FRC and EtO_2 attainment	Significant atelectasis with preserved hemodynamic stability (e.g., obesity, prolonged recumbence, post-anesthesia)	Risk of hypotension due to reduced venous return; not suitable for hemodynamic instability or barotrauma risk

(continued)

Table 8.5 (continued)

Adjunct	Mechanism/ physiological effect	Key benefits	Optimal clinical context	Limitations/ considerations
Dual oxygenation (low-flow nasal cannula + face mask or HFNC + NIV)	Provides continuous oxygen delivery before, during, and after induction without interfering with other devices or techniques; enables apneic oxygenation	Extends safe apnea time; mitigates transient hypoventilation; adds redundancy if mask seal deteriorates	Should be strongly considered in high-risk airways, anticipated difficult intubation, and time-critical scenarios	Requires additional oxygen source; flow-dependent effectiveness

Adjunctive strategies targeting lung volume, alveolar recruitment, and continuous oxygen delivery can substantially enhance preoxygenation effectiveness and should be routinely considered in patients at increased risk of hypoxemia. Comparative network analyses suggest that the effectiveness of preoxygenation is not determined by the oxygen-delivery device alone, but by the interaction between device, patient position, and the application of positive airway pressure, all of which modulate functional residual capacity

8.7 High-risk Patients for Hypoxemia

Several clinical conditions reduce the effectiveness of conventional preoxygenation and increase the likelihood of oxyhemoglobin desaturation during apnea, thereby raising the risk of life-threatening complications. In parallel, certain patient populations exhibit a diminished physiological tolerance to hypoxia, including those with cerebrovascular disease, epilepsy, or coronary artery disease. In addition, transient oxyhemoglobin desaturation has been reported in approximately 10–30% of patients undergoing rapid sequence intubation [23].

Severe desaturation is associated with a substantial increase in morbidity and mortality. Accordingly, understanding the underlying pathophysiological mechanisms of each condition is essential to individualize preoxygenation strategies and align them with patient-specific vulnerabilities [33]. From a practical standpoint, clinicians should systematically consider key questions before airway management [34]: Is difficulty with ventilation or intubation anticipated? How rapidly is desaturation likely to occur? What degree of desaturation can be safely tolerated? In these patients, combined strategies—integrating patient positioning, noninvasive ventilation for preoxygenation, and high-flow nasal oxygen for apneic oxygenation—should be considered standard practice to maximize oxygen reserve and reduce peri-intubation hypoxemia (Grade B). These patients exemplify the concept of the physiologically difficult airway introduced earlier, in which hypoxemia and limited physiological reserve, rather than anatomical complexity alone, drive airway-related risk. Figure 8.1 summarizes the principal conditions associated with an increased risk of desaturation during airway management, together with the recommended preoxygenation and apneic oxygenation strategies.

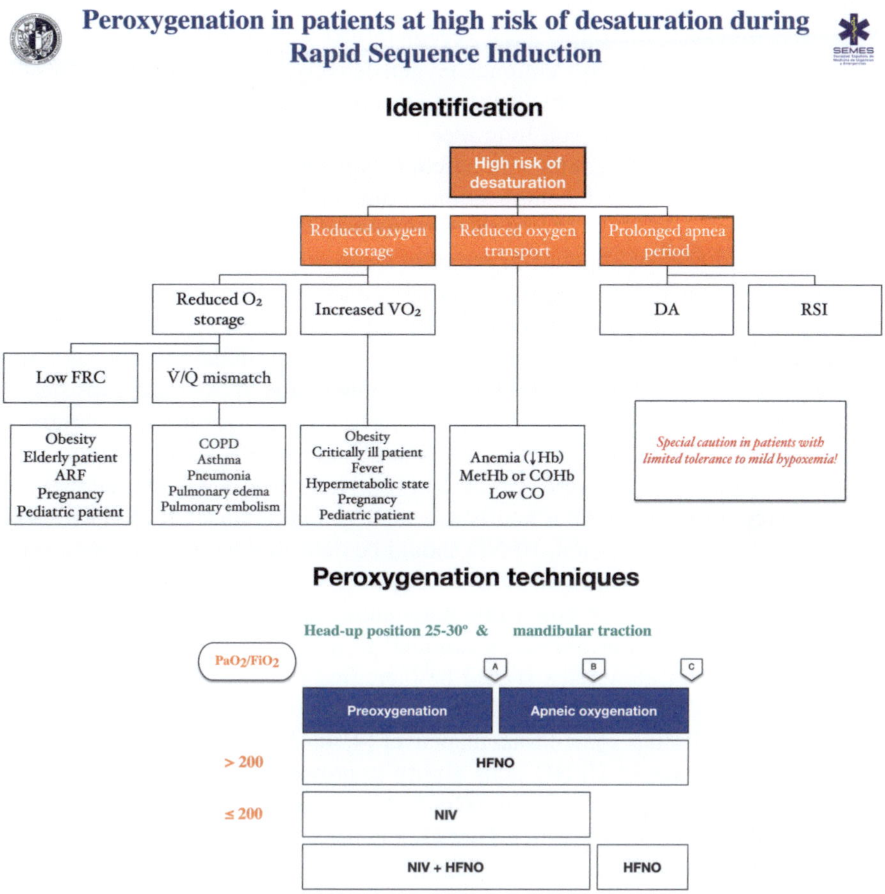

Fig. 8.1 Theoretical and educational tool developed by the Spanish Society of Anesthesiology, Reanimation and Pain Therapy (SEDAR), the Spanish Society of Emergency and Emergency Medicine (SEMES), and the Spanish Society of Otolaryngology and Head and Neck Surgery (SEORL-CCC) for the identification of patients at high risk of oxygen desaturation and for the selection of recommended preoxygenation and apneic oxygenation techniques during rapid sequence induction (RSI). This figure illustrates the two physiological strategies used to increase pulmonary oxygen reserves: preoxygenation and apneic oxygenation. Preoxygenation refers to the administration of oxygen before anesthetic induction, with the aim of maximizing alveolar oxygen content through nitrogen washout and expansion of functional residual capacity (FRC). Apneic oxygenation refers to the continuous delivery of oxygen after the loss of spontaneous ventilation, exploiting the physiological mass flow of oxygen into the alveoli during apnea to prolong safe apnea time. Patients at high risk of desaturation are characterized by reduced oxygen storage, reduced oxygen transport, increased oxygen consumption, impaired gas exchange, or a prolonged apnea period. The figure integrates clinical risk factors with physiology-based oxygenation strategies, including patient positioning, facemask oxygenation, high-flow nasal oxygen, noninvasive ventilation, and dual oxygenation techniques. Abbreviations: RSI, rapid sequence induction; COPD, chronic obstructive pulmonary disease; Hb, hemoglobin; O_2, oxygen; FRC, functional residual capacity; NIV, noninvasive ventilation; HFNO, high-flow nasal oxygen; PaO_2/FiO_2, arterial oxygen partial pressure to inspired oxygen fraction ratio

High-flow Nasal Oxygen (HFNO)

Preoxygenation using high-flow nasal oxygen (HFNO) has been increasingly investigated as an alternative to conventional oxygen delivery, with heterogeneous results across different clinical settings. Earlier studies reported variable efficacy, particularly in patients with preserved lung mechanics. However, accumulating clinical evidence indicates that, in adults with baseline hypoxemia, HFNO reduces the incidence of intubation-related complications compared with conventional oxygen therapy (Grade B) [35–37]. Several randomized trials and systematic reviews suggest that HFNO may be superior to standard facemask oxygenation in prolonging safe apnea time and improving oxygenation (Grade A). However, it appears less effective than NIV in patients with significant shunt physiology (Grade A) [7, 37–46]. By contrast, recent meta-analyses in obese patients undergoing elective surgery suggest that, while HFNO prolongs safe apnea time, it does not consistently reduce the incidence or severity of peri-intubation desaturation when compared with facemask-based strategies, likely reflecting inadequate alveolar recruitment in the absence of positive pressure (Grade B) [40]. Nevertheless, HFNO represents a valuable alternative when NIV is poorly tolerated or contraindicated [26, 35, 37, 47].

For optimal preoxygenation, HFNO should be delivered with 100% FiO_2, starting at an initial flow of approximately 30 $L{\cdot}min^{-1}$, with patients instructed to perform nasal vital-capacity breaths while maintaining strict mouth closure for about 3 min. Proper cannula positioning is essential to minimize room-air entrainment. Following induction, flow rates should be increased to 60–70 $L{\cdot}min^{-1}$ and maintained throughout laryngoscopy and tracheal intubation, while airway patency is actively preserved using a jaw-thrust maneuver [4, 48–50].

A major advantage of HFNO is its ability to provide effective apneic oxygenation during airway instrumentation (Grade A). Apneic oxygen delivery is likely the principal mechanism by which HFNO attenuates oxygen desaturation during laryngoscopy, rather than superior denitrogenation alone (Grade B) [38–40, 51–53]. Recent network meta-analyses clarify that high-flow nasal oxygen primarily prolongs apnea time and, when combined with a head-up position, ranks among the most effective strategies for extending safe apnea (Grade A), whereas noninvasive ventilation more effectively preserves arterial oxygenation, particularly in patients with reduced functional residual capacity or shunt-dominant physiology (Grade A) [8, 35].

Despite these benefits, HFNO has limitations. Accurate monitoring of EtO_2 is unreliable during HFNO, complicating objective assessment of preoxygenation adequacy [48, 54]. Additionally, HFNO may interfere with laryngoscopic conditions in some scenarios, potentially due to high gas flows or patient discomfort [36, 55]. Concerns regarding gastric insufflation have been raised; however, recent experimental and clinical studies suggest that HFNO does not significantly increase gastric insufflation compared with conventional techniques (Grade B) [39, 40, 56, 57]. Whether these findings are fully applicable to patients with a full stomach remains uncertain [36, 58].

Based on current evidence, HFNO is recommended as a first-line preoxygenation strategy in patients with mild hypoxemia (Grade B). In the specific context of rapid sequence induction for emergency surgery, recent meta-analyses show that high-flow nasal oxygen improves post-intubation PaO_2 and prolongs apnea time (Grade A), but does not consistently reduce peri-intubation desaturation or aspiration risk (Grade B), underscoring the distinction between improved oxygen reserves and clinically meaningful oxygenation [36].

Noninvasive Ventilation (NIV)

Noninvasive ventilation is particularly advantageous in patients with reduced FRC, where conventional preoxygenation techniques often fail. Multiple studies demonstrate that NIV maximizes preoxygenation efficacy in obese and critically ill patients by simultaneously increasing alveolar oxygen fraction and lung volume (Grade A) [4, 7, 32, 38, 48, 49, 59, 60]. Current evidence suggests that the efficacy of preoxygenation strategies largely depends on the amount of recruitable functional residual capacity: when FRC can be reopened, noninvasive ventilation provides a clear physiological advantage over flow-based techniques (Grade B) [26]. Importantly, the beneficial effects of NIV on arterial oxygenation may persist for up to 30 min after intubation, reflecting sustained alveolar recruitment and increased lung volume (Grade B) [39, 61]. In obese patients, noninvasive ventilation is superior to conventional oxygen therapy during anesthetic induction, resulting in improved oxygenation and reduced peri-intubation hypoxemia (Grade A) [26, 38].

Clinically, NIV is commonly applied using continuous positive airway pressure (CPAP) of 5–10 cmH_2O combined with assisted spontaneous breaths (tidal volume 7–10 $mL{\cdot}kg^{-1}$), a strategy shown to significantly improve oxygenation [4, 62]. NIV is typically discontinued during laryngoscopy [32, 38], making it potentially superior to HFNO during the spontaneous breathing phase of preoxygenation (Grade B) [40, 63], while HFNO may offer greater benefit during the apneic phase (Grade B) [35, 36, 64–66].

Multiple randomized trials and meta-analyses indicate that combining NIV for preoxygenation with HFNO for apneic oxygenation significantly reduces peri-intubation desaturation in critically ill patients (Grade B), with reported desaturation rates as low as 14–15% [7, 35, 38, 67–69]. A recent large network meta-analysis of randomized trials confirms that noninvasive ventilation provides the greatest reduction in peri-intubation hypoxemia in critically ill adults, outperforming both high-flow nasal oxygen and facemask-based strategies (Grade A), while HFNO remains superior to facemask oxygen alone (Grade A) [4]. Contemporary ICU reviews now consider NIV the most effective noninvasive strategy for preoxygenation in hypoxemic respiratory failure, particularly in shunt-dominant conditions [7, 26, 38].

Large pragmatic trials and contemporary emergency medicine reviews further support noninvasive ventilation as the preferred preoxygenation strategy during emergency intubation in critically ill patients, demonstrating significant reductions in peri-intubation hypoxemia without an increased risk of aspiration (Grade B), even in patients with altered mental status [5].

A recent network meta-analysis in patients with acute hypoxic respiratory failure suggests that noninvasive ventilation is most effective in reducing severe peri-intubation hypoxemia ($SpO_2 < 80\%$) (Grade A), whereas high-flow nasal oxygen may be associated with fewer intubation-related complications (Grade B), highlighting a trade-off between maximal oxygenation and overall procedural safety [70].

In elective surgical populations, evidence from randomized trials and meta-analyses suggests that the superiority of NIV over conventional preoxygenation is most consistent in obese patients (Grade B), whereas benefits in nonobese patients are less robust and may not translate into clinically meaningful prolongation of safe apnea time (Grade B) [39]. Combining NIV for preoxygenation with apneic oxygenation during laryngoscopy addresses both alveolar oxygen loading and ongoing oxygen consumption, representing a physiologically complementary strategy in high-risk patients [26].

In patients unable to tolerate the NIV interface or presenting with delirium or agitation, analgosedation with dexmedetomidine or dissociative-dose ketamine (10–20 mg IV boluses) can facilitate effective preoxygenation as part of a delayed sequence intubation strategy (Grade C) [26, 36, 47, 71–73]. NIV should also be considered both before and after general anesthesia in obese patients to reduce perioperative respiratory complications (Grade B) [4, 23, 48, 74].

Despite these advantages, NIV is not without risks. Airway pressures exceeding 20 cmH_2O increase the likelihood of gastric distension, necessitating careful risk–benefit assessment in patients at risk of aspiration (Grade D). Furthermore, alternative preoxygenation strategies should be preferred in patients with facial fractures, recent laryngeal, esophageal, or gastric surgery, hemodynamic instability, pulmonary hypertension, acute pulmonary embolism, or right ventricular failure (Grade D) [26, 75].

Ultimately, safe airway management depends less on any single device than on aligning preoxygenation strategy with the patient's underlying physiology.

References

1. Gómez-Ríos MA, Sastre JA, Onrubia-Fuertes X, López T, Abad-Gurumeta A, Casans-Francés R, et al. Spanish Society of Anesthesiology, Reanimation and Pain Therapy (SEDAR), Spanish Society of Emergency and Emergency Medicine (SEMES) and Spanish Society of Otolaryngology, Head and Neck Surgery (SEORL-CCC) guideline for difficult airway management. Part I. Rev Esp Anestesiol Reanim (Engl Ed). 2024;71(3):171–206. https://doi.org/10.1016/j.redare.2024.02.001.
2. Gómez-Ríos MA, Sastre JA, Onrubia-Fuertes X, López T, Abad-Gurumeta A, Casans-Francés R, et al. Spanish Society of Anesthesiology, Reanimation and Pain Therapy (SEDAR), Spanish Society of Emergency and Emergency Medicine (SEMES) and Spanish Society of Otolaryngology, Head and Neck Surgery (SEORL-CCC) guideline for difficult airway management. Part II. Rev Esp Anestesiol Reanim (Engl Ed). 2024;71(3):207–47. https://doi.org/10.1016/j.redare.2024.02.002.
3. Ahmad I, El-Boghdadly K, Iliff H, Dua G, Higgs A, Huntington M, et al. Difficult Airway Society 2025 guidelines for management of unanticipated difficult tracheal intubation in adults. Br J Anaesth. 2025. https://doi.org/10.1016/j.bja.2025.10.006.

4. Pitre T, Liu W, Zeraatkar D, Casey JD, Dionne JC, Gibbs KW, et al. Preoxygenation strategies for intubation of patients who are critically ill: a systematic review and network meta-analysis of randomised trials. Lancet Respir Med. 2025;13(7):585–96. https://doi.org/10.1016/S2213-2600(25)00029-3.
5. Gibbs KW, Semler MW, Driver BE, Seitz KP, Stempek SB, Taylor C, et al. Noninvasive ventilation for preoxygenation during emergency intubation. N Engl J Med. 2024;390(23):2165–77. https://doi.org/10.1056/NEJMoa2313680.
6. DeMasi SC, Casey JD, Semler MW. Evidence-based emergency tracheal intubation. Am J Respir Crit Care Med. 2025;211(7):1156–64. https://doi.org/10.1164/rccm.202411-2165CI.
7. Monet C, Capdevila M, Lakbar I, Aarab Y, Pensier J, De Jong A, et al. Preoxygenation in the ICU. J Clin Med. 2025;14(20). https://doi.org/10.3390/jcm14207305.
8. Crístian de Carvalho C, Iliff HA, Santos Neto JM, Potter T, Alves MB, Blake L, et al. Effectiveness of preoxygenation strategies: a systematic review and network meta-analysis. Br J Anaesth. 2024;133(1):152–63. https://doi.org/10.1016/j.bja.2024.02.028.
9. Gómez-Ríos MÁ, Úbeda Iglesias A, Esquinas AM. Respiratory Care in Anesthesiology: pre-intubation and Upper Airways Procedure. In: Esquinas AM, AlAhmari MD, editors. Respiratory care in non invasive mechanical ventilatory support: principles and practices. New York: Nova Science Publishers, Inc.; 2021. p. 549–66.
10. Nimmagadda U, Salem MR, Crystal GJ. Preoxygenation: physiologic basis, benefits, and potential risks. Anesth Analg. 2017;124(2):507–17. https://doi.org/10.1213/ane.0000000000001589.
11. Hagberg CA. Hagberg and Benumofs airway management e-book. Elsevier Health Sciences; 2017.
12. Roberts F, Behringer EC, Patel A. Perioxygenation. In: Hagberg CA, Artime CA, Aziz MF, editors. Hagberg and Benumof's airway management. 5th ed. Philadelphia: Elsevier; 2023. p. 275–304.
13. Benumof JL. Preoxygenation: best method for both efficacy and efficiency. Anesthesiology. 1999;91(3):603–5. https://doi.org/10.1097/00000542-199909000-00006.
14. Lumb A, Thomas C. Oxygen. In: Lumb A, Thomas C, editors. Nunn and Lumb's applied respiratory physiology. 9th ed. London: Elsevier; 2021. p. 136–48.
15. Weingart SD, Levitan RM. Preoxygenation and prevention of desaturation during emergency airway management. Ann Emerg Med. 2012;59(3):165–75.e1. https://doi.org/10.1016/j.annemergmed.2011.10.002.
16. Pelosi P, Croci M, Ravagnan I, Tredici S, Pedoto A, Lissoni A, et al. The effects of body mass on lung volumes, respiratory mechanics, and gas exchange during general anesthesia. Anesth Analg. 1998;87(3):654–60. https://doi.org/10.1097/00000539-199809000-00031.
17. Hedenstierna G, Edmark L. Mechanisms of atelectasis in the perioperative period. Best Pract Res Clin Anaesthesiol. 2010;24(2):157–69. https://doi.org/10.1016/j.bpa.2009.12.002.
18. Déry R, Pelletier J, Jacques A, Clavet M, Houde J. Alveolar collapse induced by denitrogenation. Can Anaesth Soc J. 1965;12(6):531–57. https://doi.org/10.1007/BF03004416.
19. Edmark L, Kostova-Aherdan K, Enlund M, Hedenstierna G. Optimal oxygen concentration during induction of general anesthesia. Anesthesiology. 2003;98(1):28–33. https://doi.org/10.1097/00000542-200301000-00008.
20. Lyons C, Callaghan M. Uses and mechanisms of apnoeic oxygenation: a narrative review. Anaesthesia. 2019;74(4):497–507. https://doi.org/10.1111/anae.14565.
21. Kolettas A, Grosomanidis V, Kolettas V, Zarogoulidis P, Tsakiridis K, Katsikogiannis N, et al. Influence of apnoeic oxygenation in respiratory and circulatory system under general anaesthesia. J Thorac Dis. 2014;6(Suppl 1):S116–45. https://doi.org/10.3978/j.issn.2072-1439.2014.01.17.
22. Koo BS, Chung YH, Lee M, Cho SH, Jung J. Apnoeic oxygenation using high-flow oxygen: effects on partial pressure of carbon dioxide in rigid bronchoscopy. J Clin Med. 2025;14(22). https://doi.org/10.3390/jcm14228064.
23. Ball L, Dameri M, Pelosi P. Modes of mechanical ventilation for the operating room. Best Pract Res Clin Anaesthesiol. 2015;29(3):285–99. https://doi.org/10.1016/j.bpa.2015.08.003.

24. Joffe AM, Aziz MF, Posner KL, Duggan LV, Mincer SL, Domino KB. Management of difficult tracheal intubation: a closed claims analysis. Anesthesiology. 2019;131(4):818–29. https://doi.org/10.1097/aln.0000000000002815.
25. Cook TM, Woodall N, Frerk C. Major complications of airway management in the UK: results of the Fourth National Audit Project of the Royal College of Anaesthetists and the Difficult Airway Society. Part 1: anaesthesia. Br J Anaesth. 2011;106(5):617–31. https://doi.org/10.1093/bja/aer058.
26. La Via L, Cuttone G, Senussi Testa T, Duarte-Medrano G, Nuno-Lambarri N, Deana C, et al. Non-invasive positive pressure ventilation for pre-oxygenation of critically ill patients before intubation. J Clin Med. 2025;14(15). https://doi.org/10.3390/jcm14155356.
27. Baillard C, Boubaya M, Statescu E, Collet M, Solis A, Guezennec J, et al. Incidence and risk factors of hypoxaemia after preoxygenation at induction of anaesthesia. Br J Anaesth. 2019;122(3):388–94. https://doi.org/10.1016/j.bja.2018.11.022.
28. Frerk C, Mitchell VS, McNarry AF, Mendonca C, Bhagrath R, Patel A, et al. Difficult Airway Society 2015 guidelines for management of unanticipated difficult intubation in adults. Br J Anaesth. 2015;115(6):827–48. https://doi.org/10.1093/bja/aev371.
29. Bouroche G, Bourgain JL. Preoxygenation and general anesthesia: a review. Minerva Anestesiol. 2015;81(8):910–20.
30. Garzón JC, Sastre JA, Gómez-Ríos M, López T, Garzón-Sánchez A, Pandit JJ. Comparing the dynamics of changes in regional cerebral oxygen saturation with arterial oxygen partial pressure with two techniques of preoxygenation in healthy adults. J Clin Anesth. 2020;68:110091. https://doi.org/10.1016/j.jclinane.2020.110091.
31. El-Boghdadly K, Aziz MF. Face-mask ventilation: the neglected essentials? Anaesthesia. 2019;74(10):1227–30. https://doi.org/10.1111/anae.14703.
32. Cortegiani A, Accurso G, Mercadante S, Giarratano A, Gregoretti C. High flow nasal therapy in perioperative medicine: from operating room to general ward. BMC Anesthesiol. 2018;18(1):166. https://doi.org/10.1186/s12871-018-0623-4.
33. De Jong A, Futier E, Millot A, Coisel Y, Jung B, Chanques G, et al. How to preoxygenate in operative room: healthy subjects and situations "at risk". Ann Fr Anesth Reanim. 2014;33(7–8):457–61. https://doi.org/10.1016/j.annfar.2014.08.001.
34. Slinger PD. Is there anything new about preoxygenation? Duh, yeah! Anesth Analg. 2017;124(2):388–9. https://doi.org/10.1213/ANE.0000000000001764.
35. Zhong M, Xia R, Zhou J, Zhang J, Yi X, Yang A. The comparison of preoxygenation methods before endotracheal intubation: a network meta-analysis of randomized trials. Front Med (Lausanne). 2024;11:1379369. https://doi.org/10.3389/fmed.2024.1379369.
36. Tang H, Yang Y, Li H. High-flow nasal cannula for pre- and apneic oxygenation during rapid sequence induction intubation in emergency surgery: a systematic review and meta-analysis. PLoS One. 2025;20(1):e0316918. https://doi.org/10.1371/journal.pone.0316918.
37. Fong KM, Au SY, Ng GWY. Preoxygenation before intubation in adult patients with acute hypoxemic respiratory failure: a network meta-analysis of randomized trials. Crit Care. 2019;23(1):319. https://doi.org/10.1186/s13054-019-2596-1.
38. Frat JP, Grieco DL, De Jong A, Gibbs K, Carteaux G, Roca O, et al. Noninvasive respiratory supports in ICU. Intensive Care Med. 2025;51(8):1476–89. https://doi.org/10.1007/s00134-025-08036-3.
39. Chiang TL, Tam KW, Chen JT, Wong CS, Yeh CT, Huang TY, et al. Non-invasive ventilation for preoxygenation before general anesthesia: a systematic review and meta-analysis of randomized controlled trials. BMC Anesthesiol. 2022;22(1):306. https://doi.org/10.1186/s12871-022-01842-y.
40. Bright MR, Harley WA, Velli G, Zahir SF, Eley V. High-flow nasal cannula for apneic oxygenation in obese patients for elective surgery: a systematic review and meta-analysis. Anesth Analg. 2023;136(3):483–93. https://doi.org/10.1213/ANE.0000000000006304.

41. Lyons C, McElwain J, Coughlan MG, O'Gorman DA, Harte BH, Kinirons B, et al. Preoxygenation with facemask oxygen vs high-flow nasal oxygen vs high-flow nasal oxygen plus mouthpiece: a randomised controlled trial. Anaesthesia. 2022;77(1):40–5. https://doi.org/10.1111/anae.15556.
42. Sjöblom A, Broms J, Hedberg M, Lodenius Å, Furubacke A, Henningsson R, et al. Preoxygenation using high-flow nasal oxygen vs. tight facemask during rapid sequence induction. Anaesthesia. 2021;76(9):1176–83. https://doi.org/10.1111/anae.15426.
43. Mir F, Patel A, Iqbal R, Cecconi M, Nouraei SA. A randomised controlled trial comparing transnasal humidified rapid insufflation ventilatory exchange (THRIVE) pre oxygenation with facemask pre-oxygenation in patients undergoing rapid sequence induction of anaesthesia. Anaesthesia. 2017;72(4):439–43. https://doi.org/10.1111/anae.13799.
44. Lodenius Å, Piehl J, Östlund A, Ullman J, Jonsson Fagerlund M. Transnasal humidified rapid-insufflation ventilatory exchange (THRIVE) vs. facemask breathing pre-oxygenation for rapid sequence induction in adults: a prospective randomised non-blinded clinical trial. Anaesthesia. 2018;73(5):564–71. https://doi.org/10.1111/anae.14215.
45. Wong DT, Dallaire A, Singh KP, Madhusudan P, Jackson T, Singh M, et al. High-flow nasal oxygen improves safe apnea time in morbidly obese patients undergoing general anesthesia: a randomized controlled trial. Anesth Analg. 2019;129(4):1130–6. https://doi.org/10.1213/ANE.0000000000003966.
46. Li J, Jing G, Scott JB. Year in review 2019: high-flow nasal cannula oxygen therapy for adult subjects. Respir Care. 2020;65(4):545–57. https://doi.org/10.4187/respcare.07663.
47. Kornas RL, Owyang CG, Sakles JC, Foley LJ, Mosier JM, Committee SfAMsSP. Evaluation and management of the physiologically difficult airway: consensus recommendations from Society for Airway Management. Anesth Analg. 2021;132(2):395–405. https://doi.org/10.1213/ANE.0000000000005233.
48. Long B, Bridwell RE, Pourmand A, Gottlieb M. Practice changing articles: noninvasive ventilation for preoxygenation during emergency intubation. Am J Emerg Med. 2025;98:315–7. https://doi.org/10.1016/j.ajem.2025.10.011.
49. Patel A, Gilhooly M. Preoxygenation and apneic oxygenation for airway management for anesthesia. UpToDate Retrieved January. 2021.
50. Mosier JM, Hypes CD, Sakles JC. Understanding preoxygenation and apneic oxygenation during intubation in the critically ill. Intensive Care Med. 2017;43(2):226–8. https://doi.org/10.1007/s00134-016-4426-0.
51. Wong DT, Yee AJ, Leong SM, Chung F. The effectiveness of apneic oxygenation during tracheal intubation in various clinical settings: a narrative review. Can J Anaesth. 2017;64(4):416–27. https://doi.org/10.1007/s12630-016-0802-z.
52. Russotto V, Cortegiani A, Raineri SM, Gregoretti C, Giarratano A. Respiratory support techniques to avoid desaturation in critically ill patients requiring endotracheal intubation: a systematic review and meta-analysis. J Crit Care. 2017;41:98–106. https://doi.org/10.1016/j.jcrc.2017.05.003.
53. Karamchandani K, Wheelwright J, Yang AL, Westphal ND, Khanna AK, Myatra SN. Emergency airway management outside the operating room: current evidence and management strategies. Anesth Analg. 2021;133(3):648–62. https://doi.org/10.1213/ANE.0000000000005644.
54. Booth AWG, Vidhani K, Lee PK, Coman SH, Pelecanos AM, Dimeski G, et al. The effect of high-flow nasal oxygen on carbon dioxide accumulation in apneic or spontaneously breathing adults during airway surgery: a randomized-controlled trial. Anesth Analg. 2021;133(1):133–41. https://doi.org/10.1213/ANE.0000000000005002.
55. Chanques G, Jaber S. Nasal high-flow preoxygenation for endotracheal intubation in the critically ill patient? Maybe. Intensive Care Med. 2019;45(4):532–4. https://doi.org/10.1007/s00134-019-05598-x.
56. McLellan E, Lam K, Behringer E, Chan V, Bozak D, Mitsakakis N, et al. High-flow nasal oxygen does not increase the volume of gastric secretions during spontaneous ventilation. Br J Anaesth. 2020;125(1):e75–80. https://doi.org/10.1016/j.bja.2020.02.023.

57. Sud A, Athanassoglou V, Anderson EM, Scott S. A comparison of gastric gas volumes measured by computed tomography after high-flow nasal oxygen therapy or conventional facemask ventilation. Anaesthesia. 2021;76(9):1184–9. https://doi.org/10.1111/anae.15433.
58. Lam SW, Irwin MG. Pre-oxygenation for rapid sequence induction: is high-flow nasal oxygenation worth the hassle? Anaesthesia. 2021;76(9):1159–62. https://doi.org/10.1111/anae.15473.
59. Deflandre EP, Javillier BX. Preoxygenation by high-flow nasal oxygen in the non-hypoxemic patient: the early stages. Minerva Anestesiol. 2020;86(11):1121–2. https://doi.org/10.23736/S0375-9393.20.14936-8.
60. Ricard JD, Gregoretti C. Nasal high-flow preoxygenation for endotracheal intubation in the critically ill patient? Pro. Intensive Care Med. 2019;45(4):529–31. https://doi.org/10.1007/s00134-019-05588-z.
61. Baillard C, Fosse JP, Sebbane M, Chanques G, Vincent F, Courouble P, et al. Noninvasive ventilation improves preoxygenation before intubation of hypoxic patients. Am J Respir Crit Care Med. 2006;174(2):171–7. https://doi.org/10.1164/rccm.200509-1507OC.
62. Papazian L, Corley A, Hess D, Fraser JF, Frat JP, Guitton C, et al. Use of high-flow nasal cannula oxygenation in ICU adults: a narrative review. Intensive Care Med. 2016;42(9):1336–49. https://doi.org/10.1007/s00134-016-4277-8.
63. Frat JP, Ricard JD, Quenot JP, Pichon N, Demoule A, Forel JM, et al. Non-invasive ventilation versus high-flow nasal cannula oxygen therapy with apnoeic oxygenation for preoxygenation before intubation of patients with acute hypoxaemic respiratory failure: a randomised, multicentre, open-label trial. Lancet Respir Med. 2019;7(4):303–12. https://doi.org/10.1016/S2213-2600(19)30048-7.
64. Ricard JD, Roca O, Lemiale V, Corley A, Braunlich J, Jones P, et al. Use of nasal high flow oxygen during acute respiratory failure. Intensive Care Med. 2020;46(12):2238–47. https://doi.org/10.1007/s00134-020-06228-7.
65. Jhou HJ, Chen PH, Lin C, Yang LY, Lee CH, Peng CK. High-flow nasal cannula therapy as apneic oxygenation during endotracheal intubation in critically ill patients in the intensive care unit: a systematic review and meta-analysis. Sci Rep. 2020;10(1):3541. https://doi.org/10.1038/s41598-020-60636-9.
66. Ricard JD. Hazards of intubation in the ICU: role of nasal high flow oxygen therapy for preoxygenation and apneic oxygenation to prevent desaturation. Minerva Anestesiol. 2016;82(10):1098–106.
67. Jaber S, Monnin M, Girard M, Conseil M, Cisse M, Carr J, et al. Apnoeic oxygenation via high-flow nasal cannula oxygen combined with non-invasive ventilation preoxygenation for intubation in hypoxaemic patients in the intensive care unit: the single-centre, blinded, randomised controlled OPTINIV trial. Intensive Care Med. 2016;42(12):1877–87. https://doi.org/10.1007/s00134-016-4588-9.
68. Cao L, Zheng H, Xie Y, Liu S, Liu K. Effect of preoxygenation and apnoeic oxygenation during intubation in the critically ill patients: a network meta-analysis. Zhonghua Wei Zhong Bing Ji Jiu Yi Xue. 2019;31(10):1236–41. https://doi.org/10.3760/cma.j.issn.2095-4352.2019.10.011.
69. Ricard JD, Gaborieau B, Bernier J, Le Breton C, Messika J. Use of high flow nasal cannula for preoxygenation and apneic oxygenation during intubation. Ann Transl Med. 2019;7(Suppl 8):S380. https://doi.org/10.21037/atm.2019.12.106.
70. Ye N, Wei C, Deng J, Wang Y, Xie H. Preoxygenation strategies before intubation in patients with acute hypoxic respiratory failure: a network meta-analysis. Front Med (Lausanne). 2025;12:1532911. https://doi.org/10.3389/fmed.2025.1532911.
71. Mosier JM, Joshi R, Hypes C, Pacheco G, Valenzuela T, Sakles JC. The physiologically difficult airway. West J Emerg Med. 2015;16(7):1109–17. https://doi.org/10.5811/westjem.2015.8.27467.
72. Weingart SD, Trueger NS, Wong N, Scofi J, Singh N, Rudolph SS. Delayed sequence intubation: a prospective observational study. Ann Emerg Med. 2015;65(4):349–55. https://doi.org/10.1016/j.annemergmed.2014.09.025.

73. De Jong A, Myatra SN, Roca O, Jaber S. How to improve intubation in the intensive care unit. Update on knowledge and devices. Intensive Care Med. 2022;48(10):1287–98. https://doi.org/10.1007/s00134-022-06849-0.
74. Carron M, Zarantonello F, Tellaroli P, Ori C. Perioperative noninvasive ventilation in obese patients: a qualitative review and meta-analysis. Surg Obes Relat Dis. 2016;12(3):681–91. https://doi.org/10.1016/j.soard.2015.12.013.
75. Manohar C, Karamchandani K. Con: the best method to preoxygenate a patient with a physiologically difficult airway is non-invasive ventilation. J Cardiothorac Vasc Anesth. 2023. https://doi.org/10.1053/j.jvca.2023.03.028.

Chapter 9
Physiologically Difficult Airway

Graham Trevor Lubinsky, Kathleen Sheridan Lubinsky, and Kunal Karamchandani

Highlights

1. Critically ill patients often present with a physiologically difficult airway and pose multiple challenges during emergency airway management.
2. Preparation of both the patient and the procedural team is paramount to preventing patient harm during the management of a physiologically difficult airway.
3. Hemodynamic and respiratory optimization can help improve patient outcomes.
4. Device and drug selection during airway management should take into account operator expertise, patients' medical condition, and overall clinical situation.

Medical literature is replete with recommendations for the management of an anatomically difficult airway; however, it is the physiologically difficult airway (PDA) that poses a unique set of challenges. A PDA occurs when physiologic derangements place the patient at higher risk of complications with tracheal intubation and conversion to positive pressure ventilation [1]. Tracheal intubation (TI) in a critically ill patient is associated with increased morbidity and mortality; major adverse events have been observed in 45% of patients, with hemodynamic collapse and hypoxemia being the most common [2]. It has also been reported that about 1 in 40

G. T. Lubinsky (✉) · K. S. Lubinsky
Department of Anesthesiology, Advocate Illinois Masonic Medical Center, Chicago, IL, USA
e-mail: Graham.Lubinsky@aah.org; kathleen.lubinsky@aah.org

K. Karamchandani
Division of Critical Care Medicine, Department of Anesthesiology and Pain Management, University of Texas Southwestern Medical Center, Dallas, TX, USA
e-mail: Kunal.Karamchandani@utsouthwestern.edu

M. Á. Gómez-Ríos, A. van Zundert (eds.), *Evidence-based Guide to Difficult Airway Management*, https://doi.org/10.1007/978-3-032-30769-9_9

emergency TIs in a non-operating room setting result in cardiac arrest [3, 4]. Critically ill patients are already subjected to extreme physiological conditions and the combination of medications used for intubation, positive pressure ventilation, and post-intubation strategies can have severe consequences on their hemodynamics, oxygenation, and ventilation. The Fourth National Audit Project of the Royal College of Anaesthetists and Difficult Airway Society (NAP4) in the United Kingdom, identified repeated gaps in care that included poor identification of at-risk patients, poor or incomplete planning, inadequate provision of skilled staff and equipment to manage these events, delayed recognition of events, and failed rescue due to lack of or failure of interpretation of capnography [5]. Hence, it is important that airway operators understand the various challenges and the ways to mitigate complications associated with TI in patients with a PDA. In this chapter, we will discuss pre-TI planning, airway management, and post-intubation care for patients with a PDA.

9.1 Physiologically Difficult Airway

A PDA occurs when the physiologic perturbations increase the risk of cardiopulmonary, neurological, and other peri-intubation complications [1, 6]. The causes of a PDA include, but are not limited to, those outlined in Table 9.1.

Table 9.1 Conditions associated with a physiologically difficult airway

Underlying condition	Potential physiological perturbations
Hypoxia	Reduced functional residual capacity Poor pulmonary reserve Ventilation/perfusion mismatch
Hypotension	Direct cardiac effects of induction agents Loss of sympathetic tone from medications Intolerance of positive pressure ventilation
Right heart failure	Decreased RVEDP, from positive pressure Increased PVR from positive pressure Hypoxia/hypercarbia increasing PVR
Severe metabolic acidosis	Loss of respiratory compensation Inability to tolerate hypercarbia
Full stomach/significant GERD	Inability to be supine for intubation High risk for pulmonary aspiration
Increased intracranial pressure	Changes in O_2 and CO_2, leading to ICP changes Changes in MAP, ICP, or CVP leading to diminished CPP
Anterior mediastinal mass	Inability to be supine for intubation Potential airway collapse Potential hemodynamic compromise

RVEDP right ventricular end-diastolic pressure, *PVR* pulmonary vascular resistance, *ICP* intracranial pressure, *MAP* mean arterial pressure, *CVP* central venous pressure

9.2 Pre-intubation Planning

Pre-intubation history and examination are often rushed in these circumstances, but gathering as much information as possible in a short time period is paramount. Also, patients may not be cooperative enough to allow proper airway examination. If time permits, assessment of patient's medical history, airway history, and performing an airway exam are vital to success. Despite the potential pressing airway concerns, sometimes the safest course of action may be to delay TI to allow for patient optimization.

9.2.1 Patient Assessment

Patient history should include, but not be limited to, past medical history, focusing on cardiopulmonary issues, most recent labs, and current/recent changes in clinical status. This should be followed by a thorough examination of the patient, ensuring that adequate intravascular access is established before attempting induction of anesthesia and tracheal intubation. Additionally, a complete airway exam and review of past airway notes, if available, will provide vital information needed to plan for TI. Unfortunately, many of the patients undergoing emergency TI are not able to cooperate with an airway exam, and a retrospective study found that in 75% of emergency airway management procedures (excluding intubations for cardiac arrest), the patients could not be assessed for Mallampati score, neck mobility, and thyromental distance [7].

In addition to standard patient assessment, the MACOCHA (Mallampati, Apnea, Cervical, Opening, Coma, Hypoxemia, Anesthesiologist) score was developed by De Jong et al. to predict difficulty with TI [8]. This scoring system, which has been validated in numerous studies, factors in the patient's physiologic alterations, airway anatomy, and the operator's competency, yielding a score of 0–12, with 0 being easy and 12 being very difficult. A score greater than or equal to 3 is a predictor of difficult intubation (Table 9.2). However, patients with a low MACOCHA score should still be approached with caution as other factors may lead to peri-intubation difficulty.

Studies have also examined the factors associated with adverse events in emergency airway management (EAM). In their review on Airway Management in Critical Illness, Scott et al. [9] found that age > 60y, acute respiratory failure as an indication for intubation, first intubation, non-invasive ventilation required before intubation, and FiO_2 less than 70% were associated with cardiovascular collapse. They also found that systolic blood pressure less than 90 mmHg, hypoxemia, no preoxygenation, body mass index >25 kg/m^2, and age >75y were associated with cardiac arrest within 5 min of intubation. In the INTUBE Study [2], investigators also found, in a post hoc exploratory analysis, that age, history of heart failure, history of hematologic malignancy, cardiovascular instability as an indication for

Table 9.2 MACOCHA difficult intubation score

Factors predicting difficult intubation	Points
Factors related to the patient's airway	
Mallampati class III or IV	5
Obstructive sleep **apnea**	2
Reduced **cervical** spine mobility	1
Limited mouth **opening**	1
Factors related to the patient's pathology	
Coma	1
Severe **hypoxemia** ($SpO_2 < 80\%$)	1
Factors related to the operator	
Anesthesiologist	0
Non-anesthesiologist	1
Total	0–12

A total score of 3 or more predicts difficulty, and appropriate steps should be taken

intubation, and other features of hemodynamic compromise were all associated with increased rates of peri-intubation adverse events.

9.2.2 *Hypotension Prediction/Resuscitation*

One of the tools designed to predict post-intubation hypotension is the Hypotension Prediction Score (HYPS) [10], which was developed using a post hoc analysis of the HEMAIR study. [11] The HYPS factors in APACHE II score are age, sepsis diagnosis, intubation setting (respiratory, hypotension, cardiac arrest, other), diuretic use, catecholamine use, phenylephrine use, SBP, and etomidate use (protective). HYPS stratifies patients into low, moderate, high, and very high-risk categories for adverse events post-intubation.

Another factor that may lead to hemodynamic compromise is right ventricular failure. In addition to its effects on gas exchange and acid-base status, right ventricular failure increases the odds of hemodynamic collapse as a byproduct of the transition to positive pressure ventilation, which increases intrathoracic pressure [12]. In a study reviewing changes in arterial pressure during mechanical ventilation, Michard [13] observed that while the reduction of left ventricular afterload with positive pressure ventilation does have its benefits, the potentially overwhelming decrease in right ventricular function can have fatal consequences. Reduction of right ventricular end-diastolic volume and increased pulmonary vascular resistance due to changes in West zone physiology can reduce forward flow from the RV. In patients with underlying RV failure, pulmonary hypertension, or hypotension from any source, this can precipitate catastrophic RV failure.

Given the potentially fatal outcomes secondary to peri-intubation hypotension, delaying intubation to allow time for patient resuscitation and optimization may be prudent. In a survey among Canadian Emergency Medicine and Critical Care Medicine physicians, respondents favored pre-administration of fluids in patients with pneumonia or trauma and favored vasopressors in patients with heart failure as their primary diagnosis [14]. While the administration of fluids to mitigate the effects of induction medications and positive pressure ventilation does make logical sense, there is conflicting data. The PrePARE Investigators [15] and the PREPARE II Investigators [16] failed to show their benefit. In these trials, patients were randomized into receiving a 500 mL bolus or no fluid bolus before tracheal intubation with sedation and positive pressure ventilation. They concluded that among critically ill adults undergoing tracheal intubation, administration of an intravenous fluid bolus did not significantly decrease the incidence of cardiovascular collapse. However, this contrasts with the peri-intubation protocols described by Jaber et al. [17] that did show benefit to fluid loading, leading to a reduction in post-intubation complications.

Regarding the peri-intubation use of vasopressors, there is a lack of evidence to create an optimal choice and approach to vasopressor therapy [18]. Hemodynamic instability is one of the prevailing concerns in PDA management, so while there might not be concrete evidence on which vasopressor to use, they should be available in the peri-intubation period. The PREVENTION (Preventing Cardiovascular Collapse With Vasopressors During Tracheal Intubation; NCT05014581) and FLUVA (Effect of a Fluid Bolus or a Low Dose VAsopressor Infusion on Cardiovascular Collapse Among Critically Ill Adults Undergoing Tracheal Intubation; NCT05318066) trials are currently underway to assess the utility of administration of fluids and the use of vasopressors in critically ill adults undergoing TI.

9.2.3 Point-of-Care Ultrasound

If a patient has advanced hemodynamic monitoring in place, some data can be obtained regarding the patient's fluid status with measures of pulse pressure variation and central venous pressures, but the broad applicability of these numbers in isolation is questionable. Additionally, the use of adjunct technology, like the Vigileo™ (Edwards Life Sciences, Irvine, CA) and Argos™ (Retia Medical Systems, White Plains, NY) monitoring systems, can provide additional information. In the absence of advanced monitoring, point-of-care ultrasound (POCUS) is an option for the assessment of fluid status, cardiac function, and any other acute abnormality such as cardiac tamponade. Ultrasound assessment of the IVC has been used in mechanically ventilated patients to assess volume status, but the data for non-mechanically ventilated patients is heterogeneous. IVC collapsibility in the spontaneously breathing patient is an available option, but the evidence is not strong enough to be a principal determinant of fluid resuscitation. [19] POCUS can also be used to assess a patient's risk of aspiration. Asokan et al. [20] performed an observational study in which they calculated the cross-sectional area of the gastric antrum

(CSA = (AP × CC) π/4) and estimated a gastric volume using Perla's formula (GV = 27.0 + 14.6(RLD CSA) − 1.28(age)). They determined that a CSA cutoff greater than or equal to 9.27 cm^2 (sensitivity 100%, specificity 87%) and a gastric volume greater than or equal to 111.6 mL (sensitivity 100%, specificity 92%) predicted aspiration. The role of POCUS in the management of PDA has recently been discussed [21], and studies are needed to assess its impact in preventing peri-intubation adverse events.

9.2.4 Respiratory Optimization

As aforementioned, hypoxemia is the second most common adverse event associated with EAM in critically ill patients. Hence, it is vital that appropriate measures are instituted to optimize the patient's respiratory status before proceeding with TI, and steps are taken to avoid critical oxygen desaturation during the procedure. Preoxygenation and apneic oxygenation are commonly employed to address these concerns.

When circumstances allow, preoxygenation should be employed to extend the period of apneic time prior to desaturation. The principal benefit of preoxygenation is denitrogenation of the functional residual capacity, which can help increase the apnea time. The duration of pre-oxygenation has been debated, and a longer duration may not always be better. Mort et al. [22] conducted a trial to assess the effectiveness of increased preoxygenation times in preparation for emergency TI. Patients were preoxygenated with a noncollapsing resuscitator bag and mask. Blood gases were taken at times zero, 4, 6, and 8 min. There was a mean increase in PaO2 of 22 mmHg at 4 min, with a decrease in the rate of rise at 6 and 8 min. Furthermore, approximately 25% of patients had a drop in PaO2 between 4 and 8 min, potentially due to atelectasis. Overall, the authors determined that extending the preoxygenation period from the customary 4 mins to either 6 or 8 min seemed to be only marginally effective in most patients and such an extension may instead jeopardize oxygenation efforts in some patients.

There is evidence to support the use of non-invasive ventilation (NIV) for preoxygenation as evidenced by higher SpO2 values in the NIV group compared to those preoxygenated with a nonrebreather [23], but this has been disputed. A 2018 multicenter, randomized study [24] evaluated the use of delivering 100% FiO_2 by non-invasive ventilation vs. a face mask for 3 min prior to intubation. The study failed to demonstrate a difference between the two populations. However, in 2019, the FLORALI-2 trial [25] did show that patients with moderate-to-severe hypoxemia (classified as a PaO_2/FiO_2 ratio less than or equal to 200 mmHg) had less post-intubation hypoxemia when compared to patients receiving high flow nasal oxygen (HFNO). Further studies may tip the scales favoring NIV versus standard preoxygenation techniques, but there are other factors to consider, including the availability of equipment, the risk of gastric insufflation, and the necessity to remove the

NIV interface prior to intubation. Nonetheless, in patients with hypoxemia and risk of desaturation, NIV should be considered if time and resources allow.

Pre-oxygenation techniques that can be continued through the intubation procedure do have demonstrated benefits. The OPTINIV trial [26] looked at combining the use of HFNO and NIV in hypoxemic patients undergoing TI. They found that the combination group had higher SpO2 values during intubation when compared to the NIV-only group. This could be, in part, due to the benefits of apneic oxygenation. Apneic oxygenation yields benefits due to the mass flow of high FiO_2, which is aided by cardiogenic oscillations, positive airway pressure, and flushing of dead space [27]. There is a growing body of evidence suggesting that the use of HFNO can lead to a reduction in desaturations and allow longer apneic periods, without hindering CO_2 exchange or increasing the risk of aspiration of gastric contents [28, 29].

In terms of patient positioning, having a patient in a semi-recumbent, or reverse Trendelenburg position does have its theoretical advantages in improving oxygenation. Supine position leads to a reduction in functional residual capacity secondary to intraabdominal contents applying pressure to the inferior surface of the diaphragm. However, the evidence regarding the impact of a semi-recumbent position on patient outcomes is equivocal. A multicenter, randomized trial looking at the ramped versus sniffing position during endotracheal intubation in critically ill adults [30] did not find improved oxygenation in the ramped position. Furthermore, they posited that the ramped position may worsen glottic view and decrease first-pass success rates. However, the use of a suboptimal ramped position was one of the major limitations of this trial. Despite limited evidence, guidelines for TI in critically ill patients have recommended the ramped position, especially in patients at high risk of aspiration or desaturation [31, 32].

Rapid sequence intubation (RSI) with cricoid pressure (Sellick's maneuver) has been the traditional approach for TI in patients with a PDA, but doing so may decrease first-pass intubation success and worsen hypoxemia. The IRIS Trial [33], a randomized, double-blinded, noninferiority trial, looked at the use of the Sellick maneuver during RSI and observed that the application of cricoid pressure failed to prevent gastric aspiration and may worsen the quality of laryngeal exposure. In a randomized controlled trial, Casey et al. [34] evaluated the use of bag-mask ventilation for TI in critically ill adults and found that patients who received bag-mask ventilation had higher median oxygen saturations than those who did not. Additionally, the rate of operator-reported aspiration was lower in the bag-mask arm. This is a topic that will require further studies, as Casey et al. relied-on operator reporting, and the study was underpowered to make a definitive conclusion regarding aspiration. Nonetheless, in patients at low risk of aspiration, but high risk of desaturation, the delivery of positive pressure ventilation using bag-mask may be safe.

9.2.5 Assembling a Team

EAM in a non-operating room setting requires the availability of trained personnel and appropriate equipment, which will be discussed later in this chapter. Ideally, the personnel performing the intubation should be the most experienced, as studies have shown that level of experience can have a significant impact on the chances of first-pass success [35]. However, it is also important to involve the trainees in the process, so that the pool of experienced providers continues to grow. This may or may not include allowing the trainee to take the first attempt at an airway with a senior specialist as backup, but the more involved a trainee can be in these cases, the more apt they will be to handle them when needed. The shared airway provided by video laryngoscopy may also provide an opportunity for trainees to perform the procedure under the guidance of an experienced airway operator.

Human factors that affect the success of intubation in a PDA include environmental influences, team behaviors, and individual performance; human factor deficits such as lack of patient preparation, equipment checks, or protocol deviation occur in up to half of ICU critical incidents [31]. Several team compositions have also been described that include the roles of first intubator, second intubator, drug administrator, an observer of patient's clinical status, cricoid force applier (the utility of which was previously discussed), airway equipment assistant, runner, team leader, and manual in-line stabilizer (in the case of cervical spine pathology or trauma with unknown injury). Often, it is not feasible to have a team this large and the expertise of certain members of the team may require them to assume multiple roles, but a four-member team with one experienced airway specialist is often sufficient [36].

9.3 Airway Management

9.3.1 Medication Selection

The choice of induction agents for TI in critically ill patients remains a topic of debate. While etomidate and ketamine have been popular choices due to their potential ability to perform a cardiac-stable induction, their use has been contested. One of the prevailing reasons for avoiding etomidate in the critically ill is the risk of adrenal suppression. Kotani et al. [37] conducted a meta-analysis of etomidate use for endotracheal intubation in critically ill patients; they found that it is highly probable that etomidate increased mortality, as well as being associated with increased risk of adrenal insufficiency. While ketamine has sympathomimetic effects, it is also a direct myocardial depressant, so for patients in extremis with already depleted catecholamine stores, the myocardial depressant effects can become more evident. Ketamine has also been considered contraindicated in patients with closed head injuries or concern for elevated intracranial pressures; however, a recent review suggested that ketamine may be safely administered to neurologically impaired patients [38]. The EvK trial, a randomized controlled trial comparing etomidate and ketamine for TI in critically ill patients showed that seven-day survival was significantly lower in patients who received etomidate, but 28-day survival was not statistically significant [39].

Propofol, a commonly used anesthetic drug is traditionally avoided in the critically ill, due to its unfavorable hemodynamic profile. In a retrospective, single-center study evaluating 2673 critically ill patients undergoing TI over 5 years, propofol use was associated with better outcomes even after adjusting for severity of illness prior to TI [40]. However, based on the study design it is hard to exclude confounding since real-time decision-making on the receipt of propofol was based on clinical judgment and not randomization. To address the concerns of the cardiorespiratory effects of pure propofol inductions, physicians have chosen to mix it with ketamine, which is a cardiorespiratory stimulant. This combination, known as ketofol, can help maintain stable hemodynamics similar to etomidate with a reduced side effect profile [41]. Some physicians choose to forgo the etomidate, ketamine, and propofol for induction and rely on the amnestic effects of midazolam and/or fentanyl prior to TI. Miller et al. [42] reviewed the use of midazolam and fentanyl for induction of anesthesia prior to TI and found that patients who received midazolam and fentanyl were not spared from hypotension as a potential consequence of induction of anesthesia for TI. However, they noticed that it was unclear if the effect was due to sympatholysis from medication administration or the transition to positive pressure ventilation.

In addition to an induction agent, neuromuscular blockade can be used to facilitate TI. While not required for the procedure, they can help improve airway conditions and maximize the chance of first-pass success. The choice of neuromuscular agent used for EAM is limited to succinylcholine and rocuronium. Succinylcholine offers rapid intubating conditions, and has a short duration of action, making return to spontaneous ventilation faster if airway difficulty is encountered. However, succinylcholine has its inherent risks and side effects. In the critically ill patient population, the risks of hyperkalemia and the potential increase in intracranial pressure need to be balanced with the beneficial onset of succinylcholine; in patients who have upper motor neuron/spinal cord lesions, burns, rhabdomyolysis, or prolonged bed rest, this risk of hyperkalemia is increased. In contrast, rocuronium does not have the same risks. However, when given in a rapid sequence intubating dose of 0.9–1.2 mg/kg, rocuronium has a significantly longer duration of action. Studies have shown no difference in the quality of intubation conditions between rocuronium and succinylcholine [43]. The ready availability of sugammadex, which can reverse even high doses of rocuronium, has made the use of rocuronium more common.

9.3.2 Device Selection

The choice of airway device (video or direct laryngoscope) being used for TI is often at the discretion of the airway operator (considering their expertise and experience), the patient's medical status and the overall clinical situation. There is evidence to suggest that video laryngoscopy can increase first-pass success when compared to direct laryngoscopy [44]. However, video laryngoscopy may not be a one-size-fits-all approach to airway management. Success with video laryngoscopy replies on familiarity with the equipment and intubating conditions. With the wide array of options, such as the scopes that employ a Macintosh or Miller blade with the addition of a camera, or the hyperangulated video laryngoscopes, airway operators must familiarize themselves with the equipment available to them. Additionally, the camera on a video laryngoscope can be rendered useless even with minimal blood, vomitus, or secretions in the oropharynx. There is also evidence to refute the utility of video laryngoscopy in certain scenarios. A recent meta-analysis showed that video laryngoscope with an hyperangulated blade did not increase first-pass success, whereas a video laryngoscope using non-hyperangulated blade did increase first-pass success; there was also no difference in first-pass success between video and direct laryngoscopy in experienced operators [45]. Furthermore, they found that the use of video laryngoscopy was associated with a greater incidence of arterial hypotension, which may be secondary to a decrease in sympathetic/hypertensive response when compared to direct laryngoscopy. Ultimately, the choice of laryngoscope is up to the operator, but it may be reasonable to have a video laryngoscope available as a primary device or backup device.

Another factor relating to first-pass success is the use of a stylet. When using a hyperangulated video laryngoscope, the use of a preformed stylet can help mimic the curvature of the blade; however, there is mixed data when considering the use of a stylet in conjunction with direct laryngoscopy. The STYLETO (STYLET of Orotracheal intubation) trial, a multicenter, randomized controlled trial involving about 1000 patients, compared the use of a stylet versus no stylet [46], and observed a superior first-attempt intubation success rate with the use of a stylet (78.2% vs 71.5%) without a statistically significant increase in adverse events. Shortly thereafter, the BOUGIE (Bougie or Stylet in Patients Undergoing Intubation Emergently) trial randomized 1102 critically ill patients into the stylet versus bougie groups and did not find a statistically significant difference in first-pass success between the two groups. As with all equipment, the choice of stylet versus bougie should depend on the operator's comfort with the airway adjuncts.

A roadblock to successful first-pass intubation that needs to be planned for is potential airway contamination. As aforementioned, the utility of video laryngoscopy could be diminished in a patient with a soiled airway, be it from copious secretions, blood, or vomitus. Gross reflux of gastric contracts is an unfortunate but not uncommon occurrence in emergent airways. If a patient has a large-bore nasogastric tube or transcutaneous gastric tube that allows for suctioning of gastric contents, that should be done prior to attempts at intubation. However, this may not be the

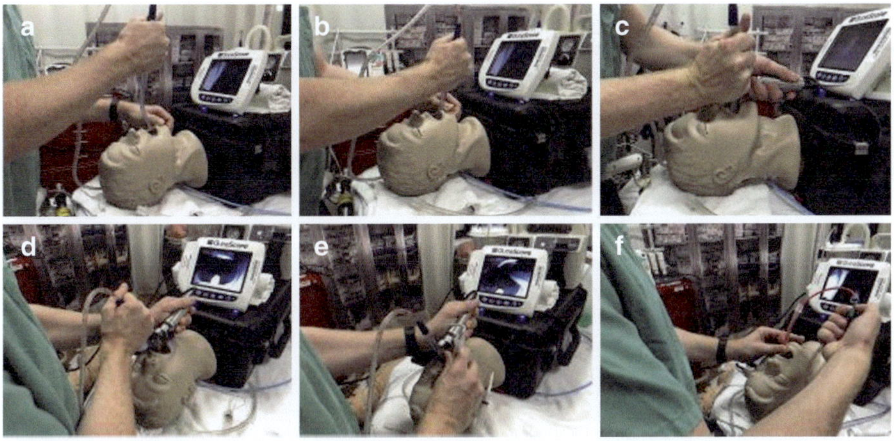

Fig. 9.1 The SALAD approach [47]. (**a**) A rigid suction catheter (RSC) is gripped in the right hand. (**b**) RSC displaces the upper airway structures. (**c**) The airway is suctioned while the laryngoscope is advanced. (**d**) RSC is repositioned to the left of the laryngoscope blade and advanced into the hypopharynx or proximal esophagus to provide continuous suctioning. (**e**) The endotracheal tube is passed through the vocal cords. (**f**) The endotracheal tube is suctioned prior to ventilation

case in a majority of patients. One technique that has been described is intentional esophageal intubation. The premise of this technique is to blindly intubate the esophagus and inflate the endotracheal tube cuff. This provides a conduit from the esophagus to outside the oropharynx, thereby decreasing the amount of vomitus in the oropharynx and allowing for adequate suctioning before the subsequent intubation attempt. Another method is the SALAD technique [47]. This technique is more widely applicable as it can be used for copious secretions, blood, or vomitus. (Fig. 9.1).

9.3.3 Backup Plans

It is vital to have backup plans in place while performing EAM in patients with PDA, similar to those that have been proposed for airway management inside the operating room [48]. Acute patient decompensation, along with situational and logistical challenges, makes this scenario overtly challenging for even the most experienced providers. Providers involved with EAM in critically ill patients must be prepared for the challenges, have practiced the procedural steps, and have adequate training to provide leadership during these stressful circumstances. Keeping calm, calling for help, and rapidly transitioning between different backup plans are the keys to success in these circumstances. A recent review proposed an algorithm for out-of-OR airway management [49], and Fig. 9.2 proposes a similar algorithm for EAM in patients with a PDA.

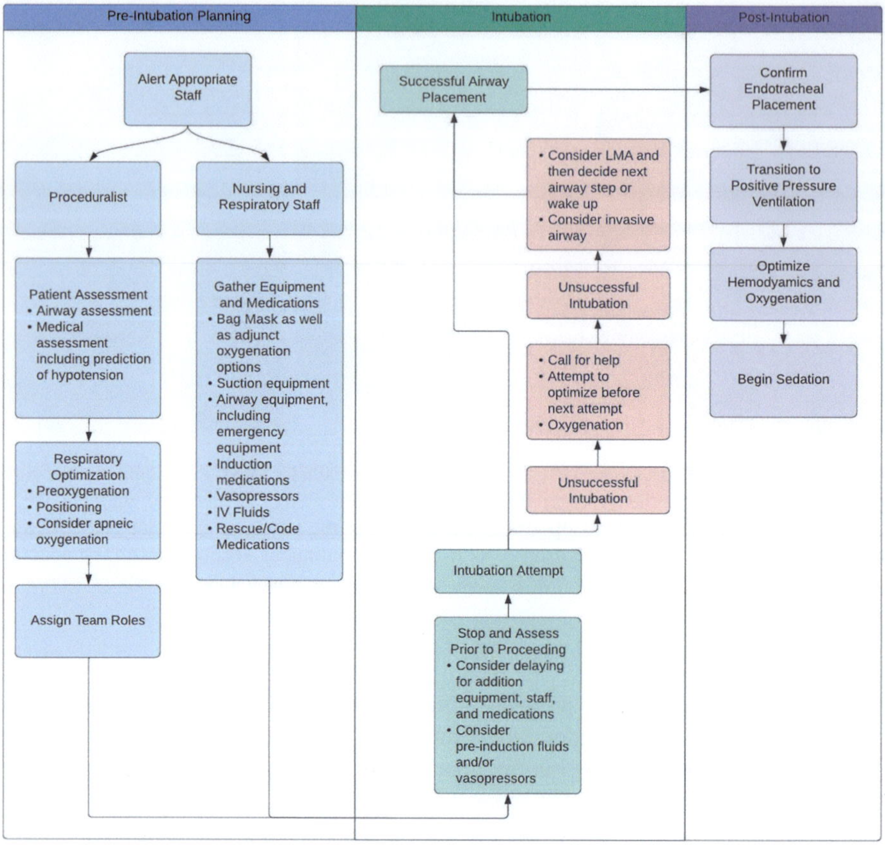

Fig. 9.2 Algorithm for emergency airway management of a physiologically difficult airway. (Reproduced with permission from [49])

After a perceived successful intubation, confirmation of the placement of the endotracheal tube in the trachea must be done prior to attention being turned elsewhere. Confirmation can be done using colorimetric end-tidal CO_2 detectors, continuous end-tidal CO_2 monitoring, auscultation, observing ventilator waveforms, bronchoscopy, and imaging. Continuous waveform capnography is considered the gold standard by many [50].

9.4 Post-TI Care

The post-intubation care of this critically ill population poses a new set of challenges that, in some instances, require complex management. Patients with PDA due to multiple causes can have conflicting treatment priorities; for example, in a patient with respiratory failure and right ventricular dysfunction, positive pressure ventilation may improve oxygenation but also increase pulmonary vascular resistance and worsen right ventricular function. Post-intubation management should include a fine balance of respiratory support and hemodynamic stability. Patients may need invasive hemodynamic monitoring and transfer to a higher level of care. Patients who receive long-acting paralytics during TI should have sedative medications administered to prevent awareness.

In 2010, Jaber et al. [17] proposed a peri-intubation algorithm to decrease the rate of complications, and over the years, the Montpellier-airway ICU Algorithm has been revisited. In a 2022 update, the authors streamlined the post-intubation care bundle to include: the use of capnography to confirm TI, vasopressor initiation for systolic blood pressure <90 mmHg and/or diastolic blood pressure <35 mmHg, initiation of long-term sedation, low airway pressure ventilation, recruitment maneuvers utilizing PEEP of 30–40 cmH_2O for 20–30 s, and maintaining cuff pressures of 25–30 cmH_2O without leak [51]. However, this was described with the caveat that attempts at increasing ventilation and mitigating hypoxemia can negatively impact post-intubation hemodynamics.

In conclusion, regardless of the thought and preparation that goes into successful TI in patients with a PDA, there is no single model or algorithm that will fit all patients. Meticulous care is important, and monitoring of the hemodynamic and respiratory changes during the procedure, and the use of algorithms and cognitive aids [31, 49, 52], can all help increase preparedness and decrease the risk of adverse events. Ultimately, it is a concerted team effort during this high-risk procedure that can help improve patient outcomes.

Important Recommendations

- Pre-intubation planning should include an assessment of the patient, which can include standard methods of airway assessment and the use of the MACOCHA score.
- Prevention of hypotension and cardiovascular collapse can be assessed using risk stratification scores and knowledge of the patient's comorbid conditions.
- The decision to present potential post-intubation hypotension with intravenous fluids or vasopressors is still a topic of research, but both should be available.
- Preoxygenation should occur to allow for increased apneic time and decrease the risk of hypoxemia. In patients with pre-existing moderate to severe hypoxemia, non-invasive ventilation has shown benefit. Apneic oxygenation can also help prevent hypoxemia.
- Patient positioning and equipment selection should be done to maximize the chance of first-pass success.
- Medication selection should be done based on the clinical scenario to minimize the effects on hemodynamics.
- Post-intubation care may require a balance between hemodynamic goals and oxygenation and should be tailored to the individual patient.

Clinical Situation

A 67 y/o female with a large pulmonary embolus in the intensive care unit requires tracheal intubation for acute hypoxemic respiratory failure. On examination, the patient is awake and alert, but in a state of panic. Her heart rate is 120 beats per minute, SpO_2 87%, and blood pressure is 136/87 mm Hg.

How To

1. Ensure the availability of appropriate personnel and equipment.
2. If feasible, perform a point-of-care ultrasound (POCUS) to identify any right ventricular dysfunction.
3. Based on the POCUS findings, consider the administration of fluids and/or vasopressors/inotropes to support the peri-intubation hemodynamics.
4. Begin oxygenating the patient, and consider the use of a high-flow nasal cannula (if available) for both pre-oxygenation and apneic oxygenation.
5. Position the patient in a ramped-up position if tolerated.
6. Choose a device (video or direct laryngoscopy) that you believe will yield the highest chance of first-pass success.
7. Confirm the correct placement of the endotracheal tube, preferably using waveform capnography.

References

1. Mosier JM, Joshi R, Hypes C, Pacheco G, Valenzuela T, Sakles JC. The physiologically difficult airway. West J Emerg Med. 2015;16:1109–17. https://doi.org/10.5811/westjem.2015.8.27467.
2. Russotto V, et al. Intubation practices and adverse peri-intubation events in critically ill patients from 29 countries. JAMA. 2021;325:1164–72. https://doi.org/10.1001/jama.2021.1727.
3. Mort TC. Emergency tracheal intubation: complications associated with repeated laryngoscopic attempts. Anesth Analg. 2004;99:607–13, table of contents. https://doi.org/10.1213/01.ANE.0000122825.04923.15.
4. De Jong A, Rolle A, Molinari N, Paugam-Burtz C, Constantin JM, Lefrant JY, Asehnoune K, Jung B, Futier E, Chanques G, Azoulay E, Jaber S. Cardiac arrest and mortality related to intubation procedure in critically ill adult patients: a multicenter cohort study. Crit Care Med. 2018;46:532–9. https://doi.org/10.1097/CCM.0000000000002925.
5. Cook TM, Woodall N, Harper J, Benger J. Major complications of airway management in the UK: results of the Fourth National Audit Project of the Royal College of Anaesthetists and the Difficult Airway Society. Part 2: intensive care and emergency departments. Br J Anaesth. 2011;106:632–42. https://doi.org/10.1093/bja/aer059.
6. Myatra SN, Divatia JV, Brewster DJ. The physiologically difficult airway: an emerging concept. Curr Opin Anaesthesiol. 2022;35(2):115–21. https://doi.org/10.1097/ACO.0000000000001102.
7. Levitan RM, Everett WW, Ochroch EA. Limitations of difficult airway prediction in patients intubated in the emergency department. Ann Emerg Med. 2004;44:307–13. https://doi.org/10.1016/j.annemergmed.2004.05.006.

8. De Jong A, Molinari N, Terzi N, Mongardon N, Arnal JM, Guitton C, et al. Early identification of patients at risk for difficult intubation in the intensive care unit: development and validation of the MACOCHA score in a multicenter cohort study. Am J Respir Crit Care Med. 2013;187(8):832–9.
9. Scott JA, Heard SO, Zayaruzny M, Walz JM. Airway management in critical illness: an update. Chest. 2020;157:877–87. https://doi.org/10.1016/j.chest.2019.10.026.
10. Smischney NJ, Surani SR, Montgomery A, Franco PM, Callahan C, Demiralp G, Tedja R, Lee S, Kumar SI, Khanna AK. Hypotension prediction score for endotracheal intubation in critically ill patients: a post hoc analysis of the HEMAIR study. J Intensive Care Med. 2022;37:1467–79. https://doi.org/10.1177/08850666221085256.
11. Smischney NJ, Kashyap R, Khanna AK, Brauer E, Morrow LE, Seisa MO, Schroeder DR, Diedrich DA, Montgomery A, Franco PM, Ofoma UR, Kaufman DA, Sen A, Callahan C, Venkata C, Demiralp G, Tedja R, Lee S, Geube M, Kumar SI, Morris P, Bansal V, Surani S. Risk factors for and prediction of post-intubation hypotension in critically ill adults: a multicenter prospective cohort study. PLoS One. 2020;15:e0233852. https://doi.org/10.1371/journal.pone.0233852.
12. Kornas RL, Owyang CG, Sakles JC, Foley LJ, Mosier JM, Terndrup T, French A, Galgon R, Friedland T, Feinleib J, Olvera DJ, Guillote C, Fuller D, Hagberg C, Steffani M, Mark L, Owyang CG. Evaluation and management of the physiologically difficult airway: consensus recommendations from Society for Airway Management. Anesth Analg. 2021;132:395–405. https://doi.org/10.1213/ANE.0000000000005233.
13. Michard F. Changes in arterial pressure during mechanical ventilation. Anesthesiology. 2005;103:419–28; quiz 449–5. https://doi.org/10.1097/00000542-200508000-00026.
14. Green RS, Fergusson DA, Turgeon AF, McIntyre LA, Kovacs GJ, Griesdale DE, Zarychanski R, Butler MB, Kureshi N, Erdogan M. Resuscitation prior to emergency endotracheal intubation: results of a national survey. West J Emerg Med. 2016;17:542–8. https://doi.org/10.5811/westjem.2016.6.30503.
15. Janz DR, Casey JD, Semler MW, et al. Effect of a fluid bolus on cardiovascular collapse among critically ill adults undergoing tracheal intubation (PrePARE): a randomised controlled trial. Lancet Respir Med. 2019;7:1039–47. https://doi.org/10.1016/S2213-2600(19)30246-2.
16. Russell DW, Casey JD, Gibbs KW, et al. Effect of fluid bolus administration on cardiovascular collapse among critically ill patients undergoing tracheal intubation: a randomized clinical trial. JAMA. 2022;328:270–9. https://doi.org/10.1001/jama.2022.9792.
17. Jaber S, Jung B, Corne P, Sebbane M, Muller L, Chanques G, Verzilli D, Jonquet O, Eledjam JJ, Lefrant JY. An intervention to decrease complications related to endotracheal intubation in the intensive care unit: a prospective, multiple-center study. Intensive Care Med. 2010;36:248–55. https://doi.org/10.1007/s00134-009-1717-8.
18. Jabaley CS. Managing the physiologically difficult airway in critically ill adults. Crit Care. 2023;27:91. https://doi.org/10.1186/s13054-023-04371-3.
19. Di Nicolò P, Tavazzi G, Nannoni L, Corradi F. Inferior vena cava ultrasonography for volume status evaluation: an intriguing promise never fulfilled. J Clin Med. 2023;12:2217. https://doi.org/10.3390/jcm12062217.
20. Asokan R, Bhardwaj BB, Agrawal N, Chauhan U, Pillai A, Shankar T, Lalneiruol DJ, Baid H, Chawang H, Patel SM. Point of care gastric ultrasound to predict aspiration in patients undergoing urgent endotracheal intubation in the emergency medicine department. BMC Emerg Med. 2023;23:111. https://doi.org/10.1186/s12873-023-00881-z.
21. Khorsand S, Chin J, Rice J, Bughrara N, Myatra SN, Karamchandani K. Role of point-of-care ultrasound in emergency airway management outside the operating room. Anesth Analg. 2023;137:124–36. https://doi.org/10.1213/ANE.0000000000006371.
22. Mort TC, Waberski BH, Clive J. Extending the preoxygenation period from 4 to 8 mins in critically ill patients undergoing emergency intubation. Crit Care Med. 2009;37:68–71. https://doi.org/10.1097/CCM.0b013e318192845e.

23. Baillard C, Fosse JP, Sebbane M, Chanques G, Vincent F, Courouble P, Cohen Y, Eledjam JJ, Adnet F, Jaber S. Noninvasive ventilation improves preoxygenation before intubation of hypoxic patients. Am J Respir Crit Care Med. 2006;174:171–7. https://doi.org/10.1164/rccm.200509-1507OC.
24. Baillard C, Prat G, Jung B, Futier E, Lefrant JY, Vincent F, Hamdi A, Vicaut E, Jaber S. Effect of preoxygenation using non-invasive ventilation before intubation on subsequent organ failures in hypoxaemic patients: a randomised clinical trial. Br J Anaesth. 2018;120:361–7. https://doi.org/10.1016/j.bja.2017.11.067.
25. Frat JP, Ricard JD, Quenot JP, et al. Non-invasive ventilation versus high-flow nasal cannula oxygen therapy with apnoeic oxygenation for preoxygenation before intubation of patients with acute hypoxaemic respiratory failure: a randomised, multicentre, open-label trial. Lancet Respir Med. 2019;7:303–12. https://doi.org/10.1016/S2213-2600(19)30048-7.
26. Jaber S, Monnin M, Girard M, Conseil M, Cisse M, Carr J, Mahul M, Delay JM, Belafia F, Chanques G, Molinari N, De Jong A. Apnoeic oxygenation via high-flow nasal cannula oxygen combined with non-invasive ventilation preoxygenation for intubation in hypoxaemic patients in the intensive care unit: the single-Centre, blinded, randomised controlled OPTINIV trial. Intensive Care Med. 2016;42:1877–87. https://doi.org/10.1007/s00134-016-4588-9.
27. Lyons C, Callaghan M. Uses and mechanisms of apnoeic oxygenation: a narrative review. Anaesthesia. 2019;74:497–507. https://doi.org/10.1111/anae.14565.
28. Lodenius Å, Piehl J, Östlund A, Ullman J, Jonsson Fagerlund M. Transnasal humidified rapid-insufflation ventilatory exchange (THRIVE) vs. facemask breathing pre-oxygenation for rapid sequence induction in adults: a prospective randomised non-blinded clinical trial. Anaesthesia. 2018;73:564–71. https://doi.org/10.1111/anae.14215.
29. Mir F, Patel A, Iqbal R, Cecconi M, Nouraei SA. A randomised controlled trial comparing transnasal humidified rapid insufflation ventilatory exchange (THRIVE) pre-oxygenation with facemask pre-oxygenation in patients undergoing rapid sequence induction of anaesthesia. Anaesthesia. 2017;72:439–43. https://doi.org/10.1111/anae.13799.
30. Semler MW, Janz DR, Russell DW, et al. A multicenter, randomized trial of ramped position vs sniffing position during endotracheal intubation of critically ill adults. Chest. 2017;152:712–22. https://doi.org/10.1016/j.chest.2017.03.061.
31. Higgs A, McGrath BA, Goddard C, Rangasami J, Suntharalingam G, Gale R, Cook TM. Guidelines for the management of tracheal intubation in critically ill adults. Br J Anaesth. 2018;120:323–52. https://doi.org/10.1016/j.bja.2017.10.021.
32. Myatra SN, Ahmed SM, Kundra P, Garg R, Ramkumar V, Patwa A, Shah A, Raveendra US, Shetty SR, Doctor JR, Pawar DK, Ramesh S, Das S, Divatia JV. Republication: all India difficult airway association 2016 guidelines for tracheal intubation in the intensive care unit. Indian J Crit Care Med. 2017;21:146–53. https://doi.org/10.4103/ijccm.IJCCM_57_17.
33. Birenbaum A, Hajage D, Roche S, Ntouba A, Eurin M, Cuvillon P, Rohn A, Compere V, Benhamou D, Biais M, Menut R, Benachi S, Lenfant F, Riou B. Effect of cricoid pressure compared with a sham procedure in the rapid sequence induction of anesthesia: the IRIS randomized clinical trial. JAMA Surg. 2019;154:9–17. https://doi.org/10.1001/jamasurg.2018.3577.
34. Casey JD, Janz DR, Russell DW, et al. Bag-mask ventilation during tracheal intubation of critically ill adults. N Engl J Med. 2019;380:811–21. https://doi.org/10.1056/NEJMoa1812405.
35. Schulte TE, Ringenberg KJ, Lisco SJ, Sayles H, Shillcutt SK. Trainee experience and success of urgent airway management. J Clin Anesth. 2016;35:536–42. https://doi.org/10.1016/j.jclinane.2016.07.041.
36. Cook TM, El-Boghdadly K, McGuire B, McNarry AF, Patel A, Higgs A. Consensus guidelines for managing the airway in patients with COVID-19: guidelines from the Difficult Airway Society, the Association of Anaesthetists the Intensive Care Society, the Faculty of Intensive Care Medicine and the Royal College of Anaesthetists. Anaesthesia. 2020;75:785–99. https://doi.org/10.1111/anae.15054.

37. Kotani Y, Piersanti G, Maiucci G, Fresilli S, Turi S, Montanaro G, Zangrillo A, Lee TC, Landoni G. Etomidate as an induction agent for endotracheal intubation in critically ill patients: a meta-analysis of randomized trials. J Crit Care. 2023;77:154317. https://doi.org/10.1016/j.jcrc.2023.154317.
38. Himmelseher S, Durieux ME. Revising a dogma: ketamine for patients with neurological injury. Anesth Analg. 2005;101:524–34. https://doi.org/10.1213/01.ANE.0000160585.43587.5B.
39. Matchett G, Gasanova I, Riccio CA, et al. Etomidate versus ketamine for emergency endotracheal intubation: a randomized clinical trial. Intensive Care Med. 2022;48:78–91. https://doi.org/10.1007/s00134-021-06577-x.
40. Wan C, Hanson AC, Schulte PJ, Dong Y, Bauer PR. Propofol, ketamine, and etomidate as induction agents for intubation and outcomes in critically ill patients: a retrospective cohort study. Crit Care Explor. 2021;3:e0435. https://doi.org/10.1097/CCE.0000000000000435.
41. Tarwade P, Smischney NJ. Endotracheal intubation sedation in the intensive care unit. World J Crit Care Med. 2022;11:33–9. https://doi.org/10.5492/wjccm.v11.i1.33.
42. Miller M, Groombridge CJ, Lyon R. Haemodynamic changes to a midazolam-fentanyl-rocuronium protocol for pre-hospital anaesthesia following return of spontaneous circulation after cardiac arrest. Anaesthesia. 2017;72:585–91. https://doi.org/10.1111/anae.13809.
43. Hristovska AM, Duch P, Allingstrup M, Afshari A. Efficacy and safety of sugammadex versus neostigmine in reversing neuromuscular blockade in adults. Cochrane Database Syst Rev. 2017;8:CD012763. https://doi.org/10.1002/14651858.CD012763.
44. Trent SA, Kaji AH, Carlson JN, McCormick T, Haukoos JS, Brown CA. Video laryngoscopy is associated with first-pass success in emergency department intubations for trauma patients: a propensity score matched analysis of the National Emergency Airway Registry. Ann Emerg Med. 2021;78:708–19. https://doi.org/10.1016/j.annemergmed.2021.07.115.
45. Arulkumaran N, Lowe J, Ions R, Mendoza M, Bennett V, Dunser MW. Videolaryngoscopy versus direct laryngoscopy for emergency orotracheal intubation outside the operating room: a systematic review and meta-analysis. Br J Anaesth. 2018;120:712–24. https://doi.org/10.1016/j.bja.2017.12.041.
46. Jaber S, Rollé A, Godet T, et al. Effect of the use of an endotracheal tube and stylet versus an endotracheal tube alone on first-attempt intubation success: a multicentre, randomised clinical trial in 999 patients. Intensive Care Med. 2021;47:653–64. https://doi.org/10.1007/s00134-021-06417-y.
47. Root CW, Mitchell OJL, Brown R, Evers CB, Boyle J, Griffin C, West FM, Gomm E, Miles E, McGuire B, Swaminathan A, St George J, Horowitz JM, DuCanto J. Suction Assisted Laryngoscopy and Airway Decontamination (SALAD): a technique for improved emergency airway management. Resusc Plus. 2020;1-2:100005. https://doi.org/10.1016/j.resplu.2020.100005.
48. Apfelbaum JL, Hagberg CA, Connis RT, Abdelmalak BB, Agarkar M, Dutton RP, Fiadjoe JE, Greif R, Klock PA, Mercier D, Myatra SN, O'Sullivan EP, Rosenblatt WH, Sorbello M, Tung A. 2022 American Society of Anesthesiologists practice guidelines for management of the difficult airway. Anesthesiology. 2022;136:31–81. https://doi.org/10.1097/ALN.0000000000004002.
49. Karamchandani K, Wheelwright J, Yang AL, Westphal ND, Khanna AK, Myatra SN. Emergency airway management outside the operating room: current evidence and management strategies. Anesth Analg. 2021;133:648–62. https://doi.org/10.1213/ANE.0000000000005644.
50. Chrimes N, Higgs A, Hagberg CA, Baker PA, Cooper RM, Greif R, Kovacs G, Law JA, Marshall SD, Myatra SN, O'Sullivan EP, Rosenblatt WH, Ross CH, Sakles JC, Sorbello M, Cook TM. Preventing unrecognised oesophageal intubation: a consensus guideline from the Project for Universal Management of Airways and international airway societies. Anaesthesia. 2022;77:1395–415. https://doi.org/10.1111/anae.15817.

51. De Jong A, Myatra SN, Roca O, Jaber S. How to improve intubation in the intensive care unit. Update on knowledge and devices. Intensive Care Med. 2022;48:1287–98. https://doi.org/10.1007/s00134-022-06849-0.
52. Corl KA, Dado C, Agarwal A, Azab N, Amass T, Marks SJ, Levy MM, Merchant RC, Aliotta J. A modified Montpellier protocol for intubating intensive care unit patients is associated with an increase in first-pass intubation success and fewer complications. J Crit Care. 2018;44:191–5. https://doi.org/10.1016/j.jcrc.2017.11.014.

Chapter 10
Awake Tracheal Intubation

Neel Desai and El-Boghdadly Kariem

Highlights

- Awake tracheal intubation is underutilized but must be considered if difficult airway management is predicted.
- Preparation, conduct, and management of complications should account for oxygenation, topicalization, sedation, and procedural performance.
- Supplemental oxygen should be delivered whenever awake tracheal intubation is performed, regardless of whether sedation is used or not.
- Topicalization is key to successful awake tracheal intubation. It should be performed and tested meticulously before attempting awake tracheal intubation. Dosing of lidocaine should be less than 9 mg per kg of lean body weight.
- If indicated, minimal sedation should be used cautiously, and ideally delivered, titrated, and monitored by an independent practitioner.
- Awake tracheal intubation can be performed with a videolaryngoscope or flexible bronchoscope, and the principles for each are the same.
- Performance of awake tracheal intubation should include minimizing the number of attempts to three, with a fourth one by a more experienced operator. A two-point check of visual confirmation and capnography should be undertaken before induction of general anesthesia following awake tracheal intubation.

N. Desai (✉) · E.-B. Kariem
Guy's and St Thomas' NHS Foundation Trust, London, UK
e-mail: neel.desai4@nhs.net; kariem.el-boghdadly@nhs.net

M. Á. Gómez-Ríos, A. van Zundert (eds.), *Evidence-based Guide to Difficult Airway Management*, https://doi.org/10.1007/978-3-032-30769-9_10

10.1 Introduction

Airway management in an anesthetized patient can be difficult. The incidence of difficult facemask ventilation, difficult supraglottic airway device (SAD) placement or ventilation, difficult tracheal intubation and difficult facemask ventilation and tracheal intubation, respectively, has been reported to be 0.66–2.5% [1–4], 0.5–4.7% [5–9], 1.9–10% [1, 4, 10–12], and 0.3–0.4% [4]. If facemask ventilation, SAD placement or ventilation, or tracheal intubation are predicted to be difficult, then a strategy for safe airway management, such as awake tracheal intubation (ATI), is likely to be indicated. Awake tracheal intubation is a procedure in which a trachea tube is inserted in an awake patient with the use of flexible bronchoscopy (ATI:FB) or videolaryngoscopy (ATI:VL) [13]. Safety is maintained with the preservation of spontaneous ventilation and intrinsic airway tone [14–18], and the potential risks of difficult airway management in the anesthetized patient are therefore obviated [19]. In this chapter, we will consider the indications, consent, procedural set-up, oxygenation, sedation and topicalization strategy, and performance of ATI in adults, with further discussion of the management of complications and unsuccessful ATI. Importantly, we will base many of these principles on the guidelines from the Difficult Airway Society (DAS) on ATI [20], highlighting key areas that have developed since.

10.2 Indications

Airway assessment, which includes history, examination, and review of investigations, must be carried out in all patients (Grade D) [21–24]. Characteristics of patients who are likely to need ATI are: morbid obesity; decreased mouth opening; limited neck extension; obstructive sleep apnea; head and neck pathology such as malignancy or previous radiotherapy and surgery; and progressive airway compromise [15, 16, 18, 25, 26]. The indicators of difficult airway management, however, are not reliable [1, 10, 27] and the evidence for individual predictive assessment tools is modest. That said, if indicators of difficult airway management are present, then ATI should be considered (Grade D). In the elective setting, the patient should be fasted (Grade D), and it is important to consider that the nonfasted patient can still regurgitate or aspirate their gastric contents with ATI. The relative contraindications to ATI include the presence of airway bleeding, local anesthetic allergy and the uncooperative patient; however, the only absolute contraindication is patient refusal.

10.3 Consent

Consent is an opportunity for the anesthesiologist to establish a rapport with the patient and prepare them psychologically, potentially increasing the confidence and cooperation of the patient with ATI should they consent to it (Grade D). It is essential that patients are provided with information, ideally including a patient information leaflet, in a timely manner [28]. The rationale, benefits, complications, and risks of and alternatives to ATI should be discussed, and their informed consent thus obtained. They should be forewarned of the unpleasant flavor of local anesthetic, comparing it to the taste of old banana or tonic water, and be readied to participate actively in the process of ATI, including the taking of deep breaths, gargling, and swallowing.

10.4 Procedural Set-Up

Awake tracheal intubation is associated with significant operator physical and psychological stress [29], which can be associated with adverse complications [30, 31]. Thus, having a competent and well-trained assistant present is important. Moreover, using a cognitive aid can improve performance and outcomes [32] and should be considered (Grade D). Safety must be preserved at all times and not threatened by the perception of time pressure.

The ideal environment in which to perform ATI is the operating room, as the necessary equipment, drugs, and skilled assistance are readily accessible (Grade D). Minimum equipment should ideally include a difficult airway cart, patient monitor, oxygen delivery system, suction, drugs and their delivery systems, and resuscitation equipment. In the high-risk patient, who may have airway obstruction, respiratory failure, hypoxia, or otherwise challenging ATI, the operating room may be preferable to the anesthetic or pre-operative preparation room as it is more spacious and has the potential for immediate surgical support [21, 33]. As a minimum, it is recommended that ECG, noninvasive blood pressure, pulse oximetry, and, if possible, continuous end-tidal carbon dioxide monitoring are used (Grade C) [34]. Complications in ATI that may be detected by monitoring following the administration of medications for topicalization and sedation include airway obstruction and hypoventilation due to oversedation [16–18, 35], and perturbations of cardiac rhythm and blood pressure [18, 36–38]. Utilization of processed electroencephalogram depth of anesthesia monitoring, such as bispectral index, can decrease the risk of oversedation and should be weighed against the risk of increased cognitive load for the operator. The ergonomics of the workplace, including optimizing the position of the patient, operator, and assistants as well as the location of the equipment and monitor, can influence conduct and safety of ATI (Grade D) [33, 39]. It is important, e.g., for the operator to have a direct and unobstructed line of sight to the FB or VL monitor. There is no consensus on the ideal operator or patient position

[40–43], but sitting up the patient may have anatomical and physiologic advantages such as reduced upper airway collapsibility, increased functional residual capacity and longer safe apnea time in the obese patient [44–46].

Choosing an appropriate route for tracheal intubation, a visualization device, and tracheal tube is important. First, the route for ATI should consider the patient anatomy, surgical access and plan for tracheal extubation. In the patient with limited mouth opening, the nasal approach may be the only option, and in the patient scheduled for nasal surgery, the oral approach might be preferred. If both routes of tracheal intubation are possible, then there remains no robust data or agreement indicating the superiority of one approach over the other [16–18, 40, 47]. Second, ATI:FB was found to have a similar first pass success rate to ATI:VL in a systematic review with no differences in regard to the incidence of esophageal intubation, requirement for change of airway technique, oxygen desaturation, airway bleeding, or the rate of hoarseness and sore throat [48]. Given this, selecting between these ATI techniques is influenced by the availability of equipment, patient factors, and operator skills. In the patient, for example, with fixed flexion deformity of the neck, a large tongue or poor mouth opening, ATI:FB may be more appropriate. In the patient, for instance, with airway bleeding, ATI:VL might be more suitable. If the selected ATI technique is not successful, then operators should consider an alternative, such as ATI:FB should ATI:VL be unsuccessful (Grade D). FB and VL can be combined in a unified approach to ATI in the setting of complex clinical scenarios (Grade D) [49–51]. Single-use and reusable FBs have been shown to have a similar safety profile [52]. Operators should therefore consider local availability and personal experience in determining which FB to use (Grade B). Similarly, there is still no evidence or agreement among experts to support the superiority of any individual VL for ATI. In view of this, operators are advised to utilize VLs with which they are most familiar (Grade B). Third, the nature of the tracheal tube selection and design is fundamental to the success of ATI, including consideration of its internal and external diameter, length, material, shape, and tip design. For ATI:VL, the selection of an appropriate tracheal tube is similar to that in an anesthetized patient and is influenced by the VL in question. With respect to ATI:FB, the reinforced tracheal tubes and Parker Flex-Tip™ (Bridgwater, CN, USA) and intubating laryngeal mask (LMA® Fastrach™ ETT, Teleflex, Beaconsfield, UK) tracheal tubes have been shown to be superior to standard polyvinylchloride tracheal tubes for advancing the tracheal tube over the FB, decreasing laryngeal impingement and increasing ease of tracheal intubation [53–61]. The use of a standard polyvinylchloride tracheal tube is thus not recommended (Grade A). Impingement may be mitigated by the utilization of the smallest appropriate external diameter tracheal tube (Grade B) and posterior positioning of the bevel of the tracheal tube [55, 57, 61].

In the event of unsuccessful ATI, the next step, be it postponement, front-of-neck airway, or high-risk general anesthesia, should be discussed and agreed on by all members of the team prior to embarking upon the ATI.

10.5 Oxygenation

In patients who receive sedation, the administration of oxygen compared to air has been demonstrated to decrease the incidence of oxygen desaturation [62–66]. Regardless of sedation used, application of supplemental oxygen during ATI is advised (Grade B) and should be commenced on patient arrival for the procedure and continued throughout the procedure (Grade D). If low-flow techniques of less than 30 L of oxygen per minute are used for ATI, the incidence of arterial oxygen desaturation ($SpO_2 \leq 90\%$) has been reported to be 12–16% [35, 67, 68]. In the presence of high-flow, humidified and warmed nasal oxygen, the incidence of oxygen desaturation has been shown to be 0–1.5% [16, 69]. Should it be available, high-flow nasal oxygen should therefore be the technique of choice, particularly as it can not only oxygenate but also provide continuous positive airway pressure and open soft tissue airway passages and support the distribution of local anesthetic.

10.6 Airway Topicalization

Understanding the innervation of the upper airway is essential to adequately anesthetize the relevant structures. The nose is innervated by branches of the trigeminal nerve. The septum and anterior parts of the nasal cavity are innervated by the anterior ethmoidal nerve, a branch of the ophthalmic nerve. The rest of the nasal cavity is supplied by the greater and lesser palatine nerves, branches of the maxillary nerve. The posterior third of the tongue, tonsils, vallecula, and anterior surface of the vallecula are innervated by the tonsillar nerve, a branch of the glossopharyngeal nerve, and the posterior and lateral wall of the pharynx is supplied by the pharyngeal nerve, a branch of the vagus nerve. In regard to the larynx, the posterior surface of the epiglottis, arytenoids, and aryepiglottic folds are innervated by the internal branch of the superior laryngeal nerve, a branch of the vagus nerve, and the vocal cords and structures inferior to the vocal cords are supplied by the recurrent laryngeal nerve, a branch of the vagus nerve.

Importantly, successful ATI relies on the effective topical application of local anesthetic to the airway. Lidocaine is the most commonly used local anesthetic for ATI and has a favorable cardiovascular and systemic toxicity risk profile [70]. Given that plasma levels exceeding toxic concentrations and clinical toxicity have been demonstrated with doses of lidocaine of 6–9.3 mg per kg of lean body weight [71–75], the dose of topical lidocaine has been advised not to be in excess of 9 mg per kg (Grade C) [76]. This, however, is not a target to aspire to but a maximum dose that operators should tend to find is rarely needed. The total dose of local anesthetic administered for ATI and other anesthetic and surgical interventions, including regional anesthesia and surgical infiltration, must be considered (Grade D). Studies have found lower concentrations of lidocaine to be as effective as higher concentrations [73, 77–79], although the latter may be associated with a more rapid onset of airway anesthesia. In case of local anesthetic systemic toxicity, emergency drugs, such as intralipid emulsion, must be readily available and emergency protocols should be in place [80–82].

The passage of the FB and tracheal tube can give rise to bleeding, and vasoconstriction of the nasal passage decreases the incidence of epistaxis [83, 84]. Before nasal tracheal intubation, the use of topical nasal vasoconstrictors should be considered (Grade A). Cocaine for topicalization and vasoconstriction may result in cardiovascular complications [85–88], and its efficacy during nasal tracheal tube insertion is not superior to co-phenylcaine [89], which is constituted by lidocaine 5% and phenylephrine 0.5%. Hence, in ATI, cocaine is not advised and co-phenylcaine is recommended for airway topicalization (Grade A).

Absorption of local anesthetic tends to vary based on the delivery method [90], although this should not influence the maximal dose calculation. There are insufficient data or expert agreement to indicate any individual topicalization technique, such as mucosal atomization, nebulization, spray as you go, or transtracheal injection, to be superior [91]. Nebulized lidocaine can be used, but its effectiveness and absorption, when delivered in this manner, is variable [92]. In the case of transtracheal injection, if it is performed with a suitable cannula, this can be utilized for rescue oxygenation or to provide a conduit for the passage of a guidewire to facilitate percutaneous tracheostomy. Glossopharyngeal and superior laryngeal nerve blockade, however, has been related to increased plasma concentration of local anesthetic, local anesthetic systemic toxicity, and reduced patient comfort [93–95]. In view of this, invasive techniques such as these should only be used by those with expertise in their performance (Grade B). The Difficult Airway Society's suggested airway topicalization regimen has been illustrated in Fig. 10.1. Once the airway is thought to be anesthetized, this may be tested in an atraumatic way with a soft suction catheter or rigid sucker [96], resulting in the simultaneous suction of residual local anesthetic and secretions (Grade D). If the patient gags, anesthesia of the glossopharyngeal nerve is inadequate, and should the patient cough, anesthesia of the superior laryngeal nerve is insufficient, presenting an opportunity to provide further local anesthetic topicalization.

Using antisialogogues, such as atropine, glycopyrronium, and hyoscine, can be associated with a decrease in airway secretions and an improvement in topical anesthesia, but may also cause undesirable consequences such as tachycardia, dizziness, and sedation [97]. In the anesthetized patient, the visual clarity through the FB may be improved [98], although limited evidence supports their use in ATI. If it is used, and in the absence of sufficient data on the intravenous route in this setting, intramuscular antisialogogues should be injected between 40–60 min prior to performing ATI to achieve the peak mucosal drying effect in a timely manner.

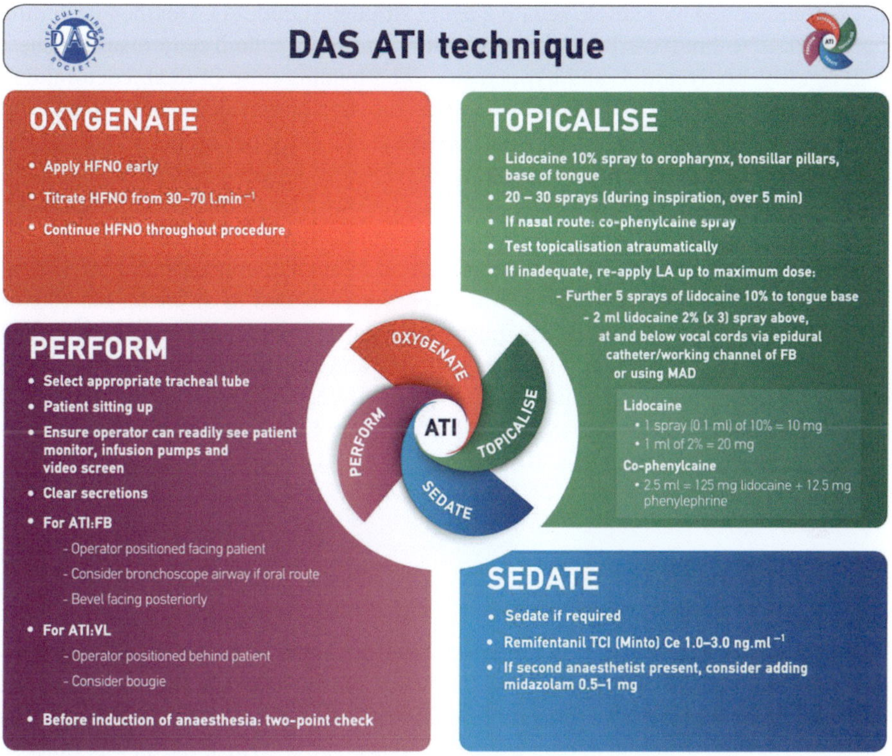

Fig. 10.1 The approach to ATI as recommended by the Difficult Airway Society. (Reproduced with permission. © Difficult Airway Society. *ATI* awake tracheal intubation, *Ce* effect site concentration, *DAS* Difficult Airway Society, *FB* flexible bronchoscopy, *HFNO* high flow nasal oxygen, *LA* local anesthetic, *MAD* mucosal atomizing device, *TCI* target controlled infusion, *VL* videolaryngoscopy)

10.7 Sedation

Sedation is not required for safe and effective ATI [16, 36, 37], but may decrease the anxiety and discomfort of the patient and hence increase their tolerance of the procedure [99]. If required, the cautious use of minimal sedation is advised (Grade D). Oversedation is a risk and its sequelae include respiratory depression, hypoxia, aspiration, loss of the airway, and cardiovascular instability. It is therefore desirable to have an independent and second anesthesiologist delivering, monitoring, and titrating sedation (Grade D), and this has the potential to decrease the cognitive load for the operator responsible for the performance of ATI. Importantly, sedation must not be used as a substitute for inadequate airway topicalization (Grade D) [91].

In terms of individual sedative medications, dexmedetomidine, and remifentanil are associated with reduced oversedation and airway obstruction and increased patient satisfaction [99]. Of interest, patient satisfaction with remifentanil persists even with the significant incidence of recall reported when it is used as a sole sedative medication. Dexmedetomidine or remifentanil is thus safest for the nonexpert and recommended as a single sedative agent strategy (Grade A). Dexmedetomidine can give rise to bradycardia and hypotension, and remifentanil may result in chest wall rigidity, bradycardia, and hypotension. The loading dose of dexmedetomidine is 1 μg per kg over 10–20 min followed by an infusion commencing at 0.7 μg per kg per h and titrated to the desired clinical effect at 0.2–1 μg per kg per h. One of the drawbacks of dexmedetomidine remains its relatively longer onset time. The loading dose of remifentanil is 0.05–0.1 μg per kg followed by an infusion titrated to the desired clinical effect at 0.03–0.1 μg per kg per min. Remifentanil can otherwise be provided as a target-controlled infusion with an effect site concentration of 1–3 ng per mL. In comparison to remifentanil, propofol is related to an increased risk of oversedation, coughing, and airway obstruction and is not recommended as the sole sedative agent (Grade A) [100–102]. Midazolam and remifentanil are reversible and can be utilized as part of a dual sedative agent strategy, recognizing the increased risk of oversedation with two synergistic drugs. The DAS-suggested sedation regimen has been illustrated in Fig. 10.1.

10.8 Performance

To conduct effective and safe ATI, familiarity with airway anatomy requires an optimal view and skillful manipulation of the FB or VL and tracheal tube. The optimal view can be gained and maintained if the FB tip is placed close to the center of the airspace. Further, whiteout occurs when the FB is positioned near the airway mucosa and may be seen in airway obstruction. If the view becomes obscured by secretions, this may be cleared by either asking the patient to swallow or gentle flexion of the FB tip against the airway mucosa. Fogging due to condensation may be decreased by either dabbing the FB tip on the tongue of the patient or placing it in warm water before commencing ATI:FB. For skillful manipulation, the FB should be inserted in the line of the airway, be it along the floor of the nose for the nasal approach or the mucosa of the tongue for the oral approach. Downward movement on the angulation control lever elevates the FB tip, placing it in the direction of the upper field of view, and upward movement on the angulation control lever depresses the FB tip, placing it in the direction of the lower field of view. Given that the angulation only moves the FB tip in one plane, rotation of the FB has the potential to facilitate sideways movement. Either the control section of the FB with one hand and its distal anchored part controlled with the contralateral hand near the patient's face can be rotated equally and simultaneously, or the control section of the FB can be rotated with one hand and the contralateral hand grip on its distal anchored part loosened to result in translation of the rotational movement to the FB tip.

In nasal ATI:FB, the following sequential steps can be followed:

– It is the authors' preference to face the patient who is placed in a sitting position with the legs slightly elevated when performing FB, and the size 5.5 or 6.0 nasal tracheal tube should be preloaded onto the FB.

- Hold the control section of the FB and advance its distal portion into the vestibule of the nose that the patient feels is subjectively more patent on sniffing.
- Follow the airspace between the floor of the nose and the inferior turbinate along the base of the septum in the irregularly shaped nasal cavity. Flexible bronchoscopy is likely to be more challenging between the inferior and middle turbinates due to variation in the anatomy and the presence of polyps. Further, damage to the middle turbinate can give rise to avulsion, epistaxis and trauma to the cribriform plate, which the ethmoid bone of the middle turbinate interfaces with, can result in cerebrospinal fluid rhinorrhea and olfactory nerve injury.
- If the nasopharyngeal isthmus seems to be closed, then the patient should be asked to breathe through their nose, as this maneuver should open up the airway. It is possible to lift the epiglottis by requesting the patient to phonate, stick out their tongue, or through the application of jaw thrust.
- Once the FB is advanced over the epiglottis, the arytenoids, and vocal cords should come into view. The FB should be passed so that the junction of the epiglottis and vocal cords is placed in the center of the field of view, and the view of the tracheal lumen may be lost as the FB tip passes over the arytenoid processes. At this point, the FB tip should be angled caudally in the line of the trachea, and the lumen of the trachea should reappear, recognized by the presence of a flattened posterior wall, that is the trachealis muscle, with longitudinal ridges and the presence of tracheal rings. Visualization of the carina is recommended (Grade D).
- Prior to passing the preloaded trachea tube over the FB, the tip of the FB should be stabilized to lie two to three tracheal rings superior to the carina.

In oral ATI:FB, the following sequential steps may be followed:

- It is the authors' preference to face the patient who is placed in a sitting position with the legs slightly elevated when performing FB, and the size 6.0 or 7.0 oral tracheal tube in women and men, respectively, should be preloaded onto the FB.
- Hold the control section of the FB, measure the distance from the angle of the mouth to the tragus and advance the distal portion of the FB that corresponds to this measured distance into the oral cavity in one movement.
- Identify the tongue, avoiding contact with it, and maintain the FB in the midline. It is possible for whiteout to occur if the operator deviates from the midline or the airway is obstructed. In the case of the former, the FB can either be rotated to the left or right or otherwise withdrawn until a recognizable view is obtained. If the airway is obstructed, as can occur should the tongue abut against the posterior pharyngeal wall, then the patient should be asked to open their mouth and stick out their tongue.
- If available, an intubating oral airway may be used to act as a midline conduit for the FB to bypass the oral cavity.
- The distance between the soft palate and the larynx is generally short, and the epiglottis should come into view as the oral cavity is navigated. It is possible to lift the epiglottis by requesting the patient to phonate and stick out their tongue or through the application of jaw thrust.

- Once the FB is advanced over the epiglottis, the arytenoids and vocal cords should come into view. The FB should be passed in such a manner that the junction of the epiglottis and vocal cords is placed in the center of the field of view, and the view of the tracheal lumen may be lost as the FB tip passes over the arytenoid processes. It is at this point that the FB tip should be angled caudally in the line of the trachea and the lumen of the trachea should reappear, recognized by the presence of a flattened posterior wall, that is, the trachealis muscle, with longitudinal ridges and the presence of tracheal rings. Visualization of the carina is recommended (Grade D).
- Prior to passing the preloaded trachea tube over the FB, the tip of the FB should be stabilized to lie two to three tracheal rings superior to the carina.

To pass the tracheal tube over the FB, the following sequential steps can be followed:

- Maintain the position of the FB with a view of the carina and gently pass the tracheal tube over the FB in a rotational manner.
- It is not uncommon for difficulties to be encountered at this point, the incidence of which has been estimated to be 0–90%, and this is due to the deviation of the course of the tracheal tube from that of the FB secondary to the physical gap present between these two [103].
- In the oral approach to ATI, the tracheal tube may tend to move posterior to the larynx, such as onto the arytenoid cartilage or esophageal inlet. The right arytenoid cartilage is more likely than the left arytenoid cartilage to obstruct the passage of the tracheal tube [104–106], and this is explained by the bevel and tip of the preformed tracheal tube, respectively, facing the left and right.
- In the nasal approach to ATI, the presence of a narrowed nasal passage, resulting from deviation of the septum, a nasal septal spur, or mucosal thickening of inflamed turbinates, and the epiglottis and arytenoid cartilages can obstruct the passage of the tracheal tube [47, 107, 108].
- Maneuvers to overcome the resistance to passage of the tracheal tube include: application of cricoid pressure as the esophageal inlet is then occluded, encouraging the tracheal tube to move anteriorly; flexion of the neck to relieve impingement of the tracheal tube on the anterior and internal surface of the subglottic area; release of jaw thrust if applied as the larynx is then shifted posteriorly and the esophageal inlet is narrowed; rotation of the conventional polyvinylchloride tracheal tube, particularly 90° in the anticlockwise direction, as the bevel should face posteriorly and the tip of the tube anteriorly; withdrawal of the tracheal tube followed by its rotation as it may have threatened to already enter the esophageal inlet; use of a flexible tracheal tube as it can change its direction more easily to follow the curve of the FB; utilization of the Parker Flex-Tip™ tracheal tube (Bridgewater, CN, USA) as it has a flexible tip positioned towards the center of its distal lumen, reducing the physical gap between the FB and the tube, and its bevel faces posteriorly rather than to the left, equivalent to the conventional tracheal tube being rotated 90° in the anticlockwise

direction; and use of the intubating laryngeal mask tracheal tube as it exhibits increased flexibility, and has a hemispherical and softer bevel with its leading edge in the midline [103].

In oral ATI:VL, the VL must be gently inserted, and the manufacturer's instructions regarding the operation of the channeled or unchanneled VL should be followed. It has been suggested, however, that channeled VLs may be preferable as unchanneled VLs such as the GlideScope™ might not be optimal as the operator is unable to visualize the distal tip of the blade, resulting in inadvertent distal placement and stimulation of gagging and coughing in the awake patient, and the stylets and tracheal introducers of unchanneled VL have been associated with airway trauma such as palatal and pharyngeal injuries [109, 110]. There is no consensus on the ideal positioning for performing oral ATI:VL, but there are benefits to the operator standing facing the patient. It should be noted that with this orientation, the VL image will be inverted to what is usually expected. In other words, the epiglottis may appear at the bottom of the screen. Thus, this may require some modifications to the handling of the tracheal tube and repositioning of the VL blade.

10.9 Confirmation of Tracheal Tube Placement

In ATI, the tracheal tube can be incorrectly placed in the pharynx, esophagus, or bronchus. Even though capnography has a sensitivity and specificity of 100% in the identification of the position of the tracheal tube in patients whose lungs are ventilated [111, 112], a capnographic trace may be present if the tracheal tube is placed in the supraglottic area or bronchus in the spontaneously breathing patient. In order to confirm the position of the tracheal tube, it is advised that a two-point check must be carried out. This consists of: first, the visualization of the tracheal lumen and carina with ATI:FB or the tracheal tube through the vocal cords with ATI:VL; and second, the presence of capnography to exclude esophageal intubation (Grade C).

Once the FB is in the trachea, the carina can be identified before advancing the tracheal tube over the FB to decrease the risk of misplacement (Grade D). It is important to evaluate the distance between the end of the tracheal tube and the carina prior to removing the FB (Grade D). On removal of the FB or VL, the correct position of the tracheal tube should be maintained. The timing of inflation of the tracheal tube cuff is influenced by the risk of aspiration, patient coughing, and movement and displacement of the tracheal tube (Grade D). If there are concerns, however, related to a possible tear of the tracheal tube cuff, then gentle inflation to check its integrity before induction of anesthesia is recommended (Grade D). General anesthesia should only be induced when the two-point check has been performed and verified the correct placement of the trachea tube in the trachea and not in the pharynx, esophagus, or bronchus.

10.10 Modifications of ATI Technique

In specific clinical circumstances, the individual components of ATI, namely oxygenation, topicalization, sedation, and performance, should be adapted, and these recommended modifications have been detailed in Table 10.1.

10.10.1 Management of Complications

In ATI, complications occur due to inadequate or suboptimal oxygenation, topicalization, sedation, and performance and have a frequency of up to 18% [16–18, 35, 113–115]. In the event of a complication, the cause should be determined to facilitate further management.

Table 10.1 Clinical circumstances with special considerations and recommendations of modifications to sedation, topicalization, oxygen and performance in order to achieve ATI in an effective and safe manner

Special circumstances	Considerations	How to do it
Critically ill	Increased respiratory secretions Limited physiologic reserve Increased oxygen demand and decreased oxygen reserve Increased cardiorespiratory sensitivity to sedative medications Increased risk of local anesthetic systemic toxicity Unstable for transfer to operating theater	Oxygenation: supplemental oxygen Topicalization: cautious use of local anesthetic; gentle suction of airway before commencement of ATI Sedation: avoid or minimize sedation Performance: do not transfer patient but maintain same standards of equipment, monitoring and staff support; and perform ATI in time critical manner
Obstetrics	Increased upper airway edema Increased risk of epistaxis Increased difficulty with FONA Increased oxygen demand and decreased oxygen reserve Increased risk of local anesthetic systemic toxicity Fetus at risk of sedation with benzodiazepines, long-acting opioids, and propofol	Oxygenation: supplemental oxygen Topicalization: cautious use of local anesthetic; use of prepregnancy lean body weight for local anesthetic dosing Sedation: consider sedation with dexmedetomidine or remifentanil; inform neonatologist of use of sedative medications Performance: oral approach to ATI; early identification and marking of cricothyroid membrane with use of airway ultrasound

(continued)

Table 10.1 (continued)

Special circumstances	Considerations	How to do it
Morbid obesity	Increased difficulty with FONA Increased oxygen demand and decreased oxygen reserve Presence of diaphragmatic splinting and decreased functional residual capacity Increased adverse sequelae to sedative medications Increased risk of local anesthetic systemic toxicity	Oxygenation: supplemental oxygen Topicalization: use lean body weight for local anesthetic dosing Sedation: avoid or minimize sedation Performance: sitting or reverse trendelenburg position to increase functional residual capacity; early identification and marking of cricothyroid membrane with use of airway ultrasound
Trauma	Airway soiling from hemorrhage, secretions, tissue edema, and vomitus Increased oxygen demand and decreased oxygen reserve Increased adverse sequelae to sedative medications Possible base of skull or facial fracture Unstable for transfer to operating theater	Oxygenation: avoid high flow nasal oxygen; supplemental oxygen Topicalization: gentle suction of airway before administration of local anesthetic Sedation: avoid or minimize sedation Performance: do not transfer patient but maintain same standards of equipment, monitoring, and staff support; oral approach to ATI; and consider ATI:VL
Trismus	Limited mouth opening Increased oxygen demand Increased adverse sequelae to sedative medications	Oxygenation: supplemental oxygen Topicalization: consider nebulized lidocaine, transtracheal lidocaine injection, or spray-as-you-go technique Sedation: avoid or minimize sedation Performance: nasal approach to ATI
Stridor	Airway obstruction Presence of narrowed airway Risk of laryngospasm Increased adverse sequelae to sedative medications	Oxygenation: consider high flow nasal oxygen Topicalization: consider lower concentration of lidocaine and nebulized lidocaine Sedation: avoid or minimize sedation Performance: most experienced operator to do ATI; use smaller tracheal tube; and prepare for FONA

Complications of ATI include airway trauma, bleeding, airway obstruction, and unsuccessful ATI. Given this, the operator should consider if they need more experienced support before commencing ATI (Grade D), ensure that oxygenation, topicalization, sedation, and performance is optimized (Grade D), and minimize the number of attempts at ATI (Grade D). Each unsuccessful attempt has been defined as the unplanned removal of the FB, VL, or tracheal tube from the airway. The Difficult Airway Society in the United Kingdom has advised that if unsuccessful at the first attempt, the operator should reassess, optimize inadequate oxygenation, topicalization, sedation, and performance, and call for help (Grade D). Strategies to optimize oxygenation, topicalization, sedation, and performance include clear airway obstruction, change mode of oxygen delivery, increase fractional inspired concentration of oxygen, and decrease or reverse sedation for oxygenation; additional topicalization to a maximum of 9 mg per kg of lean body weight for lidocaine; review of sedation regimen and consideration of reversal agents for sedation; and seeking more experienced help, use of airway suction or alternative tracheal intubation route or device, and changing the type of tracheal tube. Further, if the operator is still unsuccessful at the second attempt, then a third may be considered only if the oxygenation, topicalization, sedation and performance conditions are still amenable to further improvement (Grade D). Changing the airway device, such as switching from the FB to the VL, should be tallied in the total number of attempts. The fourth and final attempt at ATI should be undertaken by a more experienced operator and this may include a surgeon (Grade D).

10.10.2 Management of Unsuccessful ATI

It is rare not to achieve ATI after 3 + 1 attempts, but when it does occur, the unsuccessful ATI algorithm illustrated in Fig. 10.2 and recommended by DAS should be followed. Immediate actions include calling for help, applying 100% oxygen, and stopping and, if needed, reversing the effect of previously administered sedative medications (Grade D). In the event of unsuccessful ATI, the standard next step should be to postpone the procedure (Grade D), although immediate airway management may be required in some circumstances, such as those where airway patency, ventilation, or neurology is compromised, clinical deterioration is expected, or urgent or immediate surgery is needed.

If immediate airway management is required after unsuccessful ATI:FB or ATI:VL, securing the airway should be ATI with front-of-neck airway (ATI:FONA) using cricothyroidotomy or tracheostomy (Grade D). Awake tracheal intubation with FONA should be performed by the most skilled clinician (Grade C). Should ATI:FONA be unsuccessful, the next step is high-risk general anesthesia. The formulation of the airway management strategy at this juncture should take into consideration the Difficult Airway Society's guidelines for the unanticipated difficult tracheal intubation [22], and the reasons underlying the previous unsuccessful attempts at ATI. Moreover, the high-risk general anesthesia strategy should include the intravenous induction of anesthesia, full neuromuscular blockade and the use of a VL by the most skilled clinician at the first attempt at tracheal intubation [22, 116].

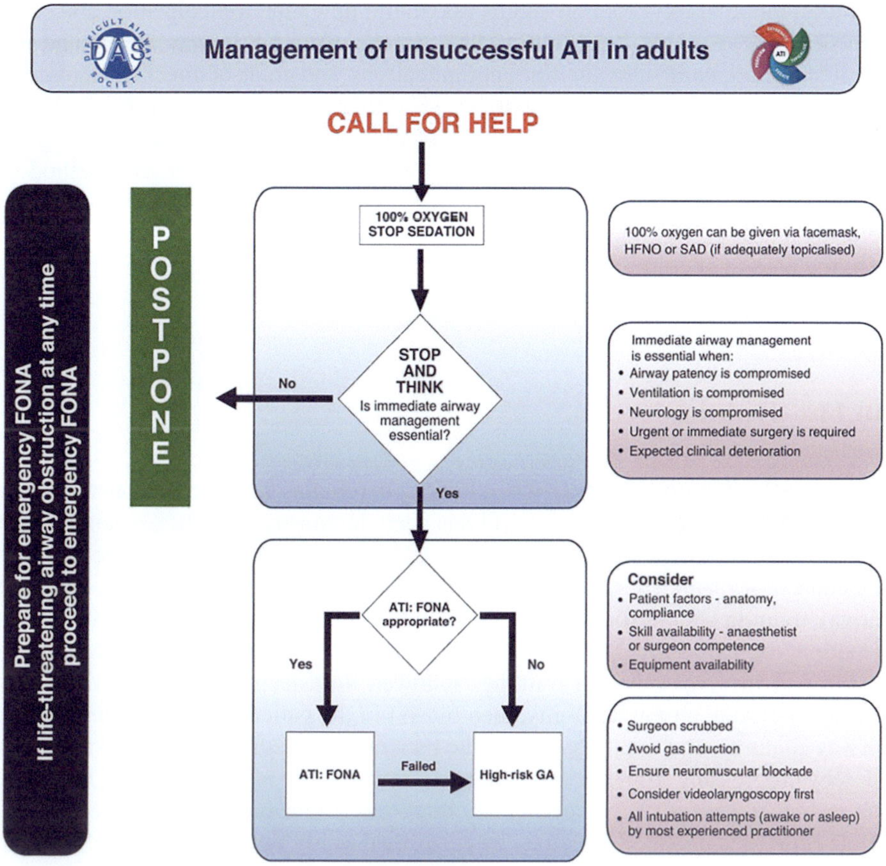

Fig. 10.2 The management of unsuccessful ATI as recommended by the Difficult Airway Society. (Reproduced with permission. © Difficult Airway Society. *GA* general anesthesia, *HFNO* high flow nasal oxygen)

10.10.3 Management of the Patient Following Tracheal Intubation

The patient who has had an ATI for predicted difficult airway management remains at high risk of adverse events and complications at tracheal extubation [21] and needs an appropriate tracheal extubation strategy [117]. Direct or videolaryngoscopy may be used to support the risk stratification of tracheal extubation. Importantly, the view at laryngoscopy may be modified by the presence of a tracheal tube, and the laryngoscopy grade or percentage of glottic opening can rule out but not rule in easy subsequent asleep tracheal intubation.

In order to inform and guide future patient management, detailed documentation in the clinical records is required [21]. The suggested minimum documented dataset includes: mode of oxygenation and its maximum flow rate; topicalization and sedation strategy; approach, be it oral, right nasal, or left nasal; airway device and tracheal tube used; number of attempts; complications; and grade of direct laryngoscopy or percentage of glottic opening with VL prior to tracheal extubation (Grade D).

The lidocaine used for airway topicalization has a dose-dependent analgesic duration of up to 40 min, and this varies with the concentration and method of administration [118, 119]. It may be a longer period of time before the laryngeal reflexes return [120] and, as the terminal elimination half-life of lidocaine is up to 2 h, the patient should remain nil by mouth for at least this period of time subsequent to topicalization.

10.11 Training

Awake tracheal intubation, even when indicated, remains an underused airway technique. Successful performance of ATI has been demonstrated to be associated with experience rather than seniority [16]. The technical aspects of ATI can be learnt in the context of manikins, simulators, cadavers, and patients [36, 121–126], and such airway training should focus on the fundamental components of ATI, namely oxygenation, topicalization, sedation, and performance. A stepwise approach to training in ATI involves manikin training, followed by asleep FB in the patient with predicted normal airway anatomy, then by ATI in the patient with predicted normal airway anatomy, and finally by ATI in the patient with predicted abnormal anatomy, thereby progressing from settings of lower stress to those of higher stress [127]. The nontechnical aspects of ATI are equally important and should be developed (Grade B). If consent is obtained, ATI may be performed solely for the purposes of training (Grade D), and team training in ATI should include anesthetic assistants, operating department practitioners, theater staff, and surgeons.

10.12 Conclusions and Future Directions

The fundamental components of ATI, that is, oxygenation, topicalization, sedation and procedural performance, are equally important. Optimization of these individual components increases the success rate of ATI. Specific clinical circumstances, such as in the setting of the critically ill or obstetric patient, require modifications to the technique to reduce risk and result in successful and uneventful tracheal intubation. The two-point check to confirm tracheal tube placement must be performed prior to induction of general anesthesia.

Future research should be performed to improve clinical and patient-centered outcomes [13]. The optimal airway topicalization and sedation strategy has not yet been confirmed. Novel technology should be developed to facilitate improved capnography and patient monitoring. Moreover, training in the nontechnical aspects of ATI has not been sufficiently explored.

References

1. Nørskov AK, Rosenstock CV, Wetterslev J, Astrup G, Afshari A, Lundstrøm LH. Diagnostic accuracy of anaesthesiologists' prediction of difficult airway management in daily clinical practice: a cohort study of 188 064 patients registered in the Danish Anaesthesia Database. Anaesthesia. 2015;70(3):272–81.
2. Nørskov AK, Wetterslev J, Rosenstock CV, Afshari A, Astrup G, Jakobsen JC, et al. Prediction of difficult mask ventilation using a systematic assessment of risk factors vs. existing practice – a cluster randomised clinical trial in 94,006 patients. Anaesthesia. 2017;72(3):296–308.
3. Kheterpal S, Martin L, Shanks AM, Tremper KK. Prediction and outcomes of impossible mask ventilation: a review of 50,000 anesthetics. Anesthesiology. 2009;110(4):891–7.
4. Kheterpal S, Han R, Tremper KK, Shanks A, Tait AR, O'Reilly M, et al. Incidence and predictors of difficult and impossible mask ventilation. Anesthesiology. 2006;105(5):885–91.
5. Verghese C, Brimacombe JR. Survey of laryngeal mask airway usage in 11,910 patients: safety and efficacy for conventional and nonconventional usage. Anesth Analg. 1996;82(1):129–33.
6. Saito T, Liu W, Chew STH, Ti LK. Incidence of and risk factors for difficult ventilation via a supraglottic airway device in a population of 14,480 patients from South-East Asia. Anaesthesia. 2015;70(9):1079–83.
7. Francksen H, Renner J, Hanss R, Scholz J, Doerges V, Bein B. A comparison of the i-gel with the LMA-Unique in non-paralysed anaesthetised adult patients. Anaesthesia. 2009;64(10):1118–24.
8. Rose DK, Cohen MM. The airway: problems and predictions in 18,500 patients. Can J Anaesth. 1994;41(5 Pt 1):372–83.
9. Cook TM, Trümpelmann P, Beringer R, Stedeford J. A randomised comparison of the Portex Softseal laryngeal mask airway with the LMA-Unique during anaesthesia. Anaesthesia. 2005;60(12):1218–25.
10. Shiga T, Wajima Z, Inoue T, Sakamoto A. Predicting difficult intubation in apparently normal patients: a meta-analysis of bedside screening test performance. Anesthesiology. 2005;103(2):429–37.
11. Lundstrøm LH, Møller AM, Rosenstock C, Astrup G, Gätke MR, Wetterslev J. A documented previous difficult tracheal intubation as a prognostic test for a subsequent difficult tracheal intubation in adults. Anaesthesia. 2009;64(10):1081–8.
12. Detsky ME, Jivraj N, Adhikari NK, Friedrich JO, Pinto R, Simel DL, et al. Will this patient be difficult to intubate?: the rational clinical examination systematic review. JAMA J Am Med Assoc. 2019;321(5):493–503.
13. Ahmad I, El-Boghdadly K, Bhagrath R, Hodzovic I, McNarry AF, Mir F, et al. Difficult Airway Society guidelines for awake tracheal intubation (ATI) in adults. Anaesthesia. 2019;75(4):509–28.
14. Alhomary M, Ramadan E, Curran E, Walsh SR. Videolaryngoscopy vs. fibreoptic bronchoscopy for awake tracheal intubation: a systematic review and meta-analysis. Anaesthesia. 2018;73(9):1151–61.
15. Ajay S, Singhania A, Akkara AG, Shah A, Adalja M. A study of flexible fiberoptic bronchoscopy aided tracheal intubation for patients undergoing elective surgery under general anesthesia. Indian J Otolaryngol Head Neck Surg. 2013;65(2):116–9.
16. El-Boghdadly K, Onwochei DN, Cuddihy J, Ahmad I. A prospective cohort study of awake fibreoptic intubation practice at a tertiary centre. Anaesthesia. 2017;72(6):694–703.
17. Law JA, Morris IR, Brousseau PA, de la Ronde S, Milne AD. The incidence, success rate, and complications of awake tracheal intubation in 1,554 patients over 12 years: an historical cohort study. Can J Anesth Can d'anesthésie. 2015;62(7):736–44.
18. Joseph TT, Gal JS, DeMaria S, Lin H, Levine AI, Hyman JB. A retrospective study of success, failure, and time needed to perform awake intubation. Anesthesiology. 2016;125(1):105–14.
19. Cook TM. Strategies for the prevention of airway complications – a narrative review. Anaesthesia. 2018;73(1):93–111.

20. Ahmad I, El-Boghdadly K, Bhagrath R, Hodzovic I, McNarry AF, Mir F, et al. Difficult Airway Society guidelines for awake tracheal intubation (ATI) in adults. Anaesthesia. 2020;75(4):509–28.
21. Cook T, Woodall N, Frerk C, behalf of the Fourth National Audit Project. Major complications of airway management in the UK: results of the Fourth National Audit Project of the Royal College of Anaesthetists and the Difficult Airway Society. Part 1: Anaesthesia. Br J Anaesth. 2011;106:617–31.
22. Frerk C, Mitchell VS, McNarry AF, Mendonca C, Bhagrath R, Patel A, et al. Difficult Airway Society 2015 guidelines for management of unanticipated difficult intubation in adults. Br J Anaesth. 2015;115(6):827–48.
23. Law JA, Broemling N, Cooper RM, Drolet P, Duggan LV, Griesdale DE, et al. The difficult airway with recommendations for management—part 2—the anticipated difficult airway. Can J Anesth Can d'anesthésie. 2013;60(11):1119–38.
24. Apfelbaum JL, Hagberg CA, Caplan RA, Connis RT, Nickinovich DG, Benumof JL, et al. Practice guidelines for management of the difficult airway: an updated report by the American Society of Anesthesiologists Task Force on Management of the Difficult Airway. Anesthesiology. 2013;118(2):251–70.
25. Benumof JL. Obstructive sleep apnea in the adult obese patient: implications for airway management. Anesthesiol Clin North Am. 2002;20(4):789–811.
26. Petrini F, Di Giancinto I, Cataldo R, Esposito C, Pavoni V, Donato P, et al. Perioperative and periprocedural airway management and respiratory safety for the obese patient: 2016 SIAARTI Consensus. Minerva Anestesiol. 2016;82(12):1314–35.
27. Roth D, Pace NL, Lee A, Hovhannisyan K, Warenits AM, Arrich J, et al. Airway physical examination tests for detection of difficult airway management in apparently normal adult patients. Cochrane Database Syst Rev. 2018;2018(5):CD008874.
28. Yentis SM, Hartle AJ, Barker IR, Barker P, Bogod DG, Clutton-Brock TH, et al. AAGBI: consent for anaesthesia 2017. Anaesthesia. 2017;72(1):93–105.
29. Weinger MB, Vredenburgh AG, Schumann CM, Macario A, Williams KJ, Kalsher MJ, et al. Quantitative description of the workload associated with airway management procedures. J Clin Anesth. 2000;12(4):273–82.
30. Reason J. Human error: models and management. Br Med J. 2000;320(7237):770.
31. Rall M, Dieckmann P. Safety culture and crisis resource management in airway management: general principles to enhance patient safety in critical airway situations. Best Pract Res Clin Anaesthesiol. 2005;19(4):539–57.
32. Greig PR, Zolger D, Onwochei DN, Thurley N, Higham H, Desai N. Cognitive aids in the management of clinical emergencies: a systematic review. Anaesthesia. 2022;78:343.
33. Davis M, Hignett S, Hillier S, Hames N, Hodder S. Safer anaesthetic rooms: human factors/ergonomics analysis of work practices. J Perioper Pract. 2016;26(12):274–80.
34. Klein AA, Meek T, Allcock E, Cook TM, Mincher N, Morris C, et al. Recommendations for standards of monitoring during anaesthesia and recovery 2021: guideline from the Association of Anaesthetists. Anaesthesia. 2021;76(9):1212–23.
35. Rosenstock CV, Thøgersen B, Afshari A, Christensen AL, Eriksen C, Gätke MR. Awake fiberoptic or awake video laryngoscopic tracheal intubation in patients with anticipated difficult airway management: a randomized clinical trial. Anesthesiology. 2012;116(6):1210–6.
36. Woodall NM, Harwood RJ, Barker GL. Complications of awake fibreoptic intubation without sedation in 200 healthy anaesthetists attending a training course. Br J Anaesth. 2008;100(6):850–5.
37. Patil V, Barker GL, Harwood RJ, Woodal NM. Training course in local anaesthesia of the airway and fibreoptic intubation using course delegates as subjects. Br J Anaesth. 2002;89(4):586–93.
38. Sun Y, Liu JX, Jiang H, Zhu YS, Xu H, Huang Y. Cardiovascular responses and airway complications following awake nasal intubation with blind intubation device and fibreoptic bronchoscope: a randomized controlled study. Eur J Anaesthesiol. 2010;27(5):461–7.

39. Carayon P, Xie A, Kianfar S. Human factors and ergonomics as a patient safety practice. Br Med J Qual Saf. 2014;23(3):196–205.
40. Ovassapian A, Tuncbilek M, Weitzel EK, Joshi CW. Airway management in adult patients with deep neck infections: a case series and review of the literature. Anesth Analg. 2005;100(2):585–9.
41. Meghjee SPL, Marshall M, Redfern EJ, McGivern DV. Influence of patient posture on oxygen saturation during fibre-optic bronchoscopy. Respir Med. 2001;95(1):5–8.
42. Van Zwam JP, Kapteijns EFG, Lahey S, Smit HJM. Flexible bronchoscopy in supine or sitting position: a randomized prospective analysis of safety and patient comfort. J Bronchol Interv Pulmonol. 2010;17(1):29–32.
43. Ling IT, Piccolo F, Mulrennan SA, Phillips MJ. Posture influences patient cough rate, sedative requirement and comfort during bronchoscopy: an observational cohort study. Cough. 2011;7(1):9.
44. Altermatt FR, Muñoz HR, Delfino AE, Cortínez LI. Pre-oxygenation in the obese patient: effects of position on tolerance to apnoea. Br J Anaesth. 2005;95(5):706–9.
45. Tagaito Y, Isono S, Tanaka A, Ishikawa T, Nishino T. Sitting posture decreases collapsibility of the passive pharynx in anesthetized paralyzed patients with obstructive sleep apnea. Anesthesiology. 2010;113(4):812–8.
46. Ikeda H, Ayuse T, Oi K. The effects of head and body positioning on upper airway collapsibility in normal subjects who received midazolam sedation. J Clin Anesth. 2006;18(3):185–93.
47. Heidegger T, Gerig HJ, Ulrich B, Schnider TW. Structure and process quality illustrated by fibreoptic intubation: analysis of 1612 cases. Anaesthesia. 2003;58(8):734–9.
48. Desai N, Ratnayake G, Onwochei DN, El-Boghdadly K, Ahmad I. Airway devices for awake tracheal intubation in adults: a systematic review and network meta-analysis. Br J Anaesth. 2021;127(4):636–47.
49. Gómez-Ríos MÁ, Nieto Serradilla L. Combined use of an Airtraq® optical laryngoscope, Airtraq video camera, Airtraq wireless monitor, and a fibreoptic bronchoscope after failed tracheal intubation. Can J Anaesth. 2011;58(4):411–2.
50. Chung MY, Park B, Seo J, Kim CJ. Successful airway management with combined use of McGrath® MAC video laryngoscope and fiberoptic bronchoscope in a severe obese patient with huge goiter – a case report. Korean J Anesthesiol. 2018;71(3):232–6.
51. Liew GHC, Wong TGL, Lu A, Kothandan H. Combined use of the Glidescope and flexible fibrescope as a rescue technique in a difficult airway. Proc Singap Healthc. 2015;24(2):117–20.
52. Kristensen MS, Fredensborg BB. The disposable Ambu aScope vs. a conventional flexible videoscope for awake intubation—a randomised study. Acta Anaesthesiol Scand. 2013;57(7):888–95.
53. Brull SJ, Wiklund R, Ferris C, Connelly NR, Ehrenwerth J, Silverman DG. Facilitation of fiberoptic orotracheal intubation with a flexible tracheal tube. Anesth Analg. 1994;78(4):746–8.
54. Hakala P, Randell T, Valli H. Comparison between tracheal tubes for orotracheal fibreoptic intubation. Br J Anaesth. 1999;82(1):135–6.
55. Jafari A, Gharaei B, Kamranmanesh MR, Aghamohammadi H, Nobahar MR, Poorzamany M, et al. Wire reinforced endotracheal tube compared with Parker Flex-Tip tube for oral fiberoptic intubation: a randomized clinical trial. Minerva Anestesiol. 2014;80(3):324–9.
56. Lucas DN, Yentis SM. A comparison of the intubating laryngeal mask tracheal tube with a standard tracheal tube for fibreoptic intubation. Anaesthesia. 2000;55(4):358–61.
57. Sharma D, Bithal PK, Rath GP, Pandia MP. Effect of orientation of a standard polyvinyl chloride tracheal tube on success rates during awake flexible fibreoptic intubation. Anaesthesia. 2006;61(9):845–8.
58. Kristensen MS. The Parker Flex-Tip tube versus a standard tube for fiberoptic orotracheal intubation: a randomized double-blind study. Anesthesiology. 2003;98(2):354–8.
59. Rai MR, Scott SH, Marfin AG, Popat MT, Pandit JJ. A comparison of a flexometallic tracheal tube with the intubating laryngeal mask tracheal tube for nasotracheal fibreoptic intubation using the two-scope technique. Anaesthesia. 2009;64(12):1303–6.

60. Barker KF, Bolton P, Cole S, Coe PA. Ease of laryngeal passage during fibreoptic intubation: a comparison of three endotracheal tubes. Acta Anaesthesiol Scand. 2001;45(5):624–6.
61. Lomax SL, Johnston KD, Marfin AG, Yentis SM, Kathawaroo S, Popat MT. Nasotracheal fibreoptic intubation: a randomised controlled trial comparing the GlideRite® (Parker-Flex® Tip) nasal tracheal tube with a standard pre-rotated nasal RAE™ tracheal tube. Anaesthesia. 2011;66(3):180–4.
62. Rozario L, Sloper D, Sheridan MJ. Supplemental oxygen during moderate sedation and the occurrence of clinically significant desaturation during endoscopic procedures. Gastroenterol Nurs. 2008;31(4):281–5.
63. Reed MWR, O'leary DP, Duncan JL, Majeed AW, Wright B, Reilly CS. Effects of sedation and supplemental oxygen during upper alimentary tract endoscopy. Scand J Gastroenterol. 1993;28(4):319–22.
64. Reshef R, Schiller M, Kinberg R, Rennert H, Rennert G, Herskovits M, et al. A prospective study evaluating the usefulness of continuous supplemental oxygen in various endoscopic procedures. Isr J Med Sci. 1996;32(9):736–40.
65. Deitch K, Chudnofsky CR, Dominici P, Latta D, Salamanca Y. The utility of high-flow oxygen during emergency department procedural sedation and analgesia with propofol: a randomized, controlled trial. Ann Emerg Med. 2011;58(4):360–4.
66. Deitch K, Chudnofsky CR, Dominici P. The utility of supplemental oxygen during emergency department procedural sedation with propofol: a randomized, controlled trial. Ann Emerg Med. 2008;52(1):1–8.
67. Sidhu VS, Whitehead EM, Ainsworth QP, Smith M, Calder I. A technique of awake fibreoptic intubation. Experience in patients with cervical spine disease. Anaesthesia. 1993;48(10):910–3.
68. Fuchs G, Schwarz G, Baumgartner A, Kaltenböck F, Voit-Augustin H, Planinz W. Fiberoptic intubation in 327 neurosurgical patients with lesions of the cervical spine. J Neurosurg Anesthesiol. 1999;11(1):11–6.
69. Badiger S, John M, Fearnley RA, Ahmad I. Optimizing oxygenation and intubation conditions during awake fibre-optic intubation using a high-flow nasal oxygen-delivery system. Br J Anaesth. 2015;115(4):629–32.
70. El-Boghdadly K, Pawa A, Chin KJ. Local anesthetic systemic toxicity: current perspectives. Local Reg Anesth. 2018;11:44.
71. Milman N, Laub M, Munch EP, Angelo HR. Serum concentrations of lignocaine and its metabolite monoethylglycinexylidide during fibre-optic bronchoscopy in local anaesthesia. Respir Med. 1998;92(1):40–3.
72. Hasmoni MH, Rani MFA, Harun R, Manap RA, Tajudin NAA, Anshar FM. Randomized-controlled trial to study the equivalence of 1% versus 2% lignocaine in cough suppression and satisfaction during bronchoscopy. J Bronchol. 2008;15(2):78–82.
73. Mainland PA, Kong AS, Chung DC, Chan CHS, Lai CKW. Absorption of lidocaine during aspiration anesthesia of the airway. J Clin Anesth. 2001;13(6):440–6.
74. Efthimiou J, Higenbottam T, Holt D, Cochrane GM. Plasma concentrations of lignocaine during fibreoptic bronchoscopy. Thorax. 1982;37(1):68–71.
75. Williams KA, Barker GL, Harwood RJ, Woodall NM. Combined nebulization and spray-as-you-go topical local anaesthesia of the airway. Br J Anaesth. 2005;95(4):549–53.
76. Ingrande J, Lemmens HJ. Dose adjustment of anaesthetics in the morbidly obese. Br J Anaesth. 2010;105(S1):16–23.
77. Woodruff C, Wieczorek PM, Schricker T, Vinet B, Backman SB. Atomised lidocaine for airway topical anaesthesia in the morbidly obese: 1% compared with 2%. Anaesthesia. 2010;65(1):12–7.
78. Xue FS, Liu HP, He N, Xu YC, Yang QY, Liao X, et al. Spray-as-you-go airway topical anesthesia in patients with a difficult airway: a randomized, double-blind comparison of 2% and 4% lidocaine. Anesth Analg. 2009;108(2):536–43.

79. Wieczorek PM, Schricker T, Vinet B, Backman SB. Airway topicalisation in morbidly obese patients using atomised lidocaine: 2% compared with 4%. Anaesthesia. 2007;62(10):984–8.
80. Giordano D, Panini A, Pernice C, Raso MG, Barbieri V. Neurologic toxicity of lidocaine during awake intubation in a patient with tongue base abscess. Case report. Am J Otolaryngol. 2014;35(1):62–5.
81. Haldar R, Gyanesh P, Samanta S. Lignocaine toxicity from topical anaesthesia of airway during awake fibreoptic intubation. J Neuroanaesth Crit Care. 2014;1(2):146–7.
82. El-Boghdadly K, Chin KJ. Local anesthetic systemic toxicity: continuing professional development. Can J Anaesth. 2016;63(3):330–49.
83. Song J. A comparison of the effects of epinephrine and xylometazoline in decreasing nasal bleeding during nasotracheal intubation. J Dent Anesth Pain Med. 2017;17(4):281–7.
84. O'Hanlon J, Harper KW. Epistaxis and nasotracheal intubation-prevention with vasoconstrictor spray. Ir J Med Sci. 1994;163(2):58–60.
85. Osula S, Stockton P, Abdelaziz MM, Walshaw MJ. Intratracheal cocaine induced myocardial infarction: an unusual complication of fibreoptic bronchoscopy. Thorax. 2003;58(8):733–4.
86. Chiu YC, Brecht K, Dasgupta DS, Mhoon E. Myocardial infarction with topical cocaine anesthesia for nasal surgery. Arch Otolaryngol Head Neck Surg. 1986;112(9):988–90.
87. Higgins TS, Hwang PH, Kingdom TT, Orlandi RR, Stammberger H, Han JK. Systematic review of topical vasoconstrictors in endoscopic sinus surgery. Laryngoscope. 2011;121(2):422–32.
88. Lenders GD, Jorens PG, De Meyer T, Vandendriessche T, Verbrugghe W, Vrints CJ. Coronary spasm after the topical use of cocaine in nasal surgery. Am J Case Rep. 2013;14:76–9.
89. Cara DM, Norris AM, Neale LJ. Pain during awake nasal intubation after topical cocaine or phenylephrine/lidocaine spray. Anaesthesia. 2003;58(8):777–80.
90. Takaenoki Y, Masui K, Oda Y, Kazama T. The pharmacokinetics of atomized lidocaine administered via the trachea: a randomized trial. Anesth Analg. 2016;123(1):74–81.
91. Cabrini L, Baiardo Redaelli M, Ball L, Filippini M, Fominskiy E, Pintaudi M, et al. Awake fiberoptic intubation protocols in the operating room for anticipated difficult airway: a systematic review and meta-analysis of randomized controlled trials. Anesth Analg. 2019;128(5):971–80.
92. O'Callaghan C, Barry PW. The science of nebulised drug delivery. Thorax. 1997;52(S2):S44.
93. Reasoner DK, Warner DS, Todd MM, Hunt SW, Kirchner J. A comparison of anesthetic techniques for awake intubation in neurosurgical patients. J Neurosurg Anesthesiol. 1995;7(2):94–9.
94. Wiles JR, Kelly J, Mostafa SM. Hypotension and bradycardia following superior laryngeal nerve block. Br J Anaesth. 1989;63(1):125–7.
95. Sitzman BT, Rich GF, Rockwell JJ, Leisure GS, Durieux ME, Difazio CA. Local anesthetic administration for awake direct laryngoscopy: are glossopharyngeal nerve blocks superior? Anesthesiology. 1997;86(1):34–40.
96. Kundra P, Kutralam S, Ravishankar M. Local anaesthesia for awake fibreoptic nasotracheal intubation. Acta Anaesthesiol Scand. 2000;44(5):511–6.
97. Ali-Melkkilä T, Kaila T, Kanto J. Glycopyrrolate: pharmacokinetics and some pharmacodynamic findings. Acta Anaesthesiol Scand. 1989;33(6):513–7.
98. Brookman CA, Teh HP, Morrison LM. Anticholinergics improve fibreoptic intubating conditions during general anaesthesia. Can J Anaesth. 1997;44(2):165–7.
99. Johnston KD, Rai MR. Conscious sedation for awake fibreoptic intubation: a review of the literature. Can J Anesth. 2013;60(6):584–99.
100. Rai MR, Parry TM, Dombrovskis A, Warner OJ. Remifentanil target-controlled infusion vs propofol target-controlled infusion for conscious sedation for awake fibreoptic intubation: a double-blinded randomized controlled trial. Br J Anaesth. 2008;100(1):125–30.
101. Lallo A, Billard V, Bourgain JL. A comparison of propofol and remifentanil target-controlled infusions to facilitate fiberoptic nasotracheal intubation. Anesth Analg. 2009;108(3):852–7.

102. Zhang X, He W, Wu X, Zhou X, Huang W, Feng X. TCI remifentanil vs. TCI propofol for awake fiber-optic intubation with limited topical anesthesia. Int J Clin Pharmacol Ther. 2012;50(1):10–6.
103. Asai T, Shingu K. Difficulty in advancing a tracheal tube over a fibreoptic bronchoscope: incidence, causes and solutions. Br J Anaesth. 2004;92(6):870–81.
104. Asai T, Murao K, Johmura S, Shingu K. Effect of cricoid pressure on the ease of fibrescope-aided tracheal intubation. Anaesthesia. 2002;57(9):909–13.
105. Katsnelson T, Frost EAM, Farcon E, Goldiner PL. When the endotracheal tube will not pass over the flexible fiberoptic bronchoscope. Anesthesiology. 1992;76(1):151–2.
106. Schwartz D, Johnson C, Roberts J. A maneuver to facilitate flexible fiberoptic intubation. Anesthesiology. 1989;71(3):470–1.
107. Nakayama M, Kataoka N, Usui Y, Inase N, Takayama S, Miura H. Techniques of nasotracheal intubation with the fiberoptic bronchoscope. J Emerg Med. 1992;10(6):729–34.
108. Ovassapian A, Yelich SJ, Dykes MH, Brunner EE. Fiberoptic nasotracheal intubation – incidence and causes of failure. Anesth Analg. 1983;62(7):692–5.
109. Cooper RM. Complications associated with the use of the GlideScope videolaryngoscope. Can J Anaesth. 2007;54(1):54–7.
110. Richardson PB, Hodzovic I. Awake tracheal intubation using videolaryngoscopy: importance of blade design. Anaesthesia. 2012;67(7):798–9.
111. Silvestri S, Ladde JG, Brown JF, Roa JV, Hunter C, Ralls GA, et al. Endotracheal tube placement confirmation: 100% sensitivity and specificity with sustained four-phase capnographic waveforms in a cadaveric experimental model. Resuscitation. 2017;115:192–8.
112. Grmec Š. Comparison of three different methods to confirm tracheal tube placement in emergency intubation. Intensive Care Med. 2002;28(6):701–4.
113. Merry AF, Mitchell SJ. Complications of anaesthesia. Anaesthesia. 2018;73(S1):7–11.
114. Wahba SS, Tammam TF, Saeed AM. Comparative study of awake endotracheal intubation with Glidescope video laryngoscope versus flexible fiber optic bronchoscope in patients with traumatic cervical spine injury. Egypt J Anaesth. 2012;28(4):257–60.
115. Kramer A, Müller D, Pförtner R, Mohr C, Groeben H. Fibreoptic vs videolaryngoscopic (C-MAC® D-BLADE) nasal awake intubation under local anaesthesia. Anaesthesia. 2015;70(4):400–6.
116. Higgs A, McGrath BA, Goddard C, Rangasami J, Suntharalingam G, Gale R, et al. Guidelines for the management of tracheal intubation in critically ill adults. Br J Anaesth. 2018;120(2):323–52.
117. Popat M, Mitchell V, Dravid R, Patel A, Swampillai C, Higgs A. Difficult Airway Society guidelines for the management of tracheal extubation. Anaesthesia. 2012;67(3):318–40.
118. Kirkpatrick MB, Sanders RV, Bass JB. Physiologic effects and serum lidocaine concentrations after inhalation of lidocaine from a compressed gas-powered jet nebulizer. Am Rev Respir Dis. 1987;136(2):447–9.
119. Schønemann NK, van der Burght M, Arendt-Nielsen L, Bjerring P. Onset and duration of hypoalgesia of lidocaine spray applied to oral mucosa – a dose response study. Acta Anaesthesiol Scand. 1992;36(7):733–5.
120. Roberts MH, Gildersleve CD. Lignocaine topicalization of the pediatric airway. Paediatr Anaesth. 2016;26(4):337–44.
121. Martin KM, Larsen PD, Segal R, Marsland CP. Effective nonanatomical endoscopy training produces clinical airway endoscopy proficiency. Anesth Analg. 2004;99(3):938–44.
122. Baker PA, Weller JM, Baker MJ, Hounsell GL, Scott J, Gardiner PJ, et al. Evaluating the ORSIM® simulator for assessment of anaesthetists' skills in flexible bronchoscopy: aspects of validity and reliability. Br J Anaesth. 2016;117(S1):i87–91.
123. Casso G, Schoettker P, Savoldelli GL, Azzola A, Cassina T. Development and initial evaluation of a novel, ultraportable, virtual reality bronchoscopy simulator: the computer airway simulation system. Anesth Analg. 2019;129(5):1258–64.

124. Jiang B, Ju H, Zhao Y, Yao L, Feng Y. Comparison of the efficacy and efficiency of the use of virtual reality simulation with high-fidelity mannequins for simulation-based training of fiberoptic bronchoscope manipulation. Simul Healthc. 2018;13(2):83–7.
125. Marsland C, Larsen P, Segal R, Hunter S, Morris J, Mezzavia P, et al. Proficient manipulation of fibreoptic bronchoscope to carina by novices on first clinical attempt after specialized bench practice. Br J Anaesth. 2010;104(3):375–81.
126. Cole AFD, Mallon JS, Rolbin SH, Ananthanarayan C. Fiberoptic intubation using anesthetized, paralyzed, apneic patients. Results of a resident training program. Anesthesiology. 1996;84(5):1101–6.
127. Vora J, Leslie D, Stacey M. Awake tracheal intubation. Br J Anaesth Educ. 2022;22(8):298–305.

Chapter 11
Alternative Techniques in Expected or Known Difficult Airway

Pavel Michalek

Abbreviations

ASA	American Society of Anesthesiologists
CI	confidence interval
CICO	cannot intubate, cannot oxygenate
CMOS	complementary metal-oxide-semiconductor
CT	computed tomography
ECMO	extracorporeal membrane oxygenation
ENT	ear, nose, and throat
FONA	front of neck access
HFNO	high-flow nasal oxygen
ILMA	intubating laryngeal mask airway
LM	laryngeal mask
LMA	laryngeal mask airway
MRI	magnetic resonance imaging
RCT	randomized controlled trial
RR	relative risk
SAD	supraglottic airway device
SMD	standardized mean difference
THRIVE	transnasal humidified rapid-insufflation ventilatory exchange
VLM	video laryngeal mask

P. Michalek (✉)
General University Hospital, Prague, Czech Republic

First Medical Faculty, Charles University, Prague, Czech Republic
e-mail: Pavel.Michalek@vfn.cz

M. Á. Gómez-Ríos, A. van Zundert (eds.), *Evidence-based Guide to Difficult Airway Management*, https://doi.org/10.1007/978-3-032-30769-9_11

11.1 Introduction

Although awake tracheal intubation using either a flexible fiberoptic bronchoscope or, in recent years, also a videolaryngoscope has been recommended as a method of choice for expected difficult airways, it is not always feasible [1]. There are some situations or specific patients where an alternative technique has to be employed. Decreased levels of understanding or cooperation, such as in children, patients with a learning disability, or those with dementia or psychiatric disorders, do not allow to perform any airway management technique while awake [1]. Another reason for not selecting awake tracheal tube placement may be a lack of skills on the part of the operator or the unavailability of the appropriate equipment for awake airway management. This situation may occur with inexperienced anesthesiologists and other physicians involved in airway management in the emergency departments, intensive care units, or ambulances [2]. The appropriate equipment is now, fortunately, widely available due to an explosion in the evolution of disposable flexible fiberoptic bronchoscopes and portable and single-use videolaryngoscopes during the COVID-19 pandemic [3].

The alternative techniques and plans in the aforementioned situations include the use of awake securement of the airways with other techniques than flexible bronchoscopy, such as videolaryngoscopes or rigid/semirigid stylets [4]. Another approach involves avoiding airway management at all and offering the patient procedure under local or regional anesthesia techniques [5]. All these approaches require full understanding and cooperation from the patients. Alternative deep sedation and asleep techniques include airway management with a supraglottic airway device, videolaryngoscopy, or stylet-guided intubation under general anesthesia, and other more invasive techniques.

11.2 Awake Techniques

11.2.1 Regional Anesthesia: Avoiding Airway Management (Level of Evidence—C, D)

The use of regional anesthesia instead of securing the airways instrumentally remains rather an exception in patients with predicted or known difficult airways. No robust evidence exists on this matter, limited only to case reports and small series of patients. The use of regional or local anesthesia as a plan A should be limited only to selected minor procedures, outside of the area of the head and neck [5]. Some prerequisites should also be fulfilled prior to consenting the patient—a detailed explanation of the procedure, anesthetic plans, potential risks, and backup plans in case of regional anesthesia failure should be discussed in full. Furthermore, an anesthesiologist experienced in both regional anesthesia techniques and advanced airway management should be present in the operating room, and all equipment and support should be immediately available [6].

Regional anesthesia technique, apart from the failure, may be associated with serious complications such as high or insufficient block, risk of local anesthetic toxicity, anaphylaxis, or hemodynamic instability. Various case reports describe the failure or complications of regional anesthesia techniques in patients with a difficult airway. Prolonged surgery may lead to fading of the sufficient block with the need for precipitous airway management [7]. Epidural anesthesia may fail or become insufficient for surgery in up to 6.3% of morbidly obese parturients [8]. A relatively safe algorithm for employing regional anesthesia as a primary plan in patients with difficult airways was presented in 2020 [5] (Fig. 11.1). It recommends considering regional anesthesia only in cooperative patients, short surgical procedures with blood loss of less than 500 ml, and if there is uncomplicated access to the patient's airway.

11.2.2 Awake Videolaryngoscopy (Level of Evidence—A)

This technique is now considered an equal alternative to awake fiberoptic intubation [1]. Three meta-analyses have been published comparing awake fiberoptic intubation with awake videolaryngoscopy [9–11]. Total success rate and first attempt success rate were without any statistical difference for both nasal and oral intubation—RR 1.01, $p = 0.99$; RR 1.01, $p = 0.8$, respectively. Awake videolaryngoscopic intubation was significantly faster with a mean difference of 45.7 s (95% CI = 25.4—66.0 s). No statistical difference was present in other outcomes, such as sore throat, hoarseness, hypoxemia, or patient satisfaction with the procedure. Based on these results, awake videolaryngoscopy under topical anesthesia or mild sedation with preserved spontaneous breathing may become a method of choice for airway management in predicted or known difficult airways and thus replace intubation with a flexible fiberscope.

A meta-analysis involving 11 trials with a total of 873 patients was published in 2024 [11]. The authors concluded that videolaryngoscopy reduced intubation time significantly—SMD -1.97 (95% CI -2.78 to -1.15) and marginally decreased the risk of desaturation ($spO2 < 90\%$). Other parameters analyzed, such as incidence of failure, success rate on the first attempt, and postprocedural sore throat or hoarseness, showed no statistical difference.

Another meta-analysis compared different devices and tools used for awake securement of the airways [12]. There was no difference found in regard to the total success rate of tracheal intubation between flexible bronchoscopes, optical intubating stylets, non-channeled videolaryngoscopes, and channeled videolaryngoscopes. Total time to tracheal intubation was significantly shorter with the optical stylets, followed by non-channeled videolaryngoscopes. Intubation with the flexible bronchoscopes, and mainly with the channeled videolaryngoscopes, took a significantly longer time. Time to visualize the vocal cords was shortest with the non-channeled videolaryngoscopes, followed by the optical intubating stylets.

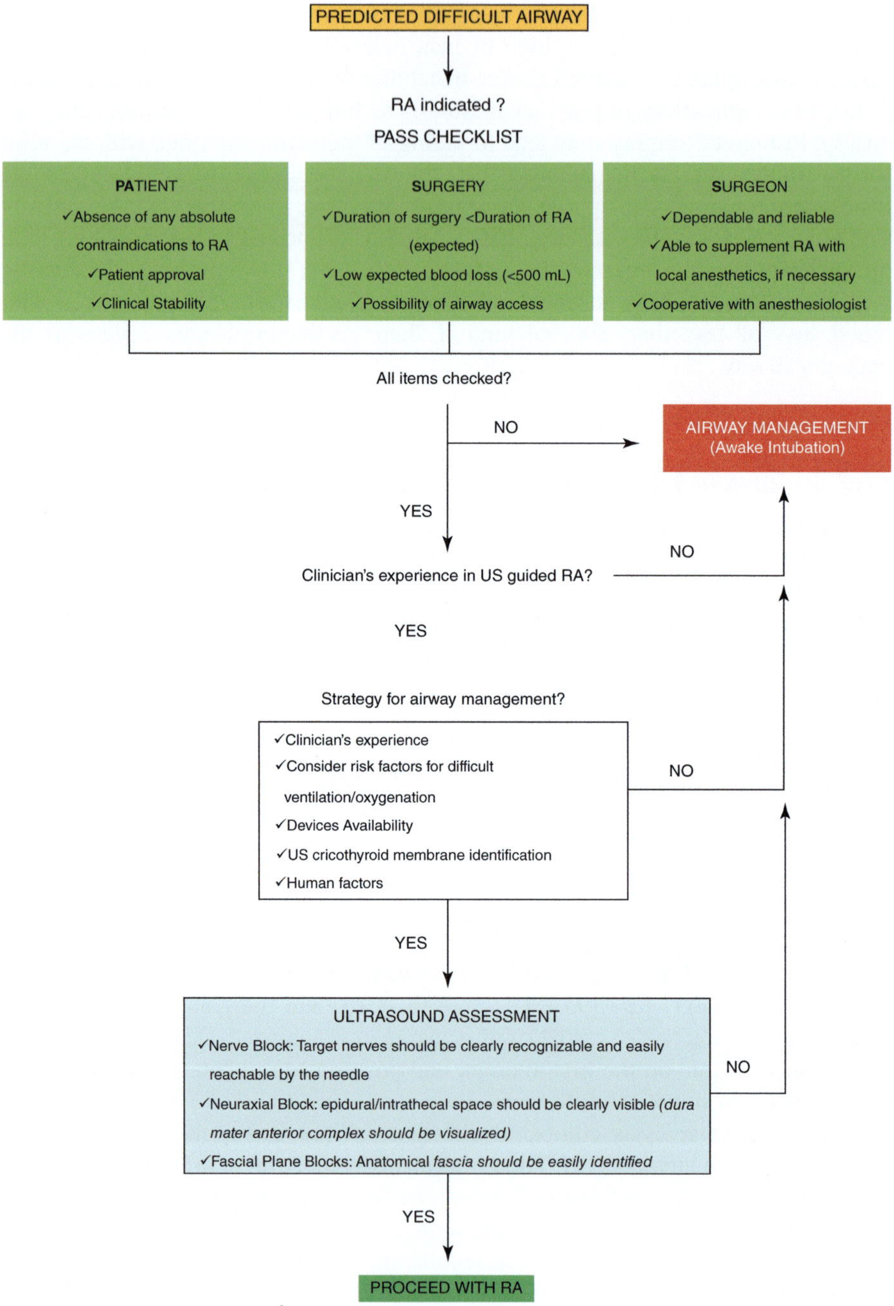

Fig. 11.1 A proposed “standard of safety” algorithm for the application of regional anesthesia in patients with predicted difficult airways (Ref. [5])

Over recent years, paradigms for tracheal intubation have changed not only in difficult airway management scenarios but also in routine intubation. Videolaryngoscopy should be considered a first-line basic technique rather than an advanced or optional tool for visualization of the larynx and insertion of an endotracheal tube [13, 14].

11.2.3 Awake Intubation Stylets (Level of Evidence—B)

The optical intubation stylets are rigid, malleable, or partially flexible devices consisting of metal or plastic tubes containing optical fibers or CMOS video chips. An endotracheal tube is mounted over the stylet prior to intubation, the laryngeal inlet is located without or with the help of a laryngoscopic blade, and finally, the tube is railroaded to the trachea under the view from the stylet camera or eyepiece. These devices were invented primarily for use in difficult airway scenarios.

The first rigid straight stylet was introduced in 1979 [15]. Its efficacy in difficult intubation was not ideal and it was often combined with the use of a Macintosh blade for removing the base of the tongue and epiglottis. The next generation of the optical stylet invented by Pierre Bonfils employed the curved rigid tip at the angle of 40 degrees, allowing direct access to the anteriorly located larynx but also the possibility of performing a novel technique of retromolar intubation [16]. This stylet, initially trialed in anesthetized children with Pierre–Robin sequence and micrognathia, showed a 99% success rate of tracheal intubation. Awake intubation with Bonfils stylet in adults was described on a cohort of 30 patients with anticipated difficult airways, while in 11 of these cases, there was previously failed intubation with Macintosh blade [17]. The total success rate was 96.6%, and one failure was managed after induction to general anesthesia with a conventional laryngoscopic technique. Similar success rates were also described in another cohort study evaluating the device in patients with ear, nose, or throat cancer [18]. Retromolar awake intubation was compared with videolaryngoscopic intubation using the Glidescope in 60 morbidly obese patients. Both devices showed a high success rate, with the Glidescope providing a slightly shorter intubation time and fewer attempts. On the other hand, patient satisfaction was better in the Bonfils group [19].

Shikani optical stylet is a device with a semimalleable tip. Its insertion is associated with lower motions of the cervical spine when compared with a Macintosh laryngoscope [20]. The stylet was compared with awake fiberoptic intubation in patients with an unstable cervical spine and showed shorter intubation time, while all other parameters, including the success rate, were without any difference [21]. Its performance was also comparable with the Glidescope videolaryngoscope in simulated difficult airway scenarios [22]. Recently, a small RCT comparing awake nasal intubation with the Shikani stylet in head and neck cancer patients with fiberoptic intubation was published [23]. Levitan FPS stylet is a shorter modification of the Shikani optical stylet developed for tracheal intubation in emergency medicine. Data describing its use in awake airway management are not available.

SensaScope represents another type of optical stylet device. SensaScope is a hybrid device consisting of an S-shaped rigid shaft and an adjustable tip. The first case series describing its application in awake intubation of 13 patients with known or predicted difficult airways was published in 2010 [24]. Subsequent studies were performed on anesthetized patients and showed unconvincing results [25]. Further clinical use of this device has not expanded worldwide.

The novel generation of optical stylets contains CMOS video chips instead of optical fibers. It is represented by various, technologically very similar devices, often with a malleable shaft or tip. The Trachway intubating stylet was first used with success for awake intubation in a patient with cervical spine subluxation [26]. The following evaluations were performed in sedated or anesthetized patients. ProVu video stylet has a maneuverable tip allowing both flection and retroflection of the device. A case study showed its feasibility as an intubation tool in three patients with a high prediction of difficult intubation [27]. Another case series described awake intubation with ProVu optical stylet in 11 morbidly obese patients [28]. The authors did not experience any failures; however, in two patients, the views were obscured by secretions, and intubation required an additional attempt after cleaning the tip of the device.

Further progress in optical stylets was achieved with the invention of a semi-flexible C-MAC device. The shaft of this device is rigid; however, its tip may be bent to an angle of 90 degrees, thus increasing the chance of visualizing even a very anteriorly positioned laryngeal inlet. A pilot evaluation of this stylet performed in 36 patients with predicted difficult intubation showed a 97% total success rate, with the first attempt success rate being 80% (mean intubation time was 45 s [29]. Other authors compared awake intubation using the C-MAC stylet with flexible fiberoptic bronchoscopy in 80 patients with expected difficult airways. Intubation with the stylet was more successful on the first attempt (90% vs. 72.5%; $p=0.04$) and significantly faster (median 45.5 s vs. 80 s; $p < 0.001$) [30]. The available level of evidence of various video intubating stylets is presented in Table 11.1.

Clinical evidence for the efficacy of other optical stylets available on the market is sparse.

Table 11.1 Optical intubating stylets and their level of evidence for awake tracheal intubation

Optical stylet	Manufacturer	Best level of evidence available for awake intubation
Bonfils stylet	Karl Storz KG, Germany	B
Shikani stylet	Clarus Medical, USA	B
Levitan FPS	Clarus Medical, USA	D
SensaScope	Acutronic Medical Systems, Switzerland	C
Trachway	Biotronic Instruments Enterprise Ltd., Taiwan, China	C
Stylet Viu	StyletViu Inc., USA	D
UE Scope	UE Medical Devices, USA	C
ProVu	Flexicare Medical Ltd., UK	C
Intular Scope	Medical Park, South Korea	D
AinCa video stylet	Anesthesia Associates Inc., USA	D
C-MAC video stylet	Karl Storz KG, Germany	B

11.2.4 Awake Insertion of Supraglottic Airway Devices (Level of Evidence—C)

Only case reports, case series, and small RCTs exist on the insertion of SAD under topical anesthesia in predicted, known, or unexpected difficult airways. The first reports on the awake insertion of laryngeal mask airway and its use as a conduit for blind insertion of a tracheal tube, Aintree exchange catheter, or fiberoptic intubation were published already in the 1990s [31, 32]. Blind intubation through an Intubating LMA (Fastrach™) (Laryngeal Mask, Mahé, Seychelles) was compared with awake flexible bronchoscopic intubation in a prospective randomized study on patients with predicted difficult airways [33]. Intubation through the Fastrach showed a higher success on the first attempt, a shorter intubation time, while total success was similar (95%) in both methods. The i-gel™ (Intersurgical Ltd., Wokingham, UK) awake insertion and subsequent fiberoptic intubation was trialed in 85 patients with predictors for difficult laryngoscopy [34]. Patients received topical anesthesia of the oropharynx and analgosedation with fentanyl and propofol. Tracheal intubation was feasible in all cases; three patients (3.5%) suffered from temporary hypoxemia ($SpO_2 < 90\%$). Other perioperative and postoperative complications were not noted. Tracheal intubation through the i-gel™ was compared with videolaryngoscopy and fiberoptic intubation in patients with a predicted difficult airway [35]. Awake insertion of a supraglottic airway and subsequent intubation was faster than fiberoptic intubation but slower than intubation with a C-MAC videolaryngoscope. AuraGain™ laryngeal mask (Ambu, Ballerup, Denmark) has been used successfully as a conduit for fiberoptic intubation in ten patients with predicted difficult airways, some of them performed by relatively inexperienced anesthesiologists [36]. In a series of cases, video laryngeal masks with an integrated camera and the availability of direct visualization of the vocal cords were used for awake/sedated insertion and subsequent tracheal intubation in patients with a history of difficult intubation or predicted difficult airway. They include CTrach™ laryngeal mask (The Laryngeal Mask Co., Singapore) [37], and SaCo VLM (UE Medical, Zhejiang, China) [38].

Awake insertion of supraglottic airway devices has also been reported in children with predicted or known difficult airways. Analysis of the Pediatric Difficult Intubation Registry (PeDI) revealed that any supraglottic airway device was inserted in 95 of 8061 (1.2%) awake children [39]. Sufficient ventilation and oxygenation were reported in 85% of cases. Successful intubation through the device was achieved in 35% on the first attempt, with a total success rate of 99%.

11.2.5 Awake Tracheostomy (Level of Evidence—C)

Surgical or percutaneous dilational tracheostomy belongs to the front of neck access (FONA). It may be used as a primary or secondary plan in expected or known difficult airways in some specific situations. The main indication is upper airway obstruction or obscured anatomical conditions due to cancer, or, less frequently, non-oncological indications such as epiglottitis, maxillofacial abscess, massive oropharyngeal bleed, angioedema, facial trauma, or burns [40].

Tracheostomy may be performed under local/regional anesthesia only or supplemented with sedation or analgosedation. Dexmedetomidine [41], remifentanil, or ketamine may be used as sedative agents [42]. The procedure should be preceded by complex imaging of the upper airway, larynx, and trachea with CT, MRI, ultrasound, and/or nasal flexible endoscopy [43]. Tracheostomy is performed by an experienced operator, most commonly by an ENT surgeon, with an anesthesiologist capable of advanced airway management techniques, maintaining oxygenation and sedation during the procedure. Oxygenation is provided using high-flow nasal oxygen (HFNO), face mask oxygenation with an oxygen reservoir, or a transnasal humidified rapid-insufflation exchange (THRIVE) system [44]. The preferred technique is open surgical or combined surgical/percutaneous. Using the ultrasound scanner, ideally, the space between the second and third tracheal ring is marked, and the subcutaneous tissue is infiltrated using 0.5% bupivacaine or 2% lidocaine with 1:200,000 adrenaline. The transversal incision is generally preferred, but some centers also employ a longitudinal approach. Following blunt preparation of the pretracheal tissue, eventually removing the thyroid isthmus caudally, the trachea is exposed, and an incision or puncture is performed between the rings. The tracheotomy cannula (size 7.0–7.5 for females, size 8.0–9.0 for males) is inserted following the dilation of the stoma. The correct position of the tube inside the trachea must be confirmed by capnography prior to induction of general anesthesia.

Acute complications of awake tracheostomy include significant bleeding (1–5%), cannula dislodgement (up to 5%), hypoxemia, and, rarely, pneumothorax, pneumomediastinum, or esophageal trauma [40, 42].

In the most risky cases, awake tracheostomy may be combined with venovenous extracorporeal oxygenation (VV-ECMO) [45].

11.3 Asleep Techniques

Techniques of securing the predicted or expected difficult airway after induction to general anesthesia are usually used only as a plan B in patients in whom awake approaches are not feasible [1]. As already described above, these include mainly uncooperative patients for any reason. The main goal is to achieve sufficient oxygenation between the intubation attempts. This may be performed using different techniques——high-flow preoxygenation, intermittent mask/SAD ventilation, oxygenation through special videolaryngoscopes, or using transnasal humidified rapid-insufflation ventilatory exchange (THRIVE).

11.3.1 Supraglottic Airway-Guided Tracheal Intubation (Level of Evidence—A, B)

One of the most frequently used asleep approaches is fiberoptic intubation through a supraglottic airway device (SAD). In the past, blind insertion of the endotracheal tube was considered a feasible option, using mainly the devices especially invented for this technique, such as the intubating laryngeal mask airway, Fastrach™ [46]. Currently recommended techniques employ confirmation of the endotracheal tube position inside the trachea using a visualization technique [47]. These involve the insertion of a flexible bronchoscope through the breathing channel of the SAD, visualization of the vocal cords, advancement of the fiberscope down to the main carina, and railroading the endotracheal tube over the fiberscope into the trachea. Another option is using a supraglottic airway device allowing direct visualization of the vocal cords, and tracheal intubation under direct vision through the supraglottic airway device.

When choosing the first option, the operator should follow some rules:

- Using the SAD routinely used in his/her clinical practice and thus minimizes the risk of failure. The SAD is used not only as a conduit for tracheal intubation but also for oxygenation and ventilation between or even during intubation attempts.
- Using the SAD, which allows higher protection against aspiration of gastric contents, means the device has an additional channel for drainage of gastric fluids (second-generation SAD).
- Use the SAD, allowing direct insertion of a reasonable-sized cuffed endotracheal tube through the SAD. For adults, this should be at least size 7.0 mm.
- Use the SAD with sufficient literature evidence as a conduit for tracheal intubation.

Table 11.2 summarizes commercially available SADs and their roles as conduits for tracheal intubation.

Relatively robust data are available for the intubating laryngeal mask airway, i-gel supraglottic airway device, and, recently, for the LMA Protector (Teleflex Medical, Westmeath, Ireland).

Blind intubation through the LMA Fastrach provided higher than 90% success, and all failures were sorted out in the next step using the fiberoptic technique [48]. A network meta-analysis evaluated the efficacy of different SADs for unassisted (blind) tracheal intubation [49]. The most effective devices were CTrach LMA (not commercially available anymore), single-use Intubating Laryngeal Mask Airway, and reusable Intubating Laryngeal Mask Airway. The Air-Q intubating laryngeal airway (Mercury Medical, Clearwater, USA) achieved almost 100% success rate as a device for oxygenation and ventilation but fiberoptic tracheal intubation failed in 8% of patients [50].

The i-gel was trialed relatively extensively in patients with predicted difficult airways. Fiberscope-guided tracheal intubation provided 96% success on the first attempt [51]. On the contrary, blind intubation through the i-gel in patients with predicted difficult airways showed a very low success rate of 15%, significantly lower than with the ILMA, and therefore should not be performed when managing known or predicted difficult airways [52]. The i-gel was also compared with the ILMA and CTrach LMA in patients with at least one predictor of difficult airway management [53]. The i-gel as a conduit was successful in all patients, providing the shortest insertion and intubation times and also the best fiberoptic visualization of the larynx. Fiberoptic intubation through the AuraGain LM was comparable in all parameters with the i-gel in a cohort of morbidly obese patients [54]. The AuraGain

Table 11.2 Available supraglottic airway devices for tracheal intubation

Device	Insertion success rate, seal pressure	Additional gastric channel	Wide breathing channel	Integrated camera/video chip	Available evidence in difficult airway management
cLMA/ uLMA	3	No	No	No	C
LMA ProSeal	2	Yes	No	No	C
LMA Supreme	1	Yes	No	No	C
ILMA/ Fastrach	2	No	Yes	No	A
LMA Protector	2	Yes	Yes	No	C
Air-Q3	2	Yes	Yes	No	?
Aura-i	2	No	Yes	No	C
Aura Gain	1	Yes	Yes	No	B
i-gel	1	Yes	Yes	No	A
i-gel Plus	1	Yes	Yes	No	C
iLTS-D	2	Yes	Yes	No	C
BlockBuster LM	2	Yes	Yes	No	B/C
CTrach LMA	2	No	Yes	Yes	A
TotalTrack VLM	1	Yes	Yes	Yes	B
SaCo VLM	1	Yes	Yes	Yes	C
SafeLM	N/A	Yes	Yes	Yes	N/A

Legend: 1—excellent, 2—very good, 3—average, 4—below average, 5—poor. N/A——not applicable

LM was also compared with the Fastrach in 116 patients [55]. Its insertion was faster, visualization of the vocal cords better, and fiberoptic intubation quicker and easier. LMA Protector (Teleflex Medical, Co., Westmeath, Ireland) was compared with the i-gel as a conduit for fiberoptic intubation in patients scheduled for elective surgery under general anesthesia [56]. Only a minority of these patients (5-10%) had predictors of difficult laryngoscopy on preoperative airway assessment. Both devices provided a good-quality visualization of the vocal cords and a high success rate of tracheal intubation. The i-gel PlusTM is an innovative version of the i-gel device, with a longer tip potentially improving the esophageal seal, wider gastric channel, and special ramp inside the bowl, facilitating tracheal intubation. The i-gel Plus has been inserted in a large prospective study, even in patients with predicted difficult airways [57], and as a conduit for tracheal intubation in embalmed cadavers [58] and in three patients with unexpected difficult laryngoscopy [59].

The disposable base of the tongue sealing supraglottic airway device, Intubating Laryngeal Tube Suction (iLTS-D, VBM Medical, Germany) had a relatively low success rate—70% for fiberscope-assisted blind intubation [60] and 96.7% for fiberoptic intubation [61]. However, in the latter study, no laryngeal structures could be visualized in 20% of patients after the device insertion. The novel supraglottic airway, BlockBusterTM laryngeal mask, has been trialed as a conduit for intubation in both adults and pediatric patients. This device achieved better performance than FastrachTM LMA in adult patients, mainly higher first-attempt insertion success and shorter intubation time [62].

Supraglottic airway devices with an integrated camera were invented directly for use in difficult airway management. The first device commercially available was a reusable CTrach™ laryngeal mask airway. The initial reports on its performance were published in 2006 [63]. The success rate of tracheal intubation through the CTrach in predicted or simulated difficult airways was similar to ILMA but significantly lower in comparison with the videolaryngoscopes Glidescope or Airtraq [64–66]. The CTrach™ was a reliable device for teaching on simulators, however, its clinical use in difficult airway scenarios was limited by a relatively frequent obstruction of the lens by secretions or epiglottis downfolding [67]. Total Track VLM (MedComflow S.A., Barcelona, Spain) is a hybrid reusable device combining the features of videolaryngoscope and video intubating laryngeal mask airway. It has also a gastric drainage channel. The TotalTrack provided good oxygenation and ventilation in obese patients, with a more than 95% success rate of tracheal intubation [68, 69]. In nine patients, the device rescued the airway following unsuccessful laryngoscopic, videolaryngoscopic, or fiberoptic attempts [70]. Novel disposable video laryngeal masks with an additional gastric drainage channel have been available since 2021. SaCo Video Laryngeal Mask Airway is a fully disposable laryngeal mask, with a wide breathing lumen and an additional gastric channel. Another side channel is designated for the placement of the optical fiber, allowing direct localization of the glottis during insertion. This device has been compared as a conduit for tracheal intubation with the i-gel and showed a 98% success rate, significantly shorter intubation time, and lower incidence of periprocedural complications [71]. The first case series describing the SaCoVLM use in predicted difficult airways after induction to general anesthesia has been published recently [72]. Another similar device, SafeLM (Magill Medical, Hunan, China) was approved for clinical use in China in 2022. The first report compared its performance with direct laryngoscopy in patients without predictors of difficult airway management and found similar results in terms of success rates and more favorable effect on hemodynamic parameters [73].

11.3.2 Videolaryngoscopy (Level of Evidence—A, B)

Videolaryngoscopic tracheal intubation after induction to general anesthesia belongs to standard techniques for securing the airway, however, it is not the best technique in patients with known or predicted difficult airways. It may be associated with severe hypoxemia due to oxygenation difficulties during and between the intubation attempts or even with the failures to intubate the trachea. A retrospective study evaluated all patients with Cormack and Lehane grade 3 or 4 on standard laryngoscopy, subsequently intubated with a videolaryngoscope [74]. In total, 20% of these patients could not be intubated with the hyperangulated videolaryngoscopic blade alone and required a combination of videolaryngoscopy and fiberoptic bronchoscopy to achieve success. Only isolated case reports are available on the efficacy of videolaryngoscopic devices, namely TruView EVO2 (Trupatek, Netanya, Israel) and Pentax AWS P-blade (Pentax, Hamburg, Germany) allowing continuous apneic oxygenation during intubation [75].

11.3.3 Intubating Stylets (Level of Evidence—B, C)

These stylets were compared with conventional laryngoscopy and videolaryngoscopy in two meta-analyses in patients with cervical spine immobilization [76, 77]. These meta-analyses compared only the results of studies in anesthetized patients. There was no statistically significant difference found between video stylets, videolaryngoscopes, and Macintosh blades in regards to the total success rate of tracheal intubation or intubation time. Intubating video stylets are generally associated with shorter intubation time when compared with flexible fiberoptic intubation [78, 79].

11.3.4 Nonconventional Techniques (Level of Evidence—C)

Other approaches may have an additive role in patients with a predicted difficult airway. They include mainly tubeless ventilation and the use of extracorporeal oxygenation techniques. Tubeless ventilation is represented by cuirass ventilation using negative pressure or biphasic (negative and positive) ventilation (Hayek RTX Respirator, United Hayek Industries Inc., Northfield, United Kingdom). This ventilation may be employed, in combination with external delivery of oxygen (Optiflow, THRIVE), in various shared airway procedures, including laryngeal and tracheal surgery [80, 81].

Extracorporeal membrane oxygenation (ECMO) circuits have been used as a planned or rescue technique in various situations of difficult airway management, including management of severe tracheal stenosis, tracheal tumor, anterior mediastinal mass, or obstruction caused by laryngeal or pharyngeal cancer [82, 83]. ECMO also should be considered in cannot intubate, cannot oxygenate (CICO) as a rescue strategy according to the last ASA guidelines [84]. However, ECMO is not available in all hospitals and its setup requires a relatively long time [85]. It is recommended that the guidewires or intravenous sheaths should be inserted in these high-risk cases prior to starting the attempts for securing the airway.

11.4 Specifics in Pediatric Anesthesia

Several guidelines and algorithms on difficult airway management in pediatric patients have been published to date [86–88]. Only one article focuses specifically on predicted difficult airway situations [89]. Children are generally not suitable patients for awake techniques of airway management, although case reports or small cohort studies exist, mainly related to newborns with the Pierre–Robin sequence [90] or cooperative adolescents [91]. Awake techniques include nasal or oral fiberoptic intubation under topical anesthesia and sedation, insertion of a supraglottic airway device with subsequent flexible fiberoptic intubation, or awake intubation with an optical stylet [91]. The most commonly used asleep technique in predicted difficult airway management is videolaryngoscopy [89]. Acceptable plan B, similar to the algorithm of an unanticipated difficult airway, includes the insertion of an SAD, which serves as an oxygenation/ventilation device and also as a conduit for fiberoptic tracheal intubation. The SADs with direct access to the trachea and protective mechanisms against aspiration of gastric contents should be preferentially used in these scenarios.

The most suitable commercially available devices include the Air-Q, AuraGain laryngeal mask, and the i-gel. The Air-Q intubating laryngeal airway was compared with the Aura-i laryngeal mask [92], and with the i-gel in preschool children scheduled for elective procedures under general anesthesia [93]. Each of these devices was reported as a feasible guide for fiberoptic intubation of the trachea. The success rate was extremely high. Fiberoptic intubation through the AuraGain achieved 100% success rate in pediatric patients while it was only 79% with the Aura-i laryngeal mask [94].

Other alternative options include the use of intubating video stylets [95] or asleep fiberoptic nasal/oral tracheal intubation with preserved spontaneous breathing [96]. This can be achieved with inhalational induction to general anesthesia using sevoflurane or with systemic application of ketamine and midazolam. The former technique is associated with environmental pollution in the operating room, while the latter one with excessive salivation and swallowing making the fiberoptic technique more difficult.

11.5 Conclusions

Any deviation from the mandatory guidelines and algorithms for the management of difficult airways must be clinically sound and justified. Both the safest and the most comfortable techniques for the patient should be chosen as plan A with reliable backup plans B and C [84]. Generally, awake airway management techniques with preserved breathing should be chosen if not contraindicated [97]. Awake videolaryngoscopy has the potential to replace awake fiberoptic intubation because it is faster and requires a more shallow learning curve although this technique is not useful in patients with severely limited mouth opening [98]. Curved video stylets may play a significant role in patients with restricted mouth opening because they may be used for retromolar intubation technique and even for nasotracheal intubation. Insertion of a supraglottic airway device, either awake or asleep, provides effective oxygenation in most cases and allows to gain time for definitive fiberoptic intubation of the trachea. Tracheostomy under local anesthesia should be reserved for the most difficult scenarios manifesting as an upper airway obstruction due to its invasivity. The last option is performing the procedure under regional anesthesia technique but this should be reserved only for peripheral surgeries with a duration shorter than two hours.

The suggested algorithm for the use of alternative airway management techniques in patients with predicted or known difficult airway management is presented in Fig. 11.2.

Subsequent cases present three different scenarios where alternative approaches were justified and applied in patients with predicted or known difficult airway management.

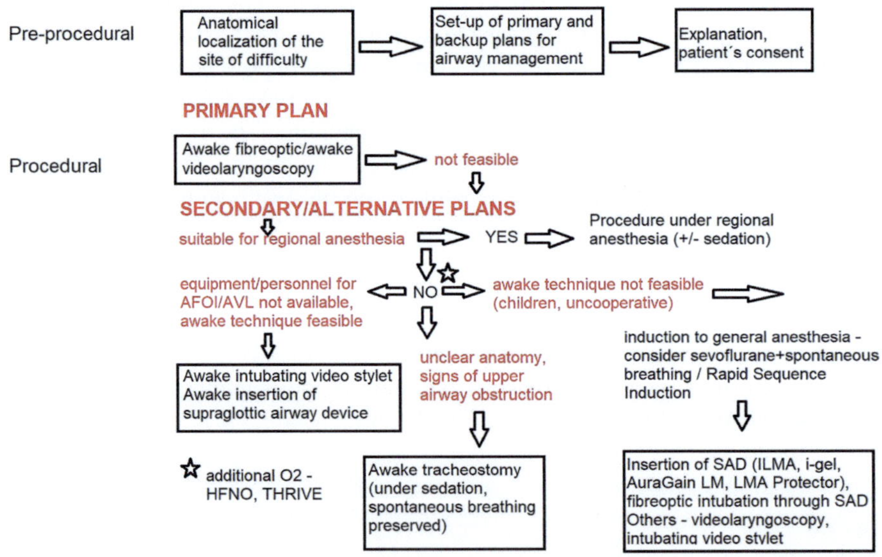

Fig. 11.2 Suggested algorithm for alternative airway management and regional anesthesia techniques in patients with known or predicted difficult airways. *AFOI* awake fiberoptic intubation, *AVL* awake videolaryngoscopy, *HFNO* high-flow nasal oxygen, *THRIVE* transnasal humidified rapid-insufflation ventilatory exchange, *SAD* supraglottic airway device, *ILMA* intubating laryngeal mask airway, *LM* laryngeal mask, *LMA* laryngeal mask airway

11.6 Case 1

A 25-year-old man, weighing 67 kg, with mucopolysaccharidosis type II was scheduled for a maxillofacial surgery. Medical history included severe learning difficulty, obstructive sleep apnea, asthma, epilepsy, dysphagia, and gastric reflux with aspirations. His anesthetic history revealed relatively easy mask ventilation, grade 3 difficult laryngoscopy, and subsequent successful LMA insertion. Preoperative airway assessment was almost impossible due to a lack of cooperation. The Mallampati score could not be evaluated, thyromental distance was 5.5 cm, and neck extension was restricted to 20 degrees. Furthermore, the patient had a short neck, a large tongue, and a small lower jaw.

Difficult airway management was predicted. The patient was not feasible for awake fiberoptic intubation due to his learning disability, definitive airway management with a supraglottic airway device was considered inappropriate due to the complex nature of surgery. Fiberoptic intubation through the i-gel supraglottic airway after preoxygenation and induction to general anesthesia was suggested as a plan A. Mask ventilation was difficult but size 4 i-gel was inserted easily, providing a good seal, ventilation, and oxygenation. A 3-mm size flexible bronchoscope was inserted through the i-gel, vocal cords were visualized immediately and a size 7.0 endotracheal tube was railroaded to the trachea over the fiberscope. The i-gel was removed with the identical technique as Fastrach LMA. All the course of the surgical procedure, extubation, and postoperative period were uncomplicated.

11.7 Case 2

A 68-yr-old woman, with a progressively growing tumor, originating from her nasopharynx was scheduled for semi-emergency tumor debulking. The procedure required the cooperation of ENT, maxillofacial, and eye surgeons. The patient had difficulties breathing, a clearly visible tumorous mass protruding out from her left nostril and mouth, and audible stridor. She was fully awake and cooperative but very anxious given the nature of her diagnosis. Her medical history included only well-controlled hypertension on medication. Apart from a local finding and impossible to evaluate the Mallampati class, her other airway examinations were normal. She agreed with a preoperative nasal flexible endoscopy and a subsequent awake tracheal intubation with a flexible bronchoscope. During the examination through the right unaffected nostril, only a mildly bleeding tumorous mass could be seen in her nasopharynx and the procedure was abandoned. Awake fiberoptic intubation or any other intubation techniques utilizing the oral or nasal cavity as a route for airway management were excluded due to uncertain anatomical conditions and the high risk of procedure-associated bleeding. Awake tracheostomy under local anesthesia and dexmedetomidine sedation with maintained spontaneous breathing was chosen as plan A and consented to by the patient. A difficult airway trolley and difficult airway management team were present in the theatre during the procedure. The patient was continuously oxygenated using high-flow nasal oxygen through the right nostril and surgical tracheostomy was performed by a maxillofacial surgeon without any complications. Following confirmation of effective ventilation with capnography, auscultation, and measurement of expiratory volumes, the patient was induced into general anesthesia, and surgical procedure was initiated. The tracheostomy was left in situ for postoperative care.

11.8 Case 3

A 77-yr-old male, weighing 83 kg, with a history of ankylosing spondylitis and previous very difficult awake fiberoptic intubation was scheduled for the left knee joint replacement. On preoperative assessment, his airway was graded as Mallampati IV, thyreomental distance 5 cm, mouth opening 3 cm with his neck in fixed flexion, with the chin almost touching the sternum and almost no mobility. Considering the nature of the surgery, the relatively predictable time of procedure up to 2 h, and his previous negative experience with awake airway management, the patient was offered spinal anesthesia. The backup plans included awake fiberoptic nasal intubation, the use of video stylet, general anesthesia with maintained spontaneous breathing using the mixture of ketamine and midazolam, and insertion of the flexible laryngeal mask airway. Subarachnoid space was located on the second attempt at L3-L4 intervertebral space with the 25 G spinal needle and a mixture of 3 ml of 0,5% hyperbaric bupivacaine and 0.1 mg of purified morphine was administered. The patient received 2 mg of midazolam i.v. throughout the course of the procedure lasting 85 min and did not complain of any pain or unpleasant experience.

References

1. Ahmad I, El-Boghdadly K, Bhagrath R, Hodzovic I, McNarry AF, Mir F, et al. Difficult Airway Society guidelines for awake tracheal intubation (ATI) in adults. Anaesthesia. 2020;75:509–28. https://doi.org/10.1111/anae.14904.
2. Karamchandani K, Wheelwright J, Yang AL, Westphal ND, Khanna AK, Myatra SN. Emergency airway management outside the operating room: current evidence and management strategies. Anesth Analg. 2021;133:648–62. https://doi.org/10.1213/ANE.0000000000005644.
3. Cook TM, El-Boghdadly K, McGuire B, McNarry AF, Patel A, Higgs A. Consensus guidelines for managing the airway in patients with COVID-19. Anaesthesia. 2020;75:785–99. https://doi.org/10.1111/anae.15054.
4. Matek J, Kolek F, Klementova O, Michalek P, Vymazal T. Optical devices in tracheal intubation—state of the art in 2020. Diagnostics (Basel). 2021;11:575. https://doi.org/10.3390/diagnostics11030575.
5. Pascarella G, Costa F, Cataldo R, del Buono R, Carassiti M, Agro FE. Regional anesthesia for predicted difficult airway: US strategy for SOS (standards of safety). Reg Anesth Pain Med. 2021;46:285–6. https://doi.org/10.1136/rapm-2020-101548.

6. Khetarpal R, Chatrath V, Dhawan A, Attri JP. Regional anesthesia in difficult airway: the quest for a solution continues. Anesth Essays Res. 2016;10:178–83. https://doi.org/10.4103/0259-1162.167829.
7. Saxena N. Airway management plan in patients with difficult airways having regional anesthesia. J Anaesthesiol Clin Pharmacol. 2013;29:558–60. https://doi.org/10.4103/0970-9185.119106.
8. Hood DD, Dewan DM. Anesthetic and obstetric outcome in morbidly obese parturients. Anesthesiology. 1993;79:1210–8. https://doi.org/10.1097/00000542-199312000-00011.
9. Alhomary M, Ramadan E, Curran E, Walsh SR. Videolaryngoscopy vs. fibreoptic bronchoscopy for awake tracheal intubation: a systematic review and meta-analysis. Anaesthesia. 2018;73:1151–61. https://doi.org/10.1111/anae.14299.
10. Jiang J, Ma DX, Wu AS, Xue FS. Videolaryngoscopy versus fiberoptic bronchoscope for awake intubation—a systemic review and meta-analysis of randomized controlled trials. Ther Clin Risk Manag. 2018;14:1955–63. https://doi.org/10.2147/TCRM.S172783.
11. Merola N, Vargas M, Marra A, Buonanno P, Coviello A, Servillo G, Iacovazzo C. Videolaryngoscopy versus fiberoptic bronchoscopy for awake tracheal intubation: a systematic review and meta-analysis of randomized controlled trials. J Clin Med. 2024;13:3186. https://doi.org/10.3390/jcm13113186.
12. Desai N, Ratnayake D, Onwochei DN, El-Boghdadly K, Ahmad I. Airway devices for awake tracheal intubation in adults: a systematic review and network meta-analysis. Br J Anaesth. 2021;127:636–47. https://doi.org/10.1016/j.bja.2021.05.025.
13. Gómez-Ríos MA, van Zundert AA, McNarry AF, Law JA, Higgs A, De Jong A, et al. Guidelines on strategies for the universal implementation of videolaryngoscopy. Eur J Anaesthesiol. 2025;42:872–88. https://doi.org/10.1097/EJA.0000000000002210.
14. Gómez-Ríos MA, Michalek P, Gaszynski T, Van Zundert AA. Human factors in airway management: designing systems for safer, team-based care. J Clin Med. 2025;14:8850. https://doi.org/10.3390/jcm14248850.
15. Katz RL, Berci D. The optical stylet—a new intubation technique for adults and children with specific reference to teaching. Anesthesiology. 1979;51:251–4. https://doi.org/10.1097/00000542-197909000-00014.
16. Bonfils P. Difficult intubation in Pierre-Robin children, a new method: the retromolar route. Anaesthetist. 1983;32:363–7. (article in German)
17. Corbanese U, Possamai C. Awake intubation with the Bonfils fibrescope in patients with difficult airway. Eur J Anaesthesiol. 2009;26:837–41. https://doi.org/10.1097/EJA.0b013e32832c6076.
18. Mazeres LE, Lefranc A, Cropet C, Steghens A, Bachmann P, Perol O, et al. Evaluation of the Bonfils intubating fibrescope for predicted difficult intubation in awake patients with ear, nose, and throat cancer. Eur J Anaesthesiol. 2011;28:646–50. https://doi.org/10.1097/EJA.0b013e3283495b85.
19. Nassar M, Zanaty OM, Ibrahim M. Bonfils fibrescope vs GlideScope for awake intubation in morbidly obese patients with expected difficult airways. J Clin Anesth. 2016;32:101–5. https://doi.org/10.1016/j.jclinane.2016.01.004.
20. Turkstra TP, Pelz DM, Shaikh AA, Craen RA. Cervical spine motion: a fluoroscopic comparison of Shikani Optical Stylet vs. Macintosh laryngoscope. Can J Anaesth. 2007;54:441–7. https://doi.org/10.1007/BF03022029.
21. Mahrous RS, Ahmed AM. The Shikani Optical Stylet as an alternative to awake fiberoptic intubation in patients at risk of secondary cervical spine injury: a randomized controlled trial. J Neurosurg Anesthesiol. 2018;30:354–8. https://doi.org/10.1097/ANA.0000000000000454.
22. Phua DS, Mah CL, Wang CF. The Shikani optical stylet as an alternative to the GlideScope videolaryngoscope in simulated difficult intubations—a randomized controlled trial. Anaesthesia. 2012;67:402–6. https://doi.org/10.1111/j.1365-2044.2011.07023.x.
23. Cheng T, Wang LK, Wu HY, Yang XD, Zhang X, Jiao L. Shikani optical stylet for awake nasal intubation in patients undergoing head and neck surgery. Laryngoscope. 2021;131:319–25. https://doi.org/10.1002/lary.28763.

24. Greif R, Kleine-Brueggeney M, Theiler L. Awake tracheal intubation using the Sensascope in 13 patients with an anticipated difficult airway. Anaesthesia. 2010;65:525–8. https://doi.org/10.1111/j.1365-2044.2010.06311.x.
25. Theiler L, Greif R, Butikofer L, Arheart K, Kleine-Brueggeney M. The skill of tracheal intubation with rigid scopes—a randomised controlled trial comparing learning curves in 740 intubations. BMC Anesthesiol. 2020;20:263. https://doi.org/10.1186/s12871-020-01181-w.
26. Cheng WC, Lan CH, Lai HY. The Clarus video system (Trachway) intubating stylet for awake intubation. Anaesthesia. 2011;66:1178–80. https://doi.org/10.1111/j.1365-2044.2011.06948.x.
27. Harrison SL, Ahmad I, Elwen F, Curtis A, Dua G, Surda P, et al. Awake tracheal intubation with the ProVu™ video stylet: a case series. Anaesth Rep. 2021;9:e12102. https://doi.org/10.1002/anr3.12102.
28. Cortese G, Gassino L, Micheletto S, Sorbello M, Cataldo R, Brazzi L. Feasibility of ProVu™ Video Stylet for awake intubation of patients with severe obesity: a pilot observational study. Trends Anaesth Crit Care. 2024;55:101339. https://doi.org/10.1016/j.tacc.2024.101339.
29. Nabecker S, Ottenhausen T, Theiler L, Braun M, Greif R, Riva T. Prospective observational study evaluating the C-MAC video stylet for awake tracheal intubation: a single-center study. Minerva Anestesiol. 2021;87:873–9. https://doi.org/10.23736/S0375-9393.21.15302-7.
30. El-Aziz RA, Osman YM. Awake intubation with C-MAC video-stylet versus fibreoptic bronchoscope in predicted difficult airway patients: comparative randomised study. Egypt J Anaesth. 2022;38:650–5. https://doi.org/10.1080/11101849.2023.2186511.
31. Asai T. Use of the laryngeal mask for tracheal in patients at increased risk of aspiration of gastric contents. Anesthesiology. 1992;77:1029–30. https://doi.org/10.1097/00000542-199211000-00027.
32. Shung J, Avidan MS, Ing R, Klein DC, Pott L. Awake intubation of the difficult airway with the intubating laryngeal mask airway. Anaesthesia. 1998;53:645–9. https://doi.org/10.1046/j.1365-2044.1998.429-az0533.x.
33. Hanna SF, Mikat-Stevens M, Loo J, Uppal R, Jellish WS, Adams M. Awake tracheal intubation in anticipated difficult airways: LMA Fastrach vs flexible bronchoscope: a pilot study. J Clin Anesth. 2017;37:31–7. https://doi.org/10.1016/j.jclinane.2016.10.040.
34. Ludena JA, Bellas JJ, Alvarez-Rementeria R, Munoz LE. Assesment of awake i-gel™ insertion for fiberoptic-guided intubation in patients with predicted difficult airway: a prospective observational study. J Anaesthesiol Clin Pharmacol. 2018;34:490–5. https://doi.org/10.4103/joacp.JOACP_329_15.
35. Yilmaz M, Yuksek A, Civraz AZ, Kara MY, Candan S, Saracoglu KT, Saracoglu A. Supraglottic airway devices in awake tracheal intubation: a viable alternative to fiberoptic and video laryngoscopy. BMC Anesthesiol. 2025;25:485. https://doi.org/10.1186/s12871-025-03331-4.
36. Lim WY, Wong P. Awake supraglottic airway guided flexible bronchoscopic intubation in patients with anticipated difficult airways: a case series and narrative review. Korean J Anesthesiol. 2019;72:548–57. https://doi.org/10.4097/kja.19318.
37. López AM, Valero R, Pons M, Anglada T. Awake intubation using the LMA-CTrach in patients with difficult airways. Anaesthesia. 2009;64:387–91. https://doi.org/10.1111/j.1365-2044.2008.05797.x.
38. Sun Y, Huang L, Xu L, Zhang M, Guo Y, Wang Y. The application of a SaCoVLM™ visual intubation laryngeal mask for the management of difficult airways in morbidly obese patients: case report. Front Med (Lausanne). 2021;8:763103. https://doi.org/10.3389/fmed.2021.763103.
39. Longacre M, Park R, Staffa S, Rowland M, Meserve J, Lord C, et al. Awake supraglottic airway placement in in pediatric patients for airway obstruction or difficult intubation: insights from and international airway registry (PeDI). Anesth Analg. 2025;140:310–6. https://doi.org/10.1213/ANE.0000000000006959.
40. Sagiv D, Nachalon Y, Mansour J, Glikson E, Alon EE, Yakirevitch A, et al. Awake tracheostomy: indications, complications and outcome. World J Surg. 2018;42:2792–9. https://doi.org/10.1007/s00268-018-4578-x.

41. David MD, De Marchi L. Dexmedetomidine sedation for awake tracheotomy: case report and literature review. J Clin Anesth. 2010;22:360–2. https://doi.org/10.1016/j.jclinane.2009.04.008.
42. Kaufman MR, Alfonso KP, Burke J, Aouad RK. Awake vs sedated tracheostomies: a review and comparison at a single institution. Otolaryngol Head Neck Surg. 2018;159:830–4. https://doi.org/10.1177/0194599818789079.
43. Lasala J, Guerra-Londono CE, Truong DT, Truong AT. Airway obstruction attributable to head and cancers: awake fiberoptic intubation versus awake tracheostomy. Anesthesiology. 2021;134:937. https://doi.org/10.1097/ALN.0000000000003744.
44. Patel A, Nouraei SA. Transnasal humidified rapid-insufflation ventilatory exchange (THRIVE): a physiological method of increasing apnoea time in patients with difficult airways. Anaesthesia. 2015;70:323–9. https://doi.org/10.1111/anae.12923.
45. Liu IH, Chou AH, Chiu CH, Cheng YT, Lin HT. Tracheostomy and venovenous extracorporeal membrane oxygenation for difficult airway patient with carinal melanoma: a case report and literature review. World J Clin Cases. 2022;10:13088–98. https://doi.org/10.12998/wjcc.v10.i35.13088.
46. Gerstein NS, Braude DA, Hung O, Sanders JC, Murphy MF. The Fastrach™ intubating laryngeal mask airway: an overview and update. Can J Anesth. 2010;57:588–601. https://doi.org/10.1007/s12630-010-9272-x.
47. Wong DT, Yang JJ, Mak HY, Jagannathan N. Use of intubation introducers through a supraglottic airway to facilitate tracheal intubation: a brief review. Can J Anaesth. 2012;59:704–15. https://doi.org/10.1007/s12630-012-9714-8.
48. Ferson DZ, Rosenblatt WH, Johansen MJ, Osborn I, Ovassapian A. Use of the intubating LMA-Fastrach in 254 patients with difficult-to-manage airways. Anesthesiology. 2001;95:1175–81. https://doi.org/10.1097/00000542-200111000-00022.
49. Ahn E, Choi G, Kang H, Baek CW, Jung YH, Woo YC, Bang SR. Supraglottic airway devices as a strategy for unassisted tracheal intubation: a network meta-analysis. PLoS One. 2018;13:e0206804. https://doi.org/10.1371/journal.pone.0206804.
50. Joffe AM, Liew EC, Galgon RE, Viernes D, Treggiari MM. The second-generation air-Q intubating laryngeal mask for airway maintenance during anaesthesia in adults: a report of the first 70 uses. Anaesth Intensive Care. 2011;39:40–5. https://doi.org/10.1177/0310057X1103900106.
51. Kleine-Brueggeney M, Theiler L, Urwyler N, Vogt A, Greif R. Randomized trial comparing the i-gel and Magill tracheal tube with the single-use ILMA™ and ILMA™ tracheal tube for fibreoptic-guided intubation in anaesthetized patients with a predicted difficult airway. Br J Anaesth. 2011;107:251–7. https://doi.org/10.1093/bja/aer103.
52. Theiler L, Kleine-Brueggeney M, Urwyler N, Graf T, Luyet C, Greif R. Randomized clinical trial of the i-gel™ and Magill tracheal tube or single-use ILMA™ and ILMA™ tracheal tube for blind intubation in anaesthetized patients with a predicted difficult airway. Br J Anaesth. 2011;107:243–50. https://doi.org/10.1093/bja/aer102.
53. Michalek P, Donaldson W, McAleavey F, Abraham A, Mathers R, Telford C. The i-gel supraglottic airway as a conduit for fibreoptic tracheal intubation—a randomised comparison with the single-use intubating laryngeal mask airway and Ctrach laryngeal mask in patients with predicted difficult laryngoscopy. Prague Med Rep. 2016;117:164–75. https://doi.org/10.14712/23362936.2016.17.
54. Moser B, Keller C, Audigé L, Dave MH, Bruppacher HR. Fiberoptic intubation of severely obese patients through supraglottic airway: A prospective, randomized trial of the Ambu AuraGain™ laryngeal mask vs. the i-gel™ airway. Acta Anaesthesiol Scand. 2019;63:187–94. https://doi.org/10.1111/aas.13242.
55. Preece G, Ng I, Lee K, Mezzavia P, Krieser R, Williams DL, et al. A randomised controlled trial comparing fibreoptic-guided tracheal intubation through two supraglottic devices: Ambu AuraGain laryngeal mask and LMA Fastrach™. Anaesth Intensive Care. 2018;46:474–9. https://doi.org/10.1177/0310057X1804600508.

56. Mendonca C, Tourville CC, Jefferson H, Nowicka A, Patteril M, Athanassoglou V. Fibreoptic-guided tracheal intubation through i-gel and LMA Protector™ supraglottic airway devices—a randomised comparison. Anaesthesia. 2019;74:203–10. https://doi.org/10.1111/anae.14475.
57. Werner J, Klementova O, Bruthans J, Macoun J, Gaszynski T, Henlin T, et al. Evaluation of the i-gel Plus supraglottic airway device in elective surgery: a prospective international multicentre study. Anaesthesia. 2024;79:1284–91. https://doi.org/10.1111/anae.16401.
58. Chaki T, Tachibana S, Kumita S, Sato S, Hirahata T, Ikeshima Y, et al. I-gel Plus acts as a superior conduit for fiberoptic intubation than standard i-gel. Sci Rep. 2023;13:18381. https://doi.org/10.1038/s41598-023-45631-0.
59. Prabha R, Shaikh FZ, Gupta A, Rastogi S. I-gel Plus as a rescue device after failure to manage airway: a case series. J Trauma Intensive Care STIC. 2024;1:15–6. https://doi.org/10.5005/jtric-11018-0005.
60. Zuercher M, Casso G, Krugel V, Potie A, Barry MP, Schoettker P. Tracheal intubation using intubating laryngeal tube iLTS-D™ and LMA Fastrach™ in 99 adult patients: a prospective multicentric randomised non-inferiority study. J Clin Anesth. 2022;78:110671. https://doi.org/10.1016/j.jclinane.2022.110671.
61. Bergold MN, Kahle S, Schultzik T, Bücheler T, Byhahn C. Intubating laryngeal tube suction disposable: Initial clinical experiences with a novel device for endotracheal intubation. Anaesthetist. 2016;65:30–5. (In German). https://doi.org/10.1007/s00101-015-0100-0.
62. Arora S, Ansari S, Longani S. Comparison of success rate of Blockbuster versus Fastrach laryngeal mask airway as a conduit for blind tracheal intubation. J Sci Soc. 2025;52:208–12. https://doi.org/10.4103/jss.jss_394_24.
63. Liu EH, Goy RW, Chen FG. The LMA CTrach, a new laryngeal mask airway for endotracheal intubation under vision: evaluation in 100 patients. Br J Anaesth. 2006;96:396–400. https://doi.org/10.1093/bja/ael001.
64. Mathew DG, Ramachandran R, Rewari V, Trikha A, Chandralekha. Endotracheal intubation with intubating laryngeal mask airway (ILMA)™, CTrach™, and Cobra PLA™ in simulated cervical spine injury patients: a comparative study. J Anesth. 2014;28:655–61. https://doi.org/10.1007/s00540-014-1794-x.
65. Arslan ZI, Yildiz T, Baykara ZN, Solak M, Toker K. Tracheal intubation in patients with rigid collar immobilisation of the cervical spine: A comparison of Airtraq and LMA CTrach devices. Anaesthesia. 2009;64:1332–6. https://doi.org/10.1111/j.1365-2044.2009.06053.x.
66. Ng SY, Ithnin E, Lim Y. Comparison of airway management during anaesthesia using the laryngeal mask airway CTrach and Glidescope. Anaesth Intensive Care. 2007;35:736–42. https://doi.org/10.1177/0310057X0703500513.
67. Michalek P, Donaldson W, Vobrubova E, Hakl M. Complications associated with the use of supraglottic airway devices in perioperative medicine. Biomed Res Int. 2015;2015:746560. https://doi.org/10.1155/2015/746560.
68. Gaszynski T. TotalTrack video intubating laryngeal mask in super-obese patients—series of cases. Ther Clin Risk Manag. 2016;12:335–8. https://doi.org/10.2147/TCRM.S95695.
69. Gómez-Ríos MA, Freire-Vila E, Casans-Francés R, Pita-Fernández S. The Totaltrack™ video laryngeal mask: an evaluation in 300 patients. Anaesthesia. 2019;74:751–7. https://doi.org/10.1111/anae.14637.
70. Gómez-Ríos MA, Freire-Vila E, Calvo-Vecino JM. Use of the Totaltrack VLM as a rescue device following failed tracheal intubation. Eur J Anaesthesiol. 2019;36:237–9. https://doi.org/10.1097/EJA.0000000000000920.
71. Yan CL, Zhang YQ, Chen Y, Qv ZY, Zuo MZ. Comparison of SaCoVLM™ video laryngeal mask-guided intubation and i-gel combined with flexible bronchoscopy-guided intubation in airway management during general anesthesia: a non-inferiority study. BMC Anesthesiol. 2022;22:302. https://doi.org/10.1186/s12871-022-01843-x.
72. Werner J, Bruthans J, Lukes M, Tosenovska K, Vobrubova E, Michalek P. Using the SaCo video laryngeal mask airway in four different scenarios—case series. Trends Anaesth Crit Care. 2023; https://doi.org/10.1016/j.tacc.2023.101264.

73. Geng CJ, Su GL, Deng Y, Cong ZK, Feng DD, Zhang SY, et al. Use of view-adjustable video laryngeal mask versus endotracheal intubation for airway management during anaesthesia for arthroscopic surgery: a randomized trial. Ann Med. 2025;57:2519683. https://doi.org/10.1080/07853890.2025.2519683.
74. O'Mahony C, O'Sullivan MP, McBride I, Mannion S. Failure rates for endotracheal tube placement using videolaryngoscopy in patients with a difficult airway. Crit Rev Biomed Eng. 2021;49:1–8. https://doi.org/10.1615/CritRevBiomedEng.2021038359.
75. Ungureanu N, Mendonca C. Oxygenation during difficult videolaryngoscopy. Anaesthesia. 2015;70:1213–4. https://doi.org/10.1111/anae.13216.
76. Chen IW, Li YY, Hung KC, Chang YJ, Chen JY, Lin MC, et al. Comparison of video-stylet and conventional laryngoscope for endotracheal intubation in adults with cervical spine immobilization: A PRISMA-compliant meta-analysis. Medicine (Baltimore). 2022;101:e30032. https://doi.org/10.1097/MD.0000000000030032.
77. Hung KC, Chang YJ, Chen IW, Lin CM, Liao SW, Chin JC, et al. Comparison of video-stylet and video-laryngoscope for endotracheal intubation in adults with cervical neck immobilisation: a meta-analysis of randomised controlled trials. Anesth Crit Care Pain Med. 2021;40:100965. https://doi.org/10.1016/j.accpm.2021.100965.
78. Ahmad I, Bailey CR. Time to abandon awake fibreoptic intubation? Anaesthesia. 2016;71:12–6. https://doi.org/10.1111/anae.13333.
79. Amir SH, Ali QE, Bansal S. A comparative evaluation of Video Stylet and flexible fibre-optic bronchoscope in the performance of intubation in adult patients. Indian J Anaesth. 2017;61:321–5. https://doi.org/10.4103/ija.IJA_501_16.
80. Bodhey A, Bodhey M, Shallik NA, Al Nadhari M, Griess HF, Al Ani O, et al. Biphasic cuirass ventilation for airway surgeries: a comprehensive review. Cureus. 2024;16:e75477. https://doi.org/10.7759/cureus.75477.
81. Kristensen MS, Hesselfeldt R, Schmidt JF. Modern cuirass ventilation for airway surgery: unlimited access to the larynx and trachea in anaesthetised patients. Br J Anaesth. 2023;131:e106–9. https://doi.org/10.1016/j.bja.2023.07.010.
82. Porizka M, Michalek P, Votruba J, Abdelmalak BB. Extracorporeal oxygenation techniques in adult critical airway obstruction. Prague Med Rep. 2021;122:61–72. https://doi.org/10.14712/23362936.2021.7.
83. Su S, Liang L, Liu Z, Wang L, Zhang T, Chen N. Extracorporeal membrane oxygenation as life-saving bridge for patients with airway obstruction caused by neck and chest tumors to salvage procedure: an in-depth review. Int J Surg. 2025;111:1090–100. https://doi.org/10.1097/JS9.0000000000002008.
84. Apfelbaum JL, Hagberg CA, Connis RT, Abdelmalak BB, Agarkar M, Dutton RP, et al. 2022 American Society of Anesthesiologists practice guidelines for management of the difficult airway. Anesthesiology. 2022;136:31–81. https://doi.org/10.1097/ALN.0000000000004002.
85. Abdelmalak BB. The role of extracorporeal membrane oxygenation in the management of the difficult airway. J Cardiothorac Vasc Anesth. 2023;37:2660–1. https://doi.org/10.1053/j.jvca.2023.08.151.
86. Black AE, Flynn PE, Smith HL, Thomas ML, Wilkinson KA. Development of a guideline for the management of the unanticipated difficult airway in pediatric practice. Paediatr Anaesth. 2015;25:346–62. https://doi.org/10.1111/pan.12615.
87. Pawar DK, Doctor JR, Raveendra US, Ramesh S, Shetty SR, Divatia JV, et al. All India Difficult Airway Association guidelines for the management of unanticipated difficult tracheal intubation in paediatrics. Indian J Anaesth. 2016;60:906–14. https://doi.org/10.4103/0019-5049.195483.
88. Krishna SG, Bryant JF, Tobias JD. Management of the difficult airway in the pediatric patient. J Pediatr Intensive Care. 2018;7:115–25. https://doi.org/10.1055/s-0038-1624576.
89. Huang AS, Hajduk J, Rim C, Coffield S, Jagannathan N. Focused review on management of the difficult paediatric airway. Indian J Anaesth. 2019;63:428–36. https://doi.org/10.4103/ija.IJA_250_19.

90. Templeton TW, Goenaga-Diaz EJ, Runyan CM, Kiell EP, Lee AJ, Templeton LB. A generalized multistage approach to oral and nasal intubation in infants with Pierre Robin sequence: a retrospective review. Paediatr Anaesth. 2018;28:1029–34. https://doi.org/10.1111/pan.13499.
91. El-Boghdadly K, Onwochei DN, Cuddihy J, Ahmad I. A prospective cohort study of awake fibreoptic intubation practice at a tertiary centre. Anaesthesia. 2017;72:694–703. https://doi.org/10.1111/anae.13844.
92. Jagannathan N, Sohn LE, Sawardekar A, Gordon J, Shah RD, Mukherji II, et al. A randomized trial comparing the Ambu Aura-i with the Air-Q intubating laryngeal airway as conduits for tracheal intubation in children. Paediatr Anaesth. 2012;22:1197–204. https://doi.org/10.1111/pan.12024.
93. Jagannathan N, Sohn L, Ramsey M, Huang A, Sawardekar A, Sequera-Ramos L, et al. A randomized comparison between the i-gel and the Air-Q supraglottic airways when used by anesthesiology trainees as conduits for tracheal intubation in children. Can J Anaesth. 2015;62:587–94. https://doi.org/10.1007/s12630-014-0304-9.
94. Gasteiger L, Oswald E, Keplinger M, Putzer G, Luger M, Neururer S, et al. A randomized trial comparing the Ambu Aura-i™and the Ambu Aura Gain™ laryngeal mask as conduit for tracheal intubation in children. Minerva Anestesiol. 2020;86:1143–50. https://doi.org/10.23736/S0375-9393.20.14422-5.
95. Pfitzner L, Cooper MG, Ho D. The Shikani seeing stylet for difficult intubation in children: initial experience. Anaesth Intensive Care. 2002;30:462–6. https://doi.org/10.1177/0310057X0203000411.
96. Fiadjoe JE, Nishisaki A, Jagannathan N, Hunyady AI, Greenberg RS, Reynolds PI, et al. Airway management complications in children with difficult tracheal intubation from the Pediatric Difficult Intubation (PeDI) registry: a prospective cohort analysis. Lancet Respir Med. 2016;4:37–48. https://doi.org/10.1016/S2213-2600(15)00508-1.
97. Edelman DA, Perkins EJ, Brewster DJ. Difficult airway management algorithms: a directed review. Anaesthesia. 2019;74:1175–85. https://doi.org/10.1111/anae.14779.
98. Long B, Gottlieb M. Video laryngoscopy versus fiberoptic bronchoscopy for awake tracheal intubation. Acad Emerg Med. 2025;32:98–100. https://doi.org/10.1111/acem.15051.

Chapter 12
The Most Recent Airway Guidelines

Daniel Edelman and David J. Brewster

12.1 History of Airway Guidelines

Airway guidelines are a set of procedural recommendations and team strategies used to manage airways, predicted to be difficult [1, 2]. These guidelines are specifically designed to ensure safe and effective airway management in the operating room, or when emergency intubation is required in other specific patient groups, such as the critically ill, pregnant, pre-hospital, or trauma patient population [2].

Airway guidelines, often termed 'difficult airway guidelines', typically include a set of algorithms or decision-making tools that clinicians can use to assess the airway and determine the best procedural approach to maintaining safe airway management. These algorithms often include a series of steps that clinicians can follow to assess and evaluate the airway, predict potential difficulties, and plan for potential airway management challenges. The difficult airway guidelines may also include recommendations for specific airway management techniques, such as the use of specialised equipment or medications.

D. Edelman
Alfred Hospital, Melbourne, VIC, Australia

D. J. Brewster (✉)
School of Translational Medicine, Faculty of Medicine, Nursing and Health Science, Monash University, Melbourne, VIC, Australia

Intensive Care Unit, Cabrini Hospital, Melbourne, VIC, Australia

M. Á. Gómez-Ríos, A. van Zundert (eds.), *Evidence-based Guide to Difficult Airway Management*, https://doi.org/10.1007/978-3-032-30769-9_12

The American Society of Anesthesioloigsts (ASA) were the first internationally recognised airway group to publish an airway guideline in 1993 [1]. Since then, the rate of publication of airway guidelines has accelerated [2]. Prior to the development of airway management guidelines and algorithms, airway management was primarily based on an individual's learned skills. The aim of producing and distributing airway guidelines was to standardise patient care and improve patient outcomes.

Today, numerous internationally recognised airway societies in the USA, UK, Canada, Germany, Italy, and India produce difficult airway guidelines at semi-regular intervals to ensure they reflect modern clinical practice [2].

12.2 Content

Airway management skills, training, and equipment will undoubtedly vary by location and the resources available at a specific site. As such, each airway guideline will differ slightly in its recommendations for airway management. Some are focused on a specific patient demographic (obese, pregnant, or paediatric); others are focused on either anticipated or unanticipated difficulty with airway management; and, since the onset of the COVID-19 pandemic, COVID-specific guidelines have also been produced.

As these guidelines provide an overview of airway management, they include all facets of intubation, from preparation and equipment to monitoring and procedure.

12.3 Preparation

Airway guidelines provide guidance not only on the procedure of tracheal intubation but also on assessment and positioning to optimise successful intubation. This involves preoperative assessment using tools such as MACOCHA scoring to evaluate anticipated difficult airways [3], and guidance on optimal positioning and options available to the airway operator to maximise preoxygenation.

12.4 Equipment

Guidelines such as ASA 2022 [4] include tables of 'examples of appropriate airway equipment' that departments, institutions, and practitioners can compare before undergoing airway management. A summary is provided in Table 12.1.

Table 12.1 Minimum contents for anaesthetic trolley or cart

Suggested equipment for an anaesthetic cart or trolley
Self-inflating resuscitation bag
Suction tubing, Yankauers, suction catheters, and appropriate connectors
Face masks of various sizes
Oral and nasal airways of various sizes
Laryngoscope blades and handles of various sizes
Tracheal tubes of various sizes
Tracheal tube introducers (bougie)
Tracheal tube stylets (both malleable and rigid)
Equipment for emergency invasive airway management
Supraglottic airways of various sizes
Water-soluble medical lubricant
Nasal cannula and oxygen face masks
Videolaryngoscope with appropriate stylets
Standard monitoring
Anaesthetic induction, maintenance, and rescue medications

Adapted from ASA 2022 [4]

12.5 Monitoring

In their most recent guidelines, both ASA and DAS have made strong recommendations for capnography as a means to confirm tracheal intubation, with DAS describing this method as the 'gold standard' for confirming lung ventilation [4, 5].

12.6 Procedure

Regarding specific airway management procedures, airway guidelines generally follow a stepwise approach involving tracheal intubation, face-mask ventilation, and SADs. When adequate airway access is not achieved, the vast majority of guidelines detail the steps involved with invasive airway access. This stepwise approach is often depicted in a traffic-light/coloured infographic transitioning from green to red [2]. Most guidelines also detail the number of attempts an airway operator should not exceed before moving to more invasive approaches.

Nevertheless, given the wide range of variation in specific equipment, techniques, and skills, the vast majority of airway guidelines ultimately recommend a comparable stepwise methodology for airway management, culminating in emergency surgical airway rescue [2].

12.7 Human Factors

As in all areas of medicine, human factors are becoming a more recognised consideration when optimising patient outcomes in clinical medicine. This focus on human factors, initially developed in the aviation industry, has become ingrained in elements of medicine, such as surgery, through the WHO Surgical Safety Checklist, and has gained attention in recent years in critical care medicine, such as anaesthetics and intensive care [6, 7].

In keeping with this movement, airway guideline development over the last three decades has increasingly drawn upon and focused on human factors in airway management [8]. Most notably, this is seen in the publication of accompanying airway management algorithms, which summarise and condense an airway guideline into a medium suitable for reading in time-sensitive situations. Other aspects of human factors, including in recent iterations of these guidelines, include ergonomics, optimising operator space, and incorporating cognitive aids in and around airway management areas such as the operating theatre or intensive care bay.

12.8 How Are Guidelines Developed?

The development of airway guidelines varies by circumstance. Generally, they can be divided into 'airway society-produced' and 'non-airway society-produced' guidelines. Of the more widely recognised international society-produced airway guidelines, the majority are formulated through a combination of evidence-based approaches, drawn from a literature search that includes clinical trials and case reports, as well as expert consensus from leading figures in the field. Non-society-produced airway guidelines are often formulated for a specific geographical location and are generally reproductions of other guidelines with minor alterations to enhance practicality for that location.

12.9 Current Guidelines

Many airway guidelines currently exist, with the majority updated at regular intervals, and most international airway societies have produced their own version. Of all guidelines, those of the Difficult Airway Society and the American Society of Anesthesiologists remain the most commonly relied-upon and most frequently referenced in the current literature.

12.10 Difficult Airway Society (DAS)

The Difficult Airway Society in the United Kingdom releases airway guidelines on a semi-regular basis, with updated recommendations reflecting the availability of new equipment and the results of both interventional and observational studies that provide evidence for best practice.

DAS's most recent editions include an intubation guideline from 2025, an extubation guideline from 2011, an obstetric guideline from 2015, and a paediatric guideline from 2018. In 2018, in collaboration with DAS, a guideline for the management of tracheal intubation in critically ill adults was produced, and in 2020, a COVID-specific guideline was produced.

12.10.1 DAS 2025

Development Process

- *A working group commissioned a systematic review and a three-round Delhi consensus process.*

Highlighted Changes Compared to the Previous Guideline

- *Video-laryngoscopy is now integrated into Plan A.*
- *Additional emphasis on the physiologically difficult airway.*
- *Continuous oxygen delivery is established as the central organising principle throughout all phases of airway management.*

12.11 American Society of Anesthesiologists (ASA)

The American Society of Anesthesiologists released new difficult airway guidelines in 2022 and an obstetric guideline in 2016. The ASA aims to update these guidelines every 5 years.

12.11.1 ASA 2022

Development Process

- *'Six-step process' involving literature search and opinion surveys of international experts.*

Highlighted Changes Compared to the Previous Guideline

- *Recommend supplemental oxygen administration before initiating and throughout difficult airway management, including the extubation process.*
- *'Time-out' is included as part of every induction process.*

– *Additional emphasis on human factors within the airway algorithm, such as 'avoiding task fixation', with an emphasis on individual decision-making and calls for help.*
– *Recommendation to confirm tracheal intubation with capnography or end-tidal carbon dioxide monitoring.*

12.12 European Journal of Anaesthesiology (EJA): Universal Videolaryngoscopy Guideline

12.12.1 EJA 2025

Development Process

– Systematic review of the evidence assessed using GRADE methodology stratified into six domains [9].

Key Recommendations

– Videolaryngoscopy is recommended as the standard primary device for tracheal induction in both elective and emergency settings.
– Training programmes are encouraged to incorporate videolaryngoscopy into teaching curricula.

12.13 All India Difficult Airway Association (AIDAA)

The All India Difficult Airway Association previously released a guideline in 2016. This guideline was updated in 2025 [10].

12.13.1 AIDAA 2025

Development Process

– A Delphi consensus process was used to generate expert consensus statements.

Highlighted Changes Compared to the Previous Guidelines

– Importance of identifying the physiologically difficult airway, in addition to the anatomically difficult airway.
– Peri-intubation oxygenation is recommended to extend safe apnoea time during intubation attempts.

12.14 COVID-19-Specific Airway Guidelines

The COVID-19 pandemic brought about specific considerations in airway management, primarily related to personal protective equipment, ventilation, infection risk to the airway operator, and the physiological considerations of COVID-19-infected patients. Soon after the onset of the pandemic, it became widely accepted that airway management, in particular tracheal intubation, is a significant aerosol-generating procedure. Therefore, the previously long-held approaches to airway management needed to be adjusted to accommodate the rapidly changing situation.

As such, multiple airway guidelines focused on the COVID-19 pandemic were produced, taking these considerations into account. In doing so, providing clinicians around the world guidance for how to best manage their patients by utilising experiences from other parts of the world.

COVID-specific airway guidelines were first produced and published by the Safe Airway Society (Australia and New Zealand). Later editions were published by SAIDAA, DAS, and the French Society of Anaesthesia and Intensive Care Medicine (SFAR) [11–14]. These guidelines were considered highly successful, given their high uptake among healthcare providers and their improvement in staff and patient safety during airway management during the early pandemic [15].

The COVID-specific airway guidelines were adapted from previous airway guidelines, with modifications reflecting the specific considerations in the management of patients with COVID-19. The consensus paper by the Safe Airway Society included lists of potential aerosol-generating events related to airway management, as well as risk factors to be aware of and protective strategies to reduce the risk of infection among healthcare workers [13]. The DAS guidelines included guidance on airway team organisation and structure, as well as detailing the principles of personal protective equipment (PPE). In addition, elements to reduce transmission, such as 'buddy systems' and PPE checklists when donning and doffing, were added to the guideline [11].

12.15 Universal Airway Management Guidelines/Algorithms

The vast majority of airway guidelines follow a near-identical approach to airway management, one that is supported by the literature and agreed upon by expert consensus [2]. However, a paradoxical effect can occur, where, rather than simplifying and standardising the process of airway management, the multitude of airway guidelines produced at an increasing frequency, with slight variations in suggestions, definitions, and language utilised, might cause misunderstanding, disrupt widespread implementation, and reduce adherence. To prevent this, efforts such as those of the Difficult Airway Society (DAS) aim to develop a lexicon for airway management that is concise, precise, and universally consistent [16].

Additionally, the Project for Universal Management of Airways (PUMA) was formed in recent years to attempt to formulate a single, universal guideline by collaborating with international airway societies to produce principles of airway management that can be applied 'without restriction to a specific provider background, patient type or geographical region and independent of the intended airway type or other contextual factors' [17]. In 2022, the first guideline by this group was produced in collaboration with multiple airway societies, including DAS, AIDAA, Society for Airway Management, European Airway Management Society, Canadian Airway Focus Group, Safe Airway Society, and International Airway Management Society, in producing the guideline for preventing unrecognised oesophageal intubation [18].

12.16 Conclusion

Airway guidelines are an essential component of airway management, providing regularly updated recommendations. These include all aspects of airway management, from assessment, equipment, monitoring, and airway procedures. Generally, they follow similar stepwise approaches to airway management, incorporating cognitive aids such as infographics and algorithms. These guidelines are updated at regular intervals to ensure that advances in technical changes and evidence from recent literature are addressed and incorporated.

Clinical Situation

A patient with a history of severe sleep apnoea is scheduled for elective surgery requiring general anaesthesia. On examination, the patient has a short neck, a large tongue, and a Mallampati class IV airway. The anaesthesiologist anticipates difficulty with intubation and ventilation.

How to Do

Prepare for a Difficult Airway

The airway operator should have a high level of suspicion for a difficult airway in this patient and prepare accordingly. This includes having a difficult airway cart and equipment readily available, a plan for emergency airway management, and ensuring that sufficiently skilled airway operators are present.

Assess for Predictors of Difficult Intubation

The airway operator should assess for predictors of difficult intubation using the ASA Difficult Airway Algorithm. In this case, the patient's short neck, large tongue, and Mallampati class IV airway are all predictors of difficult intubation.

Formulate an Airway Management Strategy

Consideration should be made for the potential of awake intubation in this anticipated difficult airway. A plan must also be formulated for situations where the patient can be adequately ventilated but is difficult to intubate, for patients who cannot be ventilated or intubated, and for difficulty with emergency invasive airway rescue.

An awake intubation may be the safest approach for this patient.

Have a Rescue Plan

The anaesthesiologist should have a rescue plan in place in case of failed intubation or ventilation. According to most airway guidelines, this follows a stepwise approach. Plan A involves tracheal intubation via laryngoscopy. Plan B involves a Supraglottic Airway Device. Plan C involves a final attempt at face mask ventilation. Plan D is applicable if one is unable to wake up the patient or maintain oxygenation. Then, emergency front-of-neck access must be considered.

References

1. Caplan RA, Benumof JI, Berry FA, et al. Ovassapian: guidelines for management of the difficult airway. A report by the American Society of Anesthesiologists Task Force on Management of the Difficult Airway. Anesthesiology. 1993;78:597–602.
2. Edelman DA, Perkins EJ, Brewster DJ. Difficult airway management algorithms: a directed review. Anaesthesia. 2019;74:1175–85. https://doi.org/10.1111/anae.14779.
3. De Jong A, Molinari N, Terzi N, Mongardon N, Arnal JM, Guitton C, et al. Early identification of patients at risk for difficult intubation in the intensive care unit: development and validation of the MACOCHA score in a multicenter cohort study. Am J Respir Crit Care Med. 2013;187(8):832–9. https://doi.org/10.1164/rccm.201210-1851OC.
4. Apfelbaum JL, Hagberg CA, Connis RT, Abdelmalak BB, Agarkar M, Dutton RP, et al. 2022 American Society of Anesthesiologists practice guidelines for management of the difficult airway. Anesthesiology. 2022;136:31–81. https://doi.org/10.1097/ALN.0000000000004002.
5. Ahmad I, El-Boghdadly K, Iliff H, Dua G, Higgs A, Huntington M, et al. Difficult Airway Society intubation guidelines working group. Difficult Airway Society 2025 guidelines for management of unanticipated difficult intubation in adults. Br J Anaesth. 2026;136(1):9–11. https://doi.org/10.1016/j.bja.2025.11.003.
6. Jones C, Fawker-Corbett J, Groom P, Morton B, Lister C, Mercer S. Human factors in preventing complications in anaesthesia: a systematic review. Anaesthesia. 2018;73:12–24. https://doi.org/10.1111/anae.14136.
7. Marshall SD, Touzell A. Human factors and the safety of surgical and anaesthetic care. Anaesthesia. 2020;75:e34–8. https://doi.org/10.1111/anae.14830.
8. Edelman DA, Duggan LV, Lockhart SL, Marshall SD, Turner MC, Brewster DJ. Prevalence and commonality of non-technical skills and human factors in airway management guidelines: a narrative review of the last 5 years. Anaesthesia. 2022;77:1129–36. https://doi.org/10.1111/anae.15813.
9. Gómez-Ríos MÁ, Van Zundert AAJ, McNarry AF, et al. Guidelines on strategies for the universal implementation of videolaryngoscopy. Eur J Anaesthesiol. 2025;42(10):872–88. https://doi.org/10.1097/EJA.0000000000002210.

10. Myatra SN, Shah AP, Ramkumar V, et al. All India Difficult Airway Association 2025 guidelines for the management of unanticipated difficult airway in adults under general anaesthesia. Indian J Anaesth. 2025;69(11):1117–41. https://doi.org/10.4103/ija.ija_1210_25.
11. Cook TM, El-Boghdadly K, McGuire B, McNarry AF, Patel A, Higgs A. Consensus guidelines for managing the airway in patients with COVID-19: guidelines from the Difficult Airway Society, the Association of Anaesthetists the Intensive Care Society, the Faculty of Intensive Care Medicine and the Royal College of Anaesthetists. Anaesthesia. 2020;75:785–99. https://doi.org/10.1111/anae.15054.
12. Sorbello M, El-Boghdadly K, Di Giacinto I, et al. The Italian coronavirus disease 2019 outbreak: recommendations from clinical practice. Anaesthesia. 2020;75:724–32. https://doi.org/10.1111/anae.15049.
13. Brewster DJ, Chrimes N, Do TB, et al. Consensus statement: Safe Airway Society principles of airway management and tracheal intubation specific to the COVID-19 adult patient group. Med J Aust. 2020;212:472–81. https://doi.org/10.5694/mja2.50598.
14. Velly L, Gayat E, Quintard H, et al. Guidelines: anaesthesia in the context of COVID-19 pandemic. Anaesth Crit Care Pain Med. 2020;39:395–415. https://doi.org/10.1016/j.accpm.2020.05.012.
15. Brewster DJ, Nickson CP, McGloughlin S, Pilcher D, Sarode VV, Gatward JJ. Preparation for airway management in Australia and New Zealand ICUs during the COVID-19 pandemic. PLoS ONE. 2021;16(5):e0251523. https://doi.org/10.1371/journal.pone.0251523.
16. Chrimes N, Higgs A, Sakles JC. Welcome to the era of universal airway management. Anaesthesia. 2020;75:711–5. https://doi.org/10.1111/anae.14998.
17. Chrimes N, Higgs A, Law JA, Baker PA, Cooper RM, Greif R, et al. Project for Universal Management of Airways – part 1: concept and methods. Anaesthesia. 2020;75(12):1671–82. https://doi.org/10.1111/anae.15269.
18. Chrimes N, Higgs A, Hagberg CA, Baker PA, Cooper RM, Greif R, et al. Preventing unrecognised oesophageal intubation: a consensus guideline from the Project for Universal Management of Airways and international airway societies. Anaesthesia. 2022;77:1395–415. https://doi.org/10.1111/anae.15817.

Chapter 13
Rapid Sequence Induction

José Alfonso Sastre, Manuel Ángel Gómez-Ríos, and Teresa López

13.1 Background

Millions of critically ill patients undergo emergency tracheal intubation every year; nearly half of them experience life-threatening hypoxemia, hypercarbia, or hypotension and 1 in 20 suffers a cardiac arrest [1]. The Royal College of Anaesthetists National Audit Project (NAP4) reported an incidence of fatal aspiration during general anesthesia as one in 45,000 [2]. The risk of aspiration itself is estimated at one in 3000–8000 patients undergoing elective surgery, 1 per 820 patients undergoing emergency surgery and 1 in 900 in women undergoing caesarean section [3–5]; these figures are even higher (13%) in patients requiring intubation in the emergency department (ED) [6].

Rapid Sequence Induction (RSI) of anesthesia was described in 1970 by Stept and Safar to address the recognized risk of aspiration of gastric contents and avoid unnecessary morbidity and mortality due to hypoxemia and hypercarbia [7]. The traditional RSI method described by these authors is a set of actions: denitrogenation of the lungs with 100% oxygen for at least 2 min, induction using a predetermined dose of thiopentone, application of cricoid pressure (CP), administration of a predetermined dose of suxamethonium, a period of apnea with no positive pressure ventilation, tracheal intubation with a cuffed tracheal tube, and the release of CP when tube placement is successfully confirmed. This technique has been a gold-standard approach to emergency anesthesia for many years and is still widely practiced in many countries. However, currently, there is no clear evidence showing that

J. A. Sastre (✉) · T. López
Department of Anesthesiology, Complejo Asistencial Universitario de Salamanca, Salamanca, Spain

M. Á. Gómez-Ríos
Department of Anesthesia and Perioperative Medicine, Complejo Hospitalario Universitario de A Coruña, A Coruña, Spain

M. Á. Gómez-Ríos, A. van Zundert (eds.), *Evidence-based Guide to Difficult Airway Management*, https://doi.org/10.1007/978-3-032-30769-9_13

traditional RSI effectively reduces aspiration or improves outcomes [8]. Furthermore, this technique is used by clinicians across multiple medical specialties, including anesthesiologists, critical care physicians, and emergency medical personnel. Due to the notable differences in terms of the patient profile, the different degree of training of practitioners, and the different availability of devices for airway management, the consensus has rapidly declined in recent years and the literature has revealed considerable variation and controversy in how the intervention is delivered [9, 10].

13.2 The Importance of Human Factors in RSI

Physicians who perform RSI work in a complex, time-constrained, rapidly changing, and stressful environment. The concept of human factors refers to the ability of the physician to understand interactions with other elements of the system, and to adapt to them to improve performance and safety. Human factors involve considering the individual, the team, and environmental and organizational factors that influence overall system performance [11]. The importance of these factors is not negligible; NAP4 identified human factors elements in all critical incidents, with a median of four contributory factors per case [12]. During airway management in critically ill patients, individual factors like insufficient patient preparation, improper equipment check, or protocol deviation contributed to 50% of critical incidents [13]. Other individual contributing factors also implicated in the appearance of adverse outcomes were poor situation awareness with suboptimal decision making, failure to re-evaluate, inadequate skills, inadequate airway assessment, stress, and fatigue. The management of high-risk interventions such as RSI requires good teamwork, including leadership and followership [14]. Studies such as NAP4 and similar ones have shown that ineffective coordination/teamwork, role allocation ambiguity, and unclear communication are also related to the occurrence of critical incidents [13, 15, 16]. A good leader should define the roles prior to the start of the RSI and clearly communicate key points in the process (e.g., explicitly verbalizing an intubation failure). Careful assignment allocation may avoid individual and team cognitive overload in both routine and challenging situations. The use of cognitive aids, such as checklists and algorithms, can help to improve decision-making and performance in stressful situations. These tools must be adapted to the availability of equipment where the RSI is carried out and to the environmental conditions [14]. This adaptation is fundamental and allows the training and skillset of junior staff.

The working and environmental conditions can also contribute to the occurrence of adverse events during critical patient care. Among them, we can mention poorly defined material location, disorder, overcrowding, obstructed viewing of monitors, poor equipment location, inadequate lighting, and excessive ambient noise [12]. The operating room (OR) is the ideal setting for airway management; however, RSI is routinely performed in other hostile environments, such as the ED or in outpatient care. In those scenarios, the patient's clinical situation, limited space (e.g., a patient trapped inside a vehicle), and the presence of staff, monitors, and equipment may limit access to the patient. Under such complex conditions, airway equipment should be chosen carefully, avoiding the overload of devices and equipment that can limit space and, moreover, can cause cognitive overload and impair decision-making [14]. Airway equipment should be standardized across the organization, with specific adaptations to each scenario.

Organizational factors have also been pointed out as a cause of adverse incidents related to airway management during emergency care to critically ill patients, such as insufficient staff with excessive workload, deficient training and supervision, and a lack of a structure that allows the reporting and analysis of incidents [17]. High-performance healthcare systems should have structured training of the human teams involved in RSI based on locally available equipment, and using checklists and algorithms adapted to their specific characteristics [14]. A model to follow can be found in the field of Formula 1, where each member of the team (mechanics, drivers, and engineers) undergoes continuous and specific training to handle "pit-stops" (an otherwise stressful situation similar to RSI) [18].

13.3 Indications and Contraindications of RSI

RSI is indicated in patients who require endotracheal intubation and are at increased risk of aspiration of gastric contents. The technique is also indicated in those pathophysiological situations in which emergent tracheal intubation is required. Contraindications are few and usually relative (Table 13.1).

Table 13.1 Indications and contraindications for RSI

Indications for RSI
Airway protection (high risk of aspiration)
Unfasted patient (emergency surgery)
Unclear or undetermined fasting period (e.g., due to a language barrier, inability of the patient to remember when the fasting period began, or decreased level of consciousness)
Medical or physiologic conditions leading to delayed gastric emptying (e.g., diabetic gastroparesis, advanced renal or hepatic dysfunction, critical illness, multiple sclerosis, Parkinson's disease, substance abuse, pain, preoperative administration of opioids, recent trauma, or labor)
Pregnancy from the second trimester onward up to 24 hours after delivery
Gastroesophageal reflux, hiatal hernia, achalasia, Zenker's diverticulum
Gastric outlet obstruction
Previous bariatric surgery (adjustable gastric band, sleeve gastrectomy, Roux-en-Y gastric bypass)
Bowel obstruction
Increased intra-abdominal pressure (ascites, abdominal mass)
Failure to ventilate or oxygenate, leading to hypercapnic or hypoxic respiratory failure
Depressed level of consciousness (Glasgow Coma Scale <8)
Impending obstruction of airway (e.g., airway burn, penetrating neck injury)
Need for neuroprotection (e.g., brain injury leading to increased intracranial pressure)
Contraindications for RSI
Known difficult airway or impossible rescue oxygenation
Patients who might not tolerate apnea
Predictors for difficult emergency surgical airway
Team lacking training and skill with the technique

13.3.1 RSI: Procedure

RSI generally consists of several steps that can be adjusted when appropriate to fit the clinical situation: (1) preparation, (2) reducing the risk of regurgitation, (3) patient positioning, (4) preoxygenation and oxygenation during the apnea, (5) hemodynamic optimization, (6) pretreatment, (7) induction and paralysis, (8) protection, (10) placement of the endotracheal tube and confirmation, and (11) postintubation management.

13.3.2 Preparation

Emergency airway management is associated with significant complications and, hence is considered an extremely high-risk procedure, especially when required in critically ill patients and in locations outside the OR. Urgency and the reduced physiological reserve in this population contribute dramatically to increased risks of profound hypoxemia, hypotension, arrhythmia, cardiac arrest, and death during the procedure, especially when delays occur during tracheal intubation and multiple attempts at laryngoscopy. Failure of "first pass success" occurs in up to 30% of intubations in critically ill patients (significantly higher than in the OR) and severe hypoxemia is reported in up to 25% of patients [14].

The first step should be an assessment to rule out potential difficulty, including anatomic, physiological, or environmental challenges, although the urgency may limit the time available for making an in-depth evaluation. The use of scales or combined methods to evaluate the difficult airway is common in anesthesiology, but it is less frequent both in intensive care units (ICUs) and in hospital or out-of-hospital emergencies. The only validated airway assessment tool in the ICU is the MACOCHA score [19], while for the evaluation prior to intubation in the ED, as well as in the out-of-hospital emergencies, several tools have been used, such as the LEMON score or the HEAVEN criteria [20–22].

Preparation involves having all the necessary personnel, drugs, and equipment such as oxygen, suction, bag-valve mask, laryngoscopes and blades, videolaryngoscopes, endotracheal tubes (with one size larger and smaller than the anticipated endotracheal tube size), bougies and stylets, resuscitation equipment, and devices for rescue maneuvers in case of a failed intubation, like supraglottic airway devices (SAD) and a cricothyrotomy set. The patient should have an intravenous line. Standard monitoring should include oximetry, waveform capnography, blood pressure, heart rate, EKG, and, where available, end-tidal oxygen concentration (ETO_2) (recommendation grade D) [23]. The mnemonic "SOAPME" can be useful to remember the essential tools needed for RSI (Suction, Oxygen, Airway, Pharmacology, Monitoring, Equipment) [24].

The NAP4 report identified some human factors as contributory causes of medical errors and critical incidents during airway management [2]. Standard

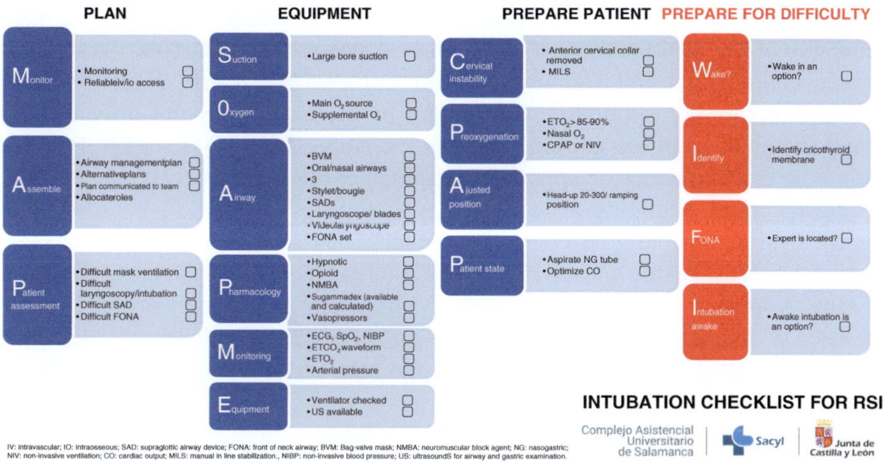

Fig. 13.1 Example of a checklist used as a cognitive aid

operating procedures and checklists have been shown to reduce error and the incidence of hypoxic events during intubation [25–27]; therefore, the use of RSI checklists adapted to each clinical situation (Fig. 13.1) and environmental conditions along with simplified algorithms (like the Vortex approach) designed to be easily recalled in situations of cognitive overload is recommended (grade of recommendation D) [14, 28].

The preparation step should be used to "MAP" (Monitor, Assemble, Patient assessment) out a treatment plan for intubation using RSI and backup alternative plans in case of an unexpected difficult airway [24]. It is important to communicate and verbalize the plan to the assistant staff as well as assign each role (e.g., leader, first and second intubators, runner, etc.).

13.4 Reducing the Risk of Regurgitation

The volume, pH, and composition of gastric contents are important in the pathophysiological process after aspiration. It is therefore important to ensure adequate fasting according to the current guidelines when possible (recommendation grade A) and, if appropriate, to make attempts to reduce gastric content and acidity before RSI [29, 30]. The current guidelines recommend that healthy patients fast for a minimum of 2 h for clear liquids, 4 h for human breastmilk, 6 h for nonhuman breastmilk infant formula or light meals, and 8 h for fried foods, fatty foods, or meat. In patients undergoing enteral feeding by nasogastric tube, an 8-h fast should be made if the tube is in the stomach, 4 h if the tube is transpyloric, and no fasting is necessary if the nasogastric tube is in the jejunum or when the patient is intubated.

An emergency procedure is one of the main risk factors for full stomach, independently of the fasting duration, with a prevalence greater than 50% [31]. In this setting, composition and volume of gastric contents are poorly predictable and should therefore be assessed before surgery by performing a point-of-care ultrasound examination of the antrum (grade of recommendation D) [31, 32]. Because there is no clear guidance on appropriate fasting periods in patients at increased risk of delayed gastric emptying, such as those with diabetes mellitus, advanced renal or hepatic dysfunction, morbid obesity, pregnancy, or recent opioid use, ultrasound assessment of the gastric antrum in these patients can help the physician in decision-making. A third group of patients in which ultrasound can be very useful is in the presence of an unclear "nil per os" (NPO) status, as seen in patients with dementia or decreased level of consciousness, language barriers, and noncompliant patients (recommendation grade D) [32].

The presence of any of the following criteria define a full stomach: (1) thick fluid or solid content in any patient position, (2) an antrum distended with clear fluid in both supine and right lateral decubitus, (3) clear fluid with an antral cross-sectional area >10 cm^2 in the right lateral decubitus for an average adult, or (4) clear fluid with an estimated gastric volume >1.5 $mL.kg^{-1}$ (Fig. 13.2); in this situation, special measures should be taken to prevent aspiration [33].

For high-risk patients, routine use of either a histamine-2-blocking agent or a proton pump inhibitor 40–60 min before induction is recommended to increase pH and reduce gastric volume (grade of recommendation B) [29, 34]. Oral premedication with a nonparticulate antacid (30 mL 0.3 M sodium citrate) immediately before induction is suggested to neutralize acidity (grade of recommendation B) [29, 34]. Prokinetic drugs like metoclopramide may be administered to patients at increased risk of pulmonary aspiration to reduce gastric contents, except if there is a contraindication like a bowel obstruction (recommendation grade D) [29, 34].

Pre-operative gastric emptying before RSI by a nasogastric tube (NG) is not recommended for routine use and it is contraindicated in patients at risk of esophageal rupture, in the presence of cervical spine, facial, or skull base fractures, or increased intracranial pressure (ICP) [35]. The indication for gastric emptying using an NG tube must be done on an individual basis, although this treatment is recommended in patients with ileus or intestinal obstruction or when the gastric volume

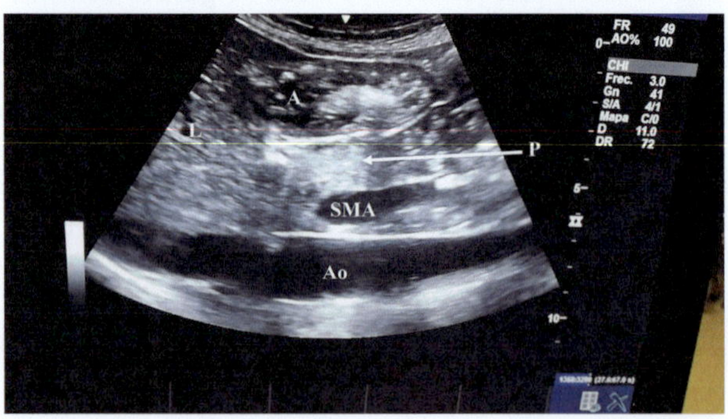

Fig. 13.2 Sonographic image of the stomach in the right lateral decubitus showing the "starry night appearance" represented by clear fluid mixed with gas bubbles. The patient had taken an indeterminate quantity of water 30 min before. *A* antrum, *Ao* aorta, *SMA* superior mesenteric artery, *P* pancreas, *L* liver

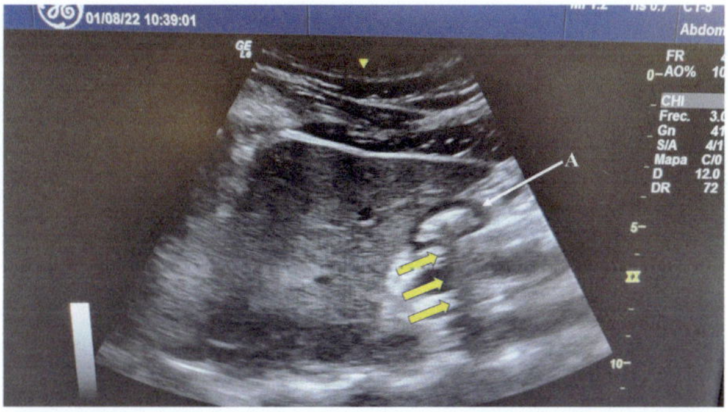

Fig. 13.3 Sonographic image of the stomach showing an empty antrum with a nasogastric tube inside, causing the typical "comet-tail" image (yellow arrows)

measured by ultrasounds is >1.5 mL.kg^{-1} (grade of recommendation D) [34–36]. If indicated, a large-bore double-lumen tube (Salem-Sump tube type) should be preferred. When the patient has a previously inserted NG tube, it should be left in place, and suction should be applied before induction and continued during the procedure. In case of doubt about the proper position of the NG tube, this can be verified by gastric ultrasound (Fig. 13.3).

13.5 Patient Positioning

Patient positioning should be tailored to their individual characteristics, as well as the skill of the person who performs RSI, and be used to optimize both anatomic and physiological parameters to increase the success of intubation and avoid complications [37]. In stable patients, tilting the patient's head up 20–30° is recommended since, although there is no evidence that this maneuver reduces the risk of aspiration [38], it prevents a reduction in the functional residual capacity (FRC), improves preoxygenation, and may reduce the risk of passive regurgitation (recommendation grade A) [39–41]. Combining a 20–30° head-up position with a sniffing position substantially improves upper airway access and reduces complication rates, including desaturation [39]. Reverse Trendelenburg and sitting positions are useful for patients with suspected cervical spine injury, while the ramping position (with the external auditory meatus situated at the same level as the sternal notch) is useful in obese patients [41–43].

If regurgitation occurs, it is recommended to adopt a Trendelenburg position to prevent gastric contents from entering the larynx, turn the head to one side, and aspirate the oropharynx and trachea before initiating positive pressure ventilation (grade of recommendation D) [44].

In patients with cervical instability, the presence of a cervical collar may limit mouth opening (and make both laryngoscopy and the insertion of an SAD more difficult or even impossible) [45]. RSI should be performed using manual-in-line stabilization (MILS) with removal of at least the anterior part of the collar to facilitate airway instrumentation, application of CP or "front of neck airway" (FONA) if necessary (recommendation grade B) [46, 47].

13.6 Preoxygenation and Oxygenation During the Apnea

The objectives of maximally preoxygenating a patient before RSI are to provide the maximum amount of time so the patient can tolerate apnea after induction of anesthesia and for the physician to solve a can-not-intubate-cannot-oxygenate (CICO) situation.

In the absence of respiratory failure, the standard recommended technique for RSI is preoxygenate using a tight-fitting facemask, with 10–15 lpm 100% oxygen for 3–5 min or eight vital capacity breaths; both techniques allow to prolong the period of apnea without desaturation and thus improve the likelihood of first attempt success. Preoxygenation with a "Hudson-type" facemask, with or without a reservoir, is not recommended, because it provides only 65–80% of the fraction of inspired oxygen (FiO_2), do not provide complete denitrogenation of the lungs, and accordingly does not maximize the duration of safe apnea (grade of recommendation A) [14, 48, 49]. Adequate preoxygenation should be measured using ETO_2, and the target should be, if possible, an $ETO_2 \geq 90\%$ [50]. A common cause of failure to reach this goal is the presence of a significant leak, which allows mixing of ambient air, causing a decrease in the effective FiO_2; the leak is detected by the absence or attenuation of the capnograph trace and can be minimized by holding the mask with a two-handed technique and using an appropriately sized facemask [51]. The addition of supplemental oxygen via a nasal cannula in the presence of mask leaks may be helpful in improving ETO_2 (recommendation grade A) [52].

Although preoxygenation techniques reduce the incidence of desaturation during tracheal intubation, they are of limited value in the scenario of prolonged difficult laryngoscopy. Furthermore, critically ill patients are especially vulnerable to hypoxemia during RSI for several reasons, including lack of time for adequate preparation, reduced FRC, increased oxygen demand, pulmonary shunting, and lack of patient cooperation. Standard methods of preoxygenation are only partially effective in those cases, in which it is impossible to obtain the target of an $ETO_2 > 90\%$, regardless of the duration of the technique, and have little impact in extending the period of apnea without desaturation [53]. Life-threatening hypoxemia is a common complication in those patients, occurring in 19–70% of intubations [54, 55].

Insufflation of continuous O_2 at 15 lpm into the pharynx through a nasal cannula (Nasal Oxygen During Efforts of Securing a Tube or NODESAT), a nasopharyngeal airway or a catheter during intubation appears to prevent or delay desaturation in patients without respiratory failure (grade of recommendation A) [56, 57]. The three key determinants for achieving effective apnea oxygenation are adequate circulation, a constant supply of fresh O_2, and a patent upper airway that allows a continuous flow of O_2 from the pharynx to the lungs during the apnea period. For this reason, it is mandatory to perform a jaw thrust after induction of anesthesia to prevent a collapse of the upper airway that impedes the free flow of oxygen.

High-flow nasal oxygen (HFNO), by delivering high flow rates (up to 60 L/min) of heated and humidified 100% O_2, may generate moderate supraglottic positive end-expiratory pressure (PEEP), and reduce the patient's respiratory effort. This technique makes it possible to hold nasal prongs in place after induction of anesthesia and during laryngoscopy to perform apneic oxygenation throughout the intubation procedure. Furthermore, tolerance of HFNO is excellent, whereas induction with a tightly applied mask can cause discomfort and claustrophobia. Current evidence suggests that HFNO applied for apneic oxygenation reduced severe desaturation in elective intubation in the OR (recommendation grade A) and in patients with mild respiratory failure ($PaO_2/FiO_2 > 200$) (recommendation grade C), but not in patients with severe respiratory failure [58–62]. Contraindications to HFNO include severe facial trauma or suspected skull base fractures [14].

Noninvasive ventilation (NIV) is the optimal technique for preoxygenation of high-risk patients (grade of recommendation A) [63–65]. With a full-face mask properly fitted, FiO_2 of 100% is assured, and no practitioner is needed to maintain the mask seal.

Apneic oxygenation should be continued during attempts, and gentle mask ventilation should be considered during RSI to prevent or treat hypoxemia. The risk/benefit of active ventilation during the apnea period must be carefully tailored in each patient. In patients at low risk for desaturation, ventilation is not usually necessary, except in the case of an unexpected difficult airway. In patients with SpO_2 between 91% and 95%, an individual assessment (including an estimation of aspiration and desaturation risks) should be made before deciding to use facemask ventilation. In hypoxemic patients ($SpO_2 \leq 90\%$), who will be unable to tolerate a brief period of apnea, low-pressure, low-volume, low-rate ventilations will be required to prevent or treat hypoxemia (grade of recommendation D) [14, 42, 66] (Table 13.2). When manual ventilation is mandatory, triple airway maneuvers (mandible advancement, neck extension, and mouth opening) with two hands in the sniffing position using an oropharyngeal or nasopharyngeal cannula is recommended (recommendation grade A) [67–69]. In patients with cervical instability, ventilation with a face mask is the maneuver that most mobilizes the cervical spine; in these patients, it would be better to perform mask ventilation using a jaw thrust maneuver to avoid excessive mobilization of the cervical spine [70]. The patient should be ventilated with the lowest pressure that allows adequate oxygenation and gas exchange (ideally <15 cmH_2O without CP and < 20 cmH_2O with CP) to prevent passage of air into the stomach and gastric distension (recommendation grade A) [71–73]. This has been referred to as *controlled RSI*. In patients at high risk of aspiration who require ventilation to prevent or treat desaturation, the application of CP can limit air passage to the stomach and prevent gastric distention (recommendation grade A) [72, 73].

Agitated patients are frequently unable to tolerate the use of a tight-fitting mask to accomplish adequate preoxygenation. In this situation, it may be necessary to carry out the RSI in a different way to achieve that objective. *Delayed sequence intubation* consists of the administration of a sedative agent, which does not alter spontaneous ventilation or airway reflexes, followed by a period of preoxygenation before the administration of a paralytic agent (grade of recommendation C) [14, 48, 74]. The currently preferred agent is ketamine because of its dissociative properties and established safety margins. Its administration in small aliquots of 0.2–0.5 mg.

Table 13.2 Preoxygenation and apneic oxygenation based on the severity of acute respiratory failure

Severity of respiratory failure[a]	Suggested preoxygenation technique (3–5 min if time permits)
No failure ($SpO_2 > 96\%$)	Standard preoxygenation using a tight-fitting facemask, with 10–15 lpm 100% O_2 for 3–5 min or 8 vital capacity breaths using an anesthesia circuit or BVM Apneic oxygenation with nasal cannula oxygen (standard or HFNO) during intubation BVM ventilation if SpO_2 drops below 90%
Mild ($PaO_2/FiO_2 > 200$ or $SpO_2 = 91–95\%$)	Standard preoxygenation using a tight-fitting facemask, with 10–15 lpm 100% O_2 for 3–5 min or 8 vital capacity breaths + CPAP 5–10 cmH_2O (when using an anesthesia circuit) or + PEEP 5–10 cm H_2O (when using BVM) HFNO Apneic oxygenation with nasal cannula oxygen (standard or HFNO) during intubation BVM ventilation if SpO_2 drops below 90%
Moderate ($PaO_2/FiO_2 \leq 200$ or $SpO_2 < 90\%$)	Noninvasive ventilation (also including CPAP) with PEEP 5–10 cmH_2O and FiO_2 100% Apneic oxygenation with nasal cannula oxygen (standard or HFNO) during intubation BVM ventilation with PEEP 5–10 cmH_2O if $SpO_{2<}$ 90%
Severe ($PaO_2/FiO_{2<}100$)	Noninvasive ventilation (also including CPAP) with PEEP 5–10 cmH_2O and FiO_2 100% Consider awake fiberoptic intubation using noninvasive ventilation, through dedicated masks Apneic oxygenation with nasal cannula oxygen (standard or HFNO) during intubation BVM ventilation with PEEP 5–10 cmH_2O if $SpO_{2<}$ 90%

Modified from Cabrini, with permission of the author [48, 66]
[a]Risk categories are based on the patient's initial response to high-flow oxygen through a tight-fitting nonrebreather mask at the time of intubation decision
BVM bag-valve-mask device, *HFNO* high-flow nasal oxygen, *NIV* noninvasive ventilation

kg^{-1} until dissociation is achieved (generally with doses of 1–1.5 $mg.kg^{-1}$) allows preoxygenation to be performed in a safe, controlled fashion. After reaching the appropriate ETO_2 target, an NMBA is administered, and RSI is continued following the usual course.

13.7 Hemodynamic Optimization

Even successful intubation in critically ill patients has a high risk of hypotension (nearly 50% of patients) [75], with cardiovascular collapse occurring in 30% of them [76]. Instability is an independent predictor of death after intubation; cardiac arrest has been reported in approximately 2% of intubations in critically ill patients and in one in eight emergency intubations outside the OR, increasing with repeated intubation attempts [77]. It is essential to stabilize the patient's hemodynamic status before RSI to avoid circulatory complications in the post-intubation period, mostly of them related to preload alterations, anesthetics, autonomic disturbances, and positive pressure ventilation.

Predicting which patients will develop hypotension is a great challenge for the physician. Aggressive free resuscitation with fluids and vasopressors was not associated with a lower risk of cardiovascular collapse and is not without risk [78, 79]; therefore, attempts have been made to find bedside tools that allow to identify those patients who would likely develop hemodynamic instability during RSI. Several studies have shown that a preintubation shock index (SI, heart rate/systolic blood pressure) >0.8–0.9 may be a useful tool for predicting postintubation hypotension (systolic blood pressure < 90 mmHg) and mortality in emergently intubated adult patients in intensive care units; despite this, still one-third of patients with a normal SI will develop postintubation hypotension [80, 81].

13.8 Pretreatment

Traditionally, lidocaine has been used to lessen the sympathetic response to intubation in patients with suspected elevations in ICP, who have asthma and are experiencing bronchospasm. The typical dose of lidocaine is 1.5 $mg.kg^{-1}$, and it has a relatively quick onset of action. It should be administered at least 3 min prior to RSI to blunt the increase in ICP; however, this could result in an unacceptable delay when emergent intubation is indicated. There is no high-quality evidence to support the use of a pretreatment dose of lidocaine in patients with head injuries requiring RSI in the emergency department; in addition, its use is not free from adverse events such as hypotension and arrhythmia [82–84]. Although lidocaine can suppress cough reflexes when administered prior to intubation, there is no clear evidence that lidocaine reduces bronchospasm [85]. Thus, the use of this drug should be considered only on an individual basis, balancing the harm and benefit (grade of recommendation D).

Precurarization or a priming dose of a nondepolarizing neuromuscular block agent (NMBA) (usually using one tenth of the normal paralyzing dose given 3 min before induction) has been commonly used in RSI. When using succinylcholine, priming doses of a NMBA have been used in order to avoid fasciculations and postoperative myalgia and to blunt the increase of intracranial, intraocular, and intragastric pressures. For nondepolarizing blocking agents, the main reason to administer a priming dose is to shorten the onset times of the NMBA used for induction and allow faster intubation. However, the existence of individual variations in sensitivity to NMBAs means that even 10% of a normal induction dose has the potential to cause harmful effects such as hypoventilation, impaired laryngeal reflexes, and muscle weakness [86–88]. Considering these facts, there is no convincing evidence supporting routine pretreatment with NMBA in RSI (recommendation grade D).

13.9 Induction and Paralysis

When Stept and Safar described the RSI in 1970, many of the induction agents currently available had not yet been introduced into clinical practice, and the technique was performed using thiopentone and suxamethonium, with doses calculated prior to induction. This technique has been associated with a high risk of accidental awareness and can result in serious hemodynamic side effects [89]; these are two of the several reasons that explain the existence of large differences between practitioners in the management of RSI nowadays [9, 10]. While appropriate and judicious resuscitation with volume and vasopressors is the mainstay of preventing postintubation hypotension, a tailored selection of anesthetics for intubation is also important to avoid cardiovascular collapse. The ideal drug for RSI should be a short-acting drug with combined sedative, analgesic, and amnesic properties and should allow adequate intubation conditions with minimal hemodynamic disturbances. However, the ideal intravenous induction agent does not exist, with individual drugs harboring benefits and disadvantages (Table 13.3). The choice of intravenous induction agent should be guided by patient's clinical condition and not by custom (grade of recommendation D) [14, 24, 90]. Propofol, for example, will provide the best intubation conditions, but its cardiovascular effects can be harmful for patients with hemodynamic instability. Predetermined dosing may be appropriate in patients at high risk of aspiration in order to minimize the time until intubation; however, this practice may increase the risk of both underdosing (which increases the probability of awareness) and also overdosing (which increases the probability of cardiovascular instability and can be life threatening). When the risk of hemodynamic disturbances will clearly outweigh the risk of aspiration, then drug choice must address the more serious problem, and administration should be titrated to effect (loss of consciousness) [91, 92]. Propofol has become the agent of choice for induction of RSI in the OR, while the use of intravenous ketamine is currently a common practice in prehospital care [9, 93, 94], because it offers a better hemodynamic profile and

Table 13.3 Induction agents in RSI

	Benefits	Disadvantages	Suggestions for use in ISR
Hypnotics (doses)			
Sodium thiopental (3–7 $mg.kg^{-1}$)	Fast onset Antiepileptic ↓ cerebral oxygen demand and ICP	Postoperative nausea and vomiting Tissue necrosis due to extravasation Antanalgesic CVS instability (i.e., hypotension, myocardial depression)	Traditionally used in obstetrics Use in hemodynamically stable patients with ↑ ICP Status epilepticus

(continued)

Table 13.3 (continued)

	Benefits	Disadvantages	Suggestions for use in ISR
Propofol (2–4 mg.kg[1])	↓ laryngeal reflexes (best intubating conditions) Anti-emetic Widespread use	CVS instability (i.e., hypotension, myocardial depression) Pain on injection	Drug of choice when intubation conditions are the main objective Drug of choice in ISR without opioids Alternative to thiopental in obstetrics (lower incidence of intraoperative awareness) Mixture of propofol and ketamine (ketofol) presents great hemodynamic stability
Etomidate (0.3 mg.kg^{-1})	CVS stability	Adrenal suppression by inhibition of 11-β-hydroxylase Pain on injection Myoclonus	Cardiovascular instability Avoid/caution in sepsis and, if used, consider supplementing with corticosteroids Not recommended for use without opioids Contraindicated for prolonged infusion
Ketamine (1–2 mg.kg^{-1})	Bronchodilator CVS stimulant: maintains cerebral perfusion pressure in hypotensive patients Maintains airway reflexes No respiratory depression Potent analgesia	↑ ICP (only if hypercapnia occurs) ↑ IOP Emergence phenomena	Asthmatic patients Shock Alternative to propofol in intubation without opioids Pre-hospital use Avoid in patients with myocardial ischemia
Midazolam (0.1–0.3 mg. kg^{-1})	Potent amnesic (↓awareness) Greater hemodynamic stability than standard induction agents	Slow onset Long acting Prolonged apnea Paradoxical agitation Delirium in elderly	No interest as sole agent for RSI Status epilepticus Unstable patients at risk of awareness

(continued)

Table 13.3 (continued)

	Benefits	Disadvantages	Suggestions for use in ISR
NMB (doses)			
Succinylcholine (1–1.5 mg.kg^{-1})	Fast onset Short acting	Life-threatening side effects (malignant hyperthermia or hyperkalemia) Fasciculations ↑ IGP and ↓ safe apnea time Highly variable duration of action due to deficiencies in plasma cholinesterase (time to recovery may exceed the period of safe apnea) Intubating conditions deteriorate quickly when the effect is wearing off	Traditional gold standard No predicted difficulty with intubation (which would otherwise require prolonged paralysis)
Rocuronium bromide (1–1.2 mg.kg^{-1})	Fast onset Longer duration of good intubating conditions Early reversion with sugammadex 16 mg. kg^{-1} (when the dose is pre-calculated and immediately available)	Prolonged action Anaphylaxis	Alternative to the traditional approach When "wake up" is not a feasible option (one-way-induction) Patient with respiratory failure Head injury ↑ ICP
Opioids (doses)			
Fentanyl (2–5 μg.kg^{-1})	Reduce sympathetic response	Respiratory depression Hypotension because of blunting of sympathetic drive in critically ill patients Muscle rigidity at high doses	Blunt intubation response specially in elevated ICP or cardiovascular disease
Alfentanil (15–40 μg.kg^{-1})	Rapid onset Reduce sympathetic response	Respiratory depression Hypotension because of blunting of sympathetic drive in critically ill patients Muscle rigidity at high doses	Blunt intubation response specially in elevated ICP or cardiovascular disease
Remifentanil (0.5–1 μg.kg^{-1})	Rapid onset Short half-life Reduce sympathetic response	Respiratory depression Hypotension because of blunting of the sympathetic drive in critically ill patients Muscle rigidity at high doses	Blunt intubation response specially in elevated ICP or cardiovascular disease

(continued)

Table 13.3 (continued)

	Benefits	Disadvantages	Suggestions for use in ISR
Sufentanil (0.1 $\mu g.kg^{-1}$)	Reduce sympathetic response	Respiratory depression Hypotension because of blunting of the sympathetic drive in critically ill patients Muscle rigidity at high doses	Blunt intubation response specially in elevated ICP or cardiovascular disease

CVS cardiovascular system, *ICP* intracranial pressure, *IOP* intraocular pressure, *IGP* intragastric pressure

conditions of intubation than thiopental [95, 96]. Etomidate and ketamine are alternatives in patients with hemodynamic instability [91, 97]. Although etomidate has been associated with adrenal insufficiency in the first 12 h after a single induction dose, it was not associated with increased mortality or organ dysfunction in the critically ill patient compared to other induction agents [98–101]. In patients with sepsis or suspected adrenal insufficiency, the theoretical risk of using etomidate must be weighed against the hemodynamic instability caused by alternative induction agents [91, 97]. The prophylactic use of empirical glucocorticoids in patients undergoing an induction with etomidate has shown conflicting results, therefore only be administered in patients with hypotension refractory to fluid resuscitation and vasopressor treatment [100, 102, 103].

Although opioid administration was not part of the original RSI protocol, currently 80% of physicians use an opioid at induction [10, 104]. Co-induction using short-acting opioids like fentanyl, remifentanil, and alfentanil allows to reduce the dose of hypnotics; they also improve intubation conditions, promoting cardiovascular stability and minimizing rises in ICP in situations where those effects could be potentially harmful (recommendation grade A) [105–112]. The choice of drug and dosage should be made balancing the risk of hypotension and the beneficial effect provided by the opioid (prevention of sympathetic discharge). Fentanyl attenuates rises in blood pressure and frequency at doses of 2 $\mu g.kg^{-1}$, but at least 5 $\mu g.kg^{-1}$ is needed to adequately blunt the hemodynamic response to intubation [106, 111, 112]. Alfentanil (15–40 $\mu g.kg^{-1}$), remifentanil (0.5–1 $\mu g.kg^{-1}$), and sufentanil (0.1 $\mu g.kg^{-1}$) provide adequate control of the response to laryngoscopy and intubation during RSI without causing excessive hypotension and bradycardia [105, 109, 113, 114].

The administration of an NMBA is considered mandatory during RSI because it improves mask ventilation and intubation conditions (by abolishing cough and laryngospasm), reduces complications, and optimizes chest wall compliance (grade of recommendation A) [115, 116]. Currently, rocuronium 1.0–1.2 $mg.kg^{-1}$ is comparable to succinylcholine 1.0–1.5 $mg.kg^{-1}$ for RSI [117–119]. Rocuronium provides a longer-lasting block, which may be advantageous if airway management difficulties arise [91], and it can be reversed more quickly than succinylcholine with sugammadex (16 mg.kg^{-1}) [120], provided that the dose of the antidote has been previously calculated and is immediately available for an assistant to prepare and administer on instructions for emergency reversal [91, 121]. Also, rocuronium has a safer clinical profile, although it may have a higher risk of anaphylaxis [122]. Succinylcholine can cause life-threatening side effects such as malignant hyperthermia or hyperkalemia, and muscular fasciculations could increase the intragastric pressure and shorten apnea time [123, 124]. Overall, the use of rocuronium is increasingly favored.

13.10 Protection

The CP maneuver was described by Sellick in 1961 based on a series of 26 patients with a high risk of aspiration [125]. Sellick's maneuver rapidly became an essential component of the RSI technique and replaced the head-up position commonly used until then. The CP has been a standard of care for almost 50 years despite the low level of evidence from the original publication. However, in the last 20 years, numerous publications have raised controversy surrounding the maneuver. Although Sellick described that CP could prevent the stomach contents from reaching the pharynx by temporary occlusion of the upper esophagus by backward pressure on the cricoid ring, magnetic resonance imaging studies showed that CP effectively compresses the hypopharynx (containing the cricopharyngeal muscle) rather than the cervical esophagus even in the presence of a nasogastric tube [126–130]. The maneuver can also be useful to avoid gastric insufflation during positive-pressure ventilation [72, 73]. For a safe use of CP, the current recommendation is to apply 10 N (1 kg) when the patient is awake and increase the force to 30 N (3 kg) once the patient loses consciousness (grade of recommendation C) [131, 132]; since gastric pressures are generally less than 25 mmHg in the supine position under general anesthesia even during emergency caesarean section with a full stomach, this force is more than enough to prevent regurgitation in most patients [131, 133, 134]. It is recommended that the personnel performing the maneuver should undergo CP simulation training to ensure that the cricoid force can be reproducible (grade of recommendation A) [135]. In the awake patient, CP may produce minor complications such as discomfort, retching, and nausea [136]. Serious complications such as esophageal rupture or fracture of the cricoid cartilage have been described but are uncommon [137, 138]. CP should be avoided in patients with retropharyngeal abscess, in patients with active vomiting, and in the presence of a sharp object in the esophagus (such as bone chips) (grade of recommendation D) [136]. There is no compelling evidence that either the BURP (Backward, Upward, Rightward Pressure) or CP maneuvers worsen neurological injury in patients with unstable cervical spine [139].

To date, the Sellick maneuver has not been shown to prevent aspiration [140–143], and a review of the scientific literature can give us some clues that explain this lack of effectiveness. One study showed that it is biomechanically impossible to maintain the recommended pressure during laryngoscopy [144]; furthermore, the CP produces a reflex reduction in the tone of the lower esophageal sphincter that can facilitate gastroesophageal reflux (the greater the applied force, the greater the reduction) [145]. On the other hand, the maneuver is not harmless. CP may increase airway obstruction [146], cause difficulty for laryngoscopy and tracheal intubation [142], and hinder facial mask ventilation [146]. CP may also compromise insertion, ventilation, and tracheal intubation through SAD [147, 148], as well as fiberoptic-guided intubation [149, 150], potentially prolonging the tracheal intubation times and increasing the rate of difficult intubation [142, 151]. By current standards, CP cannot be considered an evidence-based practice for routine use due to doubts that its benefits outweigh the risks [37, 134, 152, 153]. The maneuver can be used: (1) on an individual basis (recommendation grade D), (2) if facemask ventilation is necessary during the apnea period (to prevent gastric distension) (recommendation grade A), (3) it should be released and apply a BURP maneuver when it hinders glottic vision during laryngoscopy (recommendation grade D), and (4) it should be released before inserting a SAD if attempts of initial tracheal intubation were unsuccessful (recommendation grade D) [34, 154, 155].

Airway management is often complicated by the presence of copious secretions, blood, or massive regurgitated gastric contents, especially in cases of out-of-hospital cardiac arrest. In these circumstances, the application of the SALAD (Suction-Assisted Laryngoscopy and Airway Decontamination) technique may be useful to facilitate basic and advanced airway management [9]. This method consists of the proactive use of a rigid suction catheter (Yankauer or SSCOR DuCanto) to assist the insertion of a laryngoscope or a SAD in the manner of a laryngoscope blade itself while continuous suction of the oral cavity and hypopharynx is performed (Fig. 13.4. How to do it.). An alternative can be the use of the endotracheal tube itself as an aspirator with or without a stylet connected through a swivel adapter to a meconium aspirator or to a nasogastric tube connector (Fig. 13.5) [156].

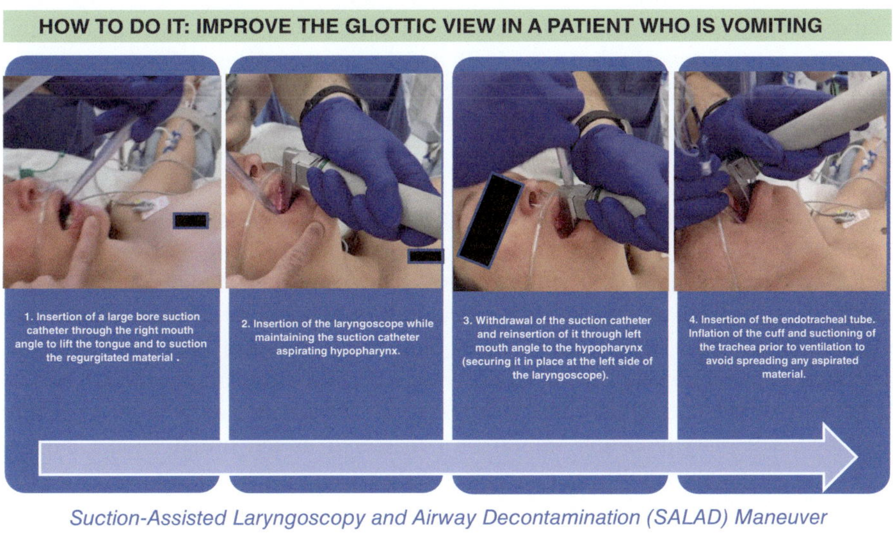

Fig. 13.4 How to do it. Steps of the SALAD maneuver

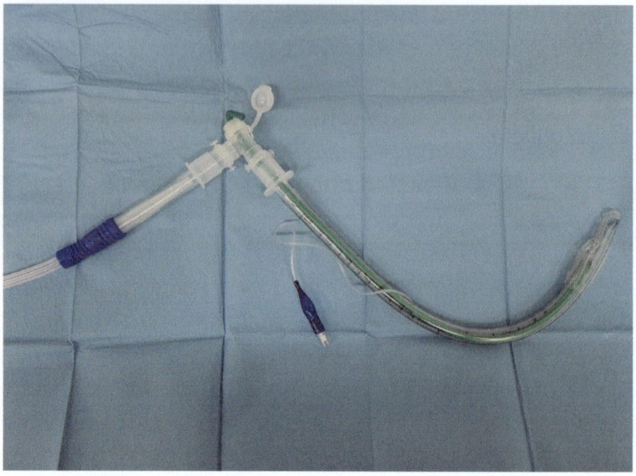

Fig. 13.5 Endotracheal tube with stylet connected to an aspirator through a swivel adapter with a perforated rubber head and a nasogastric tube connector. This technique allows both continuous removal of the vomit/blood/secretions throughout endotracheal tube placement and intubation using the same device. The trachea may then be suctioned before the aspirator is disconnected

13.11 Devices

For critically ill adults, failure to intubate the trachea on the first attempt occurs in up to 10% of cases and is associated with severe complications like hypoxemia, cardiac arrest, and death [157]. Routine use of a tracheal tube introducer (stylet or bougie) was associated with increased first-attempt success; consequently, its use is recommended for intubation in RSI (grade of recommendation A) [158–160]. Bougie or stylet is useful for Cormack-Lehane grade 2b or 3a views or when videolaryngoscopy is performed with a hyperangulated blade; on the other hand, blind efforts to pass a tracheal tube in grade 3b and 4 views are potentially traumatic and should be avoided (recommendation grade D) [161]. In patients with predictors of a difficult airway, or when this situation occurs during RSI, the use of a smaller tube (6.0 mm) may facilitate easier intubation (recommendation grade D) [14].

The use of videolaryngoscopy as the first choice of intubation has increased significantly in the last decade [162, 163]. Different observational studies [164–167], randomized clinical trials [168, 169], and even meta-analysis [170, 171] have shown that videolaryngoscopes, regardless of design, reduce rates of failed intubation and result in a higher first-attempt success rate with improved glottic views both in the OR, in ED, and also in critical care units. Macintosh-style and channeled videolaryngoscopes reduce rates of hypoxemic events, while videolaryngoscopes with a hyperangulated blade reduce rates of esophageal intubation. Based on the available evidence, videolaryngoscopy should be considered as the initial choice device, especially in patients with suspicion of a difficult airway, to maximize the likelihood of first attempt success (recommendation grade A). The first-attempt intubation rate using videolaryngoscopes with a hyperangulated blade is higher when a rigid stylet is used as an aid; therefore, the use of a stylet shaped according to the curvature of the blade is mandatory in this situation (grade of recommendation C) [172], Videolaryngoscopes can have additional benefits during RSI: (1) the existence of a screen allows a shared view of the airway facilitating team aids, and therefore can play an important role in improving human factors associated with airway management [173], (2) these devices improve intubation training for novice trainees by allowing real-time instruction [174, 175] and, (3) some models incorporate an image recording function that can serve as a useful testimony for future approaches to the airway and even serve as a legal document [176].

Patients with cervical spine instability who are intubated using the MILS maneuver may have a worse rate of glottic visualization and a higher incidence of intubation failure [177]; these patients may benefit from the combined use of a stylet and videolaryngoscope for intubation (recommendation grade B) [47]. An additional benefit of using videolaryngoscopy in these patients is that cervical spine general movements are less when compared with the direct laryngoscope, although motion is similar at the occipital—C1–C2 complex with both types of devices [178, 179].

13.12 Intubators

RSI is currently practiced by different providers, such as anesthesiologists and emergency physicians, with varying degrees of training in handling this procedure. It has been described that the experience of the intubator affects first-pass success; likewise, rescue intubation by skilled physicians is also associated with a higher probability of success at the second attempt [180, 181]. The international consensus recommends that subsequent attempts after a failed first intubation attempt be performed by experienced physicians (recommendation grade C) [155, 182].

13.12.1 Placement of the Endotracheal Tube and Confirmation

Laryngoscopy should be performed carefully, and when the larynx is visualized and the endotracheal tube placed, the stylet, if used, is then removed and the cuff inflated. CP can be discontinued on instruction from the intubator. Tube position should be confirmed by a combination of visualizing the passage of the tube between the cords, listening to both sides of the chest and the stomach and $ETCO_2$ measurement (which is the most reliable method). Failure to use capnography in ventilated patients likely contributed to more than 70% of related deaths in critically ill patients [15]. The presence of flat capnography indicates esophageal intubation or complete tracheobronchial obstruction. A frequent error is the misinterpretation of a "flat" capnography when esophageal intubation occurred in the context of a cardiac arrest or when a cardiac arrest occurred due to it. However, in cardiac arrest, the trace of capnography is not flat when the quality of chest compressions is good (an $ETCO_2$

reading >10 mmHg indicates compressions are generating perfusion) and allows differentiation of both situations [183]. Clinical practice guidelines specifically addressed "the use of waveform capnography to confirm and continuously monitor the position of an endotracheal tube in patients suffering cardiac arrest and it should be used in addition to clinical assessment; if waveform capnography is not available, a non-waveform carbon dioxide detector or esophageal detector device in addition to clinical assessment is an alternative" (grade of recommendation B) [183].

When quantitative capnography is unavailable or unreliable, point-of-care ultrasound is a valuable and highly accurate adjunct for endotracheal tube confirmation that even allows dynamic visualization in real time as the tube is introduced into the trachea or esophagus (recommendation grade A) [184, 185]. Dynamic ultrasound may not be feasible when intubation is made by only one provider, when cricoid pressure is required, and in patients with large neck masses, abnormal upper airway anatomy, soft tissue air, significant neck edema, or in the presence of a cervical collar.

13.12.2 Post-intubation Management

Pulmonary mechanics and gas exchange worsen during the induction of anesthesia due to the appearance of atelectasis. Recruitment maneuvers are potentially beneficial in hypoxic patients following intubation if hemodynamic compromise is avoided [186].

13.13 Management of the Failure

Failed intubation occurs in 10–30% in critically ill patients and is likely to result in severe hypoxemia [187]. Airway management should not be started without formulating a patient-specific strategy based on three basic elements (clinical context, the patient's history, and physical examination) to minimize the number of attempts and not compromise airway patency. Knowledge and application of airway management guidelines such as the "Vortex approach" [28], availability of and familiarization with airway devices and techniques, and a team-based approach are important factors that may improve patient safety and avoid "catastrophes."

For the first attempt, the optimal device and position should be chosen to maximize the chance of success (e.g., a videolaryngoscope may be better than a conventional laryngoscope) [176]. Limiting the number of attempts is the core principle of safe airway management [155]; additional attempts are only justified when they involve some modification that substantially improves the probability of success (e.g., the use of a different device or blade, or even the operator as necessary, use of suction, or a reduction or release of CP) [28]. External laryngeal manipulation or BURP maneuver may improve the view of the glottis. Between attempts, facemask ventilation should be verified, and an appropriate level of anesthetic depth and neuromuscular block must be maintained [155]. Neuromuscular blockade improves facemask ventilation, especially in the context of laryngeal spasm, chest wall rigidity, or obesity [188, 189]. Continue peroxygenation efforts using nasal oxygen, and facemask ventilation, or both, should be made between second-generation SAD device insertion or during intubation attempts [14, 155]. High oropharyngeal seal pressures of second-generation SADs allow adequate ventilation of poorly compliant lungs and less gastric inflation. In addition, they can vent regurgitating gastric contents via the drain tube, offering a degree of airway protection and facilitating insertion of a gastric tube.

Successful oxygenation via facemask ventilation or a SAD offers the opportunity to “stop and think,” reformulate the strategy, communicate, or even “call for help”. Once oxygenation is assured, the optimal course of action depends on the clinical situation and on the physician’s skills. The priority should be to maintain oxygenation while minimizing the risk of losing the airway, aspiration, or airway trauma. Resource to rescue facemask ventilation mandates that the team prepare for FONA while considering the most appropriate management option, including waking up the patient (rarely applicable in critically ill patients), waiting for an expert to arrive, a single attempt at fiberoptic intubation via the SAD or an endoscopy facial mask, or proceeding to FONA [14, 155].

The failure of rescue oxygenation via SAD and facemask ventilation requires declaring a CICO scenario, ensuring an adequate neuromuscular blockade, and the immediate performance of a FONA regardless of the SpO_2 value [190]. A clear and explicit declaration of airway failure facilitates practical and psychological “priming” for FONA [28]. Delayed transition to a surgical airway because of procedural reluctance is common in airway crises and is a relevant cause of morbidity and mortality (more than complications of the procedure itself) [14]. The optimal FONA technique is via the cricothyroid membrane using a scalpel-bougie-tube cricothyroidotomy technique (grade of recommendation C) [14, 155]. Transtracheal jet ventilation via a narrow bore cannula is currently not recommended because of the extremely poor outcomes related to high rates of device and technique failure [2, 191]. If a scalpel cricothyroidotomy fails, a percutaneous or surgical tracheostomy can be attempted lower in the trachea [14].

13.14 Future Directions in RSI

Traditional RSI was developed with a focus on surgical patients with a full stomach who were managed by anesthesiologists with a high level of training in airway management. However, currently this technique is frequently performed outside the OR by physicians with different levels of training and with a great variability in the availability of resources and devices; this assumes that the management of RSI is subject to multiple governance processes, which were not present in 1970 when Step and Safar developed the technique. High-performing systems should recognize that the delivery of high-quality RSI is not just a clinical activity and requires an effective team approach to apply the appropriate techniques. Accordingly, health systems must develop strategies in various areas to adapt to this new reality and deliver safer emergency management; those areas for improvement include training, supervision, development of checklists and guidelines, and incident reporting [192]. Airway management training should be an integral part of the educational curriculum of all specialties involved in RSI. Quality improvement programs for trainees, including high-fidelity simulation-based training programs, nontechnical skills (crew resource management, crisis resource management and crisis avoidance resource management), team approaches to intubation with assigned roles, and checklists may improve the odds of first attempt success and decrease complications during RSI [193, 194]. Finally, registries and databases may provide very useful information that allow us to identify key areas for improvement of the RSI process and guide quality improvement [15, 195, 196].

10 Take-Home Messages About RSI

1. Evaluate

Evaluate the airway and fasting status. If you are in doubt, use point-of-care gastric ultrasound

2. Prepare

Prepare essential equipment (suction, oxygen, airway, pharmacology, monitoring, equipment [SOAPME]) using a checklist

3. Plan

Plan each patient individually, communicate the plans to your assistants, and assign roles

4. Improve

Improve your patient's physiology by correcting hemodynamic changes and using an appropriate position for pre-oxygenation

5. Oxygenate

Oxygenate before and throughout the RSI. If your patient is at risk of desaturation, use noninvasive ventilation and consider even ventilating during apnea

6. Choose

Choose the drug, dose, and timing according to the clinical situation

7. Keep

Keep adequate neuromuscular blockade throughout the procedure

8. Optimize

Optimize the first attempt by selecting the best device and adjuvants for each patient. Remember that the first attempt is usually the best

9. Limit

Limit the number of attempts. First do no harm

10. Train

Train continuously with the team and the devices available in your work environment. Become a leader

Summary of Recommendations for Performing RSI

Recommendation	Grade
Standard monitoring for RSI should include oximetry, waveform capnography, blood pressure, heart rate, ECG, and, where available, end-tidal oxygen concentration (ETO_2)	D
Standard operating procedures, along with simplified algorithms designed to be easily recalled in situations of cognitive overload, are recommended	D
When possible, adequate fasting according to the current guidelines should be ensured before rapid sequence induction (RSI)	A
In emergencies, gastric content and volume should therefore be assessed by performing a point-of-care ultrasound examination of the antrum	D
Patients with suspicion of delayed gastric emptying or those with an unclear NPO status, an ultrasound assessment of the gastric antrum can help the physician with decision-making	D
For patients at high risk of aspiration, routine use of either a histamine-2-blocking agent or a proton pump inhibitor 40–60 min before induction is recommended to increase pH and reduce gastric volume	B
Prokinetic drugs like metoclopramide may be administered to patients at increased risk of pulmonary aspiration to reduce gastric contents	D
The indication for gastric emptying using a nasogastric tube must be done on an individual basis. However, this treatment is recommended in patients with ileus or intestinal obstruction or when the gastric volume measured by ultrasounds is >1.5 $mL.kg^{-1}$	D
Tilting the patient's head up 20–30°, reverse Trendelenburg or sitting positions (in patients with cervical spine injury), or ramping position (for obese patients) are the positions recommended before performing RSI because they may improve FRC and preoxygenation and reduce the risk of passive regurgitation	A
If regurgitation occurs, it is recommended to adopt a Trendelenburg position to prevent regurgitated gastric fluid from entering the larynx, turn the head to one side, and aspirate the oropharynx and trachea before initiating positive pressure ventilation	D
In patients with cervical instability, RSI should be performed using MILS with removal of at least the anterior part of the collar to facilitate airway instrumentation and application of CP and FONA	B
Preoxygenation with a "Hudson-type" facemask, with or without a reservoir, is not recommended	A
The addition of supplemental oxygen via a nasal cannula in the presence of mask leaks may help improve ETO_2	A
Insufflation of continuous oxygen at 15 L/min through a nasal cannula, a nasopharyngeal airway, or a catheter during the apnea period is recommended to prevent or delay desaturation in patients without respiratory failure	A
HFNO is recommended for preventing severe desaturation during the apnea period in the elective intubation of patients without respiratory failure	A
HFNO may be useful in preventing severe desaturation during the apnea period in patients with mild respiratory failure ($PaO_2/FiO_2 > 200$), but not in patients with severe respiratory failure	C

(continued)

Recommendation	Grade
Noninvasive ventilation (NIV) is the optimal technique for preoxygenation of patients at high risk of desaturation	A
In hypoxemic patients ($SpO_2 \leq 90\%$), who are unable to tolerate brief periods of apnea, low-pressure, low-volume, low-rate ventilations should be used to prevent or treat hypoxemia	D
When manual ventilation is mandatory, triple airway maneuvers (mandible advancement, neck extension, and mouth opening) with two hands in the sniffing position using an oropharyngeal or nasopharyngeal cannula are recommended	A
In patients requiring ventilation during the RSI apnea period, the lowest pressure that allows adequate oxygenation and gas exchange (ideally <15 cmH2O without CP and < 20 cmH2O with CP) should be used to prevent the passage of air into the stomach and gastric distension	A
CP may be used to limit air passage and prevent gastric distention in patients at high risk of aspiration who require ventilation to prevent or treat desaturation	A
Delayed sequence intubation should be used in uncooperative patients to allow adequate preoxygenation	C
The use of lidocaine for blunting the response to intubation in patients with increased ICP or asthma should be considered only on an individual basis, balancing the harm and benefit	D
Routine pretreatment with NMBA to avoid complications related to the use of succinylcholine or for shortening the onset times of NMBA is not recommended	D
The choice of the intravenous induction agent should be guided by the patient's hemodynamic conditions and not by custom	D
Co-induction using short-acting opioids is recommended for reducing the dose of hypnotics, improving intubation conditions, and promoting cardiovascular stability	A
The administration of an NMBA is recommended because it improves mask ventilation and intubation conditions, reduces complications, and optimizes chest wall compliance	A
The recommended force for CP is 10 N (1 kg) when the patient is awake and 30 N (3 kg) once the patient loses consciousness	C
It is recommended that the personnel performing the CP maneuver should undergo simulation training to ensure that the cricoid force can be reproducible	A
CP should be used on an individual basis	D
CP should be released and apply a BURP maneuver when it hinders laryngoscopy	D
CP should be released before inserting an SAD if attempts of initial tracheal intubation were unsuccessful	D
The use of a stylet or bougie is recommended for intubation in RSI	A
Blind efforts to pass a tracheal tube using a stylet in grade 3b and 4 views are potentially traumatic and should be avoided	D

(continued)

Recommendation	Grade
In patients with predictors of a difficult airway, or when this situation occurs during RSI, the use of a smaller tube (6.0 mm) may facilitate easier intubation (recommendation grade D)	D
Videolaryngoscopy should be considered as the initial choice device in patients with suspicion of a difficult airway to maximize the likelihood of first-attempt success	A
The use of a stylet is recommended when using videolaryngoscopes with hyperangulated blades for improving the first pass success	C
The combination of stylet and videolaryngoscope is recommended for intubation in patients with cervical spine instability	B
Subsequent attempts after a failed first intubation attempt should be performed by experienced physicians	C
Waveform capnography is recommended to confirm and continuously monitor the position of an endotracheal tube in victims of cardiac arrest, and it should be used in addition to clinical assessment	B
When quantitative capnography is unavailable or unreliable, point-of-care ultrasound is recommended for endotracheal tube confirmation	A
The optimal FONA technique is via the cricothyroid membrane using a scalpel-bougie-tube cricothyroidotomy technique	C

References

1. Seitz KP, Gandotra S, Casey JD. Emergency tracheal intubation: a procedure in need of better evidence. Am J Respir Crit Care Med. 2022;206:370–1. https://doi.org/10.1164/rccm.202204-0792ED.
2. Cook TM, Woodall N, Frerk C. Major complications of airway management in the UK: results of the Fourth National Audit Project of the Royal College of Anaesthetists' and the Difficult Airway Society. Part 1: anaesthesia. Br J Anaesth. 2011;106:617–31. https://doi.org/10.1093/bja/aer058.
3. Sun J, Wei G, Hu L, Liu C, Ding Z. Perioperative pulmonary aspiration and regurgitation without aspiration in adults: a retrospective observational study of 166,491 anesthesia records. Ann Palliat Med. 2021;10:4037–46. https://doi.org/10.21037/apm-20-2382.
4. Warner MA, Warner ME, Weber JG. Clinical significance of pulmonary aspiration during the perioperative period. Anesthesiology. 1993;78:56–62. https://doi.org/10.1097/00000542-199301000-00010.
5. Soreide E, Bjornestad E, Steen P. An audit of perioperative aspiration pneumonitis in gynaecological and obstetric patients. Acta Anaesthesiol Scand Scand. 1996;40:14–9. https://doi.org/10.1111/j.1399-6576.1996.tb04382.x.
6. Dhanapal SG, Vijay J, Amirtharaj J, Ganesan P. Aspiration during rapid sequence induction: prevalence and risk factors. Indian J Crit Care Med. 2021;25:140–5. https://doi.org/10.5005/jp-journals-10071-23714.
7. Stept WJ, Safar P. Rapid induction/intubation for prevention of gastric-content aspiration. Anesth Analg. 1970;49:633–6.

8. Neilipovitz DT, Crosby ET. No evidence for decreased incidence of aspiration after rapid sequence induction. Can J Anesth. 2007;54:748–64. https://doi.org/10.1007/BF03026872.
9. Sastre JA, López T, Gómez-Ríos MA, Garzón JC, Mariscal ML, Martínez-Hurtado E, et al. Current practice of rapid sequence induction in adults: a national survey among anesthesiologists in Spain. Rev Esp Anestesiol Reanim. 2020;67:381–90. https://doi.org/10.1016/j.redar.2020.03.007.
10. Klucka J, Kosinova M, Zacharowski K, De Hert S, Kratochvil M, Toukalkova M, et al. Rapid sequence induction. Eur J Anaesthesiol. 2020;37:435–42. https://doi.org/10.1097/EJA.0000000000001194.
11. Haerkens MH, Jenkins DH, van der Hoeven JG. Crew resource management in the ICU: the need for culture change. Ann Intensive Care. 2012;2:39. https://doi.org/10.1186/2110-5820-2-39.
12. Flin R, Fioratou E, Frerk C, Trotter C, Cook TM. Human factors in the development of complications of airway management: preliminary evaluation of an interview tool. Anaesthesia. 2013;68:817–25. https://doi.org/10.1111/anae.12253.
13. Reader T, Flin R, Lauche K, Cuthbertson BH. Non-technical skills in the intensive care unit. Br J Anaesth. 2006;96:551–9. https://doi.org/10.1093/bja/ael067.
14. Higgs A, McGrath BA, Goddard C, Rangasami J, Suntharalingam G, Gale R, et al. Guidelines for the management of tracheal intubation in critically ill adults. Br J Anaesth. 2018;120:323–52. https://doi.org/10.1016/j.bja.2017.10.021.
15. Cook TM, Woodall N, Harper J, Benger J. Chapter 6. Results of second phase of NAP4: ICU and the emergency department. In: Cook T, Woodal N, Frerk C, editors. Major complications of airway management: report and findings. London: The Royal College of Anaesthetists and the Difficult Airway Society; 2011. p. 40–51.
16. Reader T, Flin R, Cuthbertson B. Communication skills and error in the intensive care unit. Curr Opin Crit Care. 2007;13:732–6. https://doi.org/10.1097/MCC.0b013e3282f1bb0e.
17. Sexton JB, Berenholtz SM, Goeschel CA, Watson SR, Holzmueller CG, Thompson DA, et al. Assessing and improving safety climate in a large cohort of intensive care units. Crit Care Med. 2011;39:934–9. https://doi.org/10.1097/CCM.0b013e318206d26c.
18. Seamons R. 9 Lessons teams can learn from Formula 1 pit stops [Internet]. Groove. [Cited 2022 Dec 6]. Available from: https://meetgroove.com/pit-stops/
19. Luedike P, Totzeck M, Rammos C, Kindgen-Milles D, Kelm M, Rassaf T. The MACOCHA score is feasible to predict intubation failure of nonanesthesiologist intensive care unit trainees. J Crit Care. 2015;30:876–80. https://doi.org/10.1016/j.jcrc.2015.04.118.
20. Reed MJ, Dunn MJG, McKeown DW. Can an airway assessment score predict difficulty at intubation in the emergency department? Emerg Med J. 2005;22:99–102. https://doi.org/10.1136/emj.2003.008771.
21. Kuzmack E, Inglis T, Olvera D, Wolfe A, Seng K, Davis D. A novel difficult-airway prediction tool for emergency airway management: validation of the HEAVEN criteria in a large air medical cohort. J Emerg Med. 2018;54:395–401. https://doi.org/10.1016/j.jemermed.2017.12.005.
22. Nausheen F, Niknafs NP, MacLean DJ, Olvera DJ, Wolfe AC, Pennington TW, et al. The HEAVEN criteria predict laryngoscopic view and intubation success for both direct and video laryngoscopy: a cohort analysis. Scand J Trauma Resusc Emerg Med. 2019;27:1–9. https://doi.org/10.1186/s13049-019-0614-6.
23. Checketts MR, Alladi R, Ferguson K, Gemmell L, Handy JM, Klein AA, et al. Recommendations for standards of monitoring during anaesthesia and recovery 2015: Association of Anaesthetists of Great Britain and Ireland. Anaesthesia. 2016;71:85–93. https://doi.org/10.1111/anae.13316.
24. Mace SE. Challenges and advances in intubation: rapid sequence intubation. Emerg Med Clin North Am. 2008;26:1043–68. https://doi.org/10.1016/j.emc.2008.10.002.
25. Thomassen Ø, Brattebø G, Søfteland E, Lossius HM, Heltne JK. The effect of a simple checklist on frequent pre-induction deficiencies. Acta Anaesthesiol Scand. 2010;54:1179–84. https://doi.org/10.1111/j.1399-6576.2010.02302.x.

26. Turner JS, Bucca AW, Propst SL, Ellender TJ, Sarmiento EJ, Menard LM, et al. Association of checklist use in endotracheal intubation with clinically important outcomes: a systematic review and meta-analysis. JAMA Netw Open. 2020;3:1–12. https://doi.org/10.1001/jamanetworkopen.2020.9278.
27. Brindley PG, Beed M, Law JA, Hung O, Levitan R, Murphy MF, et al. Airway management outside the operating room: how to better prepare. Can J Anesth. 2017;64:530–9. https://doi.org/10.1007/s12630-017-0834-z.
28. Chrimes N. The vortex: a universal "high-acuity implementation tool" for emergency airway management. Br J Anaesth. 2016;117:i20–7. https://doi.org/10.1093/bja/aew175.
29. Practice guidelines for preoperative fasting and the use of pharmacologic agents to reduce the risk of pulmonary aspiration: application to healthy patients undergoing elective procedures: an updated report by the American Society of Anesthesiologists Tas. Anesthesiology. 2017;126:376–93. https://doi.org/10.1097/ALN.0000000000001452.
30. Folcini M, Casáis M, Fernández H, Flores L, Romero C, Rosas M, et al. Guías de la Asociación de Anestesia, Analgesia y Reanimación de Buenos Aires para el ayuno perioperatorio en pacientes adultos y pediátricos en procedimientos electivos. Rev Argentina Anestesiol. 2016;74:10–8. https://doi.org/10.1016/j.raa.2016.06.004.
31. Bouvet L, Desgranges FP, Aubergy C, Boselli E, Dupont G, Allaouchiche B, et al. Prevalence and factors predictive of full stomach in elective and emergency surgical patients: a prospective cohort study. Br J Anaesth. 2017;118:372–9. https://doi.org/10.1093/bja/aew462.
32. Perlas A, Arzola C, Van de Putte P. Point-of-care gastric ultrasound and aspiration risk assessment: a narrative review. Can J Anesth. 2018;65:437–48. https://doi.org/10.1007/s12630-017-1031-9.
33. Van de Putte P, Bouvet L. Gastric ultrasound. Image interpretation [Internet]. [cited 2022 Dec 8]. Available from: https://www.gastricultrasound.org/en/interpretation/
34. Jensen A, Callesen T, Hagemo J, Hreinsson K, Lund V, Normark J. Scandinavian clinical practice guidelines on general anaesthesia for emergency situations. Acta Anaesthesiol Scand. 2010;54:922–50. https://doi.org/10.1111/j.1399-6576.2010.02277.x.
35. Salem MR, Khorasani A, Saatee S, Crystal GJ, El-Orbany M. Gastric tubes and airway management in patients at risk of aspiration: history, current concepts, and proposal of an algorithm. Anesth Analg. 2014;118:569–79. https://doi.org/10.1213/ANE.0b013e3182917f11.
36. Mencke T, Zitzmann A, Reuter DA. New aspects of rapid sequence induction including treatment of pulmonary aspiration. Anaesthesist. 2021;70:171–84. https://doi.org/10.1007/s00101-020-00901-8.
37. Karamchandani K, Wheelwright J, Yang AL, Westphal ND, Khanna AK, Myatra SN. Emergency airway management outside the operating room: current evidence and management strategies. Anesth Analg. 2021;133:648–62. https://doi.org/10.1213/ANE.0000000000005644.
38. Jeske HC, Borovicka J, Von Goedecke A, Meyenberger C, Heidegger T, Benzer A. The influence of postural changes on gastroesophageal reflux and barrier pressure in nonfasting individuals. Anesth Analg. 2005;101:597–600. https://doi.org/10.1213/01.ANE.0000159378.97509.8D.
39. Khandelwal N, Khorsand S, Mitchell SH, Joffe AM. Head-elevated patient positioning decreases complications of emergent tracheal intubation in the ward and intensive care unit. Anesth Analg. 2016;122:1101–7. https://doi.org/10.1213/ANE.0000000000001184.
40. Ramkumar V, Umesh G, Ann Philip F. Preoxygenation with 20° head-up tilt provides longer duration of non-hypoxic apnea than conventional preoxygenation in non-obese healthy adults. J Anesth. 2011;25:189–94. https://doi.org/10.1007/s00540-011-1098-3.
41. Dixon BJ, Dixon JB, Carden JR, Burn AJ, Schachter LM, Playfair JM, et al. Preoxygenation is more effective in the 25° head-up position than in the supine position in severely obese patients: a randomized controlled study. Anesthesiology. 2005;102:1110–5. https://doi.org/10.1097/00000542-200506000-00009.
42. Weingart SD, Levitan RM. Preoxygenation and prevention of desaturation during emergency airway management. Ann Emerg Med. 2012;59:165–75.e1. https://doi.org/10.1016/j.annemergmed.2011.10.002.

43. Altermatt FR, Muñoz HR, Delfino AE, Cortínez LI. Pre-oxygenation in the obese patient: effects of position on tolerance to apnoea. Br J Anaesth. 2005;95:706–9.
44. Berkow LC. Rapid sequence induction and intubation (RSII) for anesthesia. Crowley M, editor. UpToDate. 2021.
45. Goutcher CM, Lochhead V. Reduction in mouth opening with semi-rigid cervical collars. Br J Anaesth. 2005;95:344–8. https://doi.org/10.1093/bja/aei190.
46. Crosby ET. Airway management in adults after cervical spine trauma. Anesthesiology. 2006;104:1293–318. https://doi.org/10.1097/00000542-200606000-00026.
47. Ollerton JE, Parr MJA, Harrison K, Hanrahan B, Sugrue M. Potential cervical spine injury and difficult airway management for emergency intubation of trauma adults in the emergency department – a systematic review. Emerg Med J. 2006;23:3–11. https://doi.org/10.1136/emj.2004.020552.
48. Weingart SD. Preoxygenation, reoxygenation, and delayed sequence intubation in the Emergency Department. J Emerg Med. 2011;40:661–7. https://doi.org/10.1016/j.jemermed.2010.02.014.
49. Groombridge C, Chin CW, Hanrahan B, Holdgate A, Reardon R. Assessment of common preoxygenation strategies outside of the operating room environment. Acad Emerg Med. 2016;23:342–6. https://doi.org/10.1111/acem.12889.
50. Tanoubi I, Drolet P, Donati F. Optimizing preoxygenation in adults. Can J Anesth. 2009;56:449–66. https://doi.org/10.1007/s12630-009-9084-z.
51. Benumof JL. Preoxygenation best method for both efficacy and efficiency? Anesthesiology. 1999;91:603–5. https://doi.org/10.1097/00000542-199909000-00006.
52. Hayes-Bradley C, Lewis A, Burns B, Miller M. Efficacy of nasal cannula oxygen as a preoxygenation adjunct in emergency airway management. Ann Emerg Med. 2021;68:174–80. https://doi.org/10.1016/j.annemergmed.2015.11.012.
53. Mort TC. Preoxygenation in critically ill patients requiring emergency tracheal intubation. Crit Care Med. 2005;33:2672–5. https://doi.org/10.1097/01.CCM.0000187131.67594.9E.
54. Bodily JB, Webb HR, Weiss SJ, Braude DA. Incidence and duration of continuously measured oxygen desaturation during emergency department intubation presented at the Society for Academic Emergency Medicine meeting, Atlanta, GA, May 2013. Ann Emerg Med. 2016;67:389–95. https://doi.org/10.1016/j.annemergmed.2015.06.006.
55. Griesdale DEG, Bosma TL, Kurth T, Isac G, Chittock DR. Complications of endotracheal intubation in the critically ill. Intensive Care Med. 2008;34:1835–42. https://doi.org/10.1007/s00134-008-1205-6.
56. Taha SK, Siddik-Sayyid SM, El-Khatib MF, Dagher CM, Hakki MA, Baraka AS. Nasopharyngeal oxygen insufflation following pre-oxygenation using the four deep breath technique. Anaesthesia. 2006;61:427–30. https://doi.org/10.1111/j.1365-2044.2006.04610.x.
57. Ramachandran S, Cosnowski A, Shanks A, Turner CR. Apneic oxygenation during prolonged laryngoscopy in obese patients: a randomized, controlled trial of nasal oxygen administration. J Clin Anesth. 2010;22:164–8. https://doi.org/10.1016/j.jclinane.2009.05.006.
58. Vourc'h M, Asfar P, Volteau C, Bachoumas K, Clavieras N, Egreteau PY, et al. High-flow nasal cannula oxygen during endotracheal intubation in hypoxemic patients: a randomized controlled clinical trial. Intensive Care Med. 2015;41:1538–48. https://doi.org/10.1007/s00134-015-3796-z.
59. Sjöblom A, Broms J, Hedberg M, Lodenius A, Furubacke A, Henningsson R, et al. Pre-oxygenation using high-flow nasal oxygen vs. tight facemask during rapid sequence induction. Anaesthesia. 2021;76:1176–83. https://doi.org/10.1111/anae.15426.
60. Hung KC, Ko CC, Chang PC, Wang KF, Teng IC, Lin CH, et al. Efficacy of high-flow nasal oxygenation against peri- and post-procedural hypoxemia in patients with obesity: a meta-analysis of randomized controlled trials. Sci Rep. 2022;12:1–11. https://doi.org/10.1038/s41598-022-10396-5.

61. Guitton C, Ehrmann S, Volteau C, Colin G, Maamar A, Jean-Michel V, et al. Nasal high-flow preoxygenation for endotracheal intubation in the critically ill patient: a randomized clinical trial. Intensive Care Med. 2019;45:447–58. https://doi.org/10.1007/s00134-019-05529-w.
62. Jhou HJ, Chen PH, Lin C, Yang LY, Lee CH, Peng CK. High-flow nasal cannula therapy as apneic oxygenation during endotracheal intubation in critically ill patients in the intensive care unit: a systematic review and meta-analysis. Sci Rep. 2020;10:1–11. https://doi.org/10.1038/s41598-020-60636-9.
63. Frat JP, Ricard JD, Quenot JP, Pichon N, Demoule A, Forel JM, et al. Non-invasive ventilation versus high-flow nasal cannula oxygen therapy with apnoeic oxygenation for preoxygenation before intubation of patients with acute hypoxaemic respiratory failure: a randomised, multicentre, open-label trial. Lancet Respir Med. 2019;7:303–12. https://doi.org/10.1016/S2213-2600(19)30048-7.
64. Baillard C, Fosse JP, Sebbane M, Chanques G, Vincent F, Courouble P, et al. Noninvasive ventilation improves preoxygenation before intubation of hypoxic patients. Am J Respir Crit Care Med. 2006;174:171–7. https://doi.org/10.1164/rccm.200509-1507OC.
65. Rodriguez M, Ragot S, Coudroy R, Quenot JP, Vignon P, Forel JM, et al. Noninvasive ventilation vs. high-flow nasal cannula oxygen for preoxygenation before intubation in patients with obesity: a post hoc analysis of a randomized controlled trial. Ann Intensive Care. 2021;11:1–14. https://doi.org/10.1186/s13613-021-00892-8.
66. Cabrini L, Pallanch O, Pieri M, Zangrillo A. Preoxygenation for tracheal intubation in critically ill patients: one technique does not fit all. J Thorac Dis. 2019;11:S1299–303. https://doi.org/10.21037/jtd.2019.04.67.
67. El-Boghdadly K, Aziz MF. Face-mask ventilation: the neglected essentials? Anaesthesia. 2019;74:1227–30. https://doi.org/10.1111/anae.14703.
68. Sato Y, Ikeda A, Ishikawa T, Isono S. How can we improve mask ventilation in patients with obstructive sleep apnea during anesthesia induction? J Anesth. 2013;27:152–6. https://doi.org/10.1007/s00540-012-1520-5.
69. Fei M, Blair JL, Rice MJ, Edwards DA, Liang Y, Pilla MA, et al. Comparison of effectiveness of two commonly used two-handed mask ventilation techniques on unconscious apnoeic obese adults. Br J Anaesth [Internet]; 2017;118:618–24. Available from: https://doi.org/10.1093/bja/aex035.
70. Prasarn ML, Horodyski MB, Scott NE, Konopka G, Conrad B, Rechtine GR. Motion generated in the unstable upper cervical spine during head tilt-chin lift and jaw thrust maneuvers. Spine J. 2014;14:609–14. https://doi.org/10.1016/j.spinee.2013.06.080.
71. Bouvet L, Albert ML, Augris C, Boselli E, Ecochard R, Rabilloud M, et al. Real-time detection of gastric insufflation related to facemask pressure-controlled ventilation using ultrasonography of the antrum and epigastric auscultation in nonparalyzed patients. Anesthesiology. 2014;120:326–34.
72. Vasudevan A, Srinivasan S, Vinayagam S, Ramkumar R, Senthilnathan M. Assessment of effectiveness of cricoid pressure in preventing gastric insufflation during bag and mask ventilation: a randomized controlled trial. Saudi J Anaesth. 2018;12:606–11. https://doi.org/10.4103/sja.SJA_240_18.
73. Moynihan RJ, Brock-Utne JG, Archer JH, Feld LH, Kreitzman TR. The effect of cricoid pressure on preventing gastric insufflation in infants and children. Anesthesiology. 1993;78:652–6. https://doi.org/10.1097/00000542-199304000-00007.
74. Weingart SD, Seth Trueger N, Wong N, Scofi J, Singh N, Rudolph SS. Delayed sequence intubation: a prospective observational study. Ann Emerg Med. 2015;65:349–55. https://doi.org/10.1016/j.annemergmed.2014.09.025.
75. Green RS, Turgeon AF, McIntyre LA, Fox-Robichaud AE, Fergusson DA, Doucette S, et al. Postintubation hypotension in intensive care unit patients: a multicenter cohort study. J Crit Care. 2015;30:1055–60. https://doi.org/10.1016/j.jcrc.2015.06.007.

76. Perbet S, De Jong A, Delmas J, Futier E, Pereira B, Jaber S, et al. Incidence of and risk factors for severe cardiovascular collapse after endotracheal intubation in the ICU: a multicenter observational study. Crit Care. 2015;19:1–8. https://doi.org/10.1186/s13054-015-0975-9.
77. Mort TC. The incidence and risk factors for cardiac arrest during emergency tracheal intubation: a justification for incorporating the ASA guidelines in the remote location. J Clin Anesth. 2004;16:508–16. https://doi.org/10.1016/j.jclinane.2004.01.007.
78. Janz DR, Casey JD, Semler MW, Russell DW, Dargin J, Vonderhaar DJ, et al. Effect of fluid bolus administration on cardiovascular collapse among critically ill patients undergoing tracheal intubation: a randomized clinical trial. Lancet Respir Med. 2019;7:1039–47. https://doi.org/10.1016/S2213-2600(19)30246-2.
79. Russell DW, Casey JD, Gibbs KW, Ghamande S, Dargin JM, Vonderhaar DJ, et al. Effect of fluid bolus administration on cardiovascular collapse among critically ill patients undergoing tracheal intubation: a randomized clinical trial. JAMA. 2022;328:270–9. https://doi.org/10.1001/jama.2022.9792.
80. Heffner AC, Swords DS, Nussbaum ML, Kline JA, Jones AE. Predictors of the complication of postintubation hypotension during emergency airway management. J Crit Care. 2012;27:587–93. https://doi.org/10.1016/j.jcrc.2012.04.022.
81. Trivedi S, Demirci O, Arteaga G, Kashyap R, Smischney NJ. Evaluation of preintubation shock index and modified shock index as predictors of postintubation hypotension and other short-term outcomes. J Crit Care. 2015;30:861.e1–7. https://doi.org/10.1016/j.jcrc.2015.04.013.
82. Khan FA, Ullah H. Pharmacological agents for preventing morbidity associated with the haemodynamic response to tracheal intubation. Cochrane Database Syst Rev. 2013:CD004087. https://doi.org/10.1002/14651858.CD004087.pub2.
83. Butler J, Jackson R. Towards evidence based emergency medicine: best BETs from Manchester Royal Infirmary. Lignocaine premedication before rapid sequence induction in head injuries. Emerg Med J. 2002;19:554. https://doi.org/10.1136/emj.19.6.554.
84. Robinson N, Clancy M. In patients with head injury undergoing rapid sequence intubation, does pretreatment with intravenous lignocaine/lidocaine lead to an improved neurological outcome? A review of the literature. Emerg Med J. 2001;18:453–7. https://doi.org/10.1136/emj.18.6.453.
85. Maslow AD, Regan MM, Israel E, Darvish A, Mehrez M, Boughton R, et al. Inhaled albuterol, but not intravenous lidocaine, protects against intubation-induced bronchoconstriction in asthma. Anesthesiology. 2000;93:1198–204. https://doi.org/10.1097/00000542-200011000-00011.
86. Kopman AF, Khan NA, Neuman GG. Precurarization and priming: a theoretical analysis of safety and timing. Anesth Analg. 2001;93:1253–6. https://doi.org/10.1097/00000539-200111000-00042.
87. Han TH, Martyn JAJ. Onset and effectiveness of rocuronium for rapid onset of paralysis in patients with major burns: priming or large bolus. Br J Anaesth. 2009;102:55–60. https://doi.org/10.1093/bja/aen332.
88. Mencke T, Schreiber JU, Becker C, Bolte M, Fuchs-Buder T. Pretreatment before succinylcholine for outpatient anesthesia? Anesth Analg. 2002;94:573–6. https://doi.org/10.1097/00000539-200203000-00018.
89. Pandit JJ, Cook TM. NAP5 summary of main findings and incidences. In: Pandit J, Cook T, editors. Report and findings of the 5th national audit project. London: The Royal College of Anaesthetists and the Association of Anaesthetists of Great Britain and Ireland; 2014. p. 35–43.
90. Stollings JL, Diedrich DA, Oyen LJ, Brown DR. Rapid-sequence intubation: a review of the process and considerations when choosing medications. Ann Pharmacother. 2014;48:62–76. https://doi.org/10.1177/1060028013510488.
91. Wallace C, McGuire B. Rapid sequence induction: its place in modern anaesthesia. Contin Educ Anaesth Crit Care Pain. 2014;14:130–5. https://doi.org/10.1093/bjaceaccp/mkt047.

92. El-Orbany M, Connolly LA. Rapid sequence induction and intubation: current controversy. Anesth Analg. 2010;110:1318–25. https://doi.org/10.1213/ANE.0b013e3181d5ae47.
93. Wafaisade A, Caspers M, Bouillon B, Helm M, Ruppert M, Gäßler M. Changes in anaesthetic use for trauma patients in German HEMS – a retrospective study over a ten-year period. Scand J Trauma Resusc Emerg Med. 2019;27:1–8. https://doi.org/10.1186/s13049-019-0603-9.
94. Lyon RM, Perkins ZB, Chatterjee D, Lockey DJ, Russell MQ. Significant modification of traditional rapid sequence induction improves safety and effectiveness of pre-hospital trauma anaesthesia. Crit Care. 2015;19:134. https://doi.org/10.1186/s13054-015-0872-2.
95. Hans P, Brichant JF, Hubert B, Dewandre PY, Lamy M. Influence of induction of anaesthesia on intubating conditions one minute after rocuronium administration: comparison of ketamine and thiopentone. Anaesthesia. 1999;54:276–9. https://doi.org/10.1046/j.1365-2044.1999.00703.x.
96. White PF. Comparative evaluation of intravenous agents for rapid sequence induction—thiopental, ketamine, and midazolam. Anesthesiology. 1982;57:279–84. https://doi.org/10.1097/00000542-198210000-00005.
97. Wythe S, Wittenberg M, Gilbert-Kawai E. Rapid sequence induction: an old concept with new paradigms. Br J Hosp Med. 2019;80:C58–61. https://doi.org/10.12968/hmed.2019.80.4.C58.
98. Yao Y t, He L x, Fang N x, Ma J. Anesthetic induction with etomidate in cardiac surgical patients: a PRISMA-compliant systematic review and meta-analysis. J Cardiothorac Vasc Anesth. 2021;35:1073–85. https://doi.org/10.1053/j.jvca.2020.11.068.
99. Bruder EA, Ball IM, Ridi S, Pickett W, Hohl C. Single induction dose of etomidate versus other induction agents for endotracheal intubation in critically ill patients. Cochrane Database Syst Rev. 2015:CD010225. https://doi.org/10.1002/14651858.CD010225.pub2.
100. Albert SG, Sitaula S. Etomidate, adrenal insufficiency and mortality associated with severity of illness: a meta-analysis. J Intensive Care Med. 2021;36:1124–9. https://doi.org/10.1177/0885066620957596.
101. Gäßler M, Ruppert M, Lefering R, Bouillon B, Wafaisade A, Trauma Register DGU. Prehospital emergent intubation in trauma patients: the influence of etomidate on mortality, morbidity and healthcare resource utilization. Scand J trauma Resusc Emerg Med. 2019;27:61. https://doi.org/10.1186/s13049-019-0637-z.
102. Payen JF, Dupuis C, Trouve-Buisson T, Vinclair M, Broux C, Bouzat P, et al. Corticosteroid after etomidate in critically ill patients: a randomized controlled trial. Crit Care Med. 2012;40:29–35. https://doi.org/10.1097/CCM.0b013e31822d7938.
103. Köksal GM, Erbabacan E, Tunalı Y, Karaören G, Vehid S, Öz H. Acil entübasyon sırasında tek doz etomidatın hemodinami ve adrenal korteks üzerine etkisi. Ulus Travma ve Acil Cerrahi Derg. 2015;21:358–65. https://doi.org/10.5505/tjtes.2015.06325.
104. Sajayan A, Wicker J, Ungureanu N, Mendonca C, Kimani PK. Current practice of rapid sequence induction of anaesthesia in the UK – a national survey. Br J Anaesth. 2016;117:i69–74. https://doi.org/10.1093/bja/aew017.
105. Chen P, Zeng P, Gong Y, Long X. Recommended dose of sufentanil during induction of general anesthesia to avoid coughing and drastic hemodynamic fluctuations in patients undergoing surgery. J Int Med Res. 2021;49:1–9. https://doi.org/10.1177/0300060521996143.
106. Iyer V, Russell WJ. Induction using fentanyl to suppress the intubation response in the cardiac patient: what is the optimal dose? Anaesth Intensive Care. 1988;16:411–7. https://doi.org/10.1177/0310057x8801600405.
107. Zimmerman A, Funk KJ, Tidwell JL. Propofol and alfentanil prevent the rise in intraocular pressure caused by succinylcholine and intubation during a rapid sequence induction. Anesth Analg. 1996;83:814–7. https://doi.org/10.1097/00000539-199610000-00028.
108. Min JH, Chai HS, Kim YH, Chae YK, Choi SS, Lee A, et al. Attenuation of hemodynamic responses to laryngoscopy and tracheal intubation during rapid sequence induction: remifentanil vs. lidocaine with esmolol. Minerva Anestesiol. 2010;76:188–91.
109. Alanoğlu Z, Tolu S, Yalçın Ş, Batislam Y, Özatamer O, Tüzüner F. Różne dawki remifentanylu w szybkiej indukcji znieczulenia—monitorowanie BIS i warunki intubacji [Different

remifentanil doses in rapid sequence anesthesia induction: BIS monitoring and intubation conditions]. Adv Clin Exp Med. 2013;22:47–55.
110. Chaumeron A, Castanie J, Fortier LP, Basset P, Bastide S, Alonso S, et al. Efficacy and safety of remifentanil in a rapid sequence induction in elderly patients: a three-arm parallel, double blind, randomised controlled trial. Anaesth Crit Care Pain Med. 2020;39:215–20. https://doi.org/10.1016/j.accpm.2019.09.010.
111. Chung KS, Sinatra RS, Halevy JD, Paige D, Silverman DG. A comparison of fentanyl, esmolol, and their combination for blunting the haemodynamic responses during rapid-sequence induction. Can J Anaesth. 1992;39:774–9. https://doi.org/10.1007/BF03008287.
112. Cork RC, Weiss JL, Hameroff SR, Bentley J. Fentanyl preloading for rapid-sequence induction of anesthesia. Anesth Analg. 1984;63:60–4. https://doi.org/10.1213/00000539-198401000-00012.
113. Martineau RJ, Tousignant CP, Miller DR, Hull KA. Alfentanil controls the haemodynamic response during rapid-sequence induction of anaesthesia. Can J Anaesth. 1990;37:755–61. https://doi.org/10.1007/BF03006534.
114. Abou-Arab MH, Heier T, Caldwell JE. Dose of alfentanil needed to obtain optimal intubation conditions during rapid-sequence induction of anaesthesia with thiopentone and rocuronium. Br J Anaesth. 2007;98:604–10.
115. Lundstrøm LH, Duez CHV, Nørskov AK, Rosenstock CV, Thomsen JL, Møller AM, et al. Avoidance versus use of neuromuscular blocking agents for improving conditions during tracheal intubation or direct laryngoscopy in adults and adolescents. Cochrane Database Syst Rev. 2017;5:CD009237. https://doi.org/10.1002/14651858.CD009237.pub2.
116. Wilcox SR, Bittner EA, Elmer J, Seigel TA, Nguyen NTP, Dhillon A, et al. Neuromuscular blocking agent administration for emergent tracheal intubation is associated with decreased prevalence of procedure-related complications. Crit Care Med. 2012;40:1808–13. https://doi.org/10.1097/CCM.0b013e31824e0e67.
117. Groth CM, Acquisto NM, Khadem T. Current practices and safety of medication use during rapid sequence intubation. J Crit Care. 2018;45:65–70. https://doi.org/10.1016/j.jcrc.2018.01.017.
118. de Carvalho CC, da Silva DM, de Athayde Regueira SLP, de Souza ABS, Rego CO, Ramos IB, et al. Comparison between rocuronium and succinylcholine for rapid sequence induction: a systematic review and network meta-analysis of randomized clinical trials. J Clin Anesth. 2021;72:110265. https://doi.org/10.1016/j.jclinane.2021.110265.
119. Tran D, Newton E, Mount V, Lee J, Mansour C, Wells G, et al. Rocuronium vs. succinylcholine for rapid sequence intubation: a Cochrane systematic review. Anaesthesia. 2017;72:765–77. https://doi.org/10.1111/anae.13903.
120. Sørensen MK, Bretlau C, Gätke MR, Sørensen AM, Rasmussen LS. Rapid sequence induction and intubation with rocuronium-sugammadex compared with succinylcholine: a randomized trial. Br J Anaesth. 2012;108:682–9. https://doi.org/10.1093/bja/aer503.
121. Mercer S, Moneypenny M. Can sugammadex save a patient in a simulated 'cannot intubate, cannot ventilate' situation? Anaesthesia. 2011;66:223–4. https://doi.org/10.1111/j.1365-2044.2011.06630.x.
122. Sadleir PHM, Clarke RC, Bunning DL, Platt PR. Anaphylaxis to neuromuscular blocking drugs: incidence and cross-reactivity in Western Australia from 2002 to 2011. Br J Anaesth. 2013;110:981–7. https://doi.org/10.1093/bja/aes506.
123. Taha SK, El-Khatib MF, Baraka AS, Haidar YA, Abdallah FW, Zbeidy RA, et al. Effect of suxamethonium vs rocuronium on onset of oxygen desaturation during apnoea following rapid sequence induction. Anaesthesia. 2010;65:358–61. https://doi.org/10.1111/j.1365-2044.2010.06243.x.
124. Tang L, Li S, Huang S, Ma H, Wang Z. Desaturation following rapid sequence induction using succinylcholine vs. rocuronium in overweight patients. Acta Anaesthesiol Scand. 2011;55:203–8. https://doi.org/10.1111/j.1399-6576.2010.02365.x.

125. Sellick BA. Cricoid pressure to control regurgitation of stomach contents during induction of anaesthesia. Lancet. 1961;2:404–6. https://doi.org/10.1016/s0140-6736(61)92485-0.
126. Smith KJ, Dobranowski J, Yip G. Cricoid pressure displaces the esophagus: an observational study using magnetic resonance imaging. Anesthesiology. 2003;99:60–4. https://doi.org/10.1097/00000542-200307000-00013.
127. Rice MJ, Mancuso AA, Gibbs C, Morey TE, Gravenstein N, Deitte LA. Cricoid pressure results in compression of the postcricoid hypopharynx: the esophageal position is irrelevant. Anesth Analg. 2009;109:1546–52. https://doi.org/10.1213/ane.0b013e3181b05404.
128. Zeidan AM, Salem MR, Mazoit JX, Abdullah MA, Ghattas T, Crystal GJ. The effectiveness of cricoid pressure for occluding the esophageal entrance in anesthetized and paralyzed patients: an experimental and observational glidescope study. Anesth Analg. 2014;118:580–6. https://doi.org/10.1213/ANE.0000000000000068.
129. Vanner RG, Pryle BJ. Regurgitation and oesophageal rupture with cricoid pressure: a cadaver study. Anaesthesia. 1992;47:732–5. https://doi.org/10.1111/j.1365-2044.1992.tb03248.x.
130. Vanner RG, Pryle BJ. Nasogastric tubes and cricoid pressure. Anaesthesia. 1993;48:1112–3. https://doi.org/10.1111/j.1365-2044.1993.tb07560.x.
131. Vanner R, O'Dwyer J, Pryle B, Reynolds F. Upper oesophageal sphincter pressure and the effect of cricoid pressure. Anuesthesia. 1992;47:95–100. https://doi.org/10.1111/j.1365-2044.1992.tb02001.x.
132. Vanner RG, Asai T. Safe use of cricoid pressure. Anaesthesia. 1999;54:1–3. https://doi.org/10.1046/j.1365-2044.1999.00756.x.
133. Hartsilver EL, Vanner RG, Bewley J, Clayton T. Gastric pressure during emergency caesarean section under general anaesthesia. Br J Anaesth. 1999;82:752–4. https://doi.org/10.1093/bja/82.5.752.
134. Pellrud R, Ahlstrand R. Pressure measurement in the upper esophagus during cricoid pressure: a high-resolution solid-state manometry study. Acta Anaesthesiol Scand. 2018;62:1396–402. https://doi.org/10.1111/aas.13209.
135. Johnson RL, Cannon EK, Mantilla CB, Cook DA. Cricoid pressure training using simulation: a systematic review and meta-analysis. Br J Anaesth. 2013;111:338–46. https://doi.org/10.1093/bja/aet121.
136. Salem M, Khorasani A, Zeidan A, Crystal G. Cricoid pressure controversies: narrative review. Anesthesiology. 2017;126:738–52. https://doi.org/10.1353/sym.2003.0023.
137. Ralph SJ, Wareham CA. Rupture of the oesophagus during cricoid pressure. Anaesthesia. 1991;46:40–1. https://doi.org/10.1111/j.1365-2044.1991.tb09314.x.
138. Heath KJ, Palmer M, Fletcher SJ. Fracture of the cricoid cartilage after Sellick's manoeuvre. Br J Anaesth. 1996;76:877–8. https://doi.org/10.1093/bja/76.6.877.
139. Prasarn ML, Horodyski M, Schneider P, Wendling A, Hagberg CA, Rechtine GR. The effect of cricoid pressure on the unstable cervical spine. J Emerg Med. 2016;50:427–32. https://doi.org/10.1016/j.jemermed.2015.09.009.
140. Algie CM, Mahar RK, Mahar PD, Tan HB, Ariyasinghe CP, Wasiak J. Effectiveness and risks of cricoid pressure during rapid sequence intubation. Cochrane Database Syst Rev. 2015;2015:CD011656. https://doi.org/10.1002/14651858.CD011656.
141. White L, Thang C, Hodsdon A, Melhuish T, Vlok R. Cricoid pressure during intubation: a systematic review and meta-analysis of randomised controlled trials. Hear Lung. 2020;49:175–80. https://doi.org/10.1016/j.hrtlng.2019.10.001.
142. Birenbaum A, Hajage D, Roche S, Ntouba A, Eurin M, Cuvillon P, et al. Effect of cricoid pressure compared with a sham procedure in the rapid sequence induction of anesthesia: the IRIS randomized clinical trial. JAMA Surg. 2019;154:9–17. https://doi.org/10.1001/jamasurg.2018.3577.
143. Tessarolo E, Alkhouri H, Lelos N, Sarrami P, McCarthy S. Review article: effectiveness and risks of cricoid pressure during rapid sequence induction for endotracheal intubation in the emergency department: a systematic review. Emerg Med Australas. 2022;34:484–91. https://doi.org/10.1111/1742-6723.13993.

144. Trethewy CE, Doherty SR, Burrows JM, Clausen D. Ideal cricoid pressure is biomechanically impossible during laryngoscopy. Acad Emerg Med. 2018;25:94–8. https://doi.org/10.1111/acem.13326.
145. Salem MR, Bruninga KW, Dodlapatii J, Joseph NJ. Metoclopramide does not attenuate cricoid pressure-induced relaxation of the lower esophageal sphincter in awake volunteers. Anesthesiology. 2008;109:806–10. https://doi.org/10.1097/ALN.0b013e31818a37dc.
146. Hartsilver E, Vanner R. Airway obstruction with cricoid pressure. Anaesthesia. 2000;55:208–11. https://doi.org/10.1046/j.1365-2044.2000.01205.x.
147. Aoyama K, Takenaka I, Sata T, Shigematsu A. Cricoid pressure impedes positioning and ventilation through the laryngeal mask airway. Can J Anaesth. 1996;43:1035–40. https://doi.org/10.1007/bf03011906.
148. Hashimoto Y, Asai T, Arai T, Okuda Y. Effect of cricoid pressure on placement of the I-gel™: a randomised study. Anaesthesia. 2014;69:878–82. https://doi.org/10.1111/anae.12731.
149. Asai T, Barclay K, Power I, Vaughan RS. Cricoid pressure impedes placement of the laryngeal mask airway. Br J Anaesth. 1995;74:521–5. https://doi.org/10.1093/bja/74.5.521.
150. Smith CE, Boyer D. Cricoid pressure decreases ease of tracheal intubation using fibreoptic laryngoscopy (WuScope System™). Can J Anesth. 2002;49:614–9. https://doi.org/10.1007/BF03017391.
151. Hung KC, Hung CT, Poon YY, Wu SC, Chen KH, Chen JY, et al. The effect of cricoid pressure on tracheal intubation in adult patients: a systematic review and meta-analysis. Can J Anesth. 2021;68:137–47. https://doi.org/10.1007/s12630-020-01830-1.
152. Jaber S, Jung B, Corne P, Sebbane M, Muller L, Chanques G, et al. An intervention to decrease complications related to endotracheal intubation in the intensive care unit: a prospective, multiple-center study. Intensive Care Med. 2010;36:248–55. https://doi.org/10.1007/s00134-009-1717-8.
153. Ellis DY, Harris T, Zideman D. Cricoid pressure in emergency department rapid sequence tracheal intubations: a risk-benefit analysis. Ann Emerg Med. 2007;50:653–65. https://doi.org/10.1016/j.annemergmed.2007.05.006.
154. Eichelsbacher C, Ilper H, Noppens R, Hinkelbein J, Loop T. Rapid sequence induction and intubation in patients with risk of aspiration: recommendations for action for practical management of anesthesia. Anaesthesist. 2018;67:568–83. https://doi.org/10.1007/s00101-018-0460-3.
155. Frerk C, Mitchell VS, McNarry AF, Mendonca C, Bhagrath R, Patel A, et al. Difficult Airway Society 2015 guidelines for management of unanticipated difficult intubation in adults. Br J Anaesth. 2015;115:827–48. https://doi.org/10.1093/bja/aev371.
156. Weingart SD, Bhagwan SD. A novel set-up to allow suctioning during direct endotracheal and fiberoptic intubation. J Clin Anesth. 2011;23:518–9. https://doi.org/10.1016/j.jclinane.2010.08.021.
157. Russotto V, Myatra SN, Laffey JG, Tassistro E, Antolini L, Bauer P, et al. Intubation practices and adverse peri-intubation events in critically ill patients from 29 countries. JAMA. 2021;325:1164–72. https://doi.org/10.1001/jama.2021.1727.
158. Jaber S, Rollé A, Godet T, Terzi N, Riu B, Asfar P, et al. Effect of the use of an endotracheal tube and stylet versus an endotracheal tube alone on first-attempt intubation success: a multicentre, randomised clinical trial in 999 patients. Intensive Care Med. 2021;47:653–64. https://doi.org/10.1007/s00134-021-06417-y.
159. Driver BE, Prekker ME, Klein LR, Reardon RF, Miner JR, Fagerstrom ET, et al. Effect of use of a bougie vs endotracheal tube and stylet on first-attempt intubation success among patients with difficult airways undergoing emergency intubation. JAMA. 2018;319:2179–89. https://doi.org/10.1001/jama.2018.6496.
160. Driver BE, Semler MW, Self WH, Ginde AA, Trent SA, Gandotra S, et al. Effect of use of a bougie vs endotracheal tube with stylet on successful intubation on the first attempt among critically ill patients undergoing tracheal intubation. JAMA. 2021;326:2488–97. https://doi.org/10.1001/jama.2021.22002.

161. Cook T. A new practical classification of laryngeal view. Anaesthesia. 2000;55:274–9. https://doi.org/10.1046/j.1365-2044.2000.01270.x.
162. Goto Y, Goto T, Hagiwara Y, Tsugawa Y, Watase H, Okamoto H, et al. Techniques and outcomes of emergency airway management in Japan: an analysis of two multicentre prospective observational studies, 2010–2016. Resuscitation. 2017;114:14–20. https://doi.org/10.1016/j.resuscitation.2017.02.009.
163. Brown CA, Bair AE, Pallin DJ. Techniques, success, and adverse events of emergency department adult intubations. Ann Emerg Med. 2022;65:363–70.e1. https://doi.org/10.1016/j.annemergmed.2014.10.036.
164. Hypes CD, Stolz U, Sakles JC, Joshi RR, Natt B, Malo J, et al. Video laryngoscopy improves odds of first-attempt success at intubation in the intensive care unit. Ann Am Thorac Soc. 2016;13:382–90. https://doi.org/10.1513/AnnalsATS.201508-505OC.
165. García-Pintos M, Erramouspe P, Schandera V, Murphy K, McCalla J, Taylor G, et al. Comparison of video versus direct laryngoscopy: a prospective prehospital air medical services study. Air Med J. 2021;40:45–9. https://doi.org/10.1016/j.amj.2020.10.008.
166. Okamoto H, Goto T, Wong ZS, Hagiwara Y, Watase H, Hasegawa K, et al. Comparison of video laryngoscopy versus direct laryngoscopy for intubation in emergency department patients with cardiac arrest: a multicentre study. Resuscitation. 2019;136:70–7. https://doi.org/10.1016/j.resuscitation.2018.10.005.
167. Sakles JC, Mosier JM, Patanwala AE, Dicken JM, Kalin L, Javedani PP. The C-MAC® video laryngoscope is superior to the direct laryngoscope for the rescue of failed first-attempt intubations in the emergency department. J Emerg Med. 2022;48:280–6. https://doi.org/10.1016/j.jemermed.2014.10.007.
168. Griesdale DEG, Chau A, Isac G, Ayas N, Foster D, Irwin RNC, et al. Video-laryngoscopy versus direct laryngoscopy in critically ill patients: a pilot randomized trial. Can J Anaesth Anaesth Anaesth. 2012;59:1032–9. https://doi.org/10.1007/s12630-012-9775-8.
169. Silverberg MJ, Li N, Acquah SO, Kory PD. Comparison of video laryngoscopy versus direct laryngoscopy during urgent endotracheal intubation: a randomized controlled trial. Crit Care Med. 2015;43:636–41. https://doi.org/10.1097/CCM.0000000000000751.
170. De Jong A, Molinari N, Conseil M, Coisel Y, Pouzeratte Y, Belafia F, et al. Video laryngoscopy versus direct laryngoscopy for orotracheal intubation in the intensive care unit : a systematic review and meta-analysis. Intensive Care Med. 2014;40:629–39. https://doi.org/10.1007/s00134-014-3236-5.
171. Hansel J, Rogers A, Lewis S, Cook T, Smith A. Videolaryngoscopy versus direct laryngoscopy for adults undergoing tracheal intubation (Review). Cochrane Database Syst Rev. 2022:CD011136. https://doi.org/10.1002/14651858.CD011136.pub.
172. Sakles JC, Kalin L. The effect of stylet choice on the success rate of intubation using the GlideScope video laryngoscope in the emergency department. Acad Emerg Med. 2012;19:235–8. https://doi.org/10.1111/j.1553-2712.2011.01271.x.
173. Kelly FE, Cook TM, Boniface N, Hughes J, Seller C, Simpson T. Videolaryngoscopes confer benefits in human factors in addition to technical skills. Br J Anaesth. 2015;115:132–3. https://doi.org/10.1093/bja/aev188.
174. Aseri S, Ahmad H, Vallance H. Video laryngoscopy improves endotracheal intubation training for novices. Br J Anaesth. 2015;115:133. https://doi.org/10.1093/bja/aev189.
175. Van Schuppen H, Wojciechowicz K, Hollmann MW, Preckel B. Tracheal intubation during advanced life support using direct laryngoscopy versus Glidescope® videolaryngoscopy by clinicians with limited intubation experience: a systematic review and meta-analysis. J Clin Med. 2022;11:6291. https://doi.org/10.3390/jcm11216291.
176. Natt BS, Malo J, Hypes CD, Sakles JC, Mosier JM. Strategies to improve first attempt success at intubation in critically ill patients. Br J Anaesth. 2016;117:i60–8. https://doi.org/10.1093/bja/aew061.
177. Santoni BG, Hindman BJ, Puttlitz CM, Weeks JB, Johnson N, Maktabi MA, et al. Manual in-line stabilization increases pressures applied by the laryngoscope blade during direct

laryngoscopy and orotracheal intubation. Anesthesiology. 2009;110:24–31. https://doi.org/10.1097/ALN.0b013e318190b556.
178. Turkstra TP, Craen RA, Pelz DM, Gelb AW. Cervical spine motion: a fluoroscopic comparison during intubation with lighted Stylet, GlideScope, and Macintosh laryngoscope. Anesth Analg. 2005;101:910–5. https://doi.org/10.1213/01.ane.0000166975.38649.27.
179. Paik H, Park HP. Randomized crossover trial comparing cervical spine motion during tracheal intubation with a Macintosh laryngoscope versus a C-MAC D-blade videolaryngoscope in a simulated immobilized cervical spine. BMC Anesthesiol. 2020;20:1–8. https://doi.org/10.1186/s12871-020-01118-3.
180. Kim SY, Park SO, Kim JW, Sung J, Lee KR, Lee YH, et al. How much experience do rescuers require to achieve successful tracheal intubation during cardiopulmonary resuscitation? Resuscitation. 2018;133:187–92. https://doi.org/10.1016/j.resuscitation.2018.08.032.
181. Kim JH, Kim YM, Choi HJ, Je SM, Kim E. Factors associated with successful second and third intubation attempts in the ED. Am J Emerg Med. 2013;31:1376–81. https://doi.org/10.1016/j.ajem.2013.06.018.
182. Apfelbaum JL, Hagberg CA, Connis RT, Abdelmalak BB, Agarkar M, Dutton RP, et al. 2022 American Society of Anesthesiologists practice guidelines for management of the difficult airway. Anesthesiology. 2022;136:31.
183. Deakin CD, Morrison LJ, Morley PT, Callaway CW, Kerber RE, Kronick SL, et al. Part 8: advanced life support: 2010 international consensus on cardiopulmonary resuscitation and emergency cardiovascular care science with treatment recommendations. Resuscitation. 2010;81:e93–174. https://doi.org/10.1016/j.resuscitation.2010.08.027.
184. Sahu AK, Bhoi S, Aggarwal P, Mathew R, Nayer J, Amrithanand VT, et al. Endotracheal tube placement confirmation by ultrasonography: a systematic review and meta-analysis of more than 2500 patients. J Emerg Med. 2020;59:254–64. https://doi.org/10.1016/j.jemermed.2020.04.040.
185. Gottlieb M, Holladay D, Peksa GD. Ultrasonography for the confirmation of endotracheal tube intubation: a systematic review and meta-analysis. Ann Emerg Med. 2018;72:627–36. https://doi.org/10.1016/j.annemergmed.2018.06.024.
186. Constantin JM, Futier E, Cherprenet AL, Chanques G, Guerin R, Cayot-Constantin S, et al. A recruitment maneuver increases oxygenation after intubation of hypoxemic intensive care unit patients: a randomized controlled study. Crit Care. 2010;14:R76. https://doi.org/10.1186/cc8989.
187. Bernhard M, Becker TK, Gries A, Knapp J, Wenzel V. The first shot is often the best shot: first-pass intubation success in emergency airway management. Anesth Analg. 2015;121:1389–93. https://doi.org/10.1213/ANE.0000000000000891.
188. Ikeda A, Isono S, Sato Y, Yogo H, Sato J, Ishikawa T, et al. Effects of muscle relaxants on mask ventilation in anesthetized persons with normal upper airway anatomy. Anesthesiology. 2012;117:487–93. https://doi.org/10.1097/ALN.0b013e3182668670.
189. Bennett JA, Abrams JT, Van Riper DF, Horrow JC. Difficult or impossible ventilation after sufentanil-induced anesthesia is caused primarily by vocal cord closure. Anesthesiology. 1997;87:1070–4. https://doi.org/10.1097/00000542-199711000-00010.
190. Law JA, Broemling N, Cooper RM, Drolet P, Duggan LV, Griesdale DE, et al. The difficult airway with recommendations for management – part 1 – intubation encountered in an unconscious/induced patient. Can J Anesth. 2013;60:1089–118. https://doi.org/10.1007/s12630-013-0019-3.
191. Peterson GN, Domino KB, Caplan RA, Posner KL, Lee LA, Cheney FW. Management of the difficult airway a closed claims analysis. Anesthesiology. 2005;103:35–9. https://doi.org/10.1097/01.sa.0000203217.72542.a8.
192. Avery P, Morton S, Raitt J, Lossius HM, Lockey D. Rapid sequence induction: where did the consensus go? Scand J Trauma Resusc Emerg Med. 2021;29:1–9.
193. Flin R, Maran N. Basic concepts for crew resource management and non-technical skills. Best Pract Res Clin Anaesthesiol. 2015;29:27–39. https://doi.org/10.1016/j.bpa.2015.02.002.

194. Mosier JM, Malo J, Sakles JC, Hypes CD, Natt B, Snyder L, et al. The impact of a comprehensive airway management training program for pulmonary and critical care medicine fellows: a three-year experience. Ann Am Thorac Soc. 2015;12:539–48. https://doi.org/10.1513/AnnalsATS.201501-023OC.
195. Pandit JJ, Andrade J, Bogod DG, Hitchman JM, Jonker WR, Lucas N, et al. The 5th National Audit Project (NAP5) on accidental awareness during general anaesthesia: summary of main findings and risk factors. Anaesthesia. 2014;69:1089–101.
196. National Emergency Airway Registry. [Internet]. [cited 2022 Nov 28]. Available from: http://www.nearstudy.net

Chapter 14
Facemask Ventilation

Jaideep J. Pandit

14.1 Introduction

Hand ventilation of the lungs via facemask (bag-mask ventilation, BMV) is a core skill in anaesthesia. It is part of the essential manoeuvres required for cardiopulmonary resuscitation (CPR) and, to some extent, has this same role within anaesthesia.

The need for mask ventilation arises because intravenous induction of anaesthesia invariably causes (a) collapse of the upper airway via relaxation of pharyngeal muscles and of genioglossus muscle [1]; (b) inhibition of the respiratory centre, leading to apnoea [2], compounded also by inhibition of the hypoxic chemoreflex by action at the carotid body [3, 4]. All intravenous agents also achieve this [2, 5]. Although some, like ketamine, are purported to be better at maintaining muscle tone and, to an extent, better maintain spontaneous ventilation [6], where, in fact, mask ventilation is likely needed.

As an action, mask ventilation consists of at least three important components: (a) neck extension and jaw thrust, to open the airway and counteract upper airway collapse; (b) ensuring a tight seal of the facemask with the face; (c) active ventilation of the lungs, using manual squeezing of the anaesthesia circuit bag [7].

Thus, after intravenous induction of anaesthesia, mask ventilation is needed to maintain oxygenation until a definitive airway is secured, which may be a supraglottic airway (SGA) or tracheal intubation. The latter involves prior administration of neuromuscular blockade (NMB), which can take several minutes, so mask ventilation is needed both to maintain oxygenation and anaesthesia (where volatile agents are being used).

J. J. Pandit (✉)
Nuffield Department of Anaesthetics, Oxford University Hospitals, Oxford, UK

Nuffield Department of Clinical Neuroscience, University of Oxford, Oxford, UK
e-mail: jaideep.pandit@sjc.ox.ac.uk

M. Á. Gómez-Ríos, A. van Zundert (eds.), *Evidence-based Guide to Difficult Airway Management*, https://doi.org/10.1007/978-3-032-30769-9_14

There are several issues and questions relating to mask ventilation:

1. Can we predict which patients are difficult to mask-ventilate? (and what are the consequences of predicting this?)
2. Is it important to check for the ability to mask ventilate before administering NMB? (or, what does this information tell us?)
3. What, if any, are the risks of mask ventilation? (and are there situations in which it should be avoided?)

14.2 Can we Predict Difficult Mask Ventilation?

From first principles, several patient factors are likely to predict difficult mask ventilation, based on the requirement that a good fit of the facemask is necessary, as is the need to counteract upper airway collapse. Therefore, factors that make mask ventilation difficult include: abnormal skeletal structures of the face (e.g. acromegaly); edentulous patients (who have a leak around the mouth); beards; and obesity. There is clearly an overlap between factors predicting difficult intubation. These notions from first principles are borne out in clinical studies [8, 9]. Scoring has been developed based on these principles, which is useful in research studies, but perhaps less applicable in clinical practice with perfect accuracy [10].

As a guide on what to do if there are signs of difficult mask ventilation: The anaesthetist should consider if this exists in isolation, and e.g. will be easily overcome by supraglottic airway or tracheal tube insertion, or if it forms part of a picture of a 'difficult airway'; which in practice means 'difficult oxygenation'. If this is the case, then difficult mask ventilation is arguably more important in guiding management than predicting difficult intubation, because it means that if intubation fails, the anaesthetist cannot 'fall back' on mask ventilation as a rescue. The rationale is that patients predicted to be both difficult to intubate and to mask-ventilate should not undergo induction of anaesthesia before securing the airway [11].

On the other hand, difficult mask ventilation alone in the absence of any other signs of overall difficult oxygenation (e.g. an elderly, thin, edentulous patient with good mouth opening and normal airway structure) may simply mean it is advisable to rapidly progress to tracheal intubation with minimal time spent attempting to mask ventilate.

14.3 Checking the Ability to Mask Ventilate Before Administering NMB

Some anaesthetists routinely check that they can mask-ventilate the patient's lungs before administering a long-acting neuromuscular blocking drug. However, others freely administer neuromuscular blocking drugs immediately following induction [12].

The respective logic and relative risks are as follows. It is argued that those who check do so to be informed of the patient's intrinsic ability to be easily mask-ventilated. If the patient is intrinsically difficult to mask-ventilate, and since mask ventilation is the ultimate means by which oxygen can be provided, it may be unwise to paralyse the patient, because patients who are difficult to mask-ventilate may also be difficult to tracheally intubate. And if intubation proves difficult, then it will not be possible to 'fall back' on mask ventilation.

Those who do not check apply a different rationale. They believe that NMBs make it easier to mask-ventilate, and therefore, the information provided by prior attempts without paralysis is very limited or useless.

On first principles, full neuromuscular blockade might facilitate mask ventilation by increasing chest wall compliance [13]; alternatively, it could make mask ventilation more difficult by inducing upper airway collapse [14, 15]. Clinical trials on the influence of NMBs on ease of mask ventilation are contradictory [16–21]. An emerging view, therefore, is that the impact of NMB is not as relevant as the ability to reverse it should its effect prove adverse. At induction, if mask ventilation is initially easy, the literature on balance indicates it is unlikely NMB will make it so much worse as to require urgent intervention [22]. However, an initially difficult-to-mask ventilated patient may worsen with NMB, in which case it is clearly important to reverse the NMB should the next step of intubation fail. Hitherto, only suxamethonium was available as a short-acting (self-reversible) agent. Now, rocuronium is available as a relatively rapidly acting agent that can also be reversed promptly using sugammadex. Put differently, there is little logic - as far as airway management is concerned - in using an agent other than rocuronium for induction, especially in patients whose airways (particularly with mask ventilation) may be difficult [22].

14.4 What Are the Risks of Mask Ventilation?

Other than failure to oxygenate the patient, the main risk is inflating the stomach with gas, which could cause regurgitation and then aspiration of stomach contents into the lungs. This was historically the basis for promoting the concept of 'rapid sequence induction', applied to patients already at heightened risk of regurgitation/aspiration. These include patients who have not been starved before anaesthesia (i.e. those requiring emergency surgery); those whose gastric transit time is slowed (e.g. abdominal or gastrointestinal pathology, or pregnancy); and those with symptoms of reflux (e.g. peptic ulcer disease or oesophageal motility disorders).

The components of RSI have never been formally defined in a consensual way [23], but include: preoxygenation; administering a predetermined dose of intravenous agent (i.e. not checking for effect); applying cricoid pressure (to prevent regurgitation); using a rapidly acting NMB (i.e. suxamethonium that has a clear end-point of its effect with fasciculations); and prompt tracheal intubation. However, each of these has been challenged, questioned, or modified. One stimulus for this re-analysis was the discovery that RSI is a risk factor for accidental awareness during anaesthesia (the NAP5 study) [24]. It is clear that many anaesthesiologists co-administer opiates like fentanyl with the induction. Traditionally, thiopental was the recommended agent (with sparse evidence) and is still used in obstetric anaesthesia in the UK [25], but NAP5 revealed that this promotes accidental awareness of anaesthesia (there may be inter-agent differences in mechanisms of action [26]) so there is a move towards using propofol and for checking the patient is in fact anesthetized [24]. Some anaesthetists gently check for the ability to mask-ventilate (as discussed above). The efficacy of cricoid pressure is much debated—both in terms of whether to apply it and how to apply it [27–29]. Rocuronium may have surpassed suxamethonium, especially because it can be reversed with sugammadex, and the latter also carries risks for small subpopulations with cholinesterase deficiency. Note also that an RSI is contraindicated in patients predicted to be difficult to intubate, regardless of the ability to mask ventilate, because then a failed intubation is by definition more likely and mask ventilation cannot offer rescue for the risk of stomach inflation (the reason why RSI was considered in the first place).

These considerations lead the discussion to a technique that may replace mask ventilation, and some argue that it is so effective that it may make mask ventilation redundant. High-flow nasal oxygenation HFNO is based on early physiological observations of eliminating rebreathing with prolonged very high flow (140 litres/min) oxygen delivery [30]. It has since been discovered not only to maintain oxygenation for prolonged periods (up to an hour or more) but also to prevent CO2 accumulation, in contrast to other methods of apnoeic oxygenation [31–33]. HFNO has limitations: it may, to some extent, inflate the stomach, and it appears less effective in obese patients. But in both these situations, it may nevertheless be an improvement in mask ventilation.

14.5 Conclusions

Mask ventilation remains a core skill. The development of HFNO technology is unlikely to replace it, especially in low-resource settings, but the limitations of mask ventilation, particularly in certain patient groups, warrant assessment.

Recommendations Table for Mask Ventilation

Recommendation	Grade of evidence
Prediction of difficult mask ventilation	C
Check for mask ventilation before NMB	D
Using mask ventilation as a core skill (e.g. after failed intubation)	D

References

1. Hillman DR, Platt PR, Eastwood PR. The upper airway during anaesthesia. Br J Anaesth. 2003;91(1):31–9. https://doi.org/10.1093/bja/aeg126.
2. Dahan A, Teppema LJ. Influence of anaesthesia and analgesia on the control of breathing. Br J Anaesth. 2003;91(1):40–9. https://doi.org/10.1093/bja/aeg150.
3. Pandit JJ, Buckler KJ. Differential effects of halothane and sevoflurane on hypoxia-induced intracellular calcium transients of neonatal rat carotid body type I cells. Br J Anaesth. 2009;103(5):701–10. https://doi.org/10.1093/bja/aep223.
4. Pandit JJ, Huskens N, O'Donohoe PB, Turner PJ, Buckler KJ. Competitive interactions between halothane and isoflurane at the carotid body and TASK channels. Anesthesiology. 2020;133(5):1046–59. https://doi.org/10.1097/ALN.0000000000003520.
5. O'Donohoe PB, Turner PJ, Huskens N, Buckler KJ, Pandit JJ. Influence of propofol on isolated neonatal rat carotid body glomus cell response to hypoxia and hypercapnia. Respir Physiol Neurobiol. 2019;260:17–27. https://doi.org/10.1016/j.resp.2018.10.007.
6. Mishima G, Sanuki T, Sato S, Kobayashi M, Kurata S, Ayuse T. Upper-airway collapsibility and compensatory responses under moderate sedation with ketamine, dexmedetomidine, and propofol in healthy volunteers. Physiol Rep. 2020;8(10):e14439. https://doi.org/10.14814/phy2.14439.
7. Baker P. Mask ventilation. F1000Res. 2018;7:F1000 Faculty Rev-1683. https://doi.org/10.12688/f1000research.15742.1. PMID: 30416707
8. Langeron O, Masso E, Huraux C, Guggiari M, Bianchi A, Coriat P, Riou B. Prediction of difficult mask ventilation. Anesthesiology. 2000;92(5):1229–36. https://doi.org/10.1097/00000542-200005000-00009.
9. Kheterpal S, Healy D, Aziz MF, Shanks AM, Freundlich RE, Linton F, Martin LD, Linton J, Epps JL, Fernandez-Bustamante A, Jameson LC, Tremper T, Tremper KK, Multicenter Perioperative Outcomes Group (MPOG) Perioperative Clinical Research Committee. Incidence, predictors, and outcome of difficult mask ventilation combined with difficult laryngoscopy: a report from the multicenter perioperative outcomes group. Anesthesiology. 2013;119(6):1360–9. https://doi.org/10.1097/ALN.0000435832.39353.20.
10. Lundstrøm LH, Rosenstock CV, Wetterslev J, Nørskov AK. The DIFFMASK score for predicting difficult facemask ventilation: a cohort study of 46,804 patients. Anaesthesia. 2019;74(10):1267–76. https://doi.org/10.1111/anae.14701.
11. Heidegger T. Management of the Difficult Airway. N Engl J Med. 2021;384(19):1836–47. https://doi.org/10.1056/NEJMra1916801.
12. Broomhead RH, Marks RJ, Ayton P. Confirmation of the ability to ventilate by facemask before administration of neuromuscular blocker: a non-instrumental piece of information? Br J Anaesth. 2010;104(3):313–7. https://doi.org/10.1093/bja/aep380.

13. Abrams JT, Horrow JC, Bennett JA, Van Riper D, Storella RJ. Upper airway closure. A primary source of difficult ventilation with sufentanil induction of anesthesia. Anesth Analg. 1996;83:629–32. https://doi.org/10.1097/00000539-199609000-00034.
14. Odeh M, Schnall R, Gavriely N, Oliven A. Effect of upper airway muscle contraction on supraglottic resistance and stability. Respir Physiol. 1993;92:139–50.
15. van Lunteren E, Strohl KP. The muscles of the upper airways. Clin Chest Med. 1986;7:171–88.
16. Goodwin MW, Pandit JJ, Hames K, Popat M, Yentis SM. The effect of neuromuscular blockade on the efficiency of mask ventilation of the lungs. Anaesthesia. 2003;58(1):60–3. https://doi.org/10.1046/j.1365-2044.2003.02788_3.x.
17. Warters RD, Szabo TA, Spinale FG, DeSantis SM, Reves JG. The effect of neuromuscular blockade on mask ventilation. Anaesthesia. 2011;66(3):163–7. https://doi.org/10.1111/j.1365-2044.2010.06601.x.
18. Patel A. Facemask ventilation before or after neuromuscular blocking drugs: where are we now? Anaesthesia. 2014;69(8):811–5. https://doi.org/10.1111/anae.12792.
19. offe AM, Ramaiah R, Donahue E, Galgon RE, Thilen SR, Spiekerman CF, Bhananker SM. Ventilation by mask before and after the administration of neuromuscular blockade: a pragmatic non-inferiority trial. BMC Anesthesiol. 2015;15:134. https://doi.org/10.1186/s12871-015-0111-z.
20. Soltész S, Alm P, Mathes A, Hellmich M, Hinkelbein J. The effect of neuromuscular blockade on the efficiency of facemask ventilation in patients difficult to facemask ventilate: a prospective trial. Anaesthesia. 2017;72(12):1484–90. https://doi.org/10.1111/anae.14035.
21. Min KJ, Rabinowitz AL, Hess CJ. Is it time to abandon routine mask ventilation before intubation? Anesth Analg. 2021;133(5):1353–7. https://doi.org/10.1213/ANE.0000000000005723.
22. Pandit JJ. Checking the ability to mask ventilate before administering long-acting neuromuscular blocking drugs. Anaesthesia. 2011;66(6):520–2; author reply 523-4. https://doi.org/10.1111/j.1365-2044.2011.06774_3.x.
23. Klucka J, Kosinova M, Zacharowski K, De Hert S, Kratochvil M, Toukalkova M, Stoudek R, Zelinkova H, Stourac P. Rapid sequence induction: an international survey. Eur J Anaesthesiol. 2020;37(6):435–42. https://doi.org/10.1097/EJA.0000000000001194.
24. Pandit JJ, Andrade J, Bogod DG, Hitchman JM, Jonker WR, Lucas N, Mackay JH, Nimmo AF, O'Connor K, O'Sullivan EP, Paul RG, Palmer JH, Plaat F, Radcliffe JJ, Sury MR, Torevell HE, Wang M, Hainsworth J, Cook TM, Royal College of Anaesthetists, Association of Anaesthetists of Great Britain and Ireland. 5th National Audit Project (NAP5) on accidental awareness during general anaesthesia: summary of main findings and risk factors. Br J Anaesth. 2014 Oct;113(4):549–59. https://doi.org/10.1093/bja/aeu313.
25. Odor PM, Bampoe S, Moonesinghe SR, Andrade J, Pandit JJ, Lucas DN, Pan-London Perioperative Audit and Research Network (PLAN), for the DREAMY Investigators Group. General anaesthetic and airway management practice for obstetric surgery in England: a prospective, multicentre observational study. Anaesthesia. 2021;76(4):460–71. https://doi.org/10.1111/anae.15250.
26. Pandit JJ. Monitoring (un)consciousness: the implications of a new definition of 'anaesthesia'. Anaesthesia. 2014;69(8):801–7. https://doi.org/10.1111/anae.12668.
27. Turnbull J, Patel A, Athanassoglou V, Pandit JJ. Cricoid pressure: apply—but be ready to release. Anaesthesia. 2016;71(9):999–1003. https://doi.org/10.1111/anae.13594.
28. Athanassoglou V, Pandit JJ. Cricoid pressure: the case in favour. Trends Anaesth Crit Care. 2015;5(2–3):57–60. https://doi.org/10.1016/j.tacc.2015.02.001.
29. Turnbull J, Patel A. Cricoid pressure: the argument against. Trends Anaesth Crit Care. 2015;5(2–3):52–6. https://doi.org/10.1016/j.tacc.2015.02.002.
30. Pandit JJ, Duncan T, Robbins PA. Total oxygen uptake with two maximal breathing techniques and the tidal volume breathing technique: a physiologic study of preoxygenation. Anesthesiology. 2003 Oct;99(4):841–6. https://doi.org/10.1097/00000542-200310000-00015.

31. Patel A, Nouraei SA. Transnasal humidified rapid-insufflation Ventilatory exchange (THRIVE): a physiological method of increasing apnoea time in patients with difficult airways. Anaesthesia. 2015;70(3):323–9. https://doi.org/10.1111/anae.12923.
32. Patel A, El-Boghdadly K. Apnoeic oxygenation and ventilation: go with the flow. Anaesthesia. 2020;75(8):1002–5. https://doi.org/10.1111/anae.15066.
33. Patel A, El-Boghdadly K. Facemask or high-flow nasal oxygenation: time to switch? Anaesthesia. 2022;77(1):7–11. https://doi.org/10.1111/anae.15593.

Chapter 15
Physical Characteristics of Extraglottic Devices

Tom C. R. V. Van Zundert and André van Zundert

Highlights

- More than 130 extraglottic airway devices (EADs) have been reviewed and classified, representing one of the most comprehensive technical overviews currently available.
- EADs are categorized according to key physical characteristics, including number of lumens, cuff type, intubation capability, reinforcement, bite block presence, and gastric access.
- Device development has progressed from early first-generation models to more advanced systems incorporating improved sealing, gastric drainage, and, more recently, visualization technologies.
- Appropriate cuff pressure monitoring and device sizing remain critical to minimize complications such as mucosal injury and air leakage.
- Many EADs can function as intubation conduits, supported by features such as detachable connectors and compatibility with fibreoptic or video-assisted techniques.
- Design innovations include multi-lumen configurations, integrated bite blocks, self-adjusting cuffs, and gastric drainage systems, expanding clinical applicability.

T. C. R. V. Van Zundert (✉)
Department of Emergency Medicine, Holy Heart Hospital, Mol, Belgium

A. van Zundert
Department of Anaesthesia and Perioperative Medicine, Royal Brisbane and Women's Hospital and The University of Queensland, Brisbane, QLD, Australia

M. Á. Gómez-Ríos, A. van Zundert (eds.), *Evidence-based Guide to Difficult Airway Management*, https://doi.org/10.1007/978-3-032-30769-9_15

- Device selection should be guided by clinical evidence and functional characteristics rather than regulatory marking alone.
- No single 'ideal' EAD exists; a function-based classification may better support clinical decision-making than purely structural categorization.
- Regulatory and post-marketing evaluation gaps persist; initiatives such as the DAS ADEPT project aim to improve device assessment.
- Future development should focus on standardized classification, clearer labelling, and high-quality multicentre clinical studies.

15.1 Introduction

When Archie Brain introduced the first extraglottic airway device (EAD), the Laryngeal Mask Airway (LMA-Classic™), more than four decades ago, its subsequent impact on clinical practice could not have been fully anticipated [1–4]. The device was rapidly adopted across anaesthesia, critical care, and emergency medicine due to its relative ease of use and favourable safety profile.

Since that time, the field has expanded considerably. By 2010, the National Health Service (NHS) catalogue listed 27 standard laryngeal mask devices [5], while Hernandez et al. identified 35 devices [6]. In contrast, the present review includes more than 130 EADs, reflecting both technological innovation and commercial proliferation.

This chapter aims to provide a structured comparison of the physical characteristics of EADs, highlighting both similarities and differences relevant to clinical practice [7]. While not exhaustive—owing to regional availability, discontinuation of devices, and ongoing product modifications—it emphasizes the importance of understanding device design prior to clinical use.

It is important to acknowledge that the medical device market remains highly dynamic. Mergers, acquisitions, and iterative redesigns may result in devices being reintroduced under the same or different names with modified specifications. Consequently, clinicians should remain aware that published descriptions may not always fully reflect current device versions.

This chapter does not aim to identify a 'best' EAD, nor to directly correlate specific design features with clinical performance. Decisions regarding the choice between an EAD and a tracheal tube, as well as device selection and sizing, remain dependent on clinical judgment. The limitations of individual devices are therefore not addressed in detail within this chapter.

15.2 Terminology

Terminology relating to airway devices remains inconsistent and, at times, imprecise. The term 'supraglottic airway device' is widely used to describe devices positioned above the glottis, irrespective of their sealing characteristics.

However, Brimacombe [8] argued that the term 'extraglottic airway device' is more appropriate, as many of these devices extend beyond the supraglottic region into the hypopharynx or proximal oesophagus, thereby incorporating an infraglottic component.

Strictly defined, 'supraglottic' refers to structures located above the glottis, whereas 'infraglottic' refers to structures below the vocal cords. The term 'extraglottic' encompasses both anatomical regions and more accurately reflects the functional positioning of these devices.

Accordingly, and in line with previous authors [6–9], the term 'extraglottic airway device' (EAD) will be used throughout this chapter.

15.2.1 'Classification' or 'Generation'? A Conundrum

Classification of extraglottic airway devices remains challenging due to the considerable heterogeneity in design and the continuous evolution of device features.

Over the past four decades, modifications have ranged from incremental changes—such as the transition from reusable to single-use devices or the introduction of reinforced airway tubes—to more substantial innovations, including devices designed to facilitate tracheal intubation (e.g. ILMA) and those incorporating gastric drainage channels (e.g. ProSeal™, Supreme™, Protector™).

The late 1990s and early 2000s were characterized by a rapid increase in the number of available devices. While some represented genuine innovation, others were derivative designs following patent expiration. This led to the emergence of multiple devices with similar structural concepts but variable quality and performance characteristics.

Several classification systems have been proposed, including:

1. **Brimacombe**—based on cuff presence, insertion route, and distal position [8].
2. **Miller**—based on the sealing mechanism [10]
3. **ISO standard (ISO 11712 (E))**—supralaryngeal design standard [11].
4. **Cook and Howes**—introduction of the '(second) generation' concept [5].

Despite these efforts, no universally accepted classification system has been established. Calls have been made to abandon first-generation devices in favour of more advanced second-generation models [12].

15.2.1.1 Limitations of the 'Generation' Concept

Redesigns and rebranding further complicate classification, as many devices reappear under the same name with modified features. Generally:

- **First-generation EADs** (e.g. LMA-Classic™) are simple devices with a single airway tube and cuff.
- **Second-generation EADs** (e.g. LMA-ProSeal™, i-gel®, SLIPA) include features that enhance sealing, allow gastric drainage, and support higher ventilation pressures.
- **Third-generation EADs** (e.g. Baska mask, Ambu AuraGain, videolaryngeal mask airways) incorporate additional elements like dual drain channels, sump reservoirs, bite blocks, videoscopes and intubation conduits.

The distinctions between the second and third generations remain debated. Some propose defining generations by:

1. Increasing oropharyngeal seal pressures: first: <20 cm H_2O; second: 20–30 cm H_2O; third: >30 cm H_2O.
2. Presence of effective gastric drainage systems.
3. Full-length integral bite blocks.
4. Specific functionality, such as visualisation, facilitating intubation (e.g. air-Q, Aura-i) or gastroscopy (e.g. LMA-Gastro™).

Thus, while classification remains challenging, understanding key structural and functional differences is essential for informed EAD selection.

15.3 From 'Blind' Inserted to 'Vision' Inserted SADs

Device classification is also closely related to insertion technique and the ability to achieve optimal positioning [13]. Traditionally, most first- and second-generation EADs are inserted blindly. However, studies have demonstrated that blind insertion techniques may result in suboptimal positioning, with reported malposition rates ranging from 50% to 80% [14–17].

In response to these limitations, recent developments have introduced vision-guided insertion techniques, including devices with integrated video capability. These systems allow real-time visualization during placement and have been proposed as a potential advancement in improving positioning accuracy and airway sealing.

Such devices are sometimes referred to as 'third-generation' EADs [18–21]. However, as previously discussed, this terminology remains inconsistently defined and should be interpreted cautiously.

Early clinical data on video-assisted EADs are promising, suggesting improved positioning and potentially higher success rates [19, 22–25]. Nevertheless, robust comparative data remain limited, and their definitive role relative to conventional blind insertion techniques has yet to be established.

This chapter adopts Miller's classification—cuffed perilaryngeal sealers, cuffed pharyngeal sealers, and cuffless preshaped sealers [10]—and compares EADs across 17 parameters: (1) those with multiple numbers of uses incorporated into the design; (2) number of lumens (ventilation tube); (3) presence of gastric access tube(s); (4) number of mask aperture bars; (5) cuff material; (6) tube shape/reinforcement; (7) colour coding of pilot balloon or cuff, 15 mm connector and type of EAD packaging; (8) presence of an integral bite block; (9) use as an intubation conduit; (10) detachability of the 15 mm connector; (11) reinforced tip; (12) integrated pilot tube (s); (13) availability of paediatric sizes; (14) MRI compatibility; (15) shape and anatomical fit of the laryngeal (concave) bowl and cuff; (16) method for ensuring that there is appropriate laryngeal surface sealing pressure in the cuff and design of the valve in the pilot tube(s); and (17) markings on the device tube to identify EAD depth.

15.4 Technical Overview and Device Evolution

More than 130 extraglottic airway devices (EADs), either currently available or recently described, have been identified and classified based on their technical characteristics. (Tables 15.1, 15.2, 15.3 and 15.4). This compilation represents, to our knowledge, one of the most comprehensive comparative overviews currently available.

Since the launch of the LMA-Classic™ (Fig. 15.1), numerous design enhancements have emerged to expand indications and improve safety—chiefly by increasing oropharyngeal leak pressure and functionally separating the gastrointestinal and respiratory tracts (Fig. 15.2). Modern EADs frequently incorporate dual or triple lumen designs, allowing for ventilation, gastric drainage, and, in some cases, facilitation of tracheal intubation.

Key improvements include:

- Advanced cuff materials with improved compliance.
- Anatomically preformed airway tubes.
- Integrated bite blocks.
- Anti-kinking reinforcements.
- Compatibility with fibreoptic and video-assisted intubation techniques.
- Single-use construction to mitigate cross-infection risks.

Table 15.5 summarizes the most relevant and desirable device features.

Tables 15.1, 15.2, 15.3 and 15.4 details manufacturer specifications for both reusable and disposable devices. Comparative parameters include: number of permitted uses, lumen count (1–3), material composition, tube shape, presence of bite block, size range (including paediatric options), inflation guidelines (volume/pressure), deflation valves, overinflation indicators, detachable 15 mm connectors,

Table 15.1 Cuffed perilaryngeal sealers

Company, model	Number of uses	Ventilation holes (VH)	Gastric channel	Mask aperture bars, n	Cuff material silicone (S); polyvinyl chloride (PVC)	Tube straight (S); reinforced (R); curved (C); flexible (F)	Colour coded Y/N; pilot balloon (PB); 15 mm connector (C); package (P)	Colour coded package (Y/N)	Integral bite block (Y/N)	Intubation conduit—max ETT size listed (Y/N)	Removable 15 mm connector (Y/N)	Reinforced tip (Y/N)	Integrated pilot tube (Y/N) — if yes, number of pilot tubes, n	Paediatric size available (Y/N)	MRI compatible (Y/N)
Laryngeal mask airway® the laryngeal mask company ltd, Wooburn green, bucks UK [www.lmaco.com] → Teleflex Athlone, co. Westmeath, Ireland [www.teleflex.com]															
LMA-classic™	40	1	0	2	S	S	N	N	N	N	N	N	N	Y	N
LMA-classic excel™ (N-America only)	60	1	0	EEB	S	S	N	N	N	Y	Y	N	N	N	N
LMA-unique™	1	1	0	2	PVC	S	N	Y	N	N	N	N	N	Y	N
LMA-unique™ EVO (Germany only)	1	1	0	2	PVC	C	N	Y	N	N	N	N	N	Y	N
LMA-flexible™	40	1	0	2	S	F—S	N	N	N	N	N	N	N	Y	N
LMA-flexible™ single use	1	1	0	2	S	F—S	N	N	N	N	N	N	N	Y	N
LMA-supreme™	1	2	1	2 fins	P	C	N	Y	Y	N	N	Y	N	Y	N

LMA-sure seal Precurved™	1	1	0	2	PVC	C	N	Y	Y	N	N	N	N	N	Y
LMA-ProSeal™	40	1	1	0	S	S	N	N	Y	N	N	N	N	Y	N
LMA-Fastrach™	40	1	0	EEB	S	C	N	N	Y	Y	N	N	N	N	N
LMA-Fastrach™ single use	1	1	0	EEB	PVC	C	N	N	Y	Y	N	N	N	N	N
LMA-CTrach™	40	1	0	EEB	S	C	N	N	Y	Y	N	N	N	N	N
LMA-Protector™	1	1	2	0	S	C—F	N	Y	Y	N	N	Y	N	N	Y
AES®AES black diamond, WA, USA [www.aesol.com]															
AES® ultra CPV™	1	1	0	0	S	S	Y—P	Y	N	N	N	N	N	Y	Y
AES® UltraClear CPV™	1	1	0	0	S	S	Y—P	Y	N	N	N	N	N	Y	Y
AES® UltraFlex CPV™	1	1	0	0	S	S—F—R	Y—P	Y	N	N	N	N	N	Y	N
AES® ultra™	1	1	0	0	S	S	Y—P	Y	N	Y	N	N	N	Y	N
AES® ultra MRI™	1	1	0	0	S	S	Y—P	Y	N	Y	N	N	N	Y	Y
AES® ultra clear™	1	1	0	0	S	S	Y—P	Y	N	Y	N	N	N	Y	N
AES® ultra clear MRI™	1	1	0	0	S	S	Y—P	Y	N	Y	N	N	N	Y	Y

(continued)

Table 15.1 (continued)

Company, model	Number of uses	Ventilation holes (VH)	Gastric channel	Mask aperture bars, n	Cuff material silicone (S); polyvinyl chloride (PVC)	Tube straight (S); reinforced (R); curved (C); flexible (F)	Colour coded Y/N; pilot balloon (PB); 15 mm connector (C); package (P)	Colour coded package (Y/N)	Integral bite block (Y/N)	Intubation conduit—max ETT size listed (Y/N)	Removable 15 mm connector (Y/N)	Reinforced tip (Y/N)	Integrated pilot tube (Y/N) — if yes, number of pilot tubes, n	Paediatric size available (Y/N)	MRI compatible (Y/N)
AES® ultra EX™	40	1	0	0	S	S	Y—P	Y	N	Y	N	N	N	Y	N
AES® ultra flex™	1	1	0	0	S	S—F—R	Y—P	Y	N	Y	N	N	N	Y	N
AES® ultra flex ex™	40	1	0	0	S	S—F—R	Y—P	Y	N	Y	N	N	N	Y	N
Wydeglyde CPV	1	1	0	0	S	C	N	Y	Y	Y	N	N	N	N	Y
AES Guardian CPV™	1	1	2	0	S	C	N	Y	Y	N	N	N	Y	N	Y
Ambu®Ambu A/S, Ballerup Denmark [www.ambu.com]															
Ambu® Aura 40™ reusable LM	40	1	0	0	S	C	Y—P	*Y*	N	N	N	Y	N	Y	N
Ambu® AuraFlex™ disposable LM	1	1	0	0	PVC	S—F—R	Y—P	*Y*	N	N	N	Y	Y	Y	N
Ambu® AuraOnce™ curved LMA	1	1	0	0	PVC	C	Y—P	Y	N	Y	N	Y	N	Y	N

Ambu® AuraStraight™	1	1	0	0	PVC	S	Y—P	Y	N	Y	N	Y	N	Y	Y
Ambu® Aura-i™	1	1	0	0	PVC	C	Y—P	Y	Y	Y	N	Y	N	Y	N
Ambu® AuraGain™	1	1	1	0	PVC	C	Y—P	Y	Y	Y	N	Y	N	N	Y
Armstrong medical, Coloraine Nothern Ireland [www.armstrongmedical.net]															
LaPremiere Plus®	1	1	0	0	S	S	Y—PB	N	N	N	N	Y	N	Y	Y
LaEncore Plus ®	40	1	0	0	S	S	Y—PB	N	N	N	N	Y	N	Y	Y
Cookgas® intubating laryngeal airway™ ***LLC, Saint Louis, MO*** [www.mercurymed.com]															
Air-Q® reusable masked laryngeal airway	60	1	0	KS	S	C	Y—C	N	Y	Y	Y	Y	N	Y	N
Air-Q® disposable masked laryngeal airway	1	1	0	KS	S	C	Y—C	Y	Y	Y	Y	Y	N	Y	N
Air-Q® blocker masked laryngeal airway	1	1	1	KS	S	C	Y—C	Y	Y	Y	Y	Y	N	N	N
Air-Q® SP masked laryngeal airway	1	1	0	KS	S	C	Y—C	Y	Y	Y	Y	Y	N/A	Y	Y

(continued)

Table 15.1 (continued)

Company, model	Number of uses	Venti-lation holes (VH)	Gastric channel	Mask aperture bars, n	Cuff material silicone (S); polyvinyl chloride (PVC)	Tube straight (S); rein-forced (R); curved (C); flexible (F)	Colour coded Y/N; pilot balloon (PB); 15 mm connector (C); package (P)	Colour coded package (Y/N)	Integral bite block (Y/N)	Intubation conduit—max ETT size listed (Y/N)	Remova-ble 15 mm connector (Y/N)	Rein-forced tip (Y/N)	Integrated pilot tube (Y/N)—if yes, number of pilot tubes, n	Paedia-tric size available (Y/N)	MRI compatible (Y/N)
Air-Q® SP reusable masked laryngeal airway	60	1	0	KS	S	C	Y—C	N	Y	Y	Y	Y	N/A	Y	Y
Flexicare® mountain ash, mid Glamorgan, UK [www.flexicare.com]															
LarySeal™—multiple	40	1	0	0	S	S	Y—PB	N	N	N	N	N	N	Y	N
LarySeal™—blue	1	1	0	0	S	S	Y—PB	N	N	N	N	N	N	Y	N
LarySeal™—clear	1	1	0	0	PVC	S	Y—PB	N	N	N	N	N	N	Y	N
LarySeal™—MRI	1	1	0	0	PVC	S	Y—PB	N	N	N	N	N	N	Y	Y
LarySeal™—flexi	1	1	0	0	PVC	S—F—R	Y—PB	N	N	N	N	N	N	Y	N
HSINER Taichung, Taichung City, Taiwan (R.O.C) [www.hsiner.com]															
Laryngeal airway mask	1	1	0	0	PVC	S	N	N	N	N	N	N	N	Y	N

Mallinckrodt® Tyco healthcare group LP, Nellcor puritan Bennett Devision, Pleasanton, CA															
LaryngoSeal®	1	1	1	EEB	PVC	S	N	N	N	N	N	Y	Y—1	N	N
Marshall products ltd Bath, UK [www.marshallproducts.co.uk]															
550 reusable LAD®	50	1	0	0	S	S	N	N	N	N	N	N	N	Y	N
550 flexible LAD®	50	1	0	0	S	F—R	N	N	N	N	N	N	N	Y	N
Silicone LAD®	1	1	0	0	S	S	N	N	N	N	N	N	N	Y	Y
Silicone single use flexible LAD®	1	1	0	0	S	F—R	N	N	N	N	N	N	N	Y	N
Visionary LAD®	1	1	0	0	PVC	S	N	N	N	N	N	N	N	Y	Y
Visionary flexible LAD®	1	1	0	0	PVC	F—R	N	N	N	N	N	N	N	Y	N
Tulip®	1	1	0	0	PVC	S	N	N	N	N	N	N	N	N	Y
Medsorg Mulheim/Ruhr, Germany [www.medsorg.de]															
Laryngeal airway®	1	1	0	0	PVC	S	N	N	N	N	N	Y	N	N	N
ProAct medical ltd, Corby, Northants, UK [www.proactmedical.co.uk]															
PRO-breathe® PVC disposable standard laryngeal airway	1	1	0	0	PVC	S	Y—PB	N	N	N	N	N	N	Y	N

(continued)

Table 15.1 (continued)

Company, model	Number of uses	Ventilation holes (VH)	Gastric channel	Mask aperture bars, n	Cuff material silicone (S); polyvinyl chloride (PVC)	Tube straight (S); reinforced (R); curved (C); flexible (F)	Colour coded Y/N; pilot balloon (PB); 15 mm connector (C); package (P)	Colour coded package (Y/N)	Integral bite block (Y/N)	Intubation conduit—max ETT size listed (Y/N)	Removable 15 mm connector (Y/N)	Reinforced tip (Y/N)	Integrated pilot tube (Y/N) — if yes, number of pilot tubes, n	Paediatric size available (Y/N)	MRI compatible (Y/N)
PRO-breathe® PVC disposable Armourflex® laryngeal airway	1	1	0	0	PVC	S—R	Y—PB	N	N	N	N	N	N	Y	N
PRO-breathe® silicone disposable standard laryngeal airway	1	1	0	0	S	S	Y—PB	N	N	N	N	N	N	Y	N
PRO-breathe® silicone disposable Armourflex® laryngeal airway	1	1	0	0	S	S—R	Y—PB	N	N	N	N	N	N	Y	N

PRO-breathe® silicone reusable standard laryngeal airway	40	1	0	0	S	S	Y—PB	N	N	N	N	N	N	Y	N
PRO-breathe® silicone reusable Armourflex® laryngeal airway	40	1	0	0	S	S—R	Y—PB	N	N	N	N	N	N	Y	N
Smiths medical Smiths medical international ltd, Hythe, Kent, UK [www.smiths-medical.com]															
Portex® SoftSeal® laryngeal mask	1	1	0	0	PVC	S	N	N	N	N	N	N	Y—1	Y	N
Portex® silicone laryngeal mask	1	1	0	2	S	S	N	N	N	N	N	N	N	Y	N
Intersurgical, Wokingham, Burkshire, UK [www.intersurgical.com]															
Solus® standard laryngeal mask airway	1	1	0	0	PVC	S	N	N	N	N	N	N	Y—1	Y	N
Solus® satin laryngeal mask Ariway	1	1	0	0	PVC	S	N	N	N	N	N	N	Y—1	N	N
Supra® silicone laryngeal mask airway	1	1	0	0	S	S	N	N	N	N	N	N	Y—1	Y	N

(continued)

Table 15.1 (continued)

Company, model	Number of uses	Ventilation holes (VH)	Gastric channel	Mask aperture bars, n	Cuff material silicone (S); polyvinyl chloride (PVC)	Tube straight (S); reinforced (R); curved (C); flexible (F)	Colour coded Y/N; pilot balloon (PB); 15 mm connector (C); package (P)	Colour coded package (Y/N)	Integral bite block (Y/N)	Intubation conduit—max ETT size listed (Y/N)	Removable 15 mm connector (Y/N)	Reinforced tip (Y/N)	Integrated pilot tube (Y/N) — if yes, number of pilot tubes, n	Paediatric size available (Y/N)	MRI compatible (Y/N)
Solus® flexible wire reinforced LMA	1	1	0	0	PVC	S—F—R	N	N	N	N	N	N	Y—1	Y	N
Solus® MRI-compatible LMA	1	1	0	0	PVC	S	N	N	N	N	N	N	Y—1	Y	Y
TELEFLEX, Athlone—co Westmeath, Ireland [www.teleflex.com]															
Rüsch crystal airway mask™	1	1	0	0	S	S	Y—cuff	N	N	N	N	Y	Y—1	Y	N
Sure seal® laryngeal mask with cuff pilot silicone cuff, PVC tube	1	1	0	2	S	S	P	Y	N	N	N	N	N	Y	Y
Sure seal® laryngeal mask with cuff pilot 100% silicone reinforced	1	1	0	2	S	R	P	Y	N	N	N	N	N	Y	Y

Sure seal® laryngeal mask reusable, 100% silicone	40	1	0	2	S	S	P	Y	N	N	N	N	N	Y	N
Sure seal® laryngeal mask reusable, 100% silicone, reinforced	40	1	0	2	S	R	P	Y	N	N	N	N	N	Y	N
Sure seal® laryngeal mask, 100% silicone	1	1	0	2	S	S	P	Y	N	N	N	N	N	Y	N
Sure seal® laryngeal mask, silicone cuff, PVC tube	1	1	0	2	S	S	P	Y	N	N	N	N	N	Y	N
Sure seal® laryngeal mask, 100% silicone reinforced	1	1	0	2	S	R	P	Y	N	N	N	N	N	Y	N
Sheridan laryngeal mask	1	1	0	0	PVC	S			N	N	N			Y	
Ultimate® laryngeal mask™ ultimate medical Pty ltd Richmond Victoria, Australia [www.ultimatemedical.com.au]															
Ultimate laryngeal mask™ reusable	50	1	0	2	S	S			N	N	N	N	N	Y	N

(continued)

Table 15.1 (continued)

Company, model	Number of uses	Ventilation holes (VH)	Gastric channel	Mask aperture bars, n	Cuff material silicone (S); polyvinyl chloride (PVC)	Tube straight (S); reinforced (R); curved (C); flexible (F)	Colour coded Y/N; pilot balloon (PB); 15 mm connector (C); package (P)	Colour coded package (Y/N)	Integral bite block (Y/N)	Intubation conduit—max ETT size listed (Y/N)	Removable 15 mm connector (Y/N)	Reinforced tip (Y/N)	Integrated pilot tube (Y/N) — if yes, number of pilot tubes, n	Paediatric size available (Y/N)	MRI compatible (Y/N)
Ultimate laryngeal mask™ single use	1	1	0	2	S	S	P	Y	N	N	N	N	N	Y	Y
Ultimate laryngeal mask™ with cuff pilot™	1	1	0	2	S	S	P	Y	N	N	N	N	N	Y	Y
Ultimate Flexy ™ laryngeal mask	50	1	0	2	S	S—F—R	P	Y	N	N	N	N	N	Y	N
Ultimate Flexy™ laryngeal mask with cuff pilot™	1	1	0	2	S	S—F—R	P	Y	N	N	N	N	N	y	N
Ultimate Flexy Plus laryngeal mask with cuff pilot™	1	1	0	2	S	F—R	S		N	N	N	N	N	N	N

The ultimate pre-curved with cuff pilot	1	1	0	2	S	C	N		N	N	N	N	N	Y	Y
Ultimate Clearview ™ laryngeal mask	1	1	0	2	S	S	P	Y	N	N	N	N	N	y	Y
Ultimate Clearview ™ laryngeal mask with cuff pilot™	1	1	0	2	S	S	P	Y	N	N	N	N	N	y	Y
The Guardian™ CPV laryngeal mask	1	2	2	N	S	F	N	N	Y	Y	N	N	Y—1	N	Y
All pro corporation Qingdao, China [www.allprocorporation.com]															
Reusable silicone laryngeal mask airway	40	1	0	2	S	S	N	N	N	N	Y	N	N	Y	N
Reusable silicone laryngeal mask airway	40	1	0	0	S	S	N	N	N	N	Y	N	N	Y	N
Reinforced laryngeal mask airway	1	1	0	2	S	F—R	N	N	N	N	Y	N	N	Y	N
Reinforced laryngeal mask airway	1	1	0	0	S	F—R	N	N	N	N	Y	N	N	Y	N

(continued)

Table 15.1 (continued)

Company, model	Number of uses	Venti-lation holes (VH)	Gastric channel	Mask aperture bars, n	Cuff material silicone (S); polyvinyl chloride (PVC)	Tube straight (S); rein-forced (R); curved (C); flexible (F)	Colour coded Y/N; pilot balloon (PB); 15 mm connector (C); package (P)	Colour coded package (Y/N)	Integral bite block (Y/N)	Intubation conduit—max ETT size listed (Y/N)	Remova-ble 15 mm connector (Y/N)	Rein-forced tip (Y/N)	Integrated pilot tube (Y/N) — if yes, number of pilot tubes, n	Paedia-tric size available (Y/N)	MRI compatible (Y/N)
PVC-silicone combined laryngeal mask airway	1	1	0	2	S	F—R	N	N	N	N	Y	N	N	Y	N
PVC-silicone combined laryngeal mask airway	1	1	0	0	S	F—R	N	N	N	N	Y	N	N	Y	N
Silicone laryngeal mask	1	1	0	2	S	S	N	N	N	N	Y	N	N	Y	N
Silicone laryngeal mask	1	1	0	0	S	S	N	N	N	N	Y	N	N	Y	N
Anandic medical systems, Feuerthal, Switzerland [www.anandic.com]															
Vital seal	1	1	0	0		S	N	N	N	N	N	Y	Y—1	Y	
Kindwell medical, Tianjin, China [www.kindwellmedical.com]															
Kindwell laryngeal mask airway 100% silicone	1	1	0	2	S	S	Y—cuff	Y	N	N	N	N	N	Y	Y

Kindwell laryngeal mask airway 100% silicone	1	1	0	0	S	S	Y—cuff	Y	N	N	N	N	N	Y	Y
Kindwell laryngeal mask airway PVC tube with silicone cuff	1	1	0	2	S	S	Y—cuff	Y	N	N	N	N	N	Y	Y
Kindwell laryngeal mask airway PVC tube with silicone cuff	1	1	0	0	S	S	Y—cuff	Y	N	N	N	N	N	Y	Y
Kindwell laryngeal mask airway 100% PVC	1	1	0	0	PVC	S	Y—cuff	Y	N	N	N	N	N	Y	Y
Kindwell laryngeal mask airway silicone flexible	1	1	0	2	S	F—R	Y—cuff	Y	N	N	N	N	N	Y	Y
Kindwell laryngeal mask airway silicone flexible	1	1	0	2	S	S—F—R	Y—cuff	Y	N	N	N	N	N	Y	Y

(continued)

Table 15.1 (continued)

Company, model	Number of uses	Ventilation holes (VH)	Gastric channel	Mask aperture bars, n	Cuff material silicone (S); polyvinyl chloride (PVC)	Tube straight (S); reinforced (R); curved (C); flexible (F)	Colour coded Y/N; pilot balloon (PB); 15 mm connector (C); package (P)	Colour coded package (Y/N)	Integral bite block (Y/N)	Intubation conduit—max ETT size listed (Y/N)	Removable 15 mm connector (Y/N)	Reinforced tip (Y/N)	Integrated pilot tube (Y/N)—if yes, number of pilot tubes, n	Paediatric size available (Y/N)	MRI compatible (Y/N)
Kindwell laryngeal mask airway 100% silicone reusable	40	1	0	2	S	S	Y—cuff	Y	N	N	N	N	N	Y	Y
Kindwell laryngeal mask airway 100% silicone reusable	40	1	0	0	S	S	Y—cuff	Y	N	N	N	N	N	Y	Y
Well Leed medical ltd medical, Guangzhou, China [www.welllead.com.cn]															
Disposable silicone laryngeal mask	1	1	0	0	S	S	Y—PB	N	N	N	N	N	N	Y	N
Reusable silicone laryngeal mask	40	1	0	0	S	S	Y—PB	N	N	N	N	N	N	Y	N

Disposable flexible silicone laryngeal mask	1	1	0	0	S	S—F	Y—PB	N	N	N	N	N	N	Y	N
Reusable flexible silicone laryngeal mask	40	1	0	2	S	S—F	Y—PB	N	N	N	N	N	N	Y	N
Disposable PVC laryngeal mask	1	1	0	0	PVC	S	Y—PB	N	N	N	N	N	N	Y	N
Disposable flexible PVC laryngeal mask	1	1	0	0	PVC	S	Y—C—PB	N	N	N	N	N	N	Y	N
MedCom flow Barcelona, Spain [www.medcomflow.com]															
Totaltrack VLM® (video laryngeal mask)	1	1	2	2	PVC	C	N	N	Y	Y	N	Y	Y—1	N	N

Table 15.2 Third-generation EADs video laryngeal mask airways, using a second-generation EAD + a customized videoscope (flexible optical stylet) in a special blind-ended canal + (portable) monitor (camera/light source in bowl of device)

Company, model	Number of uses	Number of lumina, n	Mask aperture bars, n	Gastric access	Cuff material silicone (S); polyvinyl chloride (PVC);; thermoplastic elastomer (TE)	Tube straight (S); reinforced (R); curved (C); flexible (F)	Colour coded (Y/N); pilot balloon (PB); 15 mm connector (C); package (P)	Colour coded package (Y/N)	Integral bite block (Y/N)	Intubation conduit max ETT size listed (Y/N)	Removable 15 mm connector Y/N	Reinforced tip (Y/N)	Integrated pilot tube (Y/N) + if yes, number of pilot tubes	Paediatric size available (Y/N)	MRI compatible (Y/N)
UE medical®, Zhejiang China [www.ueworld.com]															
SaCo video laryngeal mask™,	1	1	0	1	S	C -F	N	N	Y	Y	Y	Y	N—1	N	N
Magill medical technology®, Changsha Magill medical technology co. ltd, Hunan, China [www.magillmed.com]															
SafeLM™ video laryngeal mask	1	1	0	1	S	C—F	N	N	Y	Y	N	Y	N—1	N	N

Table 15.3 Cuffed pharyngeal sealers

Company, model	Number of uses	Number of lumina – Ventilation holes (VH)	Mask aperture bars, n	Gastric access	Cuff material silicone (S); polyvinyl chloride (PVC)	Tube straight (S); reinforced (R); curved (C); flexible (F)	Colour coded Y/N; pilot balloon (PB); 15 mm connector (C); package (P)	Integral bite block (Y/N)	Intubation conduit—max ETT size listed (Y/N)	Removable 15 mm connector (Y/N)	Reinforced tip	Integrated pilot tube (Y/N) + if yes, number of pilot tubes	Paediatric size available (Y/N)	MRI compatible (Y/N)
AMD® Nagor limited, Isle of Man; manufactured by Biosil ltd, Cumbernauld, UK														
Airway management device—AMD®	40	1	N/A	Y	S	S	N	N	N	N	N	Y—2	N	N
Pulmodyne, Indianapolis, IN [www.pulmodyne.com]														
CobraPLA®	1	1	4 6 8	0	PVC	S	N	N	Y	N	Y	N	y	N
CobraPlus®	1	1	4 6 8	0	PVC	S	N	N	Y	N	Y	N	y	N
COVIDIEN-Tyco-healthcare-Mallinckrodt Mansfield, New York [www.nellcor.com]														
Esophageal tracheal Combitube®	1	2—VH	N/A	Y	S	S	N	N	N	Y	N	Y—2	N (37Fr > 6 yrs)	N
Elisha medical technologies ltd Katzrin, Israel														
Elisha airway device—EMD®	R	3	N/A		S	C	N	Y	8		N	Y—1	N	
King systems® Noblesville, IN, USA [www.kingsystems.com]														
Silicone king LAD	1	1	N/A		S	S	N	N	N	N	N	N	Y	N
Silicone flexible king LAD	1	1	N/A		S	F	N	N	N	N	N	N	Y	N

(continued)

Table 15.3 (continued)

Company, model	Number of uses	Number of lumina – Ventilation holes (VH)	Mask aperture bars, n	Gastric access	Cuff material silicone (S); polyvinyl chloride (PVC)	Tube straight (S); reinforced (R); curved (C); flexible (F)	Colour coded Y/N; pilot balloon (PB); 15 mm connector (C); package (P)	Integral bite block (Y/N)	Intubation conduit—max ETT size listed (Y/N)	Removable 15 mm connector (Y/N)	Reinforced tip	Integrated pilot tube (Y/N) + if yes, number of pilot tubes	Paediatric size available (Y/N)	MRI compatible (Y/N)
ClearSeal king LAD			N/A						N				Y	N
Flexible ClearSeal king LAD			N/A						N				Y	N
King LT®	50	2—VH	N/A	N	S	S	Y—C—P	N	Y	Y	N	Y—1	N	N
King LT-D®	1	2—VH	N/A	N	PVC	S	Y—C—P	N	Y	N	N	Y—1	Y	N
King LTS-D®	1	2—VH	N/A	Y	PVC	S	Y—C—P	N	N	N	N	Y—1	(Y > 122 cm)	N
VBM Medizintechnik GmbH, Sulz Germany [www.vbm-medical.de]														
Lt®	50	1	N/A	N	S	S	Y—C	(*)	N	Y	N	Y—1	y	N
LTS-II®	50	2—VH	N/A	Y	S	S	Y—C	N	N	y	N	Y—1	y	N
LT-D®	1	1	N/A	N	PVC	S	Y—C	N	N	Y	N	Y—1	y	N
LTS-D®	1	2—VH	N/A	Y	PVC	S	Y—C	N	N	Y	N	Y—1	N	N
Vital signs Totowa NJ, USA [www.paxpress.nypa.hidinc.com]														
PAXpress™ pharyngeal airway	1	1	N/A		Rubber	C	N	N	N	N	Y	Y—1	N	N
Teleflex Rüsch research Triangle Park, NC, USA [www.rusch.com]														
Rusch Easytube® double lumen airway	1	2—VH	N/A	Y	PVC	S	N	N	Y	N	N	Y—2	N	N

(*): bite block optional

Table 15.4 Cuffless preshaped sealers

Company, model	Number of uses	Number of lumina, n	Mask aperture bars, n	Gastric access	Cuff material silicone (S); polyvinyl chloride (PVC); thermoplastic elastomer (TE)	Tube straight (S); reinforced (R); curved (C); flexible (F)	Colour coded (Y/N); pilot balloon (PB); 15 mm connector (C); package (P)	Colour-coded package (Y/N)	Integral bite block (Y/N)	Intubation conduit max ETT size listed (Y/N)	Removable 15 mm connector Y/N	Reinforced tip (Y/N)	Integrated pilot tube (Y/N) + if yes, number of pilot tubes	Paediatric size available (Y/N)	MRI compatible (Y/N)
Achi corporation® Achi corporation, San Jose, California USA															
ChouAirway®	1	1	N/A	0	PVC	C	N	N	N	N	N	N	N/A	N	Y
CurveAir ltd., London, UK															
SLIPA®	1	1	0	N	PVC	C	C	N	N	N	N	N	N/A	Y	Y
3gLM®	1	3	0	Y	PVC	C	N	N	Y	Y	N	Y	N/A	N	Y
Intersurgical Wokingham, Berkshire, UK [www.intersurgical.com]															
I-gel®	1	2	Epiglottic rest	Y	TE	S	P	Y	Y	Y	N	N	N/A	Y	Y
I-gel® O_2	1	2	Epiglottic rest	Y	TE	S	P	Y	Y	Y	N	N	N/A	Y	Y
Microtek medical Columbus, MS, USA [www.mdimicrotek.com/prod_salt htm]															
SALT® (Supraglottic airway laryngopharyngeal tube)	1	1	Epiglottic guard	N	N/A	C—R	N/A	N/A	Y	Y	N	Y	N/A	N/A	Y
PROACT medical systems, Frenchs Forest NSW, Australia [www.proactmedical.com.au]															

(continued)

Table 15.4 (continued)

Company, model	Number of uses	Number of lumina, n	Mask aperture bars, n	Gastric access	Cuff material silicone (S); polyvinyl chloride (PVC); thermoplastic elastomer (TE)	Tube straight (S); reinforced (R); curved (C); flexible (F)	Colour coded (Y/N); pilot balloon (PB); 15 mm connector (C); package (P)	Colour-coded package (Y/N)	Integral bite block (Y/N)	Intubation conduit max ETT size listed (Y/N)	Removable 15 mm connector Y/N	Reinforced tip (Y/N)	Integrated pilot tube (Y/N) + if yes, number of pilot tubes	Paediatric size available (Y/N)	MRI compatible (Y/N)
Baska mask® reusable	70	3	0	Y	S	S	C	N	Y	N	N	N	N/A	N	Y
Baska mask® disposable	1	3	0	Y	S	S	C	N	Y	N	N	N	N/A	N	Y
Xu BANG co. Taichung, Taiwan [http://chitsein.com]															
OPLAC™ (Oro-Pharyngo-laryngeal airway cap)	1	1	Epiglottic gliding bar	N	S	S	N/A	N	N	N	N	Y	N/A	N	Y

N/A: not applicable

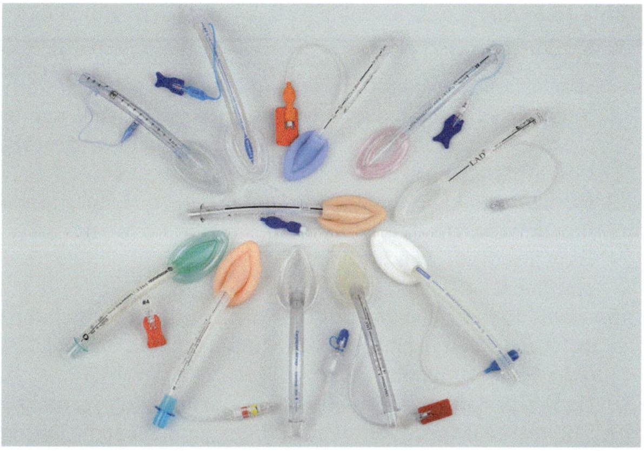

Fig. 15.1 The LMA-Classic™ (centre) and similarly designed cuffed EADs of the first generation

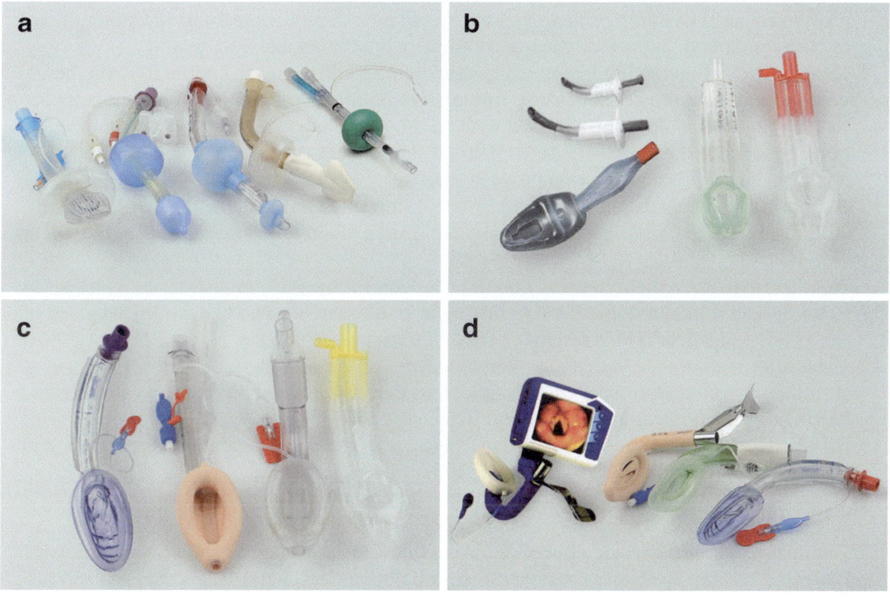

Fig. 15.2 Compilation of Extraglottic Airway Devices (from left to right): **a**) Cuffed pharyngeal sealers (Cobra-PLA, King LT, Combitube, PAXpress, Easy tube); **b**) Cuffless preshaped sealers (Chou Airway, Slipa, i-gel, Baska Mask); **c**) Multilumen EADs (air-Q Blocker, LMA ProSeal, LMA Supreme, Baska Mask); and **d**) Anatomically curved EADs (LMA CTrach, LMA Fastrach, Ambu Aura i, air-Q)

colour-coded elements, mask aperture bars, reinforced tips, and suitability for intubation. Additional factors include compatibility with MRI and laser procedures, as well as relevant size markings for tracheal tube insertion. A legend of commonly used medical symbols is provided in Fig. 15.3.

Table 15.5 Suggested desirable features of an extraglottic airway device

1. Single-use device made of quality, non-harmful, non-toxic, soft-compliant material for both spontaneous and controlled ventilation
2. Reusable versions should be robust enough to enable appropriate cleaning (minimal risk of cross-infection) and allow multiple uses without deterioration of performance. A long shelf life is desirable and adds to the cost-effectiveness
3. Devices should be suitable for routine and emergency airway management, not requiring muscle relaxants during insertion
4. Easy insertion, even by a non-anaesthetist, without the need for finger guidance, for proper placement
5. Ability to insert the device in a neutral position without the need for neck flexion or extension, even in patients with minimal mouth opening (2–3 cm), teeth problems or reduced neck mobility
6. High first attempt insertion success rate and short learning curve
7. Minimal to no need for manipulations to maintain a clear, stable hands-free airway once positioned
8. Adequate sealing quality (high oropharyngeal seal pressure, high oesophageal seal, high pharyngeal seal) enabling positive pressure ventilation at higher pressures, avoiding the risk of gastric inflation, hypoventilation, environmental pollution and drug wastage
9. Devices with a functioning integrated gastric drain tube that runs in continuity with the oesophageal inlet, protect the airway from risk of pulmonary aspiration of regurgitant matter. The stomach may be accessed with an orogastric tube via the gastric drain tube. In a boogie-guided technique, the EAD is railroaded into place over the gastric drain tube using a boogie, a suction catheter or an orogastric tube
10. A reinforced tip reduces the risk of fold-over of the cuff. The strengthened tip of the EAD cuff, formed by the distal end of the integrated gastric drain tube, further adds to the safety of EADs
11. Non-invasive (extraglottic) airway conduit. Conduit for tracheal intubation, enabling access to the airway if required. Insertion of the tracheal tube can be done blindly, light-guided or fibre optic-guided, or with a (Aintree) catheter exchange technique
12. Clear information: Size indication (colour coded—Based on weight); cuff (max insufflations volume/pressure); use (single, reusable); special requirements: Laser resistant; MRI compatible; maximum tracheal tube size
13. Standardized size-based colour coded packages, pilot tubes, cuff deflator valve and 15 mm connector for immediate identification of sizes
14. Presence of an oval-shaped short, wide-bore anatomically curved airway tube with an integral bite block and securing tools to reduce risks of displacement of the EAD
15. Minimal risk of serious side effects and lack of device-associated trauma (tongue trauma, bleeding), airway morbidity (postoperative sore throat, dysphagia, dysphonia) and serious complications (airway obstruction, loss of airway, regurgitation, laryngospasm, aspiration, neuropraxia)

15.4.1 Clinical Indications

Extraglottic airway devices are currently used across a broad spectrum of clinical settings and patient populations. Initially introduced for short-duration procedures in spontaneously breathing patients, their application has progressively expanded to include more complex surgical and non-surgical scenarios. Contemporary use now encompasses controlled ventilation, laparoscopic and open intra-abdominal

Medical Product Symbol	Explanation of reference symbol
CE	CE Mark. This symbol certifies that a product has met European Union consumer safety, health or environmental requirements
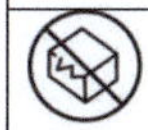	Do not use if package is opened or damaged Do not use if the product sterilization barrier or its packaging is compromised
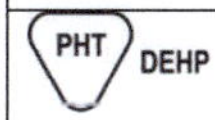	Contains phthalate–DEHP-The potential effects of phthalates on pregnant/nursing women or children have not been fully characterized and there may be concern for reproductive and developmental effects.
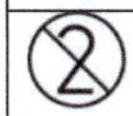	For single use only (not reusable) –Do not re-sterilise This symbol is used for disposable one-time-use products
	Reusable- maximum 40 uses
	Caution, see enclosed documentation-Please read User Manual This is a safety symbol used to highlight that there are specific warnings or precautions associated with the devices that are not otherwise found on the label.
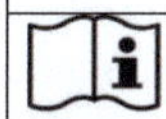	Consult instructions for use
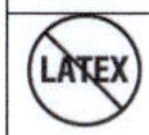	Latex free
Rx ONLY	Prescription only
STERILE R	Sterile material R = symbol for sterilized using irradiation
STERILE EO	Sterile material EO = symbol for sterilized using ethylene oxide
	Usable until- This symbol is accompanied by a date to indicate that the device should not be used after the end of the year, month or day shown.
LOT	Batch Description (Lot number or Batch number) This symbol is accompanied by the manufacturer's batch code.
	Date of Manufacture
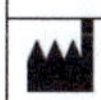	Manufacturer. This symbol is accompanied by the name and address of the manufacturer.
REF	Order Number = Reference Number = Catalogue Number
MR	MR safe. This means the item poses no known hazards in *all* magnetic resonance imaging (MRI) environments
	MR conditional. This means an item has been demonstrated to pose no known hazards in a *specified* MRI environment with *specified* conditions of use
	MR unsafe. This means an item is known to pose hazards in all MRI environments.

Fig. 15.3 List of medical product symbols printed on extraglottic airway devices

procedures, and selected cases involving obese patients, provided that appropriate device selection and monitoring are ensured.

Beyond the operating theatre, EADs have assumed an increasingly important role in emergency medicine, prehospital care, intensive care units, and obstetric practice. They are also widely incorporated into difficult airway algorithms as both primary and rescue devices [26–39].

This expansion in indications reflects both increased familiarity among clinicians and ongoing improvements in device design, particularly with respect to airway sealing and gastric drainage. However, broader applicability should not be interpreted as universal suitability. The use of an EAD must always be considered in the context of patient-specific risk factors, including aspiration risk, airway anatomy, and the anticipated need for high airway pressures. The duration of use is not inherently limited by the device itself but should be evaluated in relation to the patient's physiological status and the nature of the procedure.

Ultimately, the choice between an EAD and a tracheal tube remains a matter of clinical judgment, informed by available evidence, manufacturer recommendations, and institutional guidelines. While many modern EADs support both spontaneous and controlled ventilation, with or without neuromuscular blockade, careful patient selection remains essential to ensure safety and effectiveness.

Due to infection control concerns, many institutions now favour single-use EADs—mandatory in some regions. Additionally, device availability may vary by patent and market strategy (e.g. LMA-Excel™ is restricted to North America, while LMA-Unique EVO™ is limited to Germany).

15.4.2 Number of Uses

The original LMA-Classic™ was designed as a reusable device; however, the majority of modern EADs are now manufactured for single use. When appropriate cleaning and inspection protocols are followed, reusable devices can typically be used up to 40 times, although some manufacturers report higher durability, with up to 50 uses (e.g., Ultimate Laryngeal Mask, King LTR), 60 uses (e.g., LMA-Classic Excel, air-Q Cookgas), or even 70 uses (e.g., Baska Mask).

These reusable devices frequently incorporate reinforced airway tubes to enhance durability and are often supplied with serial numbers or tracking systems to monitor usage over time.

Nevertheless, sterilization protocols are not always described in sufficient detail, and excessive reuse may be associated with rare but clinically relevant complications. Increasing concerns regarding the transmission of prions, viruses, and other pathogens have contributed to a shift towards single-use devices, which have now become predominant in many regions. Despite their higher cost and environmental impact, disposable EADs are increasingly preferred due to their perceived safety advantages [40].

15.4.3 Material

The various components of extraglottic airway devices—including the airway tube, cuff, pilot balloon, inflation line, and mask aperture bars—are typically manufactured from medical-grade silicone, polyvinyl chloride (PVC), or combinations of these materials.

Silicone is generally preferred for cuff construction because of its softness, flexibility at body temperature, biocompatibility, and resistance to puncture and tearing. Some devices (e.g. AES Ultra-EX®) are manufactured entirely from silicone, whereas others combine a silicone cuff with a PVC airway tube in order to reduce manufacturing costs.

In an effort to approximate the mechanical properties of silicone, certain PVC-based devices incorporate softening agents (e.g., SoftSeal®, Marshall Visionary LAD®), often including plasticizers such as PHT-DEHP. Alternative materials include thermoplastic elastomers (e.g., i-gel®) and thermoplastic rubber (e.g., OPLAC®). The La Encore Plus® employs AmSil™, a medical-grade liquid silicone blend, in a single-piece cuff–tube construction.

Most contemporary EADs are latex-free; however, notable exceptions remain, such as the oesophageal tracheal Combitube (ETC), which may contain latex. It should also be noted that manufacturers do not consistently specify material composition directly on the device.

15.4.4 Correct Sizing

Selection of the appropriate EAD size depends on clinical judgment and a range of patient-specific anatomical and physiological factors. This process is complicated by inconsistent manufacturer recommendations, the diversity of available devices, and the wide range of sizes—often up to eight sizes for a single device type.

Significant challenges arise from variability in airway anatomy, body habitus, and potential ethnic differences [41–43]. Furthermore, no universal sizing system currently exists. The original LMA sizing system—size 3 for women and size 4 for men—was subsequently expanded to include size 5 for larger adults. Today, most manufacturers provide size ranges from 0.5 to 6, generally based on patient weight, following the original LMA-Classic guidelines proposed by Archie Brain [2]. However, not all manufacturers adhere to this system [44].

A variety of alternative selection criteria have been proposed, including weight or body mass index (BMI) [45], sex [46–49], age or height, and anatomical surrogates such as tongue width [50], finger width [51], or ear size in children [52]. In addition, proprietary formulas and sizing algorithms have been described [53, 54].

Berry et al. [49] proposed a pragmatic algorithm based on clinical parameters, including the number of placement attempts, oropharyngeal leak pressure, and fibreoptic assessment of positioning.

Incorrect sizing or malposition may result in air leakage, excessive intracuff pressure, or insertion-related trauma. Undersized devices are associated with higher intracuff pressures and an increased risk of mucosal injury, whereas oversized devices may provoke airway reflexes or result in folding of the cuff tip [55–58].

Although no single size will be optimal in all cases, appropriate size selection, combined with correct placement—preferably supported by visualization techniques—and careful cuff pressure monitoring, can improve the quality of the airway seal [59–61]. The development of standardized sizing systems, potentially informed by imaging modalities such as ultrasound or MRI, remains an important objective for improving safety and consistency in clinical practice.

15.4.5 Airway Tube: Number of Lumens

The original LMA and early extraglottic airway devices were designed with a single lumen, allowing ventilation and spontaneous breathing. Subsequent developments introduced dual-lumen designs, incorporating a separate channel for gastric access, as seen in devices such as the LMA-Protector™, LMA-Supreme™, LMA-ProSeal™, and i-gel®, among others.

More advanced devices may include a third channel, as observed in the Baska Mask®, 3gLM®, and Elisha Airway Device®, which can be used to facilitate tracheal intubation or enhance gastric drainage.

The gastric lumen serves several important functions. It enables placement of an orogastric tube, facilitates drainage of gastric contents—thereby potentially reducing the risk of regurgitation—and, in certain cases, allows intubation using introducers such as the Frova or similar devices.

Some devices, such as the LMA Unique EVO™, do not incorporate a gastric channel but rely on anatomical sealing at the level of the oesophageal sphincter. Others, including the LMA-Gastro™, are specifically designed to accommodate endoscopic instruments.

The use of transparent airway tubing allows visualization of condensation, secretions, or regurgitated material, which may aid in early detection of malposition or aspiration. In contrast, earlier designs relied primarily on occlusion of the oesophageal inlet by the distal cuff, which provided limited protection against aspiration, particularly under conditions of positive pressure ventilation.

Devices that incorporate separate ventilation and gastric channels generally achieve higher oropharyngeal seal pressures and improved functional separation between the respiratory and gastrointestinal tracts. Some designs, such as the SLIPA® and Baska Mask®, include sump reservoirs capable of collecting larger volumes of gastric fluid, reportedly up to 50 mL, compared with approximately 3.5 mL for the LMA-Classic™ or ProSeal™ [62, 63].

Specialized twin-lumen devices like the Combitube®, Laryngeal Tube®, and Easy-Tube® (EzT) function whether placed in the trachea or oesophagus. Ventilation is achieved through multiple apertures, depending on placement. While Combitube®

blocks fibreoptic access in oesophageal positioning, EzT allows it through its single distal lumen. The Airway Management Device® (AMD®) features dual cuffs and a forward-facing orifice, but required redesigns due to performance issues [64, 65].

Many EADs integrate a posterior bulge to enhance glottic apposition. Tubes often include colour-coded or marked guide lines (e.g. black, blue, or size-specific colours) for positioning confirmation. Integral bite blocks vary in length and material to minimize dental trauma, occlusion, and kinking. For instance, the LMA-Supreme™ has equal cuff sizes across sizes 4 and 5, but a longer bite block in the latter.

Reinforced tubes with embedded helical wires are commonly used in head, neck, or craniofacial surgery to reduce kinking and enhance stability.

15.4.6 Cuff

Cuff design remains a central element in the classification and functional performance of extraglottic airway devices. According to Miller's classification, devices may be categorized as cuffed perilaryngeal sealers, cuffed pharyngeal sealers with oesophageal components, or cuffless anatomically preshaped sealers [10]. Devices such as the i-gel®, SLIPA®, Chou Airway®, and Baska Mask® are examples of cuffless designs (Fig. 15.2b).

Effective airway protection requires the establishment of two functional seals: one at the laryngopharyngeal level (first seal) and a second at the oesophageal inlet (second seal). While most devices rely on inflatable cuffs constructed from silicone or PVC, some designs employ alternative mechanisms, such as the non-inflatable thermoplastic cuff of the i-gel® or the self-sealing membrane of the Baska Mask®.

Cuff characteristics—including thickness, compliance, and symmetry—play an important role in determining sealing performance. Malrotation or asymmetry of the cuff may impair effective sealing and compromise ventilation.

Considerable variation exists in cuff shape between devices. For example, the Guardian® features a more rectangular cuff design, whereas the LMA-Classic™ has a predominantly ovoid configuration. The LMA-ProSeal™ incorporates a deeper bowl, a posteriorly extended cuff, and a gastric drainage channel, features that contribute to increased seal pressure and improved airway security. Similarly, the LMA-Supreme™ and LMA-Protector™ include elongated cuffs with an angulation designed to align with oesophageal anatomy.

Innovative designs have also emerged, such as the Cobra PLA PLUS®, which integrates additional monitoring capabilities, including temperature and CO_2 measurement, in both adult and paediatric sizes [66].

Modern cuff designs are generally elliptical and anatomically contoured, in contrast to earlier circular or rectangular designs. In most devices, the cuff is attached to the outer rim of the mask; however, in certain devices (e.g., Cobra-PLA®, Easy-Tube®), the cuff may partially surround the airway tube itself.

Some EADs, including the Laryngeal Tube®, King Systems®, and Combitube®, employ dual-cuff systems, consisting of a proximal pharyngeal cuff and a distal oesophageal cuff, which are inflated either simultaneously or via separate pilot lines.

Finally, several devices are constructed as single-piece units (e.g., SoftSeal®, Ambu®, Baska Mask®), which may enhance structural integrity and reduce the risk of leakage at junction points. Others incorporate preformed anatomical curvature (e.g., i-gel®, Ambu Aura®, LMA Supreme™), facilitating insertion and improving positional stability.

15.4.7 Cuff Protection

Certain extraglottic airway devices—such as the LMA-Supreme™, LMA-Protector™, Ambu Aura-i®, i-gel®, SaCo VLM®, and SafeVLM®—are supplied with dedicated packaging systems that include moulded cradles designed to protect the cuff during storage and transport. These systems help preserve the anatomical shape of the airway tube and minimize deformation of the cuff prior to use.

Maintaining cuff integrity before insertion is important, as deformation or folding may adversely affect positioning, sealing, and overall device performance. Such packaging solutions, therefore, contribute to both device reliability and ease of insertion in clinical practice.

15.4.8 Cuff Deflation before Insertion and Removal

There is currently no universal consensus regarding the optimal degree of cuff inflation during insertion and removal of EADs. Some authors and manufacturers advocate complete deflation prior to insertion, thereby creating a flattened, low-profile cuff that may facilitate passage along the hard palate and posterior pharyngeal wall, reducing the likelihood of impaction at the level of the glottis or vallecula.

Certain manufacturers provide dedicated tools to assist in achieving complete cuff deflation before insertion. In contrast, other authors recommend partial inflation of the cuff, suggesting that a slightly inflated cuff may reduce insertion trauma and improve guidance of the device into position.

An alternative approach involves leaving the cuff at atmospheric pressure by venting the pilot balloon, allowing the cuff to deform naturally during insertion. Each of these techniques has potential advantages and limitations, and no single method has been definitively shown to be superior.

During removal, cuff deflation is generally recommended to minimize mucosal trauma, although clinical practice varies. Ultimately, insertion and removal techniques should be adapted to the specific device design and operator experience.

15.4.9 Cuff Pressure Monitoring

Manufacturers generally provide recommendations regarding the maximum cuff inflation volume and/or maximum intracuff pressure for extraglottic airway devices. These limits may vary considerably (e.g., up to 85 mL in Cobra-PLA, vs. 40 mL in others) depending on the specific device design, cuff material, and cuff size. In most cases, it is recommended that the intracuff pressure should not exceed 60 cm H_2O.

Despite these recommendations, cuff pressure monitoring is not routinely performed in all clinical settings, particularly in intensive care units and emergency departments. This is of concern, as intracuff pressure may change significantly during the course of anaesthesia.

Several factors contribute to increases in cuff pressure, including warming of the cuff to body temperature and the permeability of cuff materials to gases. Silicone cuffs, in particular, are more permeable than PVC cuffs, allowing diffusion of gases such as nitrous oxide into the cuff during anaesthesia. This may result in a progressive increase in intracuff pressure over time.

Nitrous oxide diffusion into the cuff has been reported to increase cuff pressure significantly during anaesthesia [67]. If the cuff is initially inflated to the maximum recommended volume, intracuff pressure may increase substantially during the procedure.

When nitrous oxide is not used, as is increasingly the case in modern anaesthetic practice, the increase in cuff pressure is generally more limited. However, clinically relevant changes may still occur.

Excessive intracuff pressure may result in compression of the pharyngeal mucosa, leading to impaired perfusion and an increased risk of complications such as sore throat, dysphagia, and, in rare cases, cranial nerve injury. Conversely, insufficient cuff pressure may lead to an inadequate seal between the respiratory and gastrointestinal tracts, increasing the risk of air leakage, ineffective ventilation, and gastric insufflation [68]. For these reasons, both overinflation and underinflation of the cuff should be avoided. Regular measurement and adjustment of intracuff pressure using a cuff manometer are therefore recommended during both induction and maintenance of anaesthesia.

Some devices, like AES Ultra® and Guardian®, include built-in pressure indicators, eliminating the need for external manometers. The TruCuff® syringe offers a visual pressure scale. Alternatively, the minimal leakage technique—inflating until a seal is achieved—can help avoid overinflation while ensuring a secure fit.

15.4.10 Pilot Balloon and Pilot Tube(s)

Most cuffed extraglottic airway devices include a pilot balloon, which is typically transparent or colour-coded and may be marked with device size or recommended inflation limits; however, this information is often absent.

In several devices (e.g. SoftSeal®, Solus®, Rusch Crystal Airway Mask®, LaryngoSeal®, air-Q®, PAXpress®), the inflation line is firmly attached to the airway tube over a length of approximately 3–6 cm in order to reduce the risk of entrapment between the teeth.

Integral pilot tubes are particularly advantageous in surgical settings such as ear, nose, and throat (ENT) procedures, where they reduce the risk of accidental damage or transection. Certain models, such as the LMA-ProSeal™, incorporate a manual red vent plug that must be opened during autoclaving to prevent cuff rupture. The La Encore Plus® (Armstrong Medical) includes a clamp and plug mechanism designed to prevent leakage from the pilot balloon.

Several modern devices (e.g. AES-Cuff Pilot Valve®, Ultimate Cuff Pilot®, Teleflex Laryngeal Mask with Cuff Pilot®) have replaced traditional pilot balloons with colour-coded valve systems that allow real-time estimation of cuff pressure. The Teleflex system, for example, incorporates four colour zones:

- Green (40–60 cm H_2O): Optimal cuff pressure.
- Yellow (0–40 cm H_2O): Underinflation.
- Red (>70 cm H_2O): Overinflation and potential risk [69].

Other systems, such as the Ultimate Cuff Pilot®, simplify this concept to two zones. Standardization of colour coding and pressure ranges across devices would likely reduce confusion and improve clinical safety.

Although the pilot balloon provides a tactile indication of cuff inflation, objective measurement of intracuff pressure remains essential for accurate and safe cuff management.

15.4.11 Mask Aperture Bars

The original LMA-Classic™ included two mask aperture bars to prevent epiglottic obstruction of the airway opening [70]. Some EADs (e.g., Cobra-PLA®) incorporate up to eight bars. However, their anatomical utility remains debated, as they may contribute to herniation of pharyngeal structures and may impede blind tracheal intubation [71].

To address these limitations, various alternative design features have been developed, including:

- Longitudinal flaps or tongues that open during intubation.
- Reinforced axial ridges.
- Deeper concave bowls to minimize herniation.
- Multiple independent conduits to ensure reliable airflow.
- Fluted distal ends to enlarge the gas aperture.
- Integrated gastric conduits.
- Rectangular cuffs designed to support the epiglottis.

These innovations have reduced the need for mask aperture bar in many modern designs. Although herniation of pharyngeal structures through the bars has been documented, its clinical incidence appears to be low [63, 72–75],

Contemporary EADs demonstrate a wide range of epiglottic control mechanisms, including:

- Epiglottic elevating bars (e.g., LaryngoSeal®, LMA-Fastrach™).
- Modified bars with distal openings (e.g., LMA-C-Trach™).
- Fins (e.g., LMA-Supreme™).
- Epiglottic rests or guards (e.g., i-gel®, SALT®).
- Built-in blockers (e.g., OPLAC®).
- Absence of bars altogether (e.g., LMA-ProSeal™, AES®, SoftSeal®), often combined with deeper bowls to reduce the risk of obstruction.

Barless designs may facilitate easier cleaning, improved access for suctioning, enhanced compatibility with fibreoptic intubation, and improved reusability. Notably, the spacing between the bars in the LMA-Classic™ is wider than in the disposable LMA-Unique™, despite the latter being constructed from more flexible material [76].

However, certain design elements, such as epiglottic fins in the LMA-Supreme™, may hinder fibreoptic scope or catheter navigation, depending on their configuration and position [77].

15.4.12 Reinforced Tip

The distal tip of an extraglottic airway device must be sufficiently soft to minimize the risk of pharyngeal trauma, yet adequately firm to resist folding during insertion. Devices with reinforced tips—such as the LMA-Supreme™, Ambu®, Laryngeal Airway®, LaryngoSeal®, air-Q®, and Cobra-PLA®—enhance ease of placement and help prevent cuff collapse. Partial cuff inflation during insertion may further reduce the risk of bending.

Incorporation of a gastric channel within the tip may also contribute to reinforcement, improving structural integrity and facilitating a more effective seal at the level of the oesophageal inlet, thereby helping to reduce the risk of reflux.

Tip reinforcement may help prevent several potential complications:

(a) Misplacement of the cuff over the larynx during insertion.
(b) Failure to pass orogastric tubes (e.g., Salem Sump) due to obstruction of the lumen.
(c) Accidental entry of the device into the laryngeal inlet, with a risk of vocal cord trauma.

Some manufacturers integrate reinforcement elements directly into the mask structure, thereby improving distal tip stability, particularly during insertion and during placement of orogastric tubes.

Due to patent restrictions, reinforced-tip EADs may not be marketed in certain regions, including the United States; clinicians should therefore verify product availability according to local regulatory approval.

Design improvements in both cuffed pharyngeal sealers (Fig. 15.2a) and cuffless preshaped sealers (Fig. 15.2b) further enhance device stability in situ. Devices such as the EzT®, Combitube®, King-LT®, and SLIPA® utilize relatively rigid lumens or chambers to reduce the risk of tip folding. The PAXpress®, for example, incorporates a distinctive flexible 'gilled' tip designed to provide additional stability.

15.4.13 Detachable 15 mm Connector

All extraglottic airway devices are equipped with a standard 15 mm connector. While most models have a fixed connector, some—such as the LMA-Excel™ and air-Q®—feature a detachable connector, which facilitates the passage of a tracheal tube (TT) through the ventilation channel.

In these designs, the removable connector is typically tethered to the device to prevent loss or misplacement (e.g. in the air-Q®). In addition, size-specific colour coding may assist in selecting a compatible tracheal tube, thereby enhancing both ease of use and safety during intubation procedures.

15.4.14 The EAD as an Intubation Conduit

Many extraglottic airway devices can serve as conduits for tracheal intubation, using blind, fibreoptic, or video-assisted techniques. Specific models designed for this purpose include the LMA-Fastrach™, LMA-Classic Excel™, air-Q®, Ambu Aura-i®, Ambu AuraGain®, and 3gLM® (Fig. 15.2d). These devices are characterized by a relatively short airway tube and a wide internal lumen (typically accommodating a tracheal tube of approximately 7.0 mm internal diameter), thereby facilitating direct insertion.

Intubation techniques include:

- Blind insertion (generally less preferred).
- Fibreoptic bronchoscopy (FOB).
- Videoscope-guided techniques (e.g., third-generation VLMAs) [19–25].

Some EADs that are not specifically designed for intubation may require the use of adjuncts, such as:

- Aintree Intubation Catheter.
- Cook Airway Exchange Device®.
- Bougies or guidewires.

Devices such as the SoftSeal®, which feature larger lumens and lack mask aperture bars, may accommodate tracheal tubes up to 7.5 mm internal diameter and allow easier passage. Fibreoptic-guided intubation over an Aintree catheter is generally preferred, as it enables accurate visualization of the vocal cords and facilitates safe placement of the tracheal tube [86, 87].

Only a limited number of EADs (e.g. Ambu Aura-i®) specify the maximum compatible tracheal tube or bronchoscope size. The Ambu Aura-i® incorporates a black guide line within the airway tube to assist fibreoptic navigation and reduce the risk of oesophageal misplacement.

More recent video laryngeal mask airways (VLMAs), such as the SaCoVLM™ and SafeLM™, incorporate a bowl rim designed to guide tracheal tube insertion and provide real-time visualization of the airway during intubation [19].

These hybrid devices—combining characteristics of extraglottic airway devices, tracheal tubes, and videolaryngoscopes (e.g. Totaltrack VLM®) [78–85]—may enhance both safety and efficiency, particularly in the management of difficult airways.

15.4.15 Special Requirements: Laser-Resistant and MRI-Compatible EADs

Some extraglottic airway devices have been used successfully during laser procedures without reported adverse effects. However, compatibility with magnetic resonance imaging (MRI), particularly of the upper body, is more limited. This limitation is primarily related to the presence of metallic components, such as stainless steel springs within pilot balloon valves, which may generate image artefacts.

To address this issue, manufacturers have introduced non-ferromagnetic silicone check valves, which eliminate MRI-related image distortion in devices such as the LMA-Supreme™, Ultimate Laryngeal Mask®, and LarySeal®-MRI.

Conversely, devices such as the LMA-Fastrach™, LMA-ILMA™, and reinforced flexible EADs are generally considered incompatible with MRI due to the presence of internal metallic structures. For clarity and patient safety, manufacturers are encouraged to label devices according to established MRI safety classifications:

- MR Safe: No known hazards in any MRI environment.
- MR Conditional: Safe under specified conditions.
- MR Unsafe: Known hazards in all MRI environments.

In the absence of clear labelling, the device should be assumed to be MR Unsafe. Examples include:

- MR Conditional: LMA-Classic™, LMA-Unique™, LMA-ProSeal™.
- MR Unsafe: LMA-Fastrach™.
- Specifically MR Safe: AES Ultra MRI®, AES Ultraclear MRI®, Solus® MRI-compatible LMA, LarySeal® MRI, and most modern cuffless preshaped sealers.

15.4.16 *Fixation of EADs*

Early extraglottic airway devices were characterized by round airway tubes, which allowed rotation after placement and increased the risk of loss of seal, particularly in edentulous patients. Oval-shaped airway tubes provide improved stability; however, they do not completely eliminate this problem. The incorporation of an integrated bite block contributes to device stabilization and helps prevent occlusion or damage to the airway tube.

Additional design features may further enhance fixation and security:

- Rings or loops (e.g. Baska® mask, i-gel® O2) to facilitate anchoring.
- Clip-on bite blocks and elastic neck ties (e.g. Laryngeal Tube®).
- Handles to assist with insertion and stabilization (e.g. LMA-Supreme™, LMA-Protector™, LMA-Fastrach™).

The technique of fixation is also of importance. Application of adhesive tape should begin centrally while applying gentle downward pressure, followed by securing the device to both cheeks and lips to achieve optimal stabilization.

15.5 Decision-Making and Perspectives on Extraglottic Airway Devices

This chapter presents one of the most comprehensive technical overviews to date of more than 130 extraglottic airway devices (EADs) currently in use or recently introduced. Without aiming to identify a single 'best' device, it highlights key physical characteristics in order to support evidence-based decision-making by clinicians. The list is not exhaustive, acknowledging that new devices will continue to be introduced while others are withdrawn from the market.

Extraglottic airway devices have significantly reshaped modern airway management. Initially limited to short-duration procedures in relatively stable patients, their use now extends to complex surgical procedures, emergency care, intensive care units, and difficult airway scenarios. They occupy an intermediate position between facemasks and tracheal tubes (TTs) within the airway management spectrum and are currently used in up to 60% of anaesthetic cases in the United Kingdom [3].

Trends in EAD design reflect increasing clinical and regulatory demands for:

- Disposable models, primarily driven by infection control considerations.
- Integrated gastric drainage capabilities.
- Functionality as conduits for tracheal intubation.
- Improved airway sealing and positional stability.

Features such as ease of insertion, versatility across different ventilation modes, and improved safety profiles have contributed to the widespread adoption of EADs. This growing demand has stimulated considerable commercial interest and ongoing technological innovation. However, many devices offer comparable functionality with only minor design variations, resulting in a saturated market that may create uncertainty among clinicians.

Although CE marking is required within Europe, certification of compliance with essential safety standards is performed by the manufacturer rather than by an independent regulatory authority. This has raised concerns that some devices may enter clinical practice without comprehensive performance validation. Regulatory approval alone does not necessarily ensure clinical effectiveness in real-world settings.

The Difficult Airway Society (DAS), through its ADEPT initiative [88, 89], has emphasized the importance of:

1. Evidence-based purchasing decisions.
2. Preference for devices with demonstrated safety and efficacy.
3. Greater clinician involvement in the selection and evaluation of airway equipment.

Current limitations in standardized testing protocols, incomplete publication of clinical data, and insufficient post-marketing surveillance weaken the overall safety framework. Furthermore, the absence of universally accepted performance benchmarks makes meaningful comparison between devices difficult. The frequent reintroduction of modified devices under existing product names further complicates the interpretation of the available evidence.

To address these challenges, experts such as Cook and Hagberg have proposed a structured three-stage evaluation process prior to market release:

1. Bench testing using standardized manikins.
2. Cohort studies assessing clinical effectiveness.
3. Randomized controlled trials comparing devices with a defined reference standard [90, 91],

At present, no single extraglottic airway device can be regarded as a 'gold standard'. Early scepticism regarding the LMA was ultimately overcome through rigorous development and evaluation. In contrast, many newer devices have not undergone comparable levels of validation, and published performance claims are often not supported by high-quality, peer-reviewed data [90].

Clinical practice would benefit from:

- Transparent and robust comparative research.
- Standardized numerical coding systems to track device iterations.
- Clear and consistent labelling of functional specifications.

Delays in publication and the absence of systematic device versioning contribute to confusion among both clinicians and researchers. A shift toward more complex trial designs, including multi-arm superiority trials as proposed by Parmar et al. [92], may be required to identify devices that offer meaningful clinical advantages. As emphasized by Pandit et al. and others, further development remains necessary, as current devices continue to present opportunities for improvement [93].

15.6 Final Considerations and Future Directions

While first-generation extraglottic airway devices (EADs) provided only basic functionality, the development of second-generation devices has significantly expanded their clinical applications. These newer models have improved oropharyngeal seal pressures, reduced the risk of aspiration, and enabled the insertion of gastric tubes through dedicated channels.

Currently, blind insertion remains the standard technique in approximately 250 million anaesthetic procedures performed annually. However, the introduction of third-generation video laryngeal mask airways (VLMAs), which incorporate integrated videoscopes, holds promise for more precise placement and a reduction in complications [19]. Nevertheless, further high-quality studies are required to establish their superiority over traditional second-generation devices.

Given the wide variety of EADs—now exceeding 130 models—it is not feasible for a single practitioner to gain experience with all available devices. This chapter, therefore, provides an overview of their physical characteristics and clinical applications, assisting anaesthetists in selecting the most appropriate device based on individual patient characteristics and institutional resources.

Continued technological refinement, together with classification based on functional characteristics, will be essential in progressing toward the concept of an 'ideal' EAD. Such an approach may better support clinical decision-making by aligning device performance with specific clinical indications, ultimately contributing to improved patient outcomes.

The field continues to evolve, and ongoing innovation, rigorous clinical evaluation, and thoughtful device selection remain critical in maximizing both the utility and safety of extraglottic airway devices in clinical practice.

Ongoing innovation, combined with rigorous clinical evaluation and evidence-based device selection, will remain essential in optimizing the safety and effectiveness of extraglottic airway devices in contemporary clinical practice.

References

1. Brain AIJ. The laryngeal mask—a new concept in airway management. Br J Anaesth. 1983;55:801–5.
2. Van Zundert TCRV, Brimacombe JR, Ferson DZ, Bacon DR, Wilkinson DJ. Archie Brain: celebrating 30 years of development in laryngeal mask airways. Anaesthesia. 2012;67:1375–85.
3. Fourth National Audit Project of the Royal College of Anaesthetists and Difficult Airway Society. Major complications of airway management in the United Kingdom. report and findings. London: Royal College of Anaesthetists; 2011. ISBN 4.-1-9000936-03-3. http://www.rcoa.ac.uk/nap4/. Accessed 23 Feb 2015
4. O'Sullivan E, Laffey J, Pandit JJ. A rude awakening after our fourth 'NAP': lessens for airway management. Anaesthesia. 2011;66:331–4.
5. Cook T, Howes B. Supraglottic airway devices: recent advances. Continuing Education in Anaesth Crit Care Pain. 2011;11:56–61.

6. Hernandez MR, Klock PA Jr, Ovassapian A. Evolution of the extraglottic airway: a review of its history, applications, and practical tips for success. Anesth Analg. 2012;114:349–68.
7. Van Zundert AA, Skinner MW, Van Zundert TC, Luney SR, Pandit JJ. Value of knowing physical characteristics of the airway device before using it. Br J Anaesth. 2016;117(1):12–6. https://doi.org/10.1093/bja/aew106. Epub 2016 May 4. PMID: 27147543; PMCID: PMC4913394
8. Brimacombe J. A proposed classification system for extraglottic airway devices. Anesthesiology. 2004;101:559.
9. Agro FE, Cataldo R, Mattei A. New devices and techniques for airway management. Minerva Anestesiol. 2009;75:141–9.
10. Miller DM. A proposed classification and scoring system for supraglottic sealing airways: a brief review. Anesth Analg. 2004;99:2553–9.
11. ISO 11712:2009 (E). Anaesthetic and respiratory equipment—supralaryngeal airways and connectors. Geneva: International Standard. www.iso.org. Accessed 26 Jun 2014
12. Cook TM, Kelly FE. Time to abandon the 'vintage' laryngeal mask airway and adopt second-generation supraglottic airway devices as first choice. Br J Anaesth. 2015;115(4):497–9. https://doi.org/10.1093/bja/aev156. Epub 2015 May 20. PMID: 25995266
13. Sorbello M, Petrini F. Supraglottic airway devices: the search for the best insertion technique or the time to change our point of view? Turk J Anaesthesiol Reanim. 2017;45(2):76–82. https://doi.org/10.5152/TJAR.2017.67764. Epub 2017 Apr 1. PMID: 28439437; PMCID: PMC5396902
14. Van Zundert AA, Kumar CM, Van Zundert TC. Malpositioning of supraglottic airway devices: preventive and corrective strategies. Br J Anaesth. 2016;116(5):579–82. https://doi.org/10.1093/bja/aew104. PMID: 27106958
15. Van Zundert AAJ, Gatt SP, Kumar CM, Van Zundert TCRV, Pandit JJ. 'Failed supraglottic airway': an algorithm for suboptimally placed supraglottic airway devices based on videolaryngoscopy. Br J Anaesth. 2017;118:645–9. https://doi.org/10.1093/bja/aex093. PMID: 28510747
16. Van Zundert AAJ, Gatt SP, Kumar CM, Van Zundert TCRV. Vision-guided placement of supraglottic airway device prevents airway obstruction: a prospective audit. Br J Anaesth. 2017;118(3):462–3. https://doi.org/10.1093/bja/aex010. PMID: 28203766
17. van Zundert AAJ, Wyssusek KH, Pelecanos A, Roets M, Kumar CM. A prospective randomized comparison of airway seal using the novel vision-guided insertion of LMA-supreme® and LMA-protector®. J Clin Monit Comput. 2020;34:285–94. https://doi.org/10.1007/s10877-019-00301-3.
18. Van Zundert AAJ, Kumar CM, Van Zundert TCRV, Gatt SP, Pandit JJ. The case for a 3rd generation supraglottic airway device facilitating direct vision placement. J Clin Monit Comput. 2021;35(2):217–24. https://doi.org/10.1007/s10877-020-00537-4. Epub 2020 Jun 15. PMID: 32537697; PMCID: PMC7293959
19. Van Zundert AAJ, Gatt SP, Van Zundert TCRV, Kumar CM, Pandit JJ. Features of new vision-incorporated third-generation video laryngeal mask airways. J Clin Monit Comput. 2022;36(4):921–8. https://doi.org/10.1007/s10877-021-00780-3. Epub 2021 Dec 17. PMID: 34919170
20. Van Zundert TCRV, Gatt SP, van Zundert AAJ. Videolaryngeal mask airway—a new monitor in airway management. J Clin Monit Comput. 2022;37:717.
21. Gómez-Ríos MÁ, López T, Sastre JA, Gaszyński T, Van Zundert AAJ. Video laryngeal masks in airway management. Expert Rev Med Devices. 2022:1–12. https://doi.org/10.1080/17434440.2022.2142558. Epub ahead of print. PMID: 36308748
22. Sun Y, Huang L, Xu L, Zhang M, Guo Y, Wang Y. The application of a SaCoVLM™ visual intubation laryngeal mask for the Management of Difficult Airways in morbidly obese patients: case report. Front Med (Lausanne). 2021;8:763103. https://doi.org/10.3389/fmed.2021.763103. PMID: 34869469; PMCID: PMC8637043
23. Yan CL, Chen Y, Sun P, Qv ZY, Zuo MZ. Preliminary evaluation of SaCoVLM™ video laryngeal mask airway in airway management for general anesthesia. BMC Anesthesiol.

2022;22(1):3. https://doi.org/10.1186/s12871-021-01541-0. PMID: 34979936; PMCID: PMC8722220
24. Yan CL, Zhang YQ, Chen Y, Qv ZY, Zuo MZ. Comparison of SaCoVLM™ video laryngeal mask-guided intubation and i-gel combined with flexible bronchoscopy-guided intubation in airway management during general anesthesia: a non-inferiority study. BMC Anesthesiol. 2022;22(1):302. https://doi.org/10.1186/s12871-022-01843-x. PMID: 36138363; PMCID: PMC9494909
25. Yan CL, Zhang YQ, Chen Y, Qv ZY, Zuo MZ. To compare the influence of blind insertion and up-down optimized glottic exposure manoeuvre on oropharyngeal leak pressure using SaCoVLM™ video laryngeal mask among patients undergoing general anesthesia. J Clin Monit Comput. 2022; https://doi.org/10.1007/s10877-022-00930-1. Epub ahead of print. PMID: 36308611
26. White LD, Thang C, Hodsdon A, Melhuish TM, Barron FA, Godsall MG, Vlok R. Comparison of supraglottic airway devices with endotracheal intubation in low-risk patients for cesarean delivery: systematic review and meta-analysis. Anesth Analg. 2020;131(4):1092–101. https://doi.org/10.1213/ANE.0000000000004618. PMID: 32925330
27. Carney N, Cheney T, Totten AM, Jungbauer R, Neth MR, Weeks C, Davis-O'Reilly C, Fu R, Yu Y, Chou R, Daya M. Prehospital airway management: a systematic review [internet]. Rockville: Agency for Healthcare Research and Quality (US); 2021. Report No.: 21-EHC023. PMID: 34181368
28. Carney N, Totten AM, Cheney T, Jungbauer R, Neth MR, Weeks C, Davis-O'Reilly C, Fu R, Yu Y, Chou R, Daya M. Prehospital airway management: a systematic review. Prehosp Emerg Care. 2022;26(5):716–27. https://doi.org/10.1080/10903127.2021.1940400. Epub 2021 Jul 20. PMID: 34115570
29. Shaw M, Waiting J, Barraclough L, Ting K, Jeans J, Black B, Pan-London Peri-operative Audit and Research Network. Airway events in obese vs. non-obese elective surgical patients: a cross-sectional observational study. Anaesthesia. 2021;76(12):1585–92. https://doi.org/10.1111/anae.15513. Epub 2021 Jun 22. PMID: 34156711
30. Metodiev Y, Mushambi M. Supraglottic airway devices for caesarean delivery under general anaesthesia: for all, for none, or for some? Br J Anaesth. 2020;125(1):e7–e11. https://doi.org/10.1016/j.bja.2020.02.012. Epub 2020 Mar 18. PMID: 32197776
31. Wong P, Sng BL, Lim WY. Rescue supraglottic airway devices at caesarean delivery: what are the options to consider? Int J Obstet Anesth. 2020;42:65–75. https://doi.org/10.1016/j.ijoa.2019.11.004. Epub 2019 Nov 18. PMID: 31843342
32. Wang CH, Lee AF, Chang WT, Huang CH, Tsai MS, Chou E, Lee CC, Chen SC, Chen WJ. Comparing effectiveness of initial airway interventions for out-of-hospital cardiac arrest: a systematic review and network meta-analysis of clinical controlled trials. Ann Emerg Med. 2020;75(5):627–36. https://doi.org/10.1016/j.annemergmed.2019.12.003. Epub 2020 Jan 23. PMID: 31983493
33. Gordon J, Cooper RM, Parotto M. Supraglottic airway devices: indications, contraindications and management. Minerva Anestesiol. 2018;84(3):389–97. https://doi.org/10.23736/S0375-9393.17.12112-7. Epub 2017 Oct 12. PMID: 29027772
34. Myatra SN, Doctor JR. Supraglottic airway devices: More devices and research required? J Anaesthesiol Clin Pharmacol. 2022;38(2):175–7. https://doi.org/10.4103/joacp.joacp_255_22. Epub 2022 Jul 28. PMID: 36171954; PMCID: PMC9511873
35. Thomsen JLD, Nørskov AK, Rosenstock CV. Supraglottic airway devices in difficult airway management: a retrospective cohort study of 658,104 general anaesthetics registered in the Danish Anaesthesia database. Anaesthesia. 2019;74(2):151–7. https://doi.org/10.1111/anae.14443. Epub 2018 Oct 4. PMID: 30288736
36. Copeland GB, Zilevicius DJ, Bedolla CN, Islas AL, Guerra MN, Salazar SJ, De Lorenzo RA, Schauer SG, Hood RL. Review of commercially available Supraglottic airway devices for prehospital combat casualty care. Mil Med. 2022;187(7–8):e862–76. https://doi.org/10.1093/milmed/usac021. PMID: 35253049

37. Johnston BJ, Leung AK, Hwang CW, Jones JM, Chowdhury MAB, Buck A, Fitzpatrick DE, Meurer DA, Becker TK. Medication-facilitated advanced airway management with first-line use of a supraglottic device—a one-year quality assurance review. Prehosp Disaster Med. 2022;37(4):561–5. https://doi.org/10.1017/S1049023X22000802. Epub 2022 May 19. PMID: 35587719; PMCID: PMC9280059
38. Hummel R, Wollschläger D, Baldering HJ, Engelhard K, Wittenmeier E, Epp K, Pirlich N. Big data: airway management at a university hospital over 16 years; a retrospective analysis. PLoS One. 2022;17(9):e0273549. https://doi.org/10.1371/journal.pone.0273549. PMID: 36126076; PMCID: PMC9488754
39. Apfelbaum JL, Hagberg CA, Connis RT, Abdelmalak BB, Agarkar M, Dutton RP, Fiadjoe JE, Greif R, Klock PA, Mercier D, Myatra SN, O'Sullivan EP, Rosenblatt WH, Sorbello M, Tung A. American Society of Anesthesiologists Practice Guidelines for Management of the Difficult Airway. Anesthesiology. 2022;136(1):31–81. https://doi.org/10.1097/ALN.0000000000004002. PMID: 34762729
40. Eckelman M, Mosher M, Gonzalez A, Sherman J. Comparative life cycle assessment of disposable and reusable laryngeal mask airways. Anesth Analg. 2012;114:1067–72.
41. LCH T. Children and size of laryngeal masks. Can J Anesth. 1994;41:345.
42. Goodman EJ, Eisenmann UB, Dumas SD. Correlation of pharyngeal size to body mass index in the adult. Anesth Analg. 1997;84:S584.
43. Brimacombe JR, Berry AM, Campbell RC, Verghese C. Selection of the proper size of laryngeal mask airway in adults. Anesh Analg. 1996;83:664.
44. Van Zundert TC, Hagberg CA, Cattano D. Inconsistent size nomenclature in extraglottic airway devices. Minerva Anestesiol. 2014;80:692–700.
45. Akca O, Wadhwa A, Sengupta P, Durrani J, Hanni K, Wenke M, Yukcel Y, Lenhardt R, Doufas AG, Sessler DI. The new perilaryngeal airway (CobraPLATM) is as efficient as the laryngeal mask airway (LMATM) but provides better airway sealing pressures. Anesth Analg. 2004;99:272–8.
46. Voyagis GS, Batzioulis PG, Secha-Doussaitou PN. Selection of the proper size of laryngeal mask airway in adults. Anesth Analg. 1996;83:663–4.
47. Berry AM, Brimacombe JR, McManus KF, Goldblatt M. An evaluation of the factors influencing selection of the optimal size of laryngeal mask airway in normal adults. Anaesthesia. 1998;53:565–70.
48. Brimacombe J, Keller C. Laryngeal mask airway size selection in males and females: ease of insertion, oropharyngeal leak pressure, pharyngeal mucosal pressures and anatomical position. Br J Anaesth. 1999;82:703–7.
49. Asai T, Murao K, Yukawa H, Shingu K. Re-evaluation of appropriate size of the laryngeal airway. Br J Anaesth. 1999;83:478–9.
50. Cherng C-H. Tongue width-based laryngeal mask airway size selection in male adults. Eur J Anaesthesiol. 2003;20:570–4.
51. Gallart L, Mases A, Martinez J, Montes A, Fernandez-Galinski s, Puig MM. Simple method to determine the size of the laryngeal mask airway in children. Eur J Anaesthesiol. 2003;20:570–4.
52. Zahoor A, Ahmad N, Sereche G, Riad W. A novel method for laryngeal mask airway size selection in paediatric patients. Eur J Anaesthesiol. 2012;29:386–90.
53. Kagawa T, Obara H. An easy formula to remember the laryngeal mask airway size-patient weight relationship. Anesthesiology. 2000;92:631–2.
54. Hirai S, Nkamura R, Maekawa N. Alternative formula for laryngeal mask airway size selection. Anesthesiology. 2004;100:460.
55. Brimacombe J, Costa E. Silva L. Pharyngeal necrosis with laryngeal mask airway. Eur J Anaesthesiol. 2003;20:502–3.
56. Brimacombe J, Keller C. Salivary gland swelling and lingual nerve injury with the ProSeal laryngeal mask airway. Eur J Anaesthesiol. 2005;22:954–5.
57. El Touky M, Tweedy O. Bilateral lingual nerve injury associated with classic laryngeal mask airway: a case report. Eur J Anaesthesiol. 2012;29:400–1.

58. Brimacombe J, Clarke G, Keller C. Lingual nerve injury associated with the ProSeal laryngeal mask airway: a case report and review of the literature. Br J Anaesth. 2005;95:420–3.
59. Keller C, Brimacombe JR, Keller K, Morris R. Comparison of four methods for assessing airway sealing pressure with the laryngeal mask airway in adult patients. Br J Anaesth. 1999;82(2):286–7. https://doi.org/10.1093/bja/82.2.286. PMID: 10365012
60. Kumar CM, Van Zundert TC, Seet E, Van Zundert AA. Time to consider supraglottic airway device oropharyngeal leak pressure measurement more objectively. Acta Anaesthesiol Scand. 2021;65(2):142–5. https://doi.org/10.1111/aas.13727. Epub 2020 Nov 29. PMID: 33141956
61. Acx E, Van Caelenberg E, De Baerdemaeker L, Coppens M. Laryngeal mask airway protector generates higher oropharyngeal leak pressures compared to the laryngeal mask airway supreme: A randomized clinical trial in the ambulatory surgery unit. J Anaesthesiol Clin Pharmacol. 2021;37(2):221–5. https://doi.org/10.4103/joacp.JOACP_416_19. Epub 2021 Jul 15. PMID: 34349370; PMCID: PMC8289652
62. Miller DM, Light D. Laboratory and clinical comparisons of the streamlined liner of the pharynx airway (SLIPA) with the laryngeal mask airway. Anaesthesia. 2003;58:136–42.
63. Van Zundert T, Gatt S. The Baska MaskR—a new concept in self-sealing membrane cuff extraglottic airway devices, using a sump and two gastric drains: a critical evaluation. J Obstet Anaesth Crit Care. 2012;2:23–30.
64. Chiu CL, Wang CY. An evaluation of the modified airway management device. Anaesth Intensive Care. 2004;32:77–80.
65. Cook TM, Gupta K, Gabbott DA, Nolan JP. An evaluation of the airway management device. Anaesthesia. 2001;56:660–4.
66. Szmuk P, Ghelber O, Matuszczak M. Cobra-PLA with an end tidal CO2 sampling site: differences between proximal and distal sampling sites. Anesthesiology. 2005;103:A1389.
67. Van Zundert AA, Fonck K, Al-Shaikh B, Mortier E. Comparison of the LMA-classic with the new disposable soft seal laryngeal mask in spontaneously breathing adult patients. Anesthesiology. 2003;99:1066–71.
68. Seet E, Yousaf F, Gupta S, Rajeev S, Wong DT, Chung F. Use of manometry for laryngeal mask airway reduces postoperative pharyngolaryngeal adverse events: a prospective, randomized trial. Anesthesiology. 2010;112:652–7.
69. Chan WK, Liu CY. Clinical performance comparison of LMA protector™ cuff pilot™ and LMA supreme™ when used in anesthetized, non-paralyzed patients. Cureus. 2022;14(3):e23176. https://doi.org/10.7759/cureus.23176. PMID: 35308185; PMCID: PMC8925931
70. Brain AI. The development of the Laryngeal Mask—a brief history of the invention, early clinical studies and experimental work from which the Laryngeal Mask evolved. Eur J Anaesthesiol Suppl. 1991;4:5–17.
71. Al-Shaikh B, Pilcher D. Is there a need for the epiglottic bars in the laryngeal mask airway? Can J Anesth. 2003;50:203–4.
72. Van Zundert J, Brimacombe J, Al-Shaikh B, Mortier E. Are all single-use laryngeal masks the same? Anaesthesia. 2006;61:608–9.
73. Van Zundert A, Brimacombe J, Kamphuis R, Haanschoten M. The anatomical position of three extraglottic airway devices in patients with clear airways. Anaesthesia. 2006;61:891–5.
74. Van Zundert T, Brimacombe JR, Marcus M. No contact of epiglottis with mask aperture bars of extraglottc airway devices: prevention of occluding the airway questioned. Eur J Anaesthesiol. 2011;28(S48):234.
75. Van Zundert TC, Hendrickx JF, De Witte JL, Wong DT, Cattano D, Brimacombe JR. Do mask aperture bars of extraglottic airway devices prevent prolapse of epiglottis causing airway obstruction? A randomized crossover trial in anesthetized adult patients. J Clin Anesth. 2016;31:231–7. https://doi.org/10.1016/j.jclinane.2015.12.004. Epub 2016 Apr 16. PMID: 27185718
76. John B, Linga-Nathan P, Mendonca C. Tracheal intubation through a single use laryngeal mask airway using a guidewire technique. Can J Anesth. 2007;54:775–6.

77. Greenland KB, Tan H, Edwards M. Intubation via a laryngeal mask airway with an Aintree catheter—not all laryngeal masks are the same. Anaesthesia. 2007;62:966–7.
78. Driver BE, Martel M, Lai T, Marko TA, Reardon RF. Use of the intubating laryngeal mask airway in the emergency department: a ten-year retrospective review. Am J Emerg Med. 2020;38(7):1367–72. https://doi.org/10.1016/j.ajem.2019.11.017. Epub 2019 Nov 19. PMID: 31836340
79. Lee DH, Stang J, Reardon RF, Martel ML, Driver BE, Braude DA. Rapid sequence airway with the intubating laryngeal mask in the emergency department. J Emerg Med. 2021;61(5):550–7. https://doi.org/10.1016/j.jemermed.2021.09.016. Epub 2021 Nov 1. PMID: 34736797
80. Gómez-Ríos MÁ, Freire-Vila E, Casans-Francés R, Pita-Fernández S. The Totaltrack™ video laryngeal mask: an evaluation in 300 patients. Anaesthesia. 2019;74(6):751–7. https://doi.org/10.1111/anae.14637. Epub 2019 Apr 1. PMID: 30933322
81. Gómez-Ríos MÁ, Bonome C. The totaltrack VLM: a novel video-assisted intubating laryngeal mask. Minerva Anestesiol. 2018;84(1):126–7. https://doi.org/10.23736/S0375-9393.17.12314-X. Epub 2017 Sep 11. PMID: 28895386
82. Gómez-Ríos MÁ, Freire-Vila E, Calvo-Vecino JM. Use of the Totaltrack VLM as a rescue device following failed tracheal intubation. Eur J Anaesthesiol. 2019;36(3):237–9. https://doi.org/10.1097/EJA.0000000000000920. PMID: 30694889
83. Gómez-Ríos MÁ, Freire-Vila E, Abad-Gurumeta A, Barreto-Calvo P, Calvo-Vecino JM. Use of Totaltrack VLM as a rescue device after failed ventilation and tracheal intubation with LMA Fastrach in emergent difficult airways. J Clin Anesth. 2019;52:29–30. https://doi.org/10.1016/j.jclinane.2018.08.020. Epub 2018 Aug 25. PMID: 30153542
84. Gómez-Ríos MÁ, Casans-Francés R, Freire-Vila E, Sastre JA, López T, Garzón JC. A prospective evaluation of the Totaltrack video laryngeal mask in paralyzed, anesthetized obese patients. J Clin Anesth. 2020;61:109688. https://doi.org/10.1016/j.jclinane.2019.109688. Epub 2019 Dec 10. PMID: 31836266
85. Gómez-Ríos MÁ, Silva-Carballal I, Freire-Vila E. Use of the TotalTrack VLM for endotracheal intubation in a patient with a giant thyroglossal duct cyst and airway compression. Anaesth Crit Care Pain Med. 2018;37(6):615–6. https://doi.org/10.1016/j.accpm.2017.07.007. Epub 2017 Sep 19. PMID: 28935456
86. Wong DT, Yang JJ, Mak HY, Jagannathan N. Use of intubation introducers through a supraglottic airway to facilitate tracheal intubation: a brief review. Can J Anaesth. 2012;59:704–15.
87. van Zundert TC, Wong DT, van Zundert AA. The LMA-Supreme™ as an intubation conduit in patients with known difficult airways: a prospective evaluation study. Acta Anaesthesiol Scand. 2013;57:77–81.
88. Pandit JJ, Popat MT, Cook TM, Wilkes AR, Groom P, Cooke H, Kapila A, O'Sullivan E. The difficult airway society 'ADEPT' guidance on selecting airway devices: the basis of a strategy for equipment evaluation. Anaesthesia. 2011;66:726–37.
89. Ní Eochagáin A, Athanassoglou V, Cumberworth A, Morris O, Corbett S, Jefferson H, O'Sullivan EP, Pandit JJ. Assessing a novel second generation laryngeal mask airway using the 'ADEPT' approach: results from the LMA® protector™ observational study. J Clin Monit Comput. 2022:1–8. https://doi.org/10.1007/s10877-022-00910-5. Epub ahead of print. PMID: 36063277; PMCID: PMC9441326
90. Cook TM. Novel airway devices: spoilt for choice? Anaesthesia. 2003;58:107–10.
91. Hagberg C. Benumof and Hagberg's airway management. 3rd ed. Saunders; 2012.
92. Parmar MKB, Carpenter J, Sydes MR. More multiarm randomised trials of superiority are needed. Lancet. 2014;384(9940):283–4.
93. Asai T, Hillman D. Current difficult airway management-not good enough! Anesthesiology. 2019;131(4):774–6. https://doi.org/10.1097/ALN.0000000000002885. PMID: 31335551

Chapter 16
Tracheal Intubation: Direct Laryngoscopy and Videolaryngoscopy

Jan Hansel and Haukur Týr Guðmundsson

> **Highlights**
> - Even though direct laryngoscopy is still the most prevalent technique used to facilitate tracheal intubation, videolaryngoscopy offers a demonstrably safer risk profile.
> - Universal videolaryngoscopy can provide marginal gains in terms of decreasing need for repeat laryngoscopy in patients where difficulty is not anticipated, decreasing rates of overall failure in challenging airways, and improving overall team dynamics.
> - Training in videolaryngoscopy skills requires a clear and dedicated approach to each device category and should not be assumed, as improper technique may not yield the full benefits of videolaryngoscopy to clinicians and patients.

J. Hansel (✉)
Intensive Care Medicine, University of Manchester, Manchester, UK

Acute Intensive Care Unit, Wythenshawe Hospital, Manchester University NHS Foundation Trust, Manchester, UK
e-mail: jan.hansel@manchester.ac.uk

H. T. Guðmundsson
Anaesthesiology and Intensive Care Medicine, Oslo University Hospital, Oslo, Norway
e-mail: haugud@ous-hf.no

M. Á. Gómez-Ríos, A. van Zundert (eds.), *Evidence-based Guide to Difficult Airway Management*, https://doi.org/10.1007/978-3-032-30769-9_16

16.1 Introduction

You can't live without oxygen. (John Sakles)

Securing the airway by means of a cuffed tracheal tube remains a reliable way of ensuring gas exchange and protecting the lungs from soiling, and is an essential skill in the armamentarium of any clinician expected to manage the airway. Ensuring a patent airway can pose a significant challenge in patients with predictive features of difficulty and is commonly associated with minor and, less commonly, with major complications [1–4]. The decision to intubate the trachea should take into account a number of patient, procedure, and logistical factors. Tracheal intubation may be performed under general anaesthesia or awake following airway topicalisation with local anaesthetic agents (Grade D). Indications for tracheal intubation are listed in Table 16.1, although the list is not exhaustive (Grade D) [5].

The above indications are not absolute and will vary based on the setting, patient condition, anticipated patient journey, staff skillset, and available equipment. Depending on any of the above factors, tracheal intubation might best be avoided, even if it ultimately will be required. An example might be an impending mechanical airway obstruction in the prehospital setting with maintained oxygenation and a preserved level of consciousness (e.g. infectious or malignant aetiology). The prehospital environment does not afford intubators ideal conditions in terms of equipment, skillset, or backup. Therefore, induction of anaesthesia in order to secure the airway may be ill-advised and result in patient harm.

Tracheal intubation provides a patent airway, allows for controlled ventilation with high fractions of oxygen and high airway pressures, protects the lungs from aspiration, and may facilitate tracheal toilet. Use of specialised tracheal tubes and devices also allows for lung isolation, if clinically required. More widespread use of second-generation supraglottic airway devices (SADs) continues to influence decisions on when tracheal intubation might be required, as indications for these devices broaden in elective and emergency settings with incoming evidence supporting their safety profile [6, 7].

Table 16.1 Indications for tracheal intubation

Perioperative indications	Indications outside the operating theatre
Prolonged surgery	Acute respiratory failure uncorrected by non-invasive measures
Shared airway not appropriate for supraglottic device	Reduced level of consciousness
Surgery impairing gas exchange	Airway obstruction (e.g., trauma, tumours, oedema)
Surgery requiring neuromuscular blockade	Severe haemodynamic instability (relative)
Patient position making rapid intubation difficult (e.g., prone position)	Cardiac arrest (relative)
Less invasive techniques ineffective	Facilitating the safe transfer of the unstable patient
Protection from aspiration of gastric contents or blood	

16.1.1 Safety Considerations

It is essential that a clear airway management plan is formulated prior to induction of anaesthesia. This will be influenced by current relevant professional guidelines, which the reader should be familiar with for their practice setting (Grade D). Each team member involved in airway management should have a clear understanding of role allocations and responsibilities, and the overall plan, including the rescue strategy. Failure to plan for failure has been highlighted as a contributing factor to major complications in airway management [2]. Availability of necessary equipment must be checked prior to proceeding. Establishing this shared mental model to enhance situational awareness is best achieved through the use of a pre-procedure checklist (Grade C) [8, 9].

The above points are of particular importance in high-risk airway management, where difficulty is anticipated, as an extended team will usually be required. This may include anaesthetic assistants, operating theatre nursing staff, head and neck surgeons, and additional skilled anaesthetists (Grade D). Cognitive aids to enhance performance in crises have been developed, with a notable example being the Vortex approach proposed by Chrimes et al. [10]. Elements of the Vortex approach have been incorporated into societal guidelines on airway management [11]. Each individual case should include a minimal risk assessment, which can be formalised. Various tools have been proposed for use in clinical practice [12]. For a more detailed exploration of these issues, see the chapter on human factors and ergonomics.

Finally, it is worth highlighting that both direct laryngoscopy (DL) and videolaryngoscopy (VL) require specific training with the device used. Furthermore, the various designs of videolaryngoscopes mandate a somewhat different insertion technique; hyperangulated (HA-VL) and channelled videolaryngoscopes necessitate dedicated training, distinct from other techniques [13, 14]. While some of the elements of the technique used with a given laryngoscope are transferable, there are sequences of steps unique to each, which we will cover in some detail later in the chapter. Suffice it to say, it is essential that the intubator is trained and familiar with any device used to facilitate tracheal intubation prior to clinical use (Grade D).

16.2 Direct Laryngoscopy

Even with the emergence of videolaryngoscopy, the century-old direct laryngoscope (DL) is still the most commonly used instrument for tracheal intubation. Numerous iterations of this tool have been developed since, but in its essence, it consists of a handle attached to a blade with a light source. With some manual force, the blade is used to gain ventral displacement of the tongue and other supraglottic airway tissues, with the aim of aligning the oral, pharyngeal, and laryngeal axes. This affords the intubator a direct line of sight from the mouth to the illuminated glottic opening.

DLs have seen countless design variations and modifications, but decades of refinements have produced two prevailing blade designs: the curved Macintosh blade and the straight Miller blade. Both blades are available in a variety of sizes, ranging from neonatal to adult. The Macintosh blade is designed to follow the curvature of the tongue, indirectly elevating the epiglottis with pressure on the hyoepiglottic ligament, while the straight blade is used to directly lift the epiglottis and has historically been preferred in paediatric airway management or patients with a prominent epiglottis.

Other specialised blades are available; the polio blade is a Macintosh blade mounted at 135° to the handle, while a McCoy blade incorporates a hinged distal tip that can be flexed, thereby purportedly improving the Cormack-Lehane (CL) grade by one (Grade C) [15, 16]. The use of these blades has largely been supplanted by the increased adoption of videolaryngoscopy [17, 18].

16.2.1 Preparation

Direct laryngoscopy (DL) should be performed by an appropriately skilled intubator with the help of a trained assistant. Ensure that airway equipment, medications, and monitoring equipment are available and fully functioning. The team should be briefed, and clinical roles assigned in accordance with individual skills and competence.

Always prepare for unanticipated difficulty; a complete pre-intubation evaluation must be performed before proceeding with direct laryngoscopy (see dedicated chapter). It is the authors' view that in the presence of patient factors indicating potential difficulty in airway management, it is not recommended to proceed with the use of DL alone (Grade D).

16.2.2 What Is the Optimal Patient Position?

A successful laryngoscopy is highly dependent on patient positioning. Various patient factors, such as obesity or potential cervical spine injury, will influence the primary choice of patient position. Since combining lower neck flexion with atlanto-occipital extension helps align the three airway axes, the 'sniffing position' (SP) is classically taught as the ideal patient position for direct laryngoscopy (Fig. 16.1) (Grade D). The anatomical theory may not hold true, but there remains a paucity of alternative explanations backed by higher-quality evidence [19, 20]. Head elevation beyond the SP has been consistently reported to improve glottic views [21, 22]. Ramped positioning gives a physiological advantage in terms of enhanced respiratory mechanics and has been shown to be beneficial in obese and pregnant individuals [23, 24]. However, this has not been supported by published

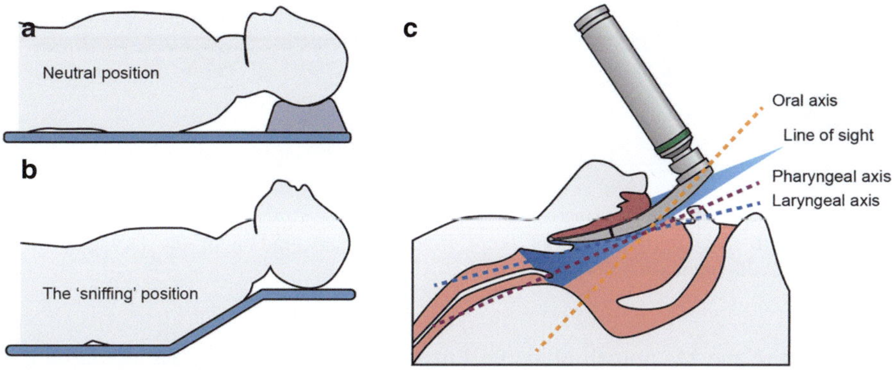

Fig. 16.1 Direct laryngoscopy with a Macintosh blade and alignment of the three axes. Panels **a** and **b** illustrate the neutral position and the more favourable sniffing position, respectively. Panel **c**: although the three axes and the two curve theories have remained contentious, there is an anatomical and practical rationale for aligning the line of sight of the intubator with the laryngeal axis, especially when using DL

evidence in general patient cohorts [25]. Some modifications may further optimise the view, but hyperextending the neck instinctively should be avoided, as it distorts the airway axes [26].

16.2.3 Manual Technique

Successful tracheal intubation using DL hinges on obtaining a view of the glottic opening before delivering the tube into the trachea. Each step has its own challenges and potential pitfalls.

16.2.3.1 Obtaining the View

The laryngoscope is held in the left hand regardless of the intubator's handedness. The handle should be held low in the hand, with the posterior end of the blade pressed against the intubator's hypothenar eminence. The intubator should be in a relaxed position, engaging the airway from a comfortable working height (see ergonomics).

- Tilt the head backwards using the right hand and open the mouth.
- Carefully insert the laryngoscope blade into the right side of the mouth, avoiding any trauma to the lips and teeth (consider using a dental guard and protecting the eyelids ahead of laryngoscopy) [27, 28] (Grade D).
- Gently sweep the tongue to the left while advancing the blade down and towards the midline.
- Track the tip of the scope as you advance until the epiglottis is identified.

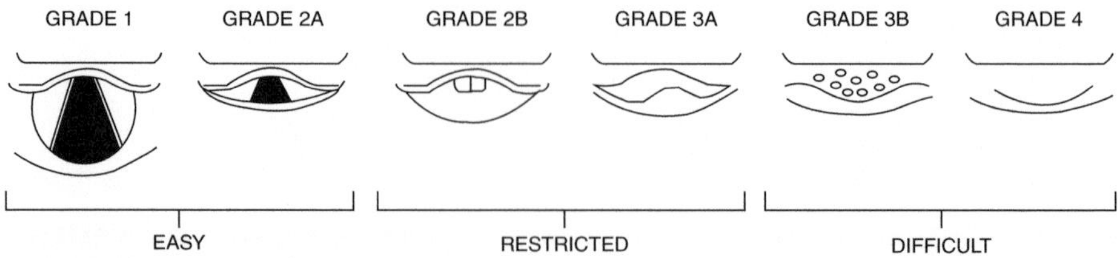

Fig. 16.2 The Cook modification of the Cormack-Lehane grading of the laryngeal view. (Reproduced with permission from [29])

The tip of the Macintosh blade will need to be placed in the vallecula before applying anterior force against the hyoepiglottic ligament, exposing the glottic opening. With a Miller blade, glottic exposure is accomplished by advancing the blade posterior to the epiglottis and directly lifting it up against the anterior larynx.

The glottic opening is then assessed. We suggest using the practical Cook modification of the CL grade (Fig. 16.2) [29]. Where an easy view (grades 1 or 2a) is encountered, intubation should be straightforward. A restricted view (grades 2b and 3a) may require the use of an adjunct, such as a stylet or bougie. Conversely, a difficult view (grades 3b and 4) will likely require the use of specialised techniques, such as a fibreoptic device or optical stylet.

16.2.3.2 Advancing the Tube

Based on the best-obtained view, the intubator must then decide how to proceed. Most airways will allow for a straightforward insertion of the tracheal tube. Typically, the intubator will maintain their view with the laryngoscope while using the right hand to pass the tube into the mouth and towards the glottic opening under direct vision. The tube is then advanced past the vocal cords, with the depth indicators (black lines) sitting at the level of the cords. The cuff is then inflated, and correct placement is confirmed using capnography to rule out oesophageal intubation. Auscultation is advised to minimise the risk of endobronchial intubation. Ideally, insertion depth should be confirmed under direct vision. However, as a general rule, securing at 21 and 23 cm at the incisors in adult women and men, respectively, should avoid endobronchial placement (Grade B) [30].

16.2.3.3 Airway Adjuncts

As previously noted, if a restricted view is encountered, the use of airway adjuncts may be required to facilitate tracheal intubation. Most often, a malleable stylet or a tracheal tube introducer (bougie) will be used.

Malleable Stylet

A stylet is a malleable rod that is inserted into the tracheal tube prior to use and shaped by the assistant or intubator. The styletted tube is often bent into a *hockey stick* shape (~30°) at its distal third. Depending on the view, a more hyperangulated shape can be chosen; however, angles exceeding 35° can make tube passage with DL more difficult [31]. The stylet is shorter than the tracheal tube, and its tip should not protrude past the length of the tracheal tube to prevent airway trauma. Once the tube's tip reaches the vocal cords, the assistant is asked to withdraw the stylet while the tube is advanced further.

The use of a stylet has been shown to improve first pass success rates and is recommended in societal guidelines (Grade B) [11, 32].

Tracheal Tube Introducer (Bougie)

A tracheal tube introducer or bougie is a 50–70 cm long, thin non-rigid rod with an angled blunt tip. Its small diameter provides high manoeuvrability, and its 30–45° angled tip is designed to facilitate navigation into the trachea in restricted views.

Use of the Bougie in Tracheal Intubation

Gently advancing the introducer along the midline with the tip angulated anteriorly will give the intubator distinctive tactile feedback, or 'clicks', as the tip slides over the tracheal rings. Note that the clicks may be absent if the tip of the bougie is rotated posteriorly. The tracheal tube is then mounted distally onto the introducer and 'railroaded' into the trachea.

Using a bougie can significantly improve first pass success rates in cases of restricted glottic views, and its routine use is commonly favoured for emergency intubations [33]. Recent evidence, however, suggests that stylets have comparable first pass success rates in these settings [34].

Risks and Precautions

Improper use of introducers carries a real risk of major airway trauma. Use gentle advancement and correct tip alignment to avoid injury. Blind insertion of the introducer in difficult views increases this risk and is unlikely to succeed. Resistance or a 'hold-up' encountered at a depth of 30–40 cm, when the distal tip lodges into a bronchus, has traditionally been used as a corroborating sign of correct placement. This practice is discouraged, as advancement beyond the carina increases risk of trauma (Grade D) [35].

Bougie with Flexible or Steerable Tip

A flexible-tip or steerable bougie—designed with a tip that can be flexed or extended by the intubator—may overcome some of the drawbacks outlined above, especially when using a hyperangulated videolaryngoscope (Grade D) [36]. Furthermore, it offers increased overall manoeuvrability to the intubator. Specific training is required for correct use.

16.2.4 Sources of Difficulty with Direct Laryngoscopy

16.2.4.1 Poor Technique

Laryngoscopy is a skill that needs to be developed through supervised practice. The novice intubator will frequently fail to recognise the epiglottis, and the narrow view of DL limits the ability of supervisors to provide meaningful feedback. This problem can be addressed by utilising Macintosh-style VL, which allows the supervisor to give real-time guidance to the trainee, who is blinded to the VL screen. Emphasis should be placed on epiglottoscopy and the recognition of known landmarks, along with optimisations in patient position.

16.2.4.2 Inability to Pass the Tube

If tube passage is difficult at the level of the arytenoids or vocal cords, especially when railroading the tube over a tracheal tube introducer, having ensured adequate neuromuscular blockade and optimal conditions, a corkscrew-like motion may be helpful. This may involve pulling the tube back by a millimetre and turning the tube anticlockwise. If a hold-up is encountered downstream from the vocal cords at the anterior tracheal structures, a clockwise turn may be more helpful.

16.2.4.3 Obstructed View

This most commonly results from suboptimal alignment of the airway axes. Unanticipated obstructive anatomy (e.g. lingual tonsillar hyperplasia), an anteriorly placed larynx, or angioedema can hinder the view. Although a retromolar technique may result in improved views, repeated attempts risk inflicting trauma to the airway, making subsequent attempts more challenging. The authors recommend following current guidelines on unanticipated difficult airway management and maintaining a low threshold for switching to HA-VL if any difficulty is encountered, if a VL was not used from the outset (Grade A).

Management of Secretions and Blood in the Airway
Small amounts of blood and secretions can be cleared with simple suction. Severe airway contamination can completely obscure the airway, making visually guided intubation extremely challenging.

No universal rescue method is recommended by current guidelines, but emerging techniques involving continuous high-calibre suction devices have been proposed

(Grade D) [37]. A second suction device may be helpful. One possible rescue technique for a flooded airway, especially with pulmonary oedema or blood, is 'following the bubbles'. This involves observing air bubbles emerging from the trachea in high-grade CL views [38]. In a fully paralysed patient this can be facilitated by a careful push on the chest by the assistant (Grade D).

External Laryngeal Manipulation

External laryngeal manipulation (ELM), also known as bi-manual laryngoscopy, involves the intubator using their right hand to simultaneously manipulate the laryngeal structures f externally during laryngoscopy to optimise their view. When an acceptable view is found, the assistant will take over and hold the view while the tracheal tube is advanced. A modified approach involves the intubator using their right hand to guide the assistant's hand and instruct them to maintain direction and force when the optimal view is found. This easy manoeuvre is highly effective, consistently yielding improved glottic views [39, 40].

The concept of 'backward upward rightward pressure' (BURP) should be distinguished from ELM; it is, in fact, associated with a worse glottic view (Grade B) [41]. If cricoid force was used as part of a rapid sequence induction, the intubator should have a low threshold for releasing it in case of a suboptimal view (Grade D).

16.2.4.4 Suboptimal Neuromuscular Blockade

Suboptimal neuromuscular blockade has been associated with increased difficulty in airway management [2]. This is especially relevant if suxamethonium was initially used for induction, and repeat attempts at airway management have resulted in its effects wearing off. Adequate neuromuscular blockade—and a sufficiently deep plane of anaesthesia—must be ensured in cases of difficulty. Quantitative neuromuscular monitoring prior to tracheal intubation is recommended (Grade C) [42].

16.3 Videolaryngoscopy

Videolaryngoscopy as a technique to facilitate tracheal intubation has grown in popularity over the past two decades. While the term *videolaryngoscopy* or *videolaryngoscope* is not ideal for describing the technique of indirect laryngoscopy in a broader sense, its ubiquitous use in the field has overtaken other descriptors. Semantically, it would be more appropriate to use rigid indirect laryngoscopy. We have opted to adhere to the term *videolaryngoscopy* (VL) throughout this text.

The scope of this chapter is to provide an overview of the techniques and devices available at the time of writing. However, it is worth emphasising that this field is rapidly developing, with new devices and innovative designs continuously entering the market. Videolaryngoscopes (VLs) use high-resolution video cameras incorporated into the blade, with the image relayed to a video display, which may be a standalone unit or attached to a handle in portable devices. The Airtraq videolaryngoscope is an exception, as it employs a series of prisms to generate the final view. In contrast to DLs, VLs provide a wide-angle view to the intubator.

16.3.1 Device Designs

VLs can broadly be classified into three distinct categories, based on the design of the blade used with the video unit:

- Macintosh-style
- Hyperangulated (HA-VL)
- Channelled

The above categorisation considers the subtle yet important differences in the technique used to successfully perform tracheal intubation with each device (Fig. 16.3) [13]. These are further expanded on in the sections below.

16.3.2 Intubation Technique Common to All VLs

The step-wise sequence of using a VL differs somewhat from the direct vision approach employed with DL. Four distinctive steps are commonly required to ensure safe and effective tracheal intubation:

1. *Look at the mouth.* Insert the videolaryngoscope either in the right corner of the mouth (Macintosh-style) or in the midline (HA-VL and channelled), taking care not to cause dental or soft tissue injury on insertion.
2. *Look at the screen.* Optimise the glottic view by slowly advancing the videolaryngoscope beyond the curvature of the tongue into the vallecula.

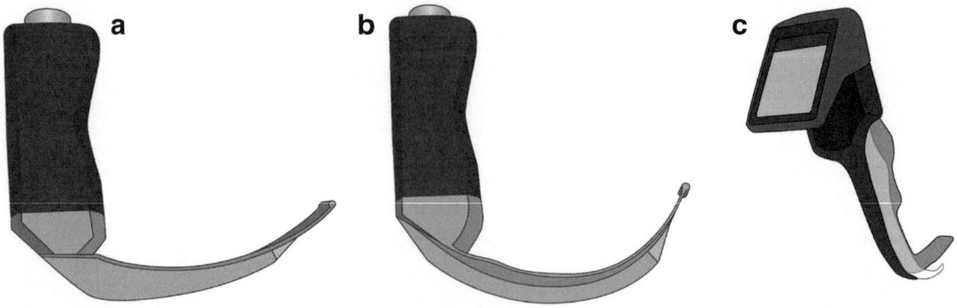

Fig. 16.3 The three main categories of videolaryngoscopes in general use. (**a**) Macintosh-style, (**b**) hyperangulated, (**c**) channelled. Note the more acute angle of the hyperangulated blade (60°), which disallows intubation under direct vision, as it makes aligning the anatomical axes significantly more challenging compared to a Macintosh-style blade (see below)

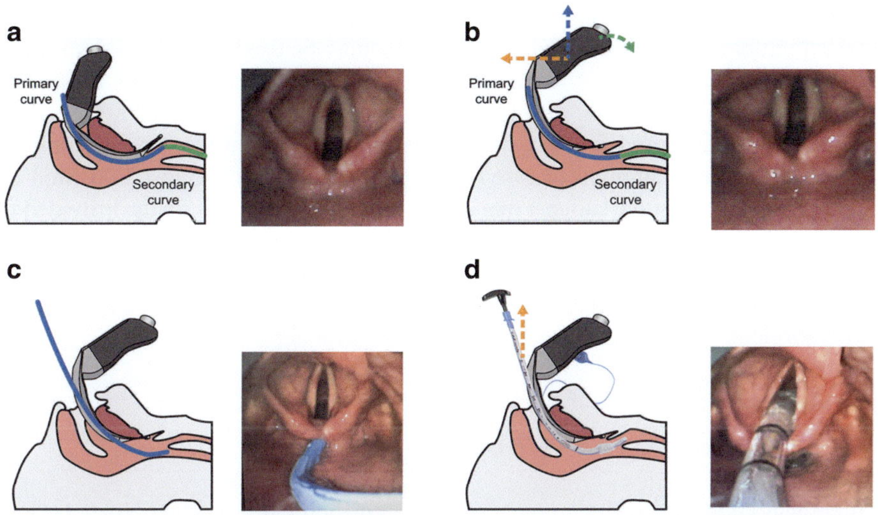

Fig. 16.4 Anatomical and technical considerations when using a hyperangulated videolaryngoscope (HA-VL). Panel **a***:* when a HA-VL is used to obtain a full view of the vocal cords, with the blade tip completely engaged in the vallecula and the handle tilted backwards, the primary curve is accentuated. Panel **b**: withdrawing the blade slightly, tilting the handle anteriorly, and lifting the base of the tongue superiorly will usually improve intubating conditions. Note the anterior commissure is partially obscured. Panel **c**: when a bougie is used, even when bent into an accentuated curve prior to insertion, it often passes posteriorly due to the above considerations. Panel **d***:* a rigid preformed stylet with the tracheal tube loaded, on the other hand, follows the blade's curvature and is more likely to engage with the glottic introitus, especially when lifted vertically by a few millimetres just before reaching the larynx

3. *Look at the mouth.* Carefully insert the tracheal tube preloaded onto a preformed rigid or malleable stylet (especially if using an HA-VL). Alternatively, a bougie or tracheal tube introducer may be used; however, it is not advised with HA-VL as difficulty is often encountered when negotiating the two curves (Fig. 16.4). Care should be taken to avoid injury to the posterior pharyngeal structures when moving the styletted tracheal tube towards the glottic opening.
4. *Look at the screen.* Advance the tube into the trachea, taking care to remove the stylet just prior to passing the vocal cords to avoid injury.

This sequence is followed by confirmation of correct tracheal tube placement with capnography [43, 44]. The specific considerations when using the three VL designs are described below.

16.3.2.1 Macintosh-Style VL (Mac-VL)

The laryngoscopy technique with a Mac-VL is similar to that of direct laryngoscopy with a Macintosh blade. The benefit to the intubator is the ability to either use the video screen or intubate using line of sight. It obviates the need for an additional attempt if a challenging view is encountered, as the intubator can switch to video-guided intubation. Adjuncts and optimisations may be used as with DL. A stylet is not required but may aid in correcting tube passage in scenarios such as an anterior larynx.

If a Mac-VL is used for DL, we suggest first looking at the screen within the same laryngoscopy attempt. In case of difficulty, even with optimised position and appropriate adjuncts, we suggest that an attempt with HA-VL is made, provided the intubator is trained in its correct use.

Examples of commonly used Mac-VLs include the C-MAC® (Storz), GlideScope® Mac (Verathon®), McGrath™ MAC (Medtronic), and i-view™ (Intersurgical®).

16.3.2.2 Hyperangulated VL (HA-VL)

Hyperangulated VLs are recommended when a difficult airway is anticipated (Grade A) [14]. Subgroup analyses of RCTs have demonstrated superior performance in this patient group. The common sequence of steps described above is the same when using an HA-VL.

The most common error when inserting an HA-VL into the mouth is advancing the blade tip too deep into the vallecula. This may produce an excellent view, but can make tube passage difficult. Withdrawing the blade slightly, tilting the handle anteriorly, and lifting the base of the tongue superiorly will usually improve intubating conditions (Fig. 16.4, panels A and B).

Another common mistake is the use of a non-rigid tracheal tube introducer/bougie. Even when bent prior to insertion into the mouth, the introducer will usually not retain this shape by the time it approaches the glottis. This, combined with deficiencies in the basic technique described above, will often result in the bougie repeatedly passing into the oesophagus (Fig. 16.4, panel C). Therefore, we do not recommend the routine use of tracheal tube introducers/bougies with HA-VL (Grade D).

When a rigid preformed stylet is used, as per manufacturer recommendations, success rates are higher. The tube loaded onto the stylet should be inserted along the same line as the HA-VL blade, with attention paid to avoid pharyngeal injury. We suggest holding the tube at the distal most portion to facilitate withdrawing the stylet with the thumb of the right hand once the glottis is reached [45]. As the tip of the tube appears on the screen, slightly lifting the styletted tube (Fig. 16.4, panel D) can improve engagement with the glottic opening (Grade D).

We suggest specific training with HA-VL beyond Mac-VL or DL, especially for experienced DL users, as the insertion technique differs markedly. Direct translation of muscle memory from DL may put intubators experienced with DL at a disadvantage (Grade D) [46].

Examples of commonly used HA-VLs include the GlideScope® LoPro (Verathon®), C-MAC® D-Blade (Storz), and the McGrath™ X-Blade/Series 5 (Medtronic).

16.3.2.3 Channelled VL

Channelled VLs are hyperangulated blades designed to match the curvature of the upper airway and incorporate a channel guide. They are bulkier than non-channelled counterparts, which can limit their usefulness in patients with restricted mouth opening. The intubation technique relies on aligning the blade with the vocal cords and advancing the tube. This design restricts the tube trajectory, as the channel guide prevents lateral movement.

Common pitfalls and reasons for failure to intubate include off-midline insertion, improper alignment with the vocal cords, excessive depth of insertion, and accidental displacement of the tracheal tube during device removal.

Examples of channelled VLs include the Airtraq® (Prodol), KingVision® (Ambu), and the Pentax AirwayScope® (Nihon Kohden).

16.3.3 Grading and Documentation

Neither the classic CL grade nor its subsequent modifications have been validated for videolaryngoscopy, as they lack several informative facets to convey any encountered difficulty [29, 47]. This potential pitfall is amplified when an HA-VL is used, where the view might be excellent, but difficulty in tube passage is encountered. The Video Classification of Intubation (VCI) score has been proposed by Chaggar et al. in 2021, incorporating information on the blade used, the percentage of glottic opening during intubation, and the overall ease of the procedure (Fig. 16.5) [48].

16.3.4 Universal Videolaryngoscopy

Although videolaryngoscopes have become increasingly available in locations where airway management is anticipated, multiple recent surveys have shown that adoption of videolaryngoscopy as a first-line approach has remained low [49, 50]. Given the mounting evidence in favour of videolaryngoscopy decreasing the incidence of major complications related to airway management, alongside other generic benefits (Table 16.2), it seems reasonable to move towards using videolaryngoscopes in preference to direct laryngoscopes for most if not all interventions [51].

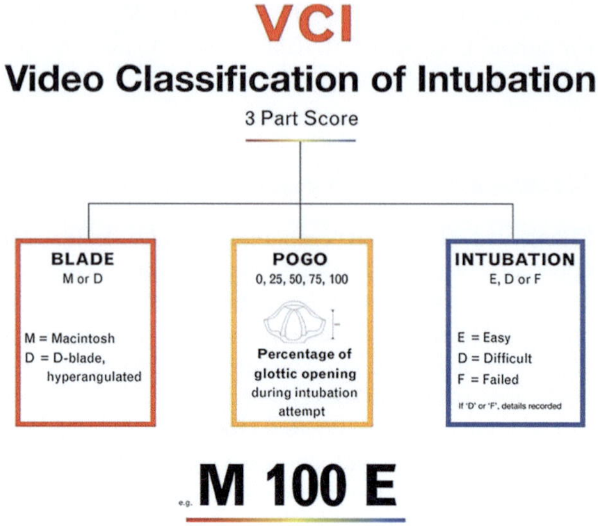

Fig. 16.5 The video classification of intubation score infographic. (Reproduced with permission from [48])

Table 16.2 Generic benefits of videolaryngoscopy

Safety	Non-technical	Other
Fewer difficult intubations	Shared mental model	Environmental implications
Fewer attempts	Improved airway assistance	Cost [52]
Fewer failures	Improved teaching of DL/VL	
Less hypoxaemia	Rescue tool always available	
Fewer oesophageal intubations		
Improved views		

The well-established safety profile of VL goes beyond just technical factors listed on the left [51]. An increase in situational awareness of the entire team yields benefits in problem-solving and improves team performance. Cost-effectiveness of videolaryngoscopy has been demonstrated in well-resourced healthcare systems

A number of departments worldwide have successfully adopted universal videolaryngoscopy, with procedural improvements noted following the shift from direct laryngoscopy [53]. This goes beyond merely universal availability of videolaryngoscopes in all locations where airway management occurs, and rather implies the whole department or organisation uses videolaryngoscopes for all tracheal intubations. The implementation of universal videolaryngoscopy can be challenging for several reasons, ranging from up-front and maintenance cost, lack of organisational buy-in, clinician resistance to change, and concerns pertaining to unintended consequences for training and skill upkeep. Cook et al. provide a template on how to overcome these barriers to implementation [54].

16.3.5 Training in the Era of Universal Videolaryngoscopy

As we transition to universal videolaryngoscopy, consideration needs to be given to skill maintenance, and the place for direct laryngoscopy in the armamentarium of the airway clinician of the future. There are arguments to be made for maintaining direct laryngoscopy skills, especially if working in environments that may not have universal access to VL. We foresee that this will become less of an issue in the coming decades as VLs will become more affordable and ubiquitous. At present, however, we need to account for the learning needs of novice intubators. We therefore propose a universal algorithm for airway management in the era of universal videolaryngoscopy, allowing both experienced and novice intubators to master direct laryngoscopy with the best available tool: a videolaryngoscope (Fig. 16.6) (Grade D).

Other benefits of using VL for DL training include allowing the supervisor to help better guide the intubator, who may have the screen obscured for practice. Finally, a human factors benefit is that the whole team is able to see the intubation ('going from me to we'), whereby the skilled airway assistant can provide better external laryngeal manipulation, reach for a given piece of equipment (e.g. a bougie/tracheal tube introducer), or help confirm tracheal placement of the tube as part of a two-person two-point check [55].

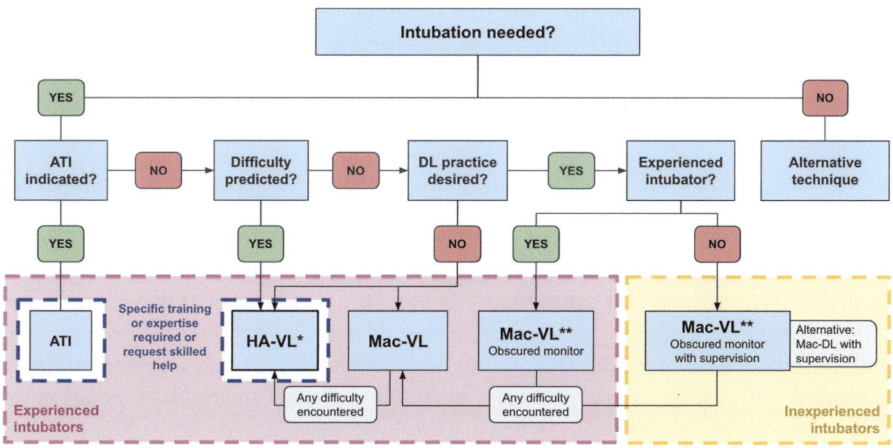

Fig. 16.6 Incorporating learning needs in transition to universal videolaryngoscopy. We present a decision-tree for airway management, where consideration is given to learning needs and skill upkeep. The yellow pane represents inexperienced/novice intubators who may benefit from direct laryngoscopy skill acquisition. They should intubate under direct supervision, and a Mac-VL with an obscured monitor is the recommended device to use. Experienced intubators (purple pane) may choose to perform direct laryngoscopy with a Mac-VL to maintain DL skills. In any case where difficulty is encountered, the monitor should be uncovered within the same attempt. If difficulty is encountered with Mac-VL, HA-VL should be considered. Training for HA-VL and other advanced techniques should be specific and distinct from Mac-VL training. *Where airway management difficulty is predicted clinically, HA-VL should be the preferred VL device used from the outset (Grade A). **Alternatively, a direct laryngoscope may be used depending on resource constraints (Grade C). *ATI* awake tracheal intubation, *DL* direct laryngoscopy, *HA-VL* hyperangulated videolaryngoscope, *Mac-DL* Macintosh direct laryngoscope, *Mac-VL* Macintosh-style videolaryngoscope

16.3.6 Myths Relating to Videolaryngoscopy

#1 You can always get a good view, but tube delivery is difficult

This is a commonly cited criticism of VL, specifically when using HA-VL. Intubators aiming to translate the same technique used for Macintosh DL onto an HA-VL will tend to struggle with this more than de novo learners who train for HA-VL and Mac-VL separately. Appropriate technique, as described above, debunks this myth.

#2 Adopting universal videolaryngoscopy will result in deskilling in DL

While it is important that clinicians involved in airway management maintain direct laryngoscopy skills to ensure they are capable of practicing in various settings, it is the view of the authors that where resources allow, videolaryngoscopy should be used routinely. The issue of skill upkeep is addressed elsewhere in this chapter, but the following point is worth highlighting: direct laryngoscopy is a skill, whereas a direct laryngoscope is a tool. Unfortunately, a direct laryngoscope is not the best available tool to teach direct laryngoscopy; it is in fact a Macintosh-style video laryngoscope.

#3 Videolaryngoscope screens can fail

All equipment can fail. Equipment failure, such as light source failure, is not uncommon in both videolaryngoscopes and direct laryngoscopes, ranging from 3% to 8% in observational studies of routine and emergency airway management [4, 56]. Planning for redundancy is essential when designing safe systems of care, and spare pieces of equipment should be available in case of failure [57]. Furthermore, all equipment needs to be checked and tested prior to use.

#4 The screen might be obscured with secretions/blood/oedema or when intubating outdoors sunlight might cause glare

There is some validity to these concerns. That said, even if the camera is obscured by secretions, one can still use a Mac-VL as a DL. Furthermore, DL is not universally successful in securing the airway in case of massive flooding of the field with pulmonary oedema or blood. Depending on the specific case and intubator skillset, a number of rescue approaches are available: change the patient position to Trendelenburg or lateral positioning, a wide-bore suction catheter (e.g. a SSCOR DuCanto Catheter®) may be inserted into the trachea to facilitate passage of a tracheal introducer, a blind digital intubation may be performed, or front-of-neck access may be employed as a last resort.

#5 Videolaryngoscopy increases success rates of novice intubators

This has not been borne out in the evidence to date [14]. That is, novice intubators perform equally well—or poorly—with VL as they do with DL. In fact, it appears that patients intubated by skilled clinicians benefit more when VLs are used. This underscores further the need for appropriate training with any device used in clinical practice.

16.3.7 *Other Techniques Using Videolaryngoscopy*

16.3.7.1 Awake Videolaryngoscopy (ATI:VL)

Awake videolaryngoscopy may be employed to facilitate airway assessment in patients with features of predicted airway difficulty [58]. If a reassuring airway is encountered, one can choose to proceed with intubation following induction of anaesthesia, otherwise, a safer approach might be an awake technique (ATI:VL). Similar principles of topicalisation and procedural sedation, if appropriate, apply as with other awake tracheal intubation (ATI) techniques [59]. One important consideration is the operator's positioning, as the patient will usually be positioned upright with the intubator facing the patient. This will result in a mirror view on the monitor—the epiglottis appearing at the bottom of the screen—and the intubator needs to account for this when performing the procedure [60].

16.3.7.2 Video-Assisted Flexible Intubation (VAFI)

Video-assisted flexible intubation (VAFI) is a two-person technique, which employs both videolaryngoscopy and flexible bronchoscopy [61–64]. The former is used to provide a wide field of view of the glottic opening, with the latter serving as a flexible introducer for the tracheal tube, which is preloaded onto the scope. It is worth thinking about the fibreoptic scope, akin to a steerable bougie, which affords the second operator increased flexibility in terms of navigating the tip into the glottic opening. This technique will most often be employed electively, but has been successfully used for securing the unanticipated difficult airway [64, 65].

Most often, the operator using the fibreoptic bronchoscope performs the intubation, while the VL operator optimises the field of view to navigate the bronchoscope into the trachea. Alternatively, the VL operator can insert the tip of the bronchoscope and use it as a bougie, while the other operator assists by flexing the tip as required [66]. The latter approach is less frequently adopted. Figure 16.7 shows a proposed layout of equipment and staff used for VAFI.

16.3.8 *Optical Stylets*

Optical stylets (OS) are rigid devices onto which a tracheal tube is loaded and provide a view from the tip to the intubator. OS can be advantageous when there is restricted mouth opening, as they can be loaded with a 5.5 mm internal diameter tracheal tube, allowing for a retromolar insertion.

The Bonfils rigid fibrescope is 40 cm long, with a fixed curvature at the distal end [67, 68]. The image can be viewed through an eyepiece or a video attachment (Fig. 16.8). The field of view is narrower than with a VL and can easily be obscured by secretions.

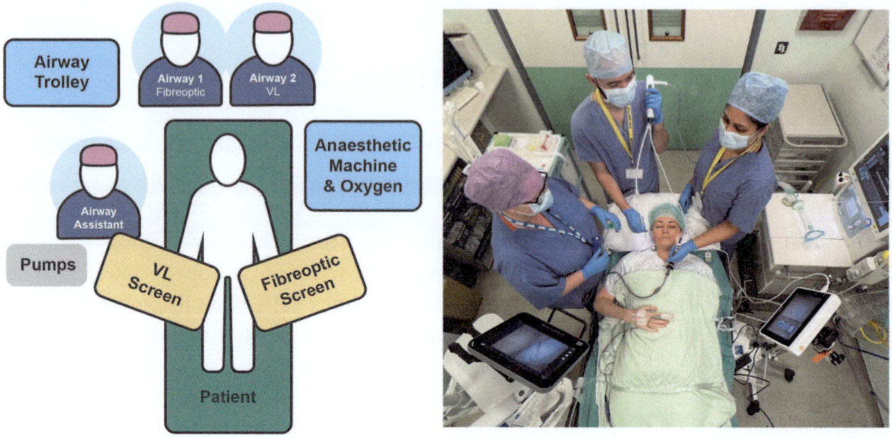

Fig. 16.7 A proposed layout of staff and equipment for video-assisted flexible intubation (VAFI) in an anaesthetised patient. Two intubators are positioned side by side, with the clinician on the left-hand side of the patient holding the VL and the clinician on the right operating the fibreoptic bronchoscope. *VL* videolaryngoscope

Fig. 16.8 The Bonfils rigid fibrescope

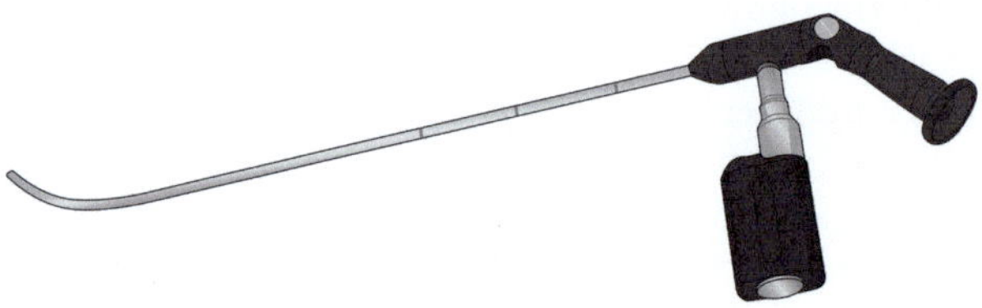

The Storz C-MAC® suite has recently added a Video Stylet, which is a modification of the original Bonfils, allowing for 60° flexion and extension of the distal tip. The recommended minimal inner diameter is 6 mm.

Clarus® produces two devices that fit into this category; the Levitan Fibreoptic Stylet uses an eyepiece at the end of a malleable stylet, whereas the Video Stylet Scope is a narrow malleable stylet with a camera at the tip and an LCD video screen at the end.

Case Vignette

A 31-year-old male, BMI 35 kg/m^2, presents with severe testicular pain while playing rugby. He ate pizza 2 h prior to being listed for operative management of suspected testicular torsion. Pre-operative clinical examination reveals no additional clinical features predicting airway difficulty. Following preoxygenation in a ramped position, a rapid sequence induction with fentanyl, propofol, and rocuronium is performed.

(continued)

Direct laryngoscopy using a Macintosh #4 blade yields a grade 3a view with optimised positioning and guided external laryngeal manipulation. An attempt is made with a bougie with no clicks felt. A tracheal tube is passed over the bougie, but there is no capnography trace on the monitor. The tube is promptly removed and facemask ventilation restarted with good gas exchange. Help is requested.

A hyperangulated VL (HA-VL) with a #4 blade is used on the second attempt. This gives an adequate view of the glottic structures. Another attempt is made with a bougie, but it repeatedly passes posteriorly into the oesophagus, even with changing the head position and external laryngeal manipulation. The airway assistant informs the intubator the SpO_2 is 91%, so facemask ventilation is restarted with adequate gas exchange.

What is the next step?

Proposed Solutions to the Above Challenge

Prior to the third attempt senior help arrives, the tracheal tube is preloaded with a rigid preformed stylet, the trachea is successfully intubated with a HA-VL, and confirmed with waveform capnography.

The case above highlights a few points worth considering:

- Improper use of specialised equipment. Specific training, beyond direct laryngoscopy, is required for the correct and successful use of HA-VL.
- Could this stressful situation have been prevented by using a Mac-VL on the first attempt?
- Not infrequently, direct laryngoscopy will fail on the initial attempt in spite of all optimisations, even in experienced hands.

Acknowledgements We would like to thank Tim Cook, James Fletcher, Gareth Jones, Fiona Kelly, Jenny Kendal, Anjali Kundu, Simon Mackie, Emma McNeill, Nils Christian Ween-Velken, and Arkadiusz Zmierczak for their input.

References

1. Cumberworth A, Lewith H, Sud A, Jefferson H, Athanassoglou V, Pandit JJ. Major complications of airway management: a prospective multicentre observational study. Anaesthesia. 2022;77(6):640–8.
2. Cook TM, Woodall N, Frerk C. Major complications of airway management in the UK: results of the Fourth National Audit Project of the Royal College of Anaesthetists and the Difficult Airway Society. Part 1: anaesthesia. Br J Anaesth. 2011;106(5):617–31.
3. Cook TM, Woodall N, Harper J, Benger J. Major complications of airway management in the UK: results of the Fourth National Audit Project of the Royal College of Anaesthetists and

the Difficult Airway Society. Part 2: intensive care and emergency departments. Br J Anaesth. 2011;106(5):632–42.
4. Huitink JM, Lie PP, Heideman I, Jansma EP, Greif R, van Schagen N, et al. A prospective, cohort evaluation of major and minor airway management complications during routine anaesthetic care at an academic medical centre. Anaesthesia. 2017;72(1):42–8.
5. Hagberg CA, Hagberg CA, Artime CA, Aziz MF. Hagberg and Benumof's airway management. 4th ed. Philadelphia: Elsevier; 2018.
6. Edelman DA, Perkins EJ, Brewster DJ. Difficult airway management algorithms: a directed review. Anaesthesia. 2019;74(9):1175–85.
7. McNarry AF, Patel A. The evolution of airway management – new concepts and conflicts with traditional practice. Br J Anaesth. 2017;119(suppl_1):i154–66.
8. De Jong A, Jaber S. Do not throw the intubation checklist out with the bath water! Chest. 2018;153(4):771–3.
9. Janz DR, Semler MW, Joffe AM, Casey JD, Lentz RJ, deBoisblanc BP, et al. A multicenter randomized trial of a checklist for endotracheal intubation of critically ill adults. Chest. 2018;153(4):816–24.
10. Chrimes N. The vortex: a universal 'high-acuity implementation tool' for emergency airway management. Br J Anaesth. 2016;117(Suppl 1):i20–7.
11. Higgs A, McGrath BA, Goddard C, Rangasami J, Suntharalingam G, Gale R, et al. Guidelines for the management of tracheal intubation in critically ill adults. Br J Anaesth. 2018;120(2):323–52.
12. Huitink JM, Bouwman RA. The myth of the difficult airway: airway management revisited. Anaesthesia. 2015;70(3):244–9.
13. Downey AW, Duggan LV, Adam Law J. A systematic review of meta-analyses comparing direct laryngoscopy with videolaryngoscopy. Can J Anaesth. 2021;68(5):706–14.
14. Hansel J, Rogers AM, Lewis SR, Cook TM, Smith AF. Videolaryngoscopy versus direct laryngoscopy for adults undergoing tracheal intubation. Cochrane Database Syst Rev. 2022;4(4):Cd011136.
15. Cook TM, Tuckey JP. A comparison between the Macintosh and the McCoy laryngoscope blades. Anaesthesia. 1996;51(10):977–80.
16. McCoy EP, Mirakhur RK. The levering laryngoscope. Anaesthesia. 1993;48(6):516–9.
17. Garg M, Shakya R, Mary Lyngdoh N, Pradhan D. Comparison between McCoy laryngoscope and C-MAC video laryngoscope in anticipated difficult airway: a prospective randomised study. Cureus. 2022;14(7):e26685.
18. Jain D, Bala I, Gandhi K. Comparative effectiveness of McCoy laryngoscope and CMAC(®) videolaryngoscope in simulated cervical spine injuries. J Anaesthesiol Clin Pharmacol. 2016;32(1):59–64.
19. Greenland KB. Two curves and three columns—a reappraisal of direct laryngoscopy. Oper Tech Otolaryngol Head Neck Surg. 2020;31(2):83–8.
20. Adnet F, Borron SW, Lapostolle F, Lapandry C. The three axis alignment theory and the "sniffing position": perpetuation of an anatomic myth? Anesthesiology. 1999;91(6):1964–5.
21. Mohta M. Head elevation beyond sniffing position – an aid to airway management. J Anaesthesiol Clin Pharmacol. 2018;34(2):247–8.
22. El-Orbany MI, Getachew YB, Joseph NJ, Salem MR, Friedman M. Head elevation improves laryngeal exposure with direct laryngoscopy. J Clin Anesth. 2015;27(2):153–8.
23. Okada Y, Nakayama Y, Hashimoto K, Koike K, Watanabe N. Ramped versus sniffing position for tracheal intubation: a systematic review and meta-analysis. Am J Emerg Med. 2021;44:250–6.
24. Collins JS, Lemmens HJ, Brodsky JB, Brock-Utne JG, Levitan RM. Laryngoscopy and morbid obesity: a comparison of the "sniff" and "ramped" positions. Obes Surg. 2004;14(9):1171–5.
25. Turner JS, Hunter BR, Haseltine ID, Motzkus CA, DeLuna HM, Cooper DD, et al. Effect of inclined positioning on first-pass success during endotracheal intubation: a systematic review and meta-analysis. Emerg Med J. 2022;40:293.
26. Hochman II, Zeitels SM, Heaton JT. Analysis of the forces and position required for direct laryngoscopic exposure of the anterior vocal folds. Ann Otol Rhinol Laryngol. 1999;108(8):715–24.

27. White E. Care of the eye during anaesthesia. Anaesth Intensive Care Med. 2004;5(9):302–3.
28. White E, Crosse MM. The aetiology and prevention of peri-operative corneal abrasions. Anaesthesia. 1998;53(2):157–61.
29. Cook TM. A new practical classification of laryngeal view. Anaesthesia. 2000;55(3):274–9.
30. Sitzwohl C, Langheinrich A, Schober A, Krafft P, Sessler DI, Herkner H, et al. Endobronchial intubation detected by insertion depth of endotracheal tube, bilateral auscultation, or observation of chest movements: randomised trial. BMJ. 2010;341:c5943.
31. Levitan RM, Pisaturo JT, Kinkle WC, Butler K, Everett WW. Stylet bend angles and tracheal tube passage using a straight-to-cuff shape. Acad Emerg Med. 2006;13(12):1255–8.
32. Jaber S, Rollé A, Godet T, Terzi N, Riu B, Asfar P, et al. Effect of the use of an endotracheal tube and stylet versus an endotracheal tube alone on first-attempt intubation success: a multicentre, randomised clinical trial in 999 patients. Intensive Care Med. 2021;47(6):653–64.
33. Driver B, Dodd K, Klein LR, Buckley R, Robinson A, McGill JW, et al. The bougie and first-pass success in the emergency department. Ann Emerg Med. 2017;70(4):473–8.e1.
34. Driver BE, Semler MW, Self WH, Ginde AA, Trent SA, Gandotra S, et al. Effect of use of a bougie vs endotracheal tube with stylet on successful intubation on the first attempt among critically ill patients undergoing tracheal intubation: a randomized clinical trial. JAMA. 2021;326(24):2488–97.
35. Marson BA, Anderson E, Wilkes AR, Hodzovic I. Bougie-related airway trauma: dangers of the hold-up sign. Anaesthesia. 2014;69(3):219–23.
36. Oxenham O, Pairaudeau C, Moody T, Mendonca C. Standard and flexible tip bougie for tracheal intubation using a non-channelled hyperangulated videolaryngoscope: a randomised comparison<sup/>. Anaesthesia. 2022;77(12):1368–75.
37. Root CW, Mitchell OJL, Brown R, Evers CB, Boyle J, Griffin C, et al. Suction assisted laryngoscopy and airway decontamination (SALAD): a technique for improved emergency airway management. Resusc Plus. 2020;1-2:100005.
38. Rosenblatt WH. Airway on demand following the bubbles to a successful intubation. Anesthesiol News; 2018. Available from: https://www.AnesthesiologyNews.com/Multimedia/Article/04-18/Airway-on-Demand-Following-the-Bubbles-to-a-Successful-Intubation/48485
39. Levitan RM, Mickler T, Hollander JE. Bimanual laryngoscopy: a videographic study of external laryngeal manipulation by novice intubators. Ann Emerg Med. 2002;40(1):30–7.
40. Hwang J, Park S, Huh J, Kim J, Kim K, Oh A, et al. Optimal external laryngeal manipulation: modified bimanual laryngoscopy. Am J Emerg Med. 2013;31(1):32–6.
41. Levitan RM, Kinkle WC, Levin WJ, Everett WW. Laryngeal view during laryngoscopy: a randomized trial comparing cricoid pressure, backward-upward-rightward pressure, and bimanual laryngoscopy. Ann Emerg Med. 2006;47(6):548–55.
42. Klein AA, Meek T, Allcock E, Cook TM, Mincher N, Morris C, et al. Recommendations for standards of monitoring during anaesthesia and recovery 2021: guideline from the Association of Anaesthetists. Anaesthesia. 2021;76(9):1212–23.
43. Chrimes N, Higgs A, Hagberg CA, Baker PA, Cooper RM, Greif R, et al. Preventing unrecognised oesophageal intubation: a consensus guideline from the Project for Universal Management of Airways and international airway societies. Anaesthesia. 2022;77:1395.
44. Kelly FE, Cook TM. Unrecognised oesophageal intubation: additional human factors and ergonomics solutions. Anaesthesia. 2022;77(6):718–9.
45. Phelan MP, Dhimar J. Techniques for improving video laryngoscopy with a hyperangulated blade. Acad Emerg Med. 2016;23(8):e15.
46. Reynolds EC, Crowther N, Corbett L, Cominos T, Thomas V, Cook TM, et al. Improving laryngoscopy technique and success with the C-MAC® D blade: development and dissemination of the 'Bath C-MAC D blade guide'. Br J Anaesth. 2020;125(1):e162–4.
47. Samsoon GL, Young JR. Difficult tracheal intubation: a retrospective study. Anaesthesia. 1987;42(5):487–90.
48. Chaggar RS, Shah SV, Berry M, Saini R, Soni S, Vaughan D. The video classification of intubation (VCI) score: a new description tool for tracheal intubation using videolaryngoscopy: a pilot study. Eur J Anaesthesiol. 2021;38(3):324–6.
49. Cook TM, Kelly FE. A national survey of videolaryngoscopy in the United Kingdom. Br J Anaesth. 2017;118(4):593–600.

50. Odor PM, Bampoe S, Moonesinghe SR, Andrade J, Pandit JJ, Lucas DN, et al. General anaesthetic and airway management practice for obstetric surgery in England: a prospective, multicentre observational study. Anaesthesia. 2021;76(4):460–71.
51. Hansel J, Rogers AM, Lewis SR, Cook TM, Smith AF. Videolaryngoscopy versus direct laryngoscopy for adults undergoing tracheal intubation: a Cochrane systematic review and meta-analysis update. Br J Anaesth. 2022;129(4):612–23.
52. Zhang J, Jiang W, Urdaneta F. Economic analysis of the use of video laryngoscopy versus direct laryngoscopy in the surgical setting. J Comp Eff Res. 2021;10(10):831–44.
53. De Jong A, Sfara T, Pouzeratte Y, Pensier J, Rolle A, Chanques G, et al. Videolaryngoscopy as a first-intention technique for tracheal intubation in unselected surgical patients: a before and after observational study. Br J Anaesth. 2022;129(4):624–34.
54. Cook TM, Boniface NJ, Seller C, Hughes J, Damen C, MacDonald L, et al. Universal videolaryngoscopy: a structured approach to conversion to videolaryngoscopy for all intubations in an anaesthetic and intensive care department. Br J Anaesth. 2018;120(1):173–80.
55. Jones L, Mulcahy K, Fox J, Cook TM, Kelly FE. C-MAC(©) videolaryngoscopy: the anaesthetic assistant's view. J Perioper Pract. 2018;28(4):83–9.
56. Jishnu M, Bhoi S, Sahu AK, Suresh S, Aggarwal P. Airway management practices among emergency physicians: an observational study. Turk J Emerg Med. 2022;22(4):186–91.
57. Gibbins M, Kelly FE, Cook TM. Airway management equipment and practice: time to optimise institutional, team, and personal preparedness. Br J Anaesth. 2020;125(3):221–4.
58. Hodzovic I, Bedreag O. Awake videolaryngoscope – guided intubation – well worth adding to your skill-mix. Rom J Anaesth Intensive Care. 2019;26(1):5–7.
59. Ahmad I, El-Boghdadly K, Bhagrath R, Hodzovic I, McNarry AF, Mir F, et al. Difficult Airway Society guidelines for awake tracheal intubation (ATI) in adults. Anaesthesia. 2020;75(4):509–28.
60. Fitzgerald E, Hodzovic I, Smith AF. 'From darkness into light': time to make awake intubation with videolaryngoscopy the primary technique for an anticipated difficult airway? Anaesthesia. 2015;70(4):387–92.
61. Koopman EM, van Emden MW, Geurts JJG, Schwarte LA, Schober P. Comparison of videolaryngoscopy alone with video-assisted fibreoptic intubation in a difficult cadaver airway model. Eur J Anaesthesiol. 2021;38(3):318–9.
62. Lenhardt R, Burkhart MT, Brock GN, Kanchi-Kandadai S, Sharma R, Akça O. Is video laryngoscope-assisted flexible tracheoscope intubation feasible for patients with predicted difficult airway? A prospective, randomized clinical trial. Anesth Analg. 2014;118(6):1259–65.
63. Sanfilippo F, Chiaramonte G, Sgalambro F. Video laryngoscopes and best rescue strategy for unexpected difficult airways: do not forget a combined approach with flexible bronchoscopy! Anesthesiology. 2017;126(6):1203.
64. Saunders TG, Gibbins ML, Seller CA, Kelly FE, Cook TM. Videolaryngoscope-assisted flexible intubation tracheal tube exchange in a patient with a difficult airway. Anaesth Rep. 2019;7(1):22–5.
65. Liew GHC, Wong TGL, Lu A, Kothandan H. Combined use of the glidescope and flexible fibrescope as a rescue technique in a difficult airway. Proc Singap Healthc. 2015;24(2):117–20.
66. Cook T, Kristensen M. Core topics in airway management. 3rd ed. Cambridge: Cambridge University Press; 2021.
67. Falcetta S, Pecora L, Orsetti G, Gentili P, Rossi A, Gabbanelli V, et al. The Bonfils fiberscope: a clinical evaluation of its learning curve and efficacy in difficult airway management. Minerva Anestesiol. 2012;78(2):176–84.
68. Thong SY, Wong TG. Clinical uses of the Bonfils Retromolar intubation fiberscope: a review. Anesth Analg. 2012;115(4):855–66.

Chapter 17
Tracheal Intubation: Fiberoptic Bronchoscopy

Hamelmal D. Kassahun and Stephen R. Collins

17.1 Introduction

Fiberoptic intubation (FOI) involves guiding a flexible fiberoptic bronchoscope under direct visualization with a light source and camera to advance an endotracheal tube into the trachea. This technique for intubation has been among the recommended strategies for managing a patient's difficult airway for the past 50 years. It is considered the "gold standard" in elective airway management of patients with anticipated difficult airways when tracheal intubation is indicated, particularly when concurrent difficult ventilation is expected. It can be performed nasally or orally in awake patients with topical or regional anesthesia alone, or in sedated or anesthetized patients.

FOI is commonly used and ideally suited in patients if difficulty is anticipated with intubation and in patients with cervical spine instability, distorted anatomy, and facial trauma. Various guidelines have been published to predict the risk of a difficult airway and to manage difficult mask ventilation and intubation [1]. In such scenarios, awake fiberoptic intubation, performed by anesthetization of the upper airway by topical local anesthesia or regional anesthesia, frequently facilitated by the administration of sedatives and analgesics while preserving spontaneous ventilation, plays a crucial role in airway management. The approach can safeguard against the risk of the "cannot intubate, cannot ventilate" scenario, as tracheal intubation can be performed prior to induction of general anesthesia with its attendant risks, including inadequate oxygenation and ventilation, loss of upper airway patency and failed intubation. For this reason, FOI is commonly considered the gold standard by national societies and experts [2–4]. Compared with direct laryngoscopy,

H. D. Kassahun · S. R. Collins (✉)
Department of Anesthesiology, University of Virginia School of Medicine, Charlottesville, VA, USA
e-mail: HK5GR@hscmail.mcc.virginia.edu; src2f@hscmail.mcc.virginia.edu

M. Á. Gómez-Ríos, A. van Zundert (eds.), *Evidence-based Guide to Difficult Airway Management*, https://doi.org/10.1007/978-3-032-30769-9_17

FOI has several advantages, including ease in visualizing a patient's entire airway (from oro- or nasopharynx to bronchi) and navigating around abnormal airway pathologies, versatility with nasal or oral approaches for intubation, ability to reduce cervical (spinal) manipulation during intubation, and less hemodynamic stimulation in sedated patients.

17.2 Indications

Fiberoptic bronchoscopes are used to facilitate endotracheal intubation via the nasal or oral route, to position endotracheal and endobronchial tubes, and to perform airway examinations or evaluations.

Tracheal intubation is often required for surgical interventions and airway protection in critically ill patients and trauma situations. A difficult airway is defined as a condition in which "a conventionally trained anesthesiologist experiences difficulty with facemask ventilation, difficulty with tracheal intubation, or both" [1]. The need for FOI may be anticipated based on the patient's history of prior difficult intubation and various anatomic features that may predict difficult laryngoscopy. These include limited mouth opening, limited thyromental distance, reduced neck mobility, inability to prognath, and oropharyngeal classification [5]. FOI may also be indicated for known or suspected cervical spine instability, anatomic malformations of the mandible or larynx, and deformities of the head and neck, either congenital or related to trauma. When airway difficulty is anticipated, the ability to mask ventilate and the need for tracheal intubation should be assessed. Awake intubation is recommended in situations where mask ventilation is anticipated to be difficult, and aspiration risk is high to minimize or avoid a "cannot intubate, cannot oxygenate" scenario.

Several studies have attempted to identify exam features or to define characteristics that predict difficult intubation. However, the reported usefulness of such predictive tests has been questioned, given their low positive predictive value [6]. A meta-analysis of over 50,000 patients with normal anatomy on pre-operative examination found difficulty with intubation in 5.8% of cases [7]. From an observational study of over 50,000 anesthetic records, an impossible mask ventilated was reported as an infrequent event (0.15%), with 25% of these patients found to be difficult to intubate [8]. Some independent predictors of difficult/impossible mask ventilation include neck radiation-induced changes, male sex, sleep apnea, Mallampati classification III or IV, and a beard [8].

FOI is an accepted standard approach in elective airway management of awake, spontaneously breathing patients with an anticipated difficult airway [2]. FOI is ideally suited for such patients because intubation can be performed prior to the induction of general anesthesia and thus provides a safer approach without loss of airway. The success of the technique, however, presupposes adequate time for preparation in a cooperative patient, a requirement for safe and successful FOI. In cases in which tracheal intubation is necessary, and mask or supraglottic ventilation (e.g.,

Table 17.1 Common indications for fiberoptic intubation

Difficult intubation Anticipated difficult airway (history of difficult intubation, physical exam findings) Unanticipated difficult airway (as a rescue of failed intubation)
Difficult ventilation Known/suspected difficult facemask ventilation Known/suspected difficult LMA placement
Unstable cervical spine
Distorted airway anatomy (tumors, abscess, trauma)
Confirmation of airway device position (endotracheal tube depth, tracheostomy insertion and positioning, and double lumen tube and bronchial blocker placement and depth assessment)

via a laryngeal mask airway [LMA]) is unlikely to be successful or poses an aspiration risk, awake FOI is a standard approach [9] (Table 17.1).

17.3 Equipment for Fiberoptic Intubation

Fiberoptic intubations require more equipment preparation than other intubating techniques. The fiberoptic bronchoscope consists of a handle, an insertion cord, and a flexible tip with an attached camera. The handle contains the control lever, working channel port, and suction connector. A control lever controls the flexible tip, which permits movement in one plane—up and down. Moving the lever down points the tip up, and moving the lever up points the tip down. Side-to-side movement is accomplished by rotation of the handle of the bronchoscope with the operator's wrist. A working channel port is used for the delivery of oxygen or a local anesthetic, which can be applied as the operator advances the fiberoptic scope. A suction connector allows clearance of any airway secretions.

17.4 Ancillary Equipment

FOI can be easily performed with the patient either in the supine or seated position. Standard airway and emergency equipment should be available. If performed orally, FOI is facilitated by an oral airway; this protects the fiberscope, keeps it in the midline position, and displaces the tongue away from the soft palate to aid in visualization of the airway. It is important to choose an appropriate size and type of endotracheal tube (ETT) to facilitate ease of intubation with a fiberoptic scope. The tube needs to be big enough to allow adequate ventilation and fit the scope, but small enough to minimize the gap between the tube and the scope and fit through the nose (if a nasal approach is planned). The larger the gap between the tube and the scope, the more likely it is to snag on tissue (e.g., epiglottis, arytenoid cartilage). Standard ETTs are acceptable, but they offer less flexibility during tube placement and may be less suitable for nasal intubation. Reinforced ETTs may facilitate easier negotiation and passage, but lack a Murphy's eye, which can cause problems if the tube becomes occluded once placed. Intubating LMA ETTs have softer tips, which may reduce the risk of trauma and a tighter fit between the ETT and the scope. Parker Flex-tip ETTs have flexible, curved, centered, and tapered distal tips, which reduce the incidence of trauma as the tube is passed through protruding features of the airway such as nasal turbinates or supraglottic tissue.

17.5 Insertion Aids

These instruments are used to assist with fiberoptic oral intubation. Ovassapian: used to protect the scope and keep it in the midline. Available in a single size. Can be opened wide to disengage it from the ETT. Berman: used to protect the scope and keep it in the midline. It is available in different sizes.

17.6 Fiberoptic Techniques

FOI can be performed orally or nasally in awake patients with topical or regional anesthetics alone, or in sedated or anesthetized patients. An awake technique is preferred in situations where mask ventilation and oxygenation may be difficult, and the risk of airway loss is significant. A nasal approach is anatomically favorable in that the laryngeal opening is more easily seen with the fiberscope as it courses past the nasopharynx with less obstruction by the tongue [10]. A nasal approach is useful for patients with redundant oral soft tissue, a large tongue, limited mouth opening, retrognathia, tracheal deviation, or when an unobstructed surgical view is preferred (e.g., a dental procedure). In addition to the high-quality optics and maneuverability of the fiberoptic scope, it also allows the application of topical anesthesia to the airway to the cords (and below). Fiberoptic tubes also have suction ports and/or working channels through which local anesthetics can be sprayed over the airway and directed evenly over the cords. This strategy allows the proceduralist to avoid a trans-laryngeal (injection) to the cords and more reliably delivers the local anesthetic to the laryngeal structures.

17.7 Setup for Fiberoptic Intubation

Before starting the procedure, it is important to ensure a working fiberoptic with a light source and video monitor, the desired ETT loaded on a lubricated insertion tube, working suction, and a reliable oxygen supply. Whether the patient is to be intubated awake or asleep, glycopyrrolate (unless contraindicated) can be administered to reduce oral secretions. Standard anxiolytic pre-medications can be titrated to effect in addition to other routinely used medications such as famotidine, metoclopramide, and sodium citrate if the patient is at risk for aspiration.

17.8 Fiberoptic Oral Intubation

17.8.1 Asleep

For oral intubations, the operator can stand either at the head of the bed (with the patient supine) or at the patient's side looking towards the patient's face (if the patient is seated). Regardless, the insertion tube must be kept as straight as possible. Sedation can be selected and administered to achieve anxiolytic effects. Once the patient has been induced and the ability to bag-mask ventilate has been confirmed, muscle relaxants can be administered. Succinylcholine is often the preferred choice unless contraindicated, as it has a short duration of action and allows the patient to resume spontaneous respiration in the rare instance that intubation is impossible and bag-mask ventilation becomes ineffective. Apneic oxygenation can be provided via nasal cannula at 3–5 L/min [11]. This can be particularly useful in patients with diminished functional residual capacity.

After the muscle relaxant takes effect, an intubating airway is inserted over the tongue with the phalange running along the base of the tongue. The intubating airway should be placed in the proper position to avoid obstruction of the oropharynx and avoid pushing the tongue further. A tongue depressor can help to flatten the tongue and place the intubating airway under direct visualization of the posterior oropharynx and the distal phalange along the base of the tongue without pushing it in too far or pushing the base of the tongue into the posterior oropharynx. Alternatively, the intubating airway can be placed about two-thirds of the way into the mouth and then a lower jaw thrust can be applied while pushing the airway in further. Alternatively, an assistant can perform a jaw thrust to gain easy access to the oropharynx. This can also be facilitated by an assistant providing a direct outward pull on the tongue to open up the oropharyngeal space. If the patient desaturates and positive pressure ventilation becomes necessary during this process, the intubating airway should be removed and replaced with a standard airway.

It is important to have an assistant provide a firm lower-jaw thrust to facilitate passage of the tip of the fiberoptic through the oropharynx. The tip of the fiberoptic should be tilted at 45 degrees (upward if intubating from the head of the bed or downward if intubating from the side of the bed). The tip of the scope can then be introduced into the mouth under direct vision. The tube is held such that the tip is directed over the phalange of the intubating airway and down towards the larynx. Once the tip of the scope has passed the intubating airway, the tip can be directed toward the cords. Normally, the tip of the insertion tube must be directed slightly downwards to get under the tip of the epiglottis, which can be facilitated by jaw thrust or tongue pulling and then up over the arytenoid cartilages and through the cords into the trachea, where the cartilaginous rings become apparent anteriorly. If it is necessary to maneuver the scope around an obstructing lesion, small wrist movements will allow fine adjustments. Once the tip of the scope enters the trachea, it is advanced to the mid-trachea, avoiding contact with the carina, as it can cause hemodynamic instability, including tachycardia, hypertension, and severe laryngospasm. Next, the ETT is guided into the trachea. Removing the intubating airway from the oral cavity will facilitate easy passage of the ETT. If the tip of the ETT becomes stuck as it passes the base of the tongue, jaw thrust can open the passage into the larynx. If the tip appears to be stuck at the level of the larynx, the ETT can be gently rotated clockwise or counterclockwise to free it from the epiglottis or the arytenoid cartilages. Choosing an appropriate size ETT that has an internal diameter close to the insertion tube can minimize the risk of the ETT getting hung up on the laryngeal structures. Once the tube is in the trachea, its position relative to the carina can be adjusted to 2–3 cm by moving the fiberoptic tube closer to the carina and withdrawing it until it reaches the tip of the ETT.

17.8.2 Awake

Glycopyrrolate is administered if not contraindicated. The patient is either seated up in the bed (if they are not able to lie flat and/or to help open the channel through the oropharynx) or can be laid down, usually with a ramp to optimize the view. Once the patient is adequately sedated and topical anesthesia has been achieved, intubation can be performed. Nasal cannula oxygen is delivered at 4–5 L/min to decrease the risk of hypoxia during sedation and intubation. The oral airway is inserted, making sure that neither the base of the tongue nor the phalange of the airway obstructs the route through the posterior oropharynx. A gentle jaw thrust is provided by an assistant, and the fiberoptic tube with the ETT loaded on it is introduced with a 45-degree bend at the tip to the back of the oral cavity. If the view is clear, the fiberoptic tube is advanced into the trachea, followed by the ETT. If the view is obstructed by redundant airway tissue, asking the patient to take a deep breath facilitates the laryngeal structures to become apparent during deep inspiration.

17.9 Nasal Fiberoptic Intubation

17.9.1 Asleep

Nasal fiberoptic intubation is useful in patients with a large tongue, limited mouth opening, a receding lower jaw, or tracheal deviation, or in surgical cases specifically to create an unobstructed surgical field. A nasal approach can be anatomically favorable as it allows easier access to the laryngeal opening with the fiberoptic tube as it courses past the nasopharynx with less obstruction by the base of the tongue. The setup for asleep fiberoptic intubation is similar to what is described above. An important step is to assess the nares and determine whether one nare is more widely patent. This can be established by asking the patient to occlude each nostril in turn and sniff rapidly. Regardless, both nares can be prepared with a vasoconstrictor to reduce the nasal mucosal vasculature as this increases the passageway for the ETT and decreases blood flow, thereby minimizing or preventing the risk of bleeding. Then, general anesthesia is induced in the standard fashion, ensuring that bag-mask ventilation is possible prior to administering a muscle relaxant.

After slow dilation of the naris with increasing-sized nasopharyngeal airways, an appropriately sized and well-lubricated ETT (usually 7.0 mm or smaller) is gently placed through the preferred nostril and passed medially and posteriorly. The goal is to place the tip of the tube into the posterior oropharynx and create a pathway to insert the fiberoptic scope into the trachea. If there is increased resistance to the advancement of the nasotracheal tube through both nares, the fiberoptic scope may be introduced prior to the nasotracheal tube, as it allows direct visualization and navigation around the turbinates, avoiding blind insertion and trauma to nasal and oral airways. A firm lower jaw thrust or pulling the tip of the tongue forward allows the base of the tongue to protrude out of the oropharynx and opens up the inlet to the larynx. A lubricated fiberoptic is then passed through the nasotracheal tube and advanced past the cords to the mid-trachea. The ETT is then gently advanced over the fiberoptic tube into the trachea. Prior to removing the fiberoptic tube, the distance to the carina can be noted. Subsequently, the scope is removed, the ETT is connected to an anesthesia circuit, and bilateral breath sounds and end-tidal CO2 are confirmed. It is important to avoid any pressure on the nasal ala when securing the nasotracheal tube, as it can cause ulcers.

17.9.2 Awake

As with asleep nasal intubations, a vasoconstrictor should be applied to the nostrils to open the nasal canals and shrink the mucosal vasculature. The most significant difference from asleep nasal intubation is the need to topicalize the nares. This can be achieved using a nasal trumpet coated with lidocaine jelly inserted into the nostrils to spread local anesthesia over the mucosal surfaces. Once the patient is sedated and adequate topical anesthesia is applied, intubation proceeds as described above. Often, the laryngeal structures come immediately into view upon passing the insertion tube beyond the tip of the ETT. If not, a deep breath by the patient opens the glottis, allowing passage of the fiberoptic tube and the ETT into the trachea.

17.10 Fiberoptic Intubation in Combination with Other Techniques

The ASA practice guidelines for the management of difficult airways were developed in 1991. In the most recent revised guideline in 2022, an LMA is included as a rescue device for ventilation and a conduit for insertion of an ETT, either blindly or guided by a fiberoptic bronchoscope. Supraglottic devices displace the tongue and epiglottis, allowing glottic exposure that may not be achieved with conventional direct laryngoscopy in difficult airways. A properly placed LMA in proximity to the glottis allows fiberoptic tube advancement [12]. The ETT size is limited by the LMA's conduit size. Previous case reports have highlighted the use of a fiberoptic scope with different types of supraglottic devices: Classic, ProSeal, Supreme, I-Gel, and iLMA to assist with intubation. The detailed description is discussed by Benumoff et al. [18].

Fiberoptic intubation can also be facilitated with direct or video laryngoscopes, such as the Airtraq, Pentax-AWS, Bullard, and GlideScope. Case reports [13, 14] and manikin studies [15] reported the use of these devices, either alone or in combination with a fiberoptic bronchoscope, to assist with intubation. A unique advantage of using a video laryngoscope with a fiberoptic is that the laryngoscope helps retract the tongue and also permits visualization of the endotracheal tube as it passes between the vocal cords, thereby limiting or avoiding trauma to glottic structures. Other reports have described modified catheter-assisted techniques [16, 17].

17.11 Regional Anesthesia Techniques

Regional airway blocks are performed to facilitate fiberoptic tracheal intubation either alone or in combination with topical anesthetics. These blocks include the glossopharyngeal nerve block, superior laryngeal nerve block, and transtracheal (transcricoid) block.

The glossopharyngeal nerve supplies sensory innervation to the posterior third of the tongue, the vallecula, the anterior surface of the epiglottis, the walls of the pharynx, and the tonsils. The glossopharyngeal nerve is most easily blocked where it crosses the palatoglossal arch. It can be blocked by spraying local anesthetics, by applying gauze or pledgets soaked in local anesthetics directly over the nerve, or by direct injection of local anesthetics around the nerve just posterior to the styloid process, where the glossopharyngeal nerve lies. This block helps to abolish the gag reflex, but it will not provide adequate conditions for awake fiberoptic intubation. The glossopharyngeal nerve blocks are no more effective than a topical application of lidocaine for awake intubation [19].

The superior laryngeal nerve provides sensation to the laryngeal structures above the vocal cords and lies inferior to the greater cornu of the hyoid bone, where it splits into the internal and external branches. The internal branch penetrates the thyrohyoid membrane below the greater cornu and continues submucosally in the piriform recess. It can be blocked by gently displacing the hyoid bone to the side where the block is to be performed, and a small needle is inserted from the lateral side of the neck, aiming toward the greater cornu. Upon contact, the needle is walked off the bone inferiorly, and local anesthetics are injected after negative aspiration. If identifying the hyoid is difficult, the superior cornu of the thyroid cartilage can be identified by locating the thyroid notch and tracing it posteriorly. This lies just inferior to the greater cornu of the hyoid. The needle can be inserted aiming for the superior cornu of the thyroid cartilage, then walked cephalad, and then local anesthetics are injected. Another approach is to place local anesthetic-soaked gauzes or pledgets in the piriform fossae.

The recurrent laryngeal nerve supplies sensory innervation to the vocal cords and trachea, and it ascends along the tracheoesophageal groove and provides motor supply to all intrinsic muscles of the larynx except the cricothyroid muscle. This nerve is blocked using the transpharyngeal block by injecting a local anesthetic in the trachea through the cricothyroid membrane.

An advantage of these airway blocks is a more rapid onset of local anesthetic action and a longer duration of action that can facilitate airway anesthesia with extubation. However, airway block complications are not insignificant and include airway obstruction, bilateral vocal cord paralysis, tracheal injury, intra-arterial injection, and hematoma formation.

17.12 Sedation

Sedative medications and supplemental oxygen are often administered while performing awake fiberoptic intubation. Sedative medications in combination with local anesthetics minimize patient anxiety and responses and also blunt reflexes to fiberoptic scope advancement and tracheal intubation, which enables hemodynamic stability. In addition, sedatives provide patient comfort and adequate anxiolysis while maintaining the patient's airway and adequate ventilation. Hypoxemia and aspiration are the most common complications associated with awake FOI [20].

A systematic review of randomized controlled trials including over 2000 patients assessing different protocols for awake FOI in patients scheduled for surgery, found a high degree of efficacy and safety with no significant differences in success rate with different sedatives [21]. Most often, benzodiazepines are combined with opioids to achieve adequate patient comfort and sedation. Midazolam is commonly used because of its rapid onset, short half-life, and ability to provide anterograde amnesia. Short-acting opioids such as fentanyl and remifentanil provide analgesia and can depress laryngeal reflexes. However, they can cause respiratory depression. Some case reports [22, 23], case series [24, 25], and randomized studies [22] have reported on dexmedetomidine for sedation and its superior characteristics in this setting. Dexmedetomidine is a selective alpha-2 adrenergic agonist with sympatholytic, analgesic, and sedative properties that does not cause significant respiratory depression within the recommended dosing ranges (0.2–0.7 mcg/kg/h). In the recent systematic review of randomized controlled trials mentioned above, dexmedetomidine resulted in fewer desaturation episodes compared to propofol and opioids with or without midazolam; occurrences of desaturation were similar with remifentanil versus propofol, while the incidence of apnea was lower with sevoflurane versus propofol [21]. There was no significant difference observed in the success rate with the different sedatives and analgesics; dexmedetomidine might offer a better safety profile compared to other sedatives.

Despite the reported safety profile and success rate, there have been some reports of upper airway obstruction using topical anesthesia approaches [26, 27]. The use of topical anesthesia combined with heavy sedation may be limited and may not provide adequate sedation and analgesia for some patients, as seen in at least one case series [28]. In patient groups with difficult airways (children, uncooperative adults, and patients with mental disabilities), general anesthesia using mask induction with sevoflurane or intravenous titration may be required.

17.13 General Anesthesia

FOI can be performed under general anesthesia, often in spontaneously ventilating patients. There are only a few studies investigating FOI in spontaneously ventilating anesthetized patients. Propofol and sevoflurane have been compared with small group differences, except that patients receiving propofol had more frequent episodes of apnea and hypoxemia [29]. Easy and titratable anesthesia was provided in both groups, with similar findings with anticipated difficult airways using sevoflurane and propofol [30, 31]. A randomized study comparing sevoflurane and propofol in patients scheduled for maxillofacial surgery who were anticipated to have difficulty intubation reported a high intubation success rate with both [32].

17.14 Contraindications and Complications Associated with Fiberoptic Intubation

Absolute contraindications include patient refusal, uncooperative patients in the case of awake fiberoptic approaches, a near-total upper airway obstruction, and a lack of endoscopic skill. Relative contraindications include the inability to tolerate apnea and blood or secretions in the airway.

Potential complications attributable to FOI include epistaxis (nasal intubation), laryngotracheal trauma, laryngospasm, aspiration of saliva, blood, or gastric contents and oversedation related to the procedure [20, 26, 33]. Most data on the specific incidence of complications are from case reports [34, 35] or small prospective investigations examining injury [36]. Rare complications include gastric distention and rupture from oxygen insufflation during FOI [34] and the development of subcutaneous emphysema and pneumomediastinum caused by tracheal perforation [37]. Placement of the ETT cuff in the larynx may cause recurrent laryngeal nerve injury if the placement is not corrected [38]. If the insertion tube is too large to fit through the ETT or it is inadequately lubricated, the outer covering of the insertion tube can be sheared off and obstruct either the ETT or the airway beyond the tip of the ETT. If the fiberoptic scope is advanced through the Murphy eye of the ETT, it can become trapped. If this occurs, the fiberoptic scope cannot be removed easily and the ETT may need to be removed with the insertion tube.

17.15 Comparison with Other Techniques, Limitations, and Advantages

FOI can be a challenging technique to learn, and continuous practice is needed to maintain the skill [39]. Heidegger and colleagues reported that anesthesiologists need at least 25 intubations to be competent with fiberoptic intubation [33] compared to only one to six intubations needed to reach the same level of competence with a video laryngoscope [40]. In a recent prospective study, awake FOI was performed in 1.7% of patients presenting for surgery under general anesthesia with a success rate of 99%, and an overall complications rate of 11% [41]. This study demonstrated a negative correlation between the number of previous awake FOIs performed by the anesthesiologist and the incidence of complications. This underscores the need for continued training to maintain the skills required to safely perform FOI. Furthermore, FOI requires additional equipment, patient preparation, and cooperation. Although the quality of evidence is lower in systematic reviews and meta-analyses, FOI can take considerable time to complete [42]. When intubation time is prolonged due to the performers' level of experience or patient factors, a further increase in time may be critical, particularly in anxious patients with respiratory compromise who are at increased risk of loss of airway patency. Additionally, tracheal tube diameter sizing is limited with fiberoptic scopes. In comparison, a video laryngoscope can provide a wider view of the airway and nearby structures [43], fewer limitations with ETT sizing, and ease of exchanging ETT sizes or preferences while maintaining an airway view.

17.16 Summary

FOI is a versatile tool in airway management and can also be used in combination with other techniques (e.g., an LMA) to aid in successful intubation. The fiberoptic bronchoscope may aid in airway inspection, nasal or oral intubation of patients with difficult airway anatomy, endotracheal tube exchange, proper positioning of bronchial blocker devices, and placement and verification of single- or double-lumen endotracheal tubes. Advantages of FOI include the ability to maintain the patient's cervical spine in a neutral position during airway management, ease in airway inspection and navigation around airway pathology during intubation, reduction in patient risk of aspiration while maintaining intact protective reflexes using awake FOI techniques, and facilitation of intubation in patients with conditions such as angioedema or limited mouth opening. FOI has become and remains a mainstay of difficult airway management, and its role is recognized in guidelines for management of both the anticipated and unanticipated difficult airway.

References

1. Apfelbaum JL, Hagberg CA, Connis RT, Abdelmalak BB, Agarkar M, Dutton RP, Fiadjoe JE, Greif R, Klock PA, Mercier D, Myatra SN, O'Sullivan EP, Rosenblatt WH, Sorbello M, Tung A. 2022 American Society of Anesthesiologists Practice Guidelines for management of the difficult airway. Anesthesiology. 2022;136:31–81.
2. Schenk A, Markus CK, Kranke P. Fiberoptische Wachintubation—Goldstandard für den erwartet schwierigen Atemweg [Awake fiberoptic intubation—gold standard for the anticipated difficult airway]. Anasthesiol Intensivmed Notfallmed Schmerzther. 2014;49(2):92–9.
3. Collins SR, Blank RS. Fiberoptic intubation: an overview and update. Respir Care. 2014;59(6):865–78; discussion 878–80
4. Wong DM, Prabhu A, Chakraborty S, Tan G, Massicotte EM, Cooper R. Cervical spine motion during flexible bronchoscopy compared with the lo-pro GlideScope. Br J Anaesth. 2009;102(3):424–30.
5. el-Ganzouri AR, McCarthy RJ, Tuman KJ, Tanck EN, Ivankovich AD. Preoperative airway assessment: predictive value of a multivariate risk index. Anesth Analg. 1996;82(6):1197–204.
6. Yentis SM. Predicting difficult intubation—worthwhile exercise or pointless ritual? Anaesthesia. 2002;57(2):105–9.
7. Shiga T, Wajima Z'i, Inoue T, Sakamoto A. predicting difficult intubation in apparently Normal patients: a meta-analysis of bedside screening test performance. Anesthesiology. 2005;103:429–37.
8. Kheterpal S, Martin L, Shanks AM, Tremper KK. Prediction and outcomes of impossible mask ventilation: a review of 50,000 anesthetics. Anesthesiology. 2009;110:891–7.
9. Koerner IP, Brambrink AM. Fiberoptic techniques. Best Pract Res Clin Anaesthesiol. 2005;19(4):611–21. https://doi.org/10.1016/j.bpa.2005.07.006. PMID: 16408537
10. Stackhouse RA, Marks JD, Bainton CR. Performing fiberoptic endotracheal intubation: clinical aspects. Int Anesthesiol Clin. 1994;32(4):57–73. https://doi.org/10.1097/00004311-199432040-00006. PMID: 7875909
11. Lee SC. Improvement of gas exchange by apneic oxygenation with nasal prong during fiberoptic intubation in fully relaxed patients. J Korean Med Sci. 1998;13(6):582–6. https://doi.org/10.3346/jkms.1998.13.6.582. PMID: 9886164; PMCID: PMC3054543
12. Benumof JL. laryngeal mask airway and the ASA difficult airway algorithm. Anesthesiology. 1996;84:686–99. https://doi.org/10.1097/00000542-199603000-00024.
13. Yuan YJ, Xue FS, Liao X, Liu JH, Wang Q. Facilitating combined use of an Airtraq® optical laryngoscope and a fiberoptic bronchoscope in patients with a difficult airway. Can J Anaesth.

2011;58(6):584–5. https://doi.org/10.1007/s12630-011-9484-8. author reply 585. Epub 2011 Mar 23. PMID: 21431451
14. Sharma D, Kim LJ, Ghodke B. Successful airway management with combined use of Glidescope videolaryngoscope and fiberoptic bronchoscope in a patient with Cowden syndrome. Anesthesiology. 2010;113(1):253–5. https://doi.org/10.1097/ALN.0b013e3181dfd334. PMID: 20526181
15. Nishikawa K, Hukuoka E, Kawagishi T, Shimodate Y, Yamakage M. Efficacy of the Airtraq(®) laryngoscope with a fiberoptic bronchoscope compared with that of Airtraq(®) alone for tracheal intubation: a manikin study. J Anesth. 2011;25(1):93–7. https://doi.org/10.1007/s00540-010-1038-7. Epub 2010 Nov 4. PMID: 21052737
16. Gosavi KSMD, Nirkhi AMMD. Exchange catheter-assisted fiberoptic nasal intubation: a modified technique. Anesth Analg. 2011;113(1):205–6. https://doi.org/10.1213/ANE.0b013e31821b106a.
17. Chu Q, Dou Z, Xie G, Yang A, Zhang W. Combined use of adult fiberoptic bronchoscope and CARTO catheter for tracheal intubation in children with known difficult airway. J Anesth. 2011;25(4):531–4. https://doi.org/10.1007/s00540-011-1149-9. Epub 2011 Apr 26. PMID: 21519926
18. Benumof JL. Use of the laryngeal mask airway to facilitate fiberscope-aided tracheal intubation. Anesth Analg. 1992;74(2):313–5. https://doi.org/10.1213/00000539-199202000-00034. PMID: 1731560
19. Sitzman BT, Rich GF, Rockwell JJ, Leisure GS, Durieux ME, DiFazio CA. Local anesthetic administration for direct laryngoscopy. Are glossopharyngeal blocks superior? Anesthesiology. 1997;86(1):34–40.
20. Ovassapian A, Yelich SJ, Dykes MH, Brunner EE. Fiberoptic nasotracheal intubation--incidence and causes of failure. Anesth Analg. 1983;62(7):692–5. PMID: 6859572
21. Cabrini L, Baiardo Redaelli M, Ball L, Filippini M, Fominskiy E, Pintaudi M, Putzu A, Votta CD, Sorbello M, Antonelli M, Landoni G, Pelosi P, Zangrillo A. Awake Fiberoptic intubation protocols in the operating room for anticipated difficult airway: a systematic review and meta-analysis of randomized controlled trials. Anesth Analg. 2019;128(5):971–80. https://doi.org/10.1213/ANE.0000000000004087. PMID: 30896601
22. Bergese SD, Khabiri B, Roberts WD, Howie MB, McSweeney TD, Gerhardt MADexmedetomidine for conscious sedation in difficult awake fiberoptic intubation cases. J Clin Anesth. 2007;19(2):141–4. https://doi.org/10.1016/j.jclinane.2006.07.005. Erratum in: J Clin Anesth 2007 19(4):323. PMID: 17379129
23. Grant SA, Breslin DS, MacLeod DB, Gleason D, Martin G. Dexmedetomidine infusion for sedation during fiberoptic intubation: a report of three cases. J Clin Anesth. 2004;16(2):124–6. https://doi.org/10.1016/j.jclinane.2003.05.010. PMID: 15110375
24. Avitsian R, Lin J, Lotto M, Ebrahim Z. Dexmedetomidine and awake fiberoptic intubation for possible cervical spine myelopathy: a clinical series. J Neurosurg Anesthesiol. 2005;17(2):97–9. https://doi.org/10.1097/01.ana.0000161268.01279.ba. PMID: 15840996
25. Abdelmalak B, Makary L, Hoban J, Doyle DJ. Dexmedetomidine as sole sedative for awake intubation in management of the critical airway. J Clin Anesth. 2007;19(5):370–3. https://doi.org/10.1016/j.jclinane.2006.09.006. PMID: 17869990
26. Ho AM, Chung DC, To EW, Karmakar MK. Total airway obstruction during local anesthesia in a non-sedated patient with a compromised airway. Can J Anaesth. 2004;51(8):838–41. https://doi.org/10.1007/BF03018461. PMID: 15470176
27. McGuire G, El-Beheiry H. Complete upper airway obstruction during awake fibreoptic intubation in patients with unstable cervical spine fractures. Can J Anaesth. 1999;46(2):176–8. https://doi.org/10.1007/BF03012553. PMID: 10083999
28. Boucek CD, Gunnerson HB, Tullock WC. Percutaneous transtracheal high-frequency jet ventilation as an aid to fiberoptic intubation. Anesthesiology. 1987;67(2):247–9. https://doi.org/10.1097/00000542-198708000-00016. PMID: 3605752
29. Bonnin M, Therre P, Albuisson E, Beaujard H, Barthelemy I, Mondie JM, Bazin JE. Comparison of a propofol target-controlled infusion and inhalational sevoflu-

rane for fibreoptic intubation under spontaneous ventilation. Acta Anaesthesiol Scand. 2007;51(1):54–9. https://doi.org/10.1111/j.1399-6576.2006.01186.x. Epub 2006 Oct 31. PMID: 17073850
30. Favier JC, Da Conceiçao M, Genco G, Bidallier I, Fassassi M, Steiner T, Pitti R. Intubation fibroscopique sous sévoflurane chez l'adulte avec un masque facial endoscopique en cas d'intubation difficile [Fiberoptic intubation in adult patients with predictive signs of difficult intubation: inhalational induction using sevoflurane and an endoscopic facial mask]. Ann Fr Anesth Reanim. 2003;22(2):96–102. https://doi.org/10.1016/s0750-7658(02)00858-4. PMID: 12706762
31. Bourgain JL, Billard V, Cros AM. Pressure support ventilation during fibreoptic intubation under propofol anaesthesia. Br J Anaesth. 2007;98(1):136–40. https://doi.org/10.1093/bja/ael317. Epub 2006 Dec 2. PMID: 17142824
32. Péan D, Floch H, Beliard C, Piot B, Testa S, Bazin V, Lejus C, Asehnoune K. Propofol versus sevoflurane for fiberoptic intubation under spontaneous breathing anesthesia in patients difficult to intubate. Minerva Anestesiol. 2010;76(10):780–6. Epub 2010 Apr 12. PMID: 20935613
33. Heidegger T, Gerig HJ, Ulrich B, Schnider TW. Structure and process quality illustrated by fibreoptic intubation: analysis of 1612 cases. Anaesthesia. 2003;58(8):734–9. https://doi.org/10.1046/j.1365-2044.2003.03200.x. PMID: 12859463
34. Hershey MD, Hannenberg AA. Gastric distention and rupture from oxygen insufflation during fiberoptic intubation. Anesthesiology. 1996;85(6):1479–80. https://doi.org/10.1097/00000542-199612000-00030. PMID: 8968196
35. Maktabi MA, Hoffman H, Funk G, From RP. Laryngeal trauma during awake fiberoptic intubation. Anesth Analg. 2002;95(4):1112–4. https://doi.org/10.1097/00000539-200210000-00061. Table of contents. PMID: 12351306
36. Johnson DM, From AM, Smith RB, From RP, Maktabi MA. Endoscopic study of mechanisms of failure of endotracheal tube advancement into the trachea during awake fiberoptic orotracheal intubation. Anesthesiology. 2005;102(5):910–4. https://doi.org/10.1097/00000542-200505000-00008. PMID: 15851876
37. Kaneko Y, Nakazawa K, Yokoyama K, Ishikawa S, Uchida T, Takahashi M, Tsunoda A, Makita K. Subcutaneous emphysema and pneumomediastinum after translaryngeal intubation: tracheal perforation due to unsuccessful fiberoptic tracheal intubation. J Clin Anesth. 2006;18(2):135–7. https://doi.org/10.1016/j.jclinane.2005.10.006. PMID: 16563333
38. Marsh NJ. easier Fiberoptic intubations. Anesthesiology. 1992;76:860. https://doi.org/10.1097/00000542-199205000-00031.
39. Fitzgerald E, Hodzovic I, Smith AF. 'From darkness into light': time to make awake intubation with videolaryngoscopy the primary technique for an anticipated difficult airway? Anaesthesia. 2015;70(4):387–92. https://doi.org/10.1111/anae.13042. PMID: 25764402
40. Mihai R, Blair E, Kay H, Cook TM. A quantitative review and meta-analysis of performance of non-standard laryngoscopes and rigid fibreoptic intubation aids. Anaesthesia. 2008;63(7):745–60. https://doi.org/10.1111/j.1365-2044.2008.05489.x. PMID: 18582261
41. El-Boghdadly K, Onwochei DN, Cuddihy J, Ahmad I. A prospective cohort study of awake fibreoptic intubation practice at a tertiary Centre. Anaesthesia. 2017;72:694–703.
42. Alhomary M, Ramadan E, Curran E, Walsh SR. Videolaryngoscopy vs. fibreoptic bronchoscopy for awake tracheal intubation: a systematic review and meta-analysis. Anaesthesia. 2018;73(9):1151–61. https://doi.org/10.1111/anae.14299. Epub 2018 Apr 17. PMID: 29687891
43. Jeyadoss J, Nanjappa N, Nemeth D. Awake intubation using Pentax AWS videolaryngoscope after failed fibreoptic intubation in a morbidly obese patient with a massive thyroid tumour and tracheal compression. Anaesth Intensive Care. 2011;39(2):311–2. PMID: 21485687

Chapter 18
Multimodal Airway Management and Adjuvants

Tomasz Gaszynski

18.1 Introduction

Available now, airway management devices are technically advanced and provide better visualization of the entrance to the larynx, so they should overcome most of the difficulties in airway management. However, there are cases when the use of a single airway device, even a very sophisticated one, may not create sufficient visualization of the glottis and therefore may fail in airway management. In such cases, a multimodal airway management approach may help.

18.2 Fiberoscope Combined with Supraglottic Airway Devices for Endotracheal Intubation

The first example of multimodal airway management techniques is the combined use of supraglottic devices and fiberscopes (or airway scopes) for intubation. Second-generation supraglottic airway devices (SADs) are designed in such a way that it is possible to intubate through their lumen. The difficult airway management guidelines "plan B" are based on the use of supraglottic devices. The use of a second-generation SAD is strongly recommended because it may be necessary to secure the patient's airway with an endotracheal intubation. In situations of unexpected difficult intubation, when a patient is already unconscious and has received muscle

T. Gaszynski (✉)
Medical University of Lodz, Lodz, Poland
e-mail: tomasz.gaszynski@umed.lodz.pl

M. Á. Gómez-Ríos, A. van Zundert (eds.), *Evidence-based Guide to Difficult Airway Management*, https://doi.org/10.1007/978-3-032-30769-9_18

relaxants, performing the fiberoptic intubation (FOI) may be difficult. The patient can not cooperate and maintain spontaneous respiration and a patent airway. There may be secretions and possible blood in the patient's mouth and pharynx, limiting the possibility of visualization of the glottis using FOI because of obstructing the view obtained with the fiberoscope. First and most important at this moment is providing oxygenation to the patient, so inserting the SAD is the recommended method in such a condition. SAD can then serve as a conduit for a fiberoscope, which allows for overcoming the abovementioned problems: the inserted SAD holds the basis of the tongue, and limits the amount of secretions in the ventilation channel, which can be suctioned. The FOI can be performed using the ventilation channel of SAD, which makes it easier and possible to perform fast, even for not very experienced FOI providers (Grade A). No special advantages of one specific second-generation SAD for FOI are observed (Grade A); however, some second-generation SAD are specially designed for facilitating FOI. Some SADs are even equipped with additional marks on the ventilation channels, helping to navigate the tip of the fiberscope. The ventilation channel of SAD guides the fiberoscope to the area of entrance to the larynx and small adjustments are necessary to visualize the glottis and to enter the larynx. Another advantage of this multimodal method is the possibility of ventilation and oxygenation of the patient with SAD during FOI intubation efforts. Removing the SAD in difficult airway patients before performing FOI may lead to loss of airway patency and the following complications. So a multimodal approach in such a situation is recommended. This opportunity of ventilation and oxygenation provides the next possible application of combined use of SAD and FOI for intubation in difficult airway cases: SAD can be inserted under local anesthesia and sedation, and after ensuring proper ventilation, the patient can be generally anaesthetized for FOI intubation. This multimodal approach can be especially useful for the intubation of patients with suspected difficult intubation but with limited possibility of cooperation during the standard awake intubation technique (Grade B). The advantage of using a SAD in such conditions is also the possibility of insertion of SAD in patients with limited mouth opening (the majority of SADs can be inserted with mouth opening >1 cm) and intubation using a fiberoscope when nasal approach for FOI is not possible for some reasons. A good example of this situation may be a patient with a history of difficult intubation requiring urgent intubation after multitrauma injury, cervical collar, and fracture of the base of the skull (Fig. 18.1).

New, third-generation SAD offers visualization of the glottis during insertion and positioning of the SAD. They are equipped with additional channels for a camera attached to the monitor. Using this third-generation SAD allows for the evaluation of the proper positioning of SAD. However, it also gives the possibility of intubation through its lumen when necessary, under the control of vision. It is also possible to use those third-generation SADs together with FOI, which increases the probability of successful intubation, furthermore in very difficult airway cases (Fig. 18.2).

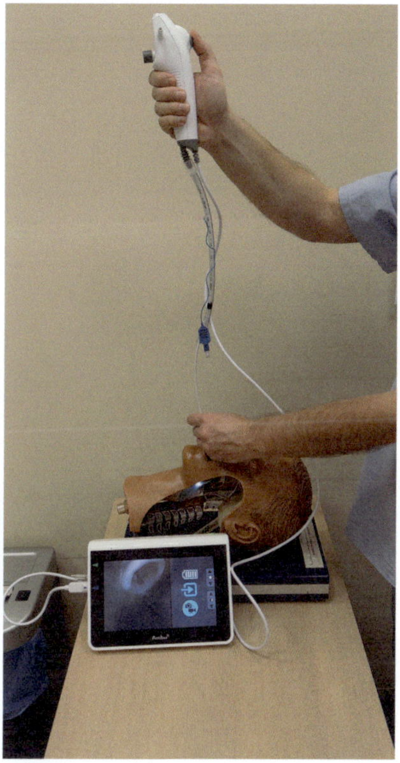

Fig. 18.1 Combination of supraglottic airway device and fiberoptic scope for endotracheal intubation

There are more and more new airway devices for visualization of the entrance of the larynx and their use combined with standard airway devices is possible. For example, optical stylets, also called rigid fiberscopes, can be used together with a standard Macintosh blade laryngoscope. They can be also used together with SADs for intubation through their lumen. However, the author's opinion of this chapter follows the clinical experience with this technique, the main limitation of combined use of optical rigid stylets for intubation through SAD is that curvature of rigid stylet may not allow for insertion to SAD ventilation channel and even if it is done, lack of mobility of tip of rigid stylet may cause failure in endotracheal intubation if entrance to larynx is not positioned centrally in the SAD's end of ventilation channel. In such cases, new optical stylets with moveable tips can be successfully used as some kind of alternative to fiberoptic scopes (Fig. 18.3).

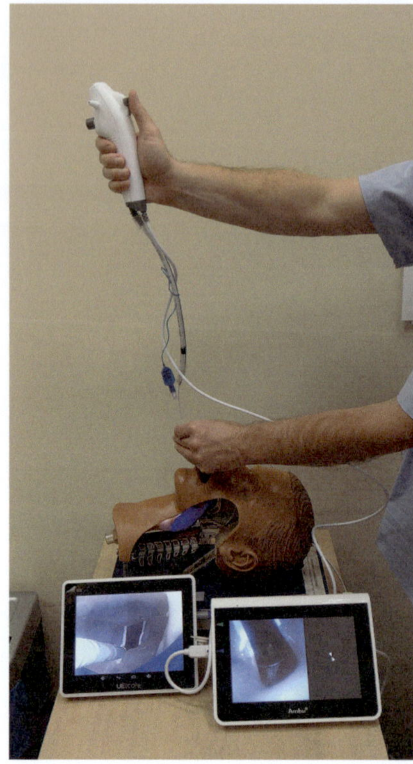

Fig. 18.2 Combined use of third-generation supraglottic video device and fiberoscope

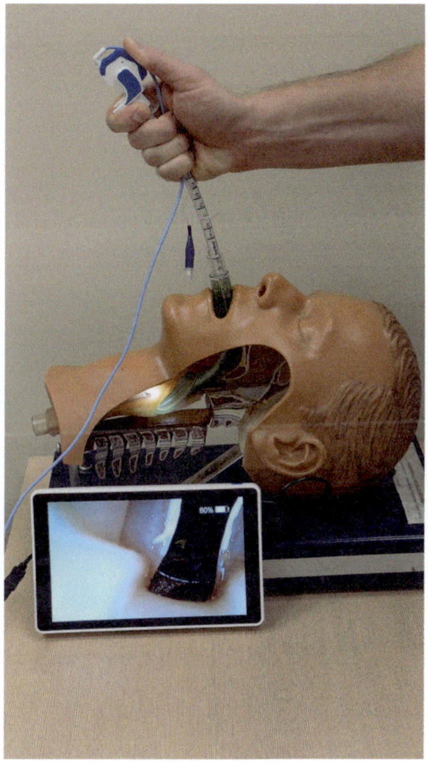

Fig. 18.3 Combined use of video intubation stylet and supraglottic airway device

18.3 Combined Use of Fiberoscope and Videolaryngoscope for Endotracheal Intubation

The next example of a multimodal approach in airway management is the combined use of fiberoptic scope with videolaryngoscopes (VL). In some cases, even the use of a videolaryngoscope may not provide sufficient visualization of the glottis. Rarely, but it may happen that achieved with VL visualization of the glottis can be estimated on the Cormack–Lehane scale 3 or 4. In such conditions, a fiberoptic scope can be used together with VL in the so-called smart stylet technique. In situations of unexpected difficult intubation, when the patient is anesthetized and relaxed, performing FOI may be difficult because of the abovementioned problems: secretions and blood in the mouth and pharynx of the patient. If VL is used and the achieved visualization is not satisfactory, then a fiberoptic scope can be used for the visualization of the glottis, using VL. VL allows for overcoming the abovementioned problems, keeps the basis of the tongue away from the posterior wall of the pharynx, and provides better visualization of anatomical landmarks in the glottis area (Grade B, C, D). The fiberscope can be inserted following the blade of VL and when approaching the glottis area can be navigated towards the entrance of the glottis by looking at VL's monitor. It is enough to visualize epiglottis with VL. Looking

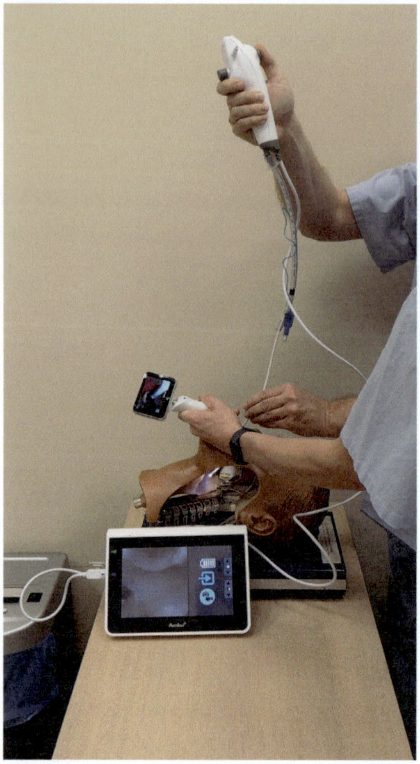

Fig. 18.4 Combined use of a videolaryngoscope and a fiberoptic scope for endotracheal intubation

at the monitor of the fiberoscope, it is possible to localize the entrance to the larynx and perform endotracheal intubation. Different VLs can be used for this technique; however, it may be more suitable to use channeled VLs, as the channel for the endotracheal tube can be used as a conduit for the fiberoptic scope, guiding the tip of the fiberoptic scope to the area of the entrance to the larynx when small adjustments are required to visualize the glottis (Fig. 18.4).

This method can also be used in patients with suspected difficult intubation when FOI alone is not effective in the "awake intubation" technique under local anesthesia (Grade C). Insertion of VL into the mouth of the patient is possible with local anesthesia and produces less gag reflex than the insertion of a standard Macintosh blade laryngoscope. In this multimodal technique for awake FOI combined with VL again, it may be more suitable to use channeled VL because they produce less gag reflex than a Macintosh blade VL.

VL can also be used in combination with a video intubation stylet, which increases visualization of the glottis (Fig. 18.5).

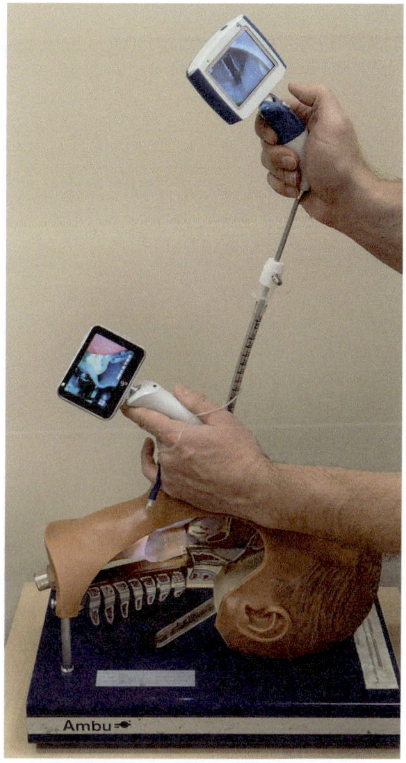

Fig. 18.5 Combined use of video intubation stylet and a videolaryngoscope

18.4 Videolaryngoscopes for Insertion of Supraglottic Airway Devices

A new and promising multimodal airway management technique is the combined use of VL and SAD. The insertion of SAD is performed without any visualization of the glottis. New studies show that in many cases, such a method of placement of SAD may not lead to the correct SAD placement and may cause air leakage during ventilation. This new method of combined use of VL and SAD can provide proper positioning of SAD because of the visualization of the entrance to the larynx (Fig. 18.6).

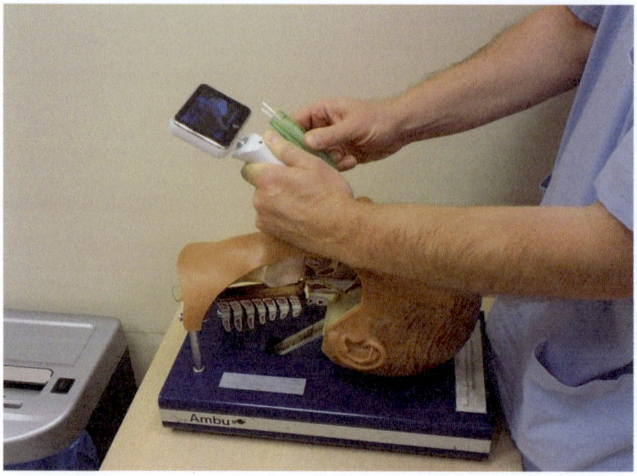

Fig. 18.6 The use of videolaryngoscope for insertion of a supraglottic airway device

18.5 Conclusion

It may be considered to use more often combined techniques of airway management because difficult airway cases consist of a combination of factors that make intubation difficult. To overcome problems, it may be useful to take advantage of the combined strengths of particular airway devices, rather than using those devices separately, which may not provide success in airway management because of specific shortcomings of every airway device used alone.

Although there is a lack of randomized control trials comparing standard airway management techniques based on the use of a single airway device with multimodal airway techniques, based on the clinical experience of many cases of multimodal airway management, this approach seems to have increasing popularity and an increasing number of probable indications to use. This multimodal airway management is especially useful for clinicians who occasionally perform FOI. Multimodal airway management techniques can be applied to an increasing number of airway devices and potentially increase the effectiveness of the procedure, the safety of the patient, and the comfort of intubation providers.

Recommendations

Combined use of a supraglottic airway device and a fiberoptic scope provides better intubation conditions than a fiberoptic scope alone in difficult airway patients (Grade A).

The combined use of videolaryngoscopy and a fiberoptic scope provides better intubation efficiency than using a fiberoptic scope alone in difficult airway patients (Grade A, C).

Further Reading

Francisco OV, Cecil BR, Aaron S, Shannan CC. Videolaryngoscope assisted fiberoptic bronchoscopy for difficult intubation in upper airway cancer. Glob J Oto. 2018;14(3):555888. https://doi.org/10.19080/GJO.2018.14.555888.

Frerk C, Mitchell VS, McNarry AF, Mendonca C, Bhagrath R, Patel A, O'Sullivan EP, Woodall NM, Ahmad I, Difficult Airway Society Intubation Guidelines Working Group. Difficult Airway Society 2015 guidelines for management of unanticipated difficult intubation in adults. Br J Anaesth. 2015;115(6):827–48. https://doi.org/10.1093/bja/aev371. Epub 2015. PMID: 26556848; PMCID: PMC4650961.

Gaszyński T. A combination of KingVision video-laryngoscope and flexible fibroscope for awake intubation in patient with laryngeal tumor—case report and literature review. Anaesthesiol Intensive Ther. 2015;47(4):433–5. https://doi.org/10.5603/AIT.a2015.0019. Epub 2015 Apr 1. PMID: 25830936.

Gómez-Ríos MA, Nieto Serradilla L. Combined use of an Airtraq® optical laryngoscope, Airtraq video camera, Airtraq wireless monitor, and a fibreoptic bronchoscope after failed tracheal intubation. Can J Anaesth. 2011;58(4):411–2. https://doi.org/10.1007/s12630-011-9460-3. Epub 2011 Jan 22. PMID: 21258974.

Jhuang B-J, Luk H-N, Qu JZ, Shikani A. Video-twin technique for airway management, combining video-intubating stylet with videolaryngoscope: a case series report and review of the literature. Healthcare. 2022;10:2175. https://doi.org/10.3390/healthcare10112175.

Koopman EM, van Emden MW, Geurts JJG, Schwarte LA, Schober P. Comparison of videolaryngoscopy alone with video-assisted fibreoptic intubation in a difficult cadaver airway model. Eur J Anaesthesiol. 2021;38(3):318–9. https://doi.org/10.1097/EJA.0000000000001333. PMID: 33538435; PMCID: PMC7932750.

Lenhardt R, Burkhart MT, Brock GN, Kanchi-Kandadai S, Sharma R, Akça O. Is video laryngoscope-assisted flexible tracheoscope intubation feasible for patients with predicted difficult airway? A prospective, randomized clinical trial. Anesth Analg. 2014;118(6):1259–65. https://doi.org/10.1213/ANE.0000000000000220. Erratum in: Anesth Analg. 2015 Feb;120(2):495. PMID: 24842175.

Metterlein T, Dintenfelder A, Plank C, Graf B, Roth G. A comparison of various supraglottic airway devices for fiberoptical guided tracheal intubation. Braz J Anesthesiol. 2017;67(2):166–71. https://doi.org/10.1016/j.bjane.2015.09.007. Epub 2016 May 26. PMID: 28236864.

Michálek P, Donaldson W, McAleavey F, Abraham A, Mathers RJ, Telford C. The i-gel supraglottic airway as a conduit for fibreoptic tracheal intubation – a randomized comparison with the single-use intubating laryngeal mask airway and CTrach laryngeal mask in patients with predicted difficult laryngoscopy. Prague Med Rep. 2016;117(4):164–75. https://doi.org/10.14712/23362936.2016.17. PMID: 27930894.

Ozgul U, Erdil FA, Erdogan MA, et al. Comparison of videolaryngoscope-guided versus standard digital insertion techniques of the ProSeal™ laryngeal mask airway: a prospective randomized study. BMC Anesthesiol. 2019;19:244. https://doi.org/10.1186/s12871-019-0915-3.

Pieters BM, Theunissen M, van Zundert AA. Macintosh blade videolaryngoscopy combined with rigid bonfils intubation endoscope offers a suitable alternative for patients with difficult airways. Anesth Analg. 2018;126(3):988–94. https://doi.org/10.1213/ANE.0000000000002739.

Sharma D, Kim LJ, Ghodke B. Successful airway management with combined use of Glidescope® videolaryngoscope and fiberoptic bronchoscope in a patient with Cowden syndrome. Anesthesiology. 2010;113:253–5. https://doi.org/10.1097/ALN.0b013e3181dfd334.

Van Zundert A, Gatt SP, Kumar CM, Van Zundert TCRV, Pandit JJ. 'Failed supraglottic airway': an algorithm for suboptimally placed supraglottic airway devices based on videolaryngoscopy. Br J Anaesth. 2017;118(5):645–9. https://doi.org/10.1093/bja/aex093.

Van Zundert AAJ, Kumar CM, Van Zundert TCRV, et al. The case for a 3rd generation supraglottic airway device facilitating direct vision placement. J Clin Monit Comput. 2021;35:217–24. https://doi.org/10.1007/s10877-020-00537-4.

Yan CL, Zhang YQ, Chen Y, Qv ZY, Zuo MZ. Comparison of SaCoVLM™ video laryngeal mask-guided intubation and i-gel combined with flexible bronchoscopy-guided intubation in airway management during general anesthesia: a non-inferiority study. BMC Anesthesiol. 2022;22(1):302. https://doi.org/10.1186/s12871-022-01843-x. PMID: 36138363; PMCID: PMC9494909.

Chapter 19
Front of Neck Airway (FONA)

Matthew Bigwood and Chris Frerk

Highlights

- Emergency front of neck airway (eFONA) is a last-resort intervention in cannot intubate, cannot oxygenate (CICO) scenarios.
- Scalpel-bougie cricothyroidotomy is the recommended technique due to its reliability and ability to provide standard ventilation.
- Cannula-based techniques require careful ventilation strategies to prevent barotrauma and complications.
- Frequent hands-on training (every 6–12 months) is crucial to maintain eFONA proficiency.
- Human factors, such as stress and equipment familiarity, significantly impact eFONA success rates.
- A structured airway strategy, including backup plans for failure to intubate or oxygenate, is essential.
- Emerging technologies, such as ultrasound and digital airway registries, may improve future airway management outcomes.

M. Bigwood (✉)
East Lancashire Hospitals, Lancashire, England, UK
e-mail: matthew.bigwood@elht.nhs.uk

C. Frerk
College of Life Sciences/Leicester Medical School, University of Leicester, Leicester, UK

University Hospitals of Northamptonshire, Northamptonshire, England, UK
e-mail: christopher.frerk@nhs.net

M. Á. Gómez-Ríos, A. van Zundert (eds.), *Evidence-based Guide to Difficult Airway Management*, https://doi.org/10.1007/978-3-032-30769-9_19

19.1 Introduction

Front of neck airway (FONA) refers to a situation where the trachea is accessed directly through the anterior aspect of the patient's neck to facilitate oxygenation and ventilation. The trachea can be accessed between the first and second or second and third tracheal rings (via a tracheostomy) or through the cricothyroid membrane (via a cricothyroidotomy).

FONA is usually a planned procedure performed as a tracheostomy, either as part of head and neck surgery or to facilitate ventilation in intensive care (see Chap. 26); rarely, it is required as an urgent or emergency procedure in order to restore or maintain oxygenation when this has proved impossible using standard techniques from above the glottis. For the rest of this chapter, we will only consider emergency FONA (eFONA), which is most commonly performed via a cricothyroidotomy by an anaesthetist in a can't intubate, can't oxygenate (CICO) scenario. This procedure, also known as "*emergency* surgical airway (ESA)", "cric" or "neck rescue", is rare in general anaesthetic practice [1, 2].

Estimates from the fourth national audit, between 1:10,000 and 1:50,000 anaesthetics [3], correlate well with data from the Danish database, showing that 27 out of 452,461 patients required an ESA, representing an incidence of 1 in 16,000 [4]. In the emergency department, where patients present with airway compromise from trauma, tumours, bleeding and infection, the rate is much higher; reports vary depending on populations included but are in the region of 1 in 300 [5]. A similarly higher rate (1 in 400) was found in one study in the intensive care setting [6], with problems encountered at initial intubation and after planned or accidental extubations.

eFONA is a lifesaving intervention, so, despite its rarity, every clinician involved in airway management should be trained and competent to perform it in a CICO situation.

19.2 History

Records indicate that the airway has been accessed through the front of the neck for a long time, with evidence of this practice dating back to ancient Egyptian times. However, it has only become a mainstream procedure in the last 50 years or so [7]. Most research into emergency cricothyroidotomy in the first 20 years of the twenty-first century utilized manikins, animal tissue models, and simulation studies, concentrating on identifying the quickest techniques for accessing the airway and preventing procedural complications, such as equipment failure, device misplacement, and posterior tracheal wall injury [8–11]. Further studies investigated technical problems and complications related to oxygen delivery.

19.2.1 Wide-Bore Cannula Devices

Wide-bore cannula over trochar devices had 15 mm connectors, allowing connection to standard anaesthetic breathing systems, and were available in both cuffed and uncuffed versions. The uncuffed versions offered no protection against aspiration and were thought likely to be associated with significant gas leaks in patients with poorly compliant lungs.

Evidence has accumulated to demonstrate that wide-bore devices are quick to insert but are associated with significant procedural complications.

Wide-bore devices were also produced commercially as Seldinger kits, which contained all the required equipment for the procedure. They were more complicated and took longer to insert than cannula-over-trochar devices [9].

19.2.2 Narrow-Bore Cannulae

By way of contrast, narrow-bore cannulae have been used for many years to provide oxygenation during planned head and neck surgery, with commercial devices produced for this purpose. They have also been recommended in guidelines as a rescue technique in the CICO situation [12].

Some anaesthetists in the past advocated the use of standard intravenous cannulae for this technique due to availability and familiarity. However, in addition to this being an "off licence" use, the lack of kink resistance and shape memory of intravenous cannulae (when compared with transtracheal cannulae) presented a significant risk of failure.

The principal problem identified with narrow-bore cannulae has been the unacceptably high complication rate associated with the high-pressure ventilation devices used for oxygen delivery (e.g. Sanders injector/Manujet). Cannula misplacement, leading to pneumothorax, pneumomediastinum, and/or subcutaneous emphysema, has been reported in more than 89% of rescues in one study [13]. Additionally, unless the upper airway is patent, expiration can only occur through the cannula, presenting a risk of hyperinflation and barotrauma.

19.2.3 Newer Devices

A variety of other devices have been developed and marketed to try to provide "high success, minimum risk" solutions for emergency cricothyroidotomy, but they have not gained widespread adoption in difficult airway carts.

19.3 Current State of Play (2026)

There are currently two eFONA techniques which have considerable support as a means of accessing the trachea through the cricothyroid membrane in a CICO emergency. These include: using a narrow-bore cannula with low-pressure oxygenation or using a scalpel and bougie to place a tracheal tube.

The narrow-bore cannula technique, as described by Heard [14], has very specific requirements regarding the choice of cannula, ventilation device, and ventilation strategy to minimize the risk of failure and complications.

The scalpel-bougie approach, advocated by the UK Difficult Airway Society [15], also has a tightly specified equipment list, but offers the benefit that ventilation can be achieved using a standard anaesthetic breathing system or a self-inflating bag, and that exhaled carbon dioxide can be measured to provide confirmation of the correct placement of the airway.

Both techniques have clearly defined, detailed steps for insertion to minimize the risk of failure. These need to be rehearsed regularly to maintain an appropriate level of procedural skill. It is beyond the scope of this chapter to describe these techniques in detail, however a brief description can be found below.

19.3.1 Narrow-Bore Cannula Cricothyroidotomy [14]

- Identify and stabilize cricothyroid membrane.
- Hold the 5 mL syringe attached to the specified cannula in the dominant hand.
- Insert the needle caudally at around 45°.
- Aspirate on the syringe throughout.
- Stop when air is freely aspirated.
- Stabilize cannula hub with the non-dominant hand.
- Stabilize the trochar against the patient with the dominant hand.
- Advance the cannula into the airway and remove the trochar.
- Check for free air aspiration from cannula to confirm placement.

19.3.2 Scalpel Cricothyroidotomy [15]

- Position neck in maximal extension and identify laryngeal anatomy.
- Non-dominant hand holds the skin in tension whilst the dominant hand performs a midline incision.

- Perform blunt dissection, stabilize larynx and identify cricothyroid membrane.
- Transverse stab incision with cutting edge towards you.
- Twist scalpel 90° so cutting edge faces caudally.
- Swap hands so the non-dominant hand holds the scalpel.
- Gently pull scalpel towards you and slide bougie along blade and into trachea.
- Remove scalpel and hold bougie with the non-dominant hand.
- Railroad size 6.0 tracheal tube over bougie, twisting as you go.
- Remove bougie and attach breathing circuit.

Studies have demonstrated that skills for a number of cricothyroidotomy techniques fade, with the decline becoming apparent after 6 months [16], supporting the call for regular retraining [17, 18] to maintain personal preparedness to perform eFONA.

19.4 Guidelines

For an emergency procedure such as eFONA, a guideline should not only describe in detail the technical skills required but also encourage recognition of the importance of human factors in influencing task performance under pressure, including the impact of reduced capacity for decision making in high-stress situations. Guidelines can be useful in including cognitive aids and recommendations for the optimal use of non-technical skills in emergency situations. Many airway algorithms and guidelines exist from individual institutions and specialist anaesthetic airway societies around the world [19–21]. The final step in all of them is "eFONA" as a final attempt to rescue a "lost" airway and save a patient's life.

Over the years, many guidelines steered clear of identifying a specific procedure for CICO, in part because of the lack of grade A evidence for the superiority of any one technique over another. Some current guidelines still give no preferred method and just instruct a "trained person" to carry out the procedure [21]. This can lead to two distinct but related problems: First, in the midst of an unfolding emergency, clinicians have to decide which technique to use (which will be difficult at a time of high cognitive load). Second, emergency airway carts become cluttered with a variety of preferred devices from different clinicians, leading to potential confusion when locating the necessary equipment in a time-critical emergency.

Until recently, human factors considerations such as these have been largely overlooked in emergency airway guidelines, with little attention given to the deterioration in personal and team performance in high-stress emergency situations

[22]. The value of reliable systems and well-designed equipment to support healthcare workers has also been underestimated [23].

Some guidelines, including the original 2004 DAS guideline [12] and the 2017 ANZCA guidelines [24], limited the choice to one of two techniques: scalpel-bougie or narrow-bore cannula. This meant that only two sets of equipment needed to be stored in the emergency airway cart. However, it still required clinicians to make a "high stakes" decision during an emergency, a time of high stress, which could potentially add extra delay before starting the procedure.

19.4.1 Guidelines Specifying One Particular Procedure in Detail

A narrow-bore cannula technique is recommended in the Royal Perth Hospital guideline [14, 25, 26]. They theorize that the familiarity of a cannula provides less of a "mental hurdle" to performing the procedure. If true, this could lead to less delay, and therefore potentially less morbidity and mortality. A scalpel-bougie approach is only required (and importantly, is still possible) if the cannula rescue fails.

The Difficult Airway Society recommends the scalpel-bougie technique as the sole rescue technique in their 2025 guidelines [15], as well as by other organizations that endorse them [27]. The guideline authors acknowledge the lack of grade A or B evidence for the superiority of any particular technique, but considered the simplicity of the equipment required and the ability to measure exhaled CO2 by connecting to standard breathing systems to make this technique appropriate.

Both of the above techniques have minimal equipment needs, reducing complexity and minimizing the time taken to gather the necessary equipment. The scalpel-bougie technique requires a scalpel (10-blade), a bougie, and a 6.0 ID cuffed tracheal tube. The cannula technique (for initial rescue) requires a non-kinking (14G Insyte) cannula, a syringe containing saline, and a "rapid O_2" ventilation device (see Fig. 19.1 [28]).

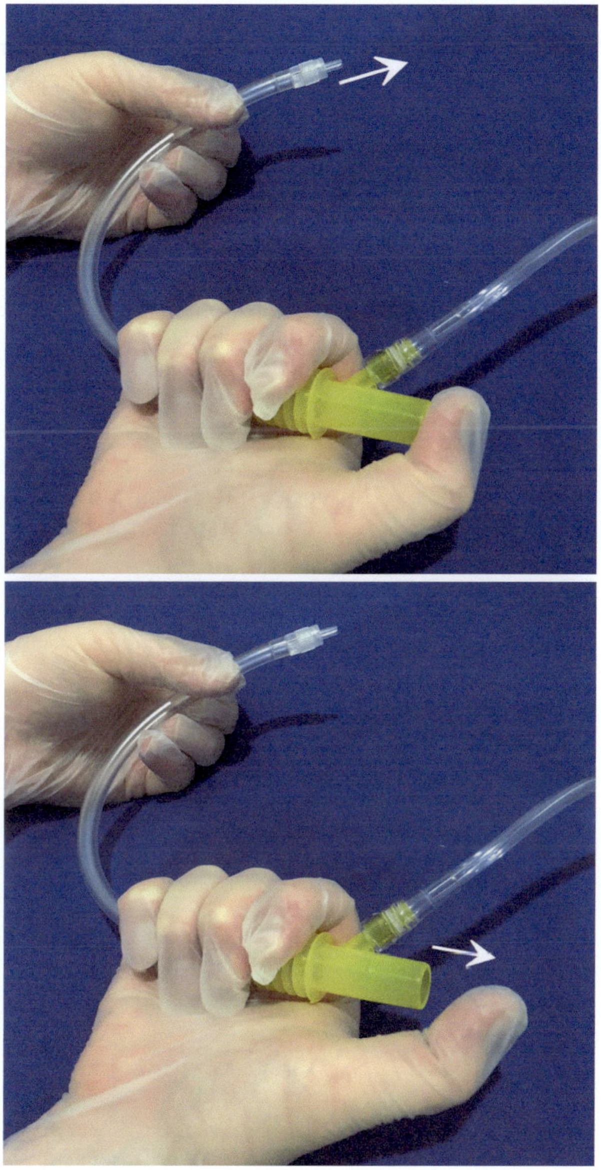

Fig. 19.1 The Meditech's rapid O_2 device

19.5 Scalpel-Bougie vs. Narrow-Bore Cannula Technique

As previously discussed, it is unknown which of these two techniques would be most effective if deployed as an organizational standard operating procedure (SOP). There have been no (and likely never will be) randomized controlled trials that can definitively determine which technique has the highest success and lowest complication rates. Published guidelines rely on expert opinion, case series reports for surgical techniques, and wet lab data for narrow-bore cannula cricothyroidotomy. Most case series originate from prehospital emergency medicine [29], where training and environmental factors differ significantly from hospital-based anaesthetic services. The wet lab data from Heard et al. demonstrated a high success rate for narrow-bore cannula cricothyroidotomy in rescuing the airway in sheep; however, its applicability to hospital-based settings remains uncertain [14, 30, 31]. However a recent case series of narrow-bore cannula technique being used in 8 patients over 19 years showed promising and safe results [32].

The key characteristics of each technique, including their advantages, disadvantages, and specific requirements, are summarized in Table 19.1. This comparison facilitates a clearer understanding of the factors to consider when selecting the most appropriate approach in an emergency situation.

For safe ventilation, the narrow-bore cannula requires specific additional equipment, such as the "rapid O_2", a purpose-designed device that connects to a standard oxygen flowmetre. This device allows an open port to be occluded with a digit to

Table 19.1 Comparison of scalpel-bougie and narrow-bore cannula techniques

Aspect	Scalpel-Bougie	Narrow-bore cannula
Technique	Stab incision with a No. 10 blade through the cricothyroid membrane. A bougie is inserted alongside the blade into the airway. A 6.0 mm cuffed tracheal tube is then railroaded over the bougie into the trachea, and the cuff is inflated	A narrow-bore cannula-over-needle is inserted through the cricothyroid membrane (or between tracheal rings) while attached to a syringe containing a small amount of saline. Continuous aspiration is used to confirm airway entry as air is aspirated into the syringe. The cannula is then threaded off the needle into the airway
Advantages and disadvantages	The cuffed tube provides a definitive airway, protecting against aspiration and enabling positive pressure ventilation, even in patients with poor lung compliance	Does not initially protect the airway but can be upgraded to a cuffed device after stabilization, either by performing a formal tracheostomy or using the Seldinger technique with a guidewire through the existing cannula
How to proceed if the cricothyroid membrane cannot be identified	8–10 cm vertical cranial-caudal incision, followed by blunt fingertip dissection to locate the larynx. The scalpel-bougie technique is then performed from this point	8–10 cm vertical cranial-caudal incision, followed by blunt fingertip dissection to locate the larynx or the trachea. The cannula technique is then performed from this point
Confirmation of device position	Same as for all tracheal intubations: observe for the presence (or absence) of sustained exhaled carbon dioxide, which is the gold standard used by anaesthetists	Stepwise confirmation: (1) aspiration of air during and after placement (2) Haptic/tactile feedback during the first ventilation attempt using the rapid O_2 device, where variations in pressure on the thumb or finger occluding the device in order to deliver oxygen can be detected (3) Rise in oxygen saturations

control oxygen delivery. Heard et al. describe a specific standard operating procedure, known as "minimal ventilation", to reduce the risk of hyperinflation and barotrauma [31, 33]. The oxygen flow is set to 15 L/min, with the first "breath" lasting 4 s (1000 mL). Subsequent two-second (500 mL) breaths should only be administered as needed, defined as when the oxygen saturations have fallen by 5% from the peak rise after the previous breath.

Both techniques can fail, particularly if procedural steps are not followed precisely. Potential failure modes include scalpel blade positioning that prevents bougie insertion if not held perpendicular to the floor, or a false-positive air aspiration sign, which can lead to misplacement of the cannula if the needle is accidentally withdrawn, even slightly, during advancement through tissues.

Bleeding is inevitable during the scalpel-bougie approach and may contaminate the airway. Nevertheless, it rarely requires surgical intervention for haemostasis. Endobronchial intubation is another well-recognized complication but is easily corrected. In contrast, bleeding is uncommon with the cannula approach, and endobronchial intubation is not a concern, as the cannula is too short to reach the carina. Kinking of the cannula may still occur, especially if inserted at a steep angle.

Other complications associated with the cannula technique include pneumothorax, pneumomediastinum, and subcutaneous emphysema. These complications are generally less severe when oxygenating with a low-pressure source compared to much of the published data, which primarily relates to high-pressure oxygen sources [13]. Posterior tracheal wall injury can occur with both techniques.

19.6 Preparing for eFONA

Nationally agreed guidelines and training standards provide a framework for organizations and clinicians. Each organization should establish a clear strategy and standard operating procedure for eFONA. Systems must ensure that all staff receive adequate training and that essential equipment is readily available for this rare, time-critical emergency. Individual clinicians are responsible for maintaining proficiency in the technical skills required by their organization's SOP and for knowing the location of the necessary equipment. Finally, clinicians must recognize and prepare for the differences in decision-making and technical execution that arise in a real CICO emergency compared to even the most realistic simulated scenarios.

19.6.1 National Strategy

Professional and regulatory bodies can mandate training requirements. The Australian and New Zealand College of Anaesthetists (ANZCA) was the first organization to mandate regular simulated eFONA management for CICO scenarios as part of revalidation requirements [34].

19.6.2 *Organizational Preparedness*

Even when eFONA training is not mandated nationally, individual hospitals and departments can still provide and encourage participation. Basic technical skills training is useful and easier to implement than running immersive multidisciplinary simulation training. However, simulation-based emergency drills offer the opportunity to develop and practise essential non-technical skills in a safe environment. In situ simulation can be integrated into any hospital setting, with the added benefit of identifying location-specific system issues.

The equipment required depends on the chosen technique; having a national standard simplifies the process for individual organizations to establish local policies on equipment availability. For example, the Difficult Airway Society national standard states that all anaesthetists should be trained in the "scalpel-bougie-tube" technique [15].

Both techniques described above require minimal equipment, allowing every anaesthesia location to have a pre-prepared eFONA pack stored in transparent packaging on the airway cart, ensuring it is "ready to go" with all necessary equipment in one place.

19.6.3 *Individual Preparedness*

Every clinician involved in airway management has a personal responsibility to learn how to use eFONA equipment and to rehearse and maintain this skill. This is best achieved through regular training sessions organized by each hospital or service. At a minimum, eFONA practice should follow national and institutional recommendations regarding technique and frequency.

Maintaining procedural competence is essential, but individual preparation should also focus on understanding and anticipating the differences between training and real-life emergencies. These differences are most apparent in decision-making, technical skill performance, bleeding, and stress management.

19.6.3.1 Decision-Making

The decision to transition from attempts to ventilate and oxygenate using facemask ventilation, a supraglottic airway, or a tracheal tube to performing an eFONA is among the most difficult decisions an anaesthetist will ever face. Several strategies exist to facilitate this transition when necessary.

The Vortex approach emphasizes that this transition should involve a gradual increase in preparedness, occurring alongside other airway management steps, such as calling for help, allocating roles, gathering, and ultimately opening equipment [19, 35]. Some steps in cricothyroidotomy are technically simple but may be overlooked, for example, ensuring complete paralysis to rule out laryngospasm as the cause of CICO, optimizing patient positioning, and maintaining oxygenation attempts through the upper airway using a facemask, supraglottic airway, or nasal high flow oxygen during eFONA.

The use of algorithms and action cards has been shown to decrease the risk of omitting critical steps [36]. Additionally, enhancing education on non-technical skills and improving situational awareness can help mitigate task fixation and loss of time perception.

Other critical steps are easy to remember but technically difficult to perform, requiring repeated practice to ensure proficiency.

19.6.3.2 Identification of the Larynx and Cricothyroid Membrane

Practising cricothyroidotomy on a plastic manikin or part-task trainer aids in technical skill acquisition, but standardized anatomy—often marked by pre-existing holes from previous training exercises—does not significantly help with the real-world challenge of identifying the larynx in patients, where clinical examination remains the mainstay.

The cricothyroid membrane (CTM) is composed of fibroelastic tissue and connects the thyroid cartilage superiorly to the cricoid cartilage inferiorly. It is laterally bordered by the bilateral cricothyroid muscles. Unfortunately, the laryngeal prominence of the thyroid cartilage is often the only visible landmark, if any, making palpation necessary.

Studies indicate that palpation alone correctly identifies the cricothyroid membrane in only 24–62% of cases [37–39]. The Laryngeal handshake, proposed by Levitan [40] is recommended by DAS as a technique to improve tactile confidence in recognizing the cone-shaped laryngeal anatomy. This method involves a firm side-to-side "handshake" with the non-dominant hand, using the thumb and middle finger to locate the hyoid, thyroid cartilage, and cricoid cartilage, followed by stabilizing the larynx and identifying the cricothyroid membrane with the index finger. A recent meta-analysis showed no significant difference in the success rate of cricothyroid membrane identification [Risk Ratio 1.09, 95% CI 0.89–1.34, $p = 0.41$] between the laryngeal handshake and palpation alone [41]. The absence of demonstrated inferiority allows the laryngeal handshake to remain a standard technique for teaching, learning, and practice until a more effective alternative is identified.

Ultrasound identification of the cricothyroid membrane is becoming increasingly common. Emerging data suggest that ultrasound is highly accurate for locating the cricothyroid membrane, but takes longer than clinical examination [42]. In the future, as ultrasound machines become ubiquitous, more mobile, and faster to power up, their use in hypoxic emergencies may be recommended in clinical guidelines.

19.6.3.3 Bleeding

Bleeding is inevitable when using the scalpel-bougie technique. The suprasternal notch can accumulate blood from subcutaneous tissue and occasionally from vessels overlying the cricothyroid membrane, making the procedure inherently blind in real-life scenarios. Therefore, it should be rehearsed with this in mind. In contrast, significant bleeding is highly unlikely with the cannula technique, meaning the technical skill required closely resembles that practiced during training.

19.6.3.4 Dealing with/Managing Stress

At the earliest opportunity, the primary airway clinician should be relieved of overall patient care responsibility. CICO situations are extremely stressful, and ongoing clinical management may become compromised. Transferring responsibility to another clinician can help maintain optimal patient safety and decision-making.

19.7 Post-procedure Management

If rescue is successful, which occurs in approximately 85% of cases [3], an urgent review by an ENT surgeon is required. At this stage, a tracheostomy may be performed, and immediate complications—such as bleeding, secondary tracheal or laryngeal injury, and formation of false passages—should be actively assessed and treated.

A chest X-ray should be performed to check for pneumothorax or pneumomediastinum. The next steps will depend on the device used and the patient's pre-existing clinical condition.

- If surgery is not immediately life-threatening, it should be postponed, and a decision should be made on whether to wake the patient or transfer them to a Critical Care Unit for further stabilization.
- If lifesaving surgery is required or the patient remains critically ill, they should remain anaesthetized, and once the airway is secured, other necessary management can proceed.

19.8 Team Debrief

A team debrief following an emergency, such as eFONA, is considered beneficial by some. However, evidence suggests that a full psychological debrief for all staff involved in a critical event may cause more harm than good [43].

Certain structured tools, facilitated by appropriately trained staff, can support an immediate "diffusion meeting". These meetings can be beneficial if they are brief and include ongoing supportive follow-up [44]. While informal peer support has long been practiced, structured peer support tools, such as Trauma Risk Management (TRiM) [45], now provide a standardized framework for managing the immediate aftermath of critical events. These tools help identify staff members who may benefit from professional psychological support and can direct them to appropriate services [46].

19.9 Follow-Up

All patients who have undergone eFONA should be followed up by the anaesthetist involved, supported by a head of department or departmental airway lead. Many healthcare systems impose a "duty of candour", requiring clinical staff to fully disclose events to patients. Even when this is not an organizational requirement, patients should be provided with a clear explanation of what happened and given the opportunity to ask questions. A summary letter should be sent to the patient, with a copy to their primary care physician. eFONA carries risks of long-term complications, including tracheal stenosis, scarring, and voice changes. If any of these complications occur, follow-up with an ENT specialist will be required.

In addition to documenting all relevant details in the patient's personal medical record, this information should be entered into local and national "difficult airway databases" whenever possible. The Difficult Airway Society maintains a database [47] that enables clinical staff to access case information, including details of difficult tracheal intubations and other serious airway events.

- Patients whose details are recorded in the system receive an alert card with information about their airway difficulties, which they can provide to healthcare staff in future encounters.
- The DAS database also serves as a "big data" source, enabling trend analysis in the management of difficult airways [48].
- Specifically for eFONA, a mobile-accessible database (the airway app) [49, 50] has been developed to capture eFONA attempts and outcomes, thereby helping to refine airway management techniques.

19.10 The Future

The airway App [49, 50] project has provided evidence that it is possible to collect and analyse eFONA data using a smartphone application. Through a series of drop-down menus, the app gathers information on patient demographics, use of muscle relaxation, oxygen saturation levels, confidence in locating the cricothyroid membrane, equipment, and oxygen delivery methods used. The app also prompts users to provide feedback on human factors associated with the event, such as teamwork and shared mental models.

Over time, this data may help determine which techniques are most effective in "real-world" CICO situations. However, since participation in the system is voluntary, there is no denominator data, making it impossible to determine incidence rates. Furthermore, reporting bias (e.g. over-reporting of successful cases, under-reporting of unsuccessful ones, or disproportionate participation from certain units) may limit the accuracy of findings on eFONA prevalence and management trends.

A collaboration between DAS and the RCoA is currently developing an eFONA registry for the United Kingdom [51]. At the time of writing, the registry had not yet been launched. Its goal is to systematically capture all eFONA cases across the United Kingdom. This initiative aims to provide more accurate data on this emergency intervention, enabling large datasets to guide future guideline development.

Recommendations

1. Institutions should establish and implement a clear standard operating procedure (SOP) for emergency front-of-neck access (eFONA), including the chosen technique, required equipment, and defined team roles (Grade D).
2. A single, standardized eFONA technique should be adopted within each institution to reduce cognitive load, variability, and delay during a crisis (Grade D).
3. When a surgical approach is selected, the scalpel-bougie-tube technique should be considered to facilitate placement of a cuffed tracheal tube, allow conventional ventilation, and enable confirmation with capnography (Grade C).
4. If a cannula technique is used, an appropriate non-kinking cannula and a low-pressure oxygen delivery system should be employed, with a predefined strategy to minimize the risk of barotrauma (Grade C).
5. Regular hands-on training in eFONA should be provided, with refresher training at least every 6–12 months to mitigate skill decay (Grade B).
6. Cognitive aids and a structured approach to escalation should be used to support a timely transition to eFONA in "cannot intubate, cannot oxygenate" situations (Grade C). Training should emphasize systematic identification of the cricothyroid membrane and include a clear alternative strategy for cases in which surface landmarks are impalpable (Grade B).
7. Ultrasound may be used to identify the cricothyroid membrane in advance when time, equipment, and expertise allow, particularly in patients at high risk of difficult anatomy (Grade B).

(continued)

8. Following successful eFONA, early otolaryngology review and structured assessment for complications should be undertaken (Grade D).
9. The eFONA event should be clearly documented, communicated to the patient and relevant healthcare providers, and recorded in airway alert or difficult airway systems where available (Grade D).
10. A structured team debrief should be conducted after an eFONA event, with access to ongoing support as required, while avoiding mandatory universal psychological debriefing (Grade B).

References

1. Nagaro T, Yorozuya T, Sotani M, et al. Survey of patients whose lungs could not be ventilated and whose trachea could not be intubated in university hospitals in Japan. J Anesth. 2003;17(4):232–40.
2. Kheterpal S, Martin L, Shanks AM, Tremper KK. Prediction and outcomes of impossible mask ventilation: a review of 50,000 anesthetics. Anesthesiology. 2009;110(4):891–7.
3. Cook TM, Woodall N, Ferk C. Major complications of airway management in the UK: results of the Fourth National Audit Project of the Royal College of Anaesthetists and the Difficult Airway Society. Part 1: Anaesthesia. Br J Anaesth. 2011;106:617–31.
4. Rosenstock CV, Nørskov AK, Wetterslev J, Lundstrøm LH, Danish Anaesthesia Database. Emergency surgical airway management in Denmark: a cohort study of 452 461 patients registered in the Danish Anaesthesia Database. Br J Anaesth. 2016;117(Suppl 1):i75–82.
5. Kwon YS, Lee CA, Park S, Ha SO, Sim YS, Baek MS. Incidence and outcomes of cricothyrotomy in the “cannot intubate, cannot oxygenate” situation. Medicine. 2019;98(42):e17713.
6. Martin LD, Mhyre JM, Shanks AM, Tremper KK, Kheterpal S. 3,423 emergency tracheal intubations at a university hospital: airway outcomes and complications. Anesthesiology. 2011;114(1):42–8.
7. McKenna P, Desai NM, Morley EJ. Cricothyrotomy. Treasure Island: StatPearls Publishing; 2022.
8. Vadodaria BS, Gandhi SD, McIndoe AK. Comparison of four different emergency airway access equipment sets on a human patient simulator. Anaesthesia. 2004;59(1):73–9.
9. Dimitriadis JC, Paoloni R. Emergency cricothyroidotomy: a randomised crossover study of four methods. Anaesthesia. 2008;63(11):1204–8.
10. Murphy C, Rooney SJ, Maharaj CH, Laffey JG, Harte BH. Comparison of three cuffed emergency percutaneous cricothyroidotomy devices to conventional surgical cricothyroidotomy in a porcine model. Br J Anaesth. 2011;106(1):57–64.
11. King W, Teare J, Vandrevala T, Cartwright S, Mohammed KB, Patel B. Evaluation of a novel Surgicric® cricothyroidotomy device for emergency tracheal access in a porcine model. Anaesthesia. 2016;71(2):177–84.
12. Henderson JJ, Popat MT, Latto IP, Pearce AC, Difficult Airway Society. Difficult Airway Society guidelines for management of the unanticipated difficult intubation. Anaesthesia. 2004;59(7):675–94.
13. Peterson GN, Domino KB, Caplan RA, Posner KL, Lee LA, Cheney FW. Management of the difficult airway: a closed claims analysis. Anesthesiology. 2005;103(1):33–9.
14. Heard AM, Green RJ, Eakins P. The formulation and introduction of a ‘can’t intubate, can’t ventilate’ algorithm into clinical practice. Anaesthesia. 2009;64(6):601–8.
15. Ahmad I, El-Boghdadly K, Iliff H. Difficult Airway Society 2025 guidelines for management of unanticipated difficult tracheal intubation in adults. Br J Anaesth. 2026;136(1):283–307.

16. GMC Skills fade: a review of the evidence that clinical and professional skills fade during time out of practice, and of how skills fade may be measured or remediated. 2014. https://www.gmc-uk.org/about/what-we-do-and-why/data-and-research/research-and-insight-archive/skills-fade-literature-review. Accessed 3 July 2025.
17. Price TM, McCoy EP. Emergency front of neck access in airway management. BJA Educ. 2019;19(8):246–53.
18. Baker PA, Weller JM, Greenland KB, Riley RH, Merry AF. Education in airway management. Anaesthesia. 2011;66(Suppl 2):101–11.
19. Chrimes N, Fritz P. The Vortex Approach to airway management. 2013. http://www.vortexapproach.org. Accessed 3 July 2025.
20. Law JA, Duggan LV, Asselin M, et al. Canadian Airway Focus Group updated consensus-based recommendations for management of the difficult airway: part 1. Difficult airway management encountered in an unconscious patient. Can J Anaesth. 2021;68(9):1373–404.
21. Apfelbaum JL, Hagberg CA, Connis RT, et al. 2022 American Society of Anesthesiologists practice guidelines for management of the difficult airway. Anesthesiology. 2022;136(1):31–81.
22. Cummings S. Inquest into the death of Glenda May Logsdail – Regulation 28: report to prevent future deaths. 2021. https://www.judiciary.UK/wp-content/uploads/2021/09/Glenda-Logsdail-Prevention-of-future-deaths-report-2021-0295_Published.pdf. Accessed 3 July 2025.
23. Edelman DA, Duggan LV, Lockhart SL, Marshall SD, Turner MC, Brewster DJ. Prevalence and commonality of non-technical skills and human factors in airway management guidelines: a narrative review of the last 5 years. Anaesthesia. 2022;77(10):1129–36.
24. ANZCA. PG61(A) guideline for the management of evolving airway obstruction: transition to the can't intubate can't oxygenate airway emergency 2017. 2017. https://www.anzca.edu.au/getattachment/71f54974-314a-4d96-bef2-c03f39c8a8e9/PG61(A)-Guideline-for-management-of-evolving-airway-obstruction-transition-to-CICO-airway-emergency. Accessed 3 July 2025.
25. Ibrahim Z, Tarrant K, Heard AM. Royal Perth Hospital airway & head and neck anesthesiology fellowship. J Head Neck Anesth. 2019;3(1):e12.
26. Heard A, Dinsmore J, Douglas S, Lacquiere D. Plan D: cannula first, or scalpel only? Br J Anaesth. 2016;117(4):533–5.
27. Higgs A, McGrath BA, Goddard C. Guidelines for the management of tracheal intubation in critically ill adults. Br J Anaesth. 2018;120:323–52.
28. Meditech. Metitech News. 2018. https://www.meditechsystems.com.au/news. Accessed 3 July 2025.
29. Lockey D, Crewdson K, Weaver A, Davies G. Observational study of the success rates of intubation and failed intubation airway rescue techniques in 7256 attempted intubations of trauma patients by pre-hospital physicians. Br J Anaesth. 2014;113(2):220–5.
30. Heard A, Gordon H, Douglas S, et al. Front-of-neck airway rescue with impalpable anatomy during a simulated cannot intubate, cannot oxygenate scenario: scalpel-finger-cannula versus scalpel-finger-bougie in a sheep model. Br J Anaesth. 2020;125(2):184–91.
31. Heard A. Percutaneous emergency oxygenation strategies in the "can't intubate, can't oxygenate" scenario. Smashworks. 2013. Available from https://www.smashwords.com/books/view/377530. Accessed 3 July 2025.
32. Heard A, Lacquiere D, Gordon H, et al. A case series of the Royal Perth Hospital cannula-first approach in the 'can't intubate, can't oxygenate' scenario. Anaesth Intensive Care. 2024;52(3):159–67.
33. DrAMBHeardAirway. 06 jet oxygenation. In: YouTube. 2013. https://www.youtube.com/watch?v=QR7ek7VBNiQ. Accessed 3 July 2025.
34. ANZCA & FPM. CPD program: emergency responses. 2022. https://libguides.anzca.edu.au/cpd/emergency. Accessed 3 July 2025.
35. Chrimes N, Higgs A, Rehak A. Lost in transition: the challenges of getting airway clinicians to move from the upper airway to the neck during an airway crisis. Br J Anaesth. 2020;125(1):e38–46.

36. Harvey R, Foulds L, Housden T, et al. The impact of didactic read-aloud action cards on the performance of cannula cricothyroidotomy in a simulated 'can't intubate can't oxygenate' scenario. Anaesthesia. 2017;72(3):343–9.
37. Aslani A. Accuracy of identification of the cricothyroid membrane in female subjects using palpation: an observational study. Anesth Analg. 2012;114:987–92.
38. Drew T, McCaul CL. Laryngeal handshake technique in locating the cricothyroid membrane: a non-randomised comparative study. Br J Anaesth. 2018;121(5):1173–8.
39. Bair AE, Chima R. The inaccuracy of using landmark techniques for cricothyroid membrane identification: a comparison of three techniques. Acad Emerg Med. 2015;22:908–14.
40. Levitan RM. Cricothyrotomy with laryngeal handshake, sternal stabilization. https://www.airwaycam.com/videos/. Accessed 3 July 2025.
41. Hung KC, Lin YT, Sun CK. Comparison between laryngeal handshake and palpation techniques in the identification of cricothyroid membrane: a meta-analysis. J Clin Monit Comput. 2021;35(5):1235–8.
42. Rai Y, You-Ten E, Zasso F, De Castro C, Ye XY, Siddiqui N. The role of ultrasound in front-of-neck access for cricothyroid membrane identification: a systematic review. J Crit Care. 2020;60:161–8.
43. Brooks SK, Rubin GJ, Greenberg N. Traumatic stress within disaster-exposed occupations: overview of the literature and suggestions for the management of traumatic stress in the workplace. Br Med Bull. 2019;129:25–34.
44. Johnson TJ, Millinchamp FJ, Kelly FE. Use of a team immediate debrief tool to improve staff well-being after potentially traumatic events. Anaesthesia. 2019;76:1001–2.
45. Greenberg N, Langston V, Jones N. Trauma risk management (TRiM) in the UK armed forces. J R Army Med Corps. 2018;154:124–7.
46. Kelly FE, Osborn M, Stacey MS. Improving resilience in anaesthesia and intensive care medicine—learning lessons from the military. Anaesthesia. 2020;75:720–3.
47. Difficult Airway Society. Difficult Airway Database. 2021. https://das.uk.com/dad. Accessed 3 July 2025.
48. Sajayan A, Nair A, McNarry AF, Mir F, Ahmad I, El-Boghdadly K. Analysis of a national difficult airway database. Anaesthesia. 2022;77(10):1081–8.
49. Duggan LV, Cook TM, Lockhart SL, O'Sullivan EP, Baker PA. Emergency front-of-neck airway: an update from the Airway App. Br J Anaesth. 2020;125(1):E212–3.
50. Duggan LV, Lockhart SL, Cook TM, O'Sullivan EP, Dare T, Baker PA. The Airway App: exploring the role of smartphone technology to capture emergency front-of-neck airway experiences internationally. Anaesthesia. 2018;73(6):703–10.
51. eFONA registry: an update. 2022 https://rcoa.ac.uk/bulletin/october-2022/efona-registry-update. Accessed 3 July 2025.

Chapter 20
Extubation of the At-Risk Airway

Sheila Nainan Myatra and Jeson Rajan Doctor

20.1 Introduction

Extubation is the purposeful removal of a tracheal tube. Extubation is an elective procedure involving the transition from an established airway to a normal natural airway [1]. Extubation should be carried out in a controlled manner with the same standards and care that are available at induction of anaesthesia and tracheal intubation [2].

Extubation failure is defined as the inability of the patient to maintain a patent airway with effective spontaneous ventilation after the purposeful removal of the previously placed tracheal tube within a specified time [1]. Majority of the problems following extubation failure are of a minor nature, but serious complications like hypoxia, brain injury, and death have been reported. The incidence of perioperative extubation failure is 0.1–0.45%, while extubation failure in the critically ill is between 0.4% and 25% [3].

The term "*difficult extubation*" is a misnomer, as, unlike tracheal intubation, removal of the tube from the trachea is not difficult. Extubation of the "*at-risk*" airway includes those conditions or situations due to which there is an increased risk of extubation failure or complications during extubation. These include but are not limited to patients who have a normal airway, but have medical conditions which require suppression of haemodynamic responses (pressor response), a difficult airway (difficult mask ventilation or tracheal intubation or difficult reintubation), delayed recovery or awakening from anaesthesia, pre-existing diseases e.g. obstructive sleep apnoea (OSA), rheumatoid arthritis, cervical spine disease, etc., surgical causes for airway compromise e.g. maxillofacial surgery, surgeries causing damage

S. N. Myatra (✉) · J. R. Doctor
Department of Anaesthesiology, Critical Care and Pain, Tata Memorial Hospital, Homi Bhabha National Institute, Mumbai, India

M. Á. Gómez-Ríos, A. van Zundert (eds.), *Evidence-based Guide to Difficult Airway Management*, https://doi.org/10.1007/978-3-032-30769-9_20

to nerves supplying the airway, spine fixation, etc., airway oedema or airway collapse [1].

In this chapter, we enumerate the various risk factors for the occurrence of extubation failure and complications during extubation. Unlike tracheal intubation, which may sometimes be required in an emergency, extubation is always an elective procedure. We describe various strategies and precautions to be taken while extubating the "at-risk" patients, in order to promote safe extubation. Various societies have issued guidelines for aiding clinicians to perform safe extubation [1, 2, 4].

20.2 Complications During Extubation [2]

1. *Altered airway reflexes*
   (a) Exaggerated airway reflexes—laryngospasm, coughing, bucking, bronchospasm, and breath holding may complicate emergence from the anaesthetic. This may be compounded by the presence of oral secretions and blood in the oral cavity.
   (b) Reduced airway reflexes—reduced pharyngeal tone (causing airway collapse) and airway obstruction are common, especially in obese patients who have a history of OSA and are sensitive to the sedative effect of opioids. Residual neuromuscular blockade and reduced laryngotracheal reflexes predispose the patients to the risk of aspiration and airway soiling. Aspiration of oral secretions, gastric secretions, and blood in the setting of reduced airway reflexes can cause aspiration pneumonitis.
2. *Pressor response:* Tachycardia and hypertension, which may result in a myocardial supply-demand mismatch [5, 6]
3. *Increased intraocular pressure*
4. *Increased intracranial pressure* [7].
5. *Depletion of oxygen stores leading to hypoxia*
   (a) Residual effects of anaesthetics, opioids, and neuromuscular blockers
   (b) Hypoventilation
   (c) Reduced functional residual capacity (FRC)
   (d) Diffusion hypoxia
   (e) Atelectasis
   (f) Shivering
6. *Airway trauma or injury:* May occur following airway instrumentation, head and neck surgery, airway edema, fluid shifts, and surgical positioning.

20.3 The "At-Risk" Airway [1, 2, 8]

This includes those patients having conditions where there is an increased risk of extubation failure or complications during extubation. Experts recommend identifying these risk factors for extubation failure prior to performing an extubation [9]. These include, but are not limited to, the following:

The normal airway in patients having medical conditions requires suppression of haemodynamic response (pressor response) to extubation.

1. Patients with *D*ifficult mask ventilation (BONES—Bearded, Obese, No Teeth, Elderly, Obstructive Sleep Apnoea, Stiff lungs with poor lung compliance)
2. Patients with *D*ifficult tracheal intubation (pre-existing)
3. Patients with *D*ifficult reintubation for e.g. head and neck/maxillofacial surgery/reconstructive surgery, interdental wiring, predicted likelihood of airway bleeding, or limited access to the airway
4. Patients with *D*elayed recovery or awakening from anaesthesia due to residual anaesthetic effect, haemodynamic instability, residual neuromuscular blockade, hypothermia, acid-base imbalance, electrolyte imbalance, coagulation abnormality, etc.
5. Airway difficulty due to pre-existing *D*iseases or conditions—obesity, OSA, Rheumatoid arthritis, cervical spine disease, post-radiotherapy, neuromuscular disease, full stomach, etc.
6. *S*urgical cause for airway compromise—anterior cervical spine surgery, maxillofacial surgery, surgeries causing nerve damage supplying the airway, pre-existing unilateral or bilateral vocal cord palsy, spine fixation, etc.
7. *S*uspected airway oedema—oedema associated with surgical handling, impaired venous drainage, multiple attempts at airway instrumentation, hematoma, massive fluid infusion, steep Trendelenburg position for long duration, pre-eclampsia, angioedema, prolonged ventilation in the Intensive Care Unit.
8. *S*uspected Airway collapse—post-excision of long-standing thyroid and neck masses causing tracheomalacia.

The causes enumerated above may be remembered as "5 D's" and "3 S's" [1].

20.4 Routine Extubation

20.4.1 Mandatory Requirements Before Proceeding with Extubation

1. Availability of an oxygen source
2. Availability of airway equipment for reintubation and bag-mask ventilation
3. Equipment for suctioning

4. Patient monitoring equipment e.g. continuous electrocardiogram, pulse-oximetry, non-invasive blood pressure monitoring, etc.
5. Patent intravenous access
6. Provision for change in patient position if required (head high and head low)
7. Equipment for cardiopulmonary resuscitation
8. Availability of trained and skilled help if needed.

20.4.2 Steps for Routine Extubation [9]

1. Ensure delivery of 100% oxygen through the endotracheal tube with a breathing system. Switch off the inhalational anaesthetic. Preoxygenation before extubation, along with recruitment manoeuvres, is helpful in situations or conditions when hypoxia is common.
2. Suction the oropharynx and remove all the secretions. Tracheal suctioning prevents lung recruitment and should preferably be avoided unless absolutely necessary.
3. Give a backup position to increase the functional residual capacity.
4. Gastric decompression by suctioning the orogastric may help in relieving the diaphragmatic splinting.
5. Antagonize the neuromuscular blockade. The train of four ratio (TOFR) should be >90% before starting NMB reversal.
6. Ensure adequate muscle tone using clinical signs such as sustained leg lift or head lift for more than 5 s.
7. Ensure regular and adequate spontaneous breathing attempts. The haemodynamic conditions should be satisfactory.
8. Wait until the patient is awake and obeys commands (unless a deep extubation to prevent coughing is planned).
9. Deflate the tracheal tube cuff and extubate. The utility of lung recruitment and positive airway pressure before extubation is debatable. [10]
10. Check that the patient maintains an unobstructed airway with regular breathing.
11. Continue oxygen supplementation and shift to the recovery room in a backup and head-elevated position.

20.5 Strategies for Extubation of the "At-Risk" Airway

Since reintubation is a source of increased morbidity and mortality, guidelines recommend adapting airway management to risk factors associated with extubation failure [9]. Patients with an "at-risk" airway are best managed in the operating room, if feasible. The presence of two healthcare professionals, with at least one experienced in airway management, can help prevent serious complications during extubation.

1. *Awake Extubation with Pharmacological Attenuation of the Pressor Response*

Patients who have undergone high-risk surgeries like cardiac surgeries, eye surgeries, and neurosurgeries need to have a smooth extubation. The vasopressor response associated with a 10–30% increase in heart rate and blood pressure and coughing during extubation needs to be avoided. The aim is to minimize the vasopressor response and rise in intraocular and intracranial pressure with coughing. Various drugs have been used to abolish this response during extubation [11]. Few of the commonly administered drugs are IV Esmolol (1.5–2 mg/kg 2–5 min prior), lignocaine IV (1 mg/kg 2 min prior), fentanyl 0.5–1 mg/kg, or Dexmedetomidine 0.75 mg/kg 10–15 min prior to extubation. Other options like remifentanil—an ultrashort-acting intravenous opioid-help in smooth extubation by attenuating the vasopressor response and cough suppressant action of opioids [12]. The use of a bite block for awake extubation may prevent biting of the tracheal tube in semiconscious patients and subsequent problems like negative pressure pulmonary oedema (NPPE) [13].

2. *The Bailey's Manoeuvre*

The Bailey's manoeuvre, an advanced airway manoeuvre, is a hybrid technique. This involves extubation in deeper planes of anaesthesia using supraglottic airways (SGAs) as a bridge to extubation [14–16]. The premise behind using this technique is that SGAs are better tolerated than a tracheal tube in lighter planes of anaesthesia. This allows smooth emergence from anaesthesia, maintaining the airway with an SGA till the patient is fully awake and then the SGA can be removed. It is useful in patients where a deep extubation strategy is needed, such as in neurosurgical patients, where coughing and bucking on a tracheal tube can lead to a rise in intracranial pressure and deleterious consequences [17]. This technique is contraindicated in conditions of a full stomach or where there is a risk of aspiration of gastric contents.

The steps involved for SGA as a bridge to deep extubation are as follows:

(a) Exchanging the tracheal tube for an SGA (when the patient is deep under anaesthesia) can be done by one of the following techniques:
   (i) Remove the ETT and insert an SGA blindly.
   (ii) Insert an SGA behind the ETT and remove the ETT.
   (iii) Remove the ETT over an Airway Exchange Catheter (AEC) and railroad an SGA over the AEC (recommended for patients with a difficult airway).
(b) Switch off the inhalational anaesthetic agent and start 100% oxygen.
(c) Reversal of neuromuscular blockade.
(d) Removal of the SGA once the breathing is regular, muscle tone is adequate, and the patient is fully awake and obeying commands.

Awake extubation with pharmacological attenuation of the pressor response or Bailey's manoeuvre may be considered in those patients with normal airways having medical conditions requiring suppression of haemodynamic response (pressor response) to extubation.

3. *Recruitment Manoeuvres and Extubation with Positive Airway Pressure*

Certain groups of patients, such as obese patients with OSA, are known to be sensitive to opioids and may have a delayed awakening. They may also have poor upper airway tone and be snorers. They need some amount of positive airway pressure, like continuous positive airway pressure (CPAP) or Bi-level positive airway pressure (BiPAP), to keep the upper airway patent. In addition, they have a shorter apnoea time and are prone to develop hypoxia due to a reduced FRC. Such patients may benefit from extubation after an alveolar recruitment with the use of non-invasive ventilation, CPAP, or high-flow nasal oxygen (HFNO), which provides positive airway pressure to keep the upper airway patent after extubation [19–21].

4. *Use of an Airway Exchange Catheter (AEC)*

Extubation over an AEC is useful in patients with difficult mask ventilation or difficult reintubation. The AEC placed in the trachea prior to extubation serves as a conduit for reintubation, in case required. AEC appears to increase the first-pass success rate in patients with known or suspected difficult airways and decrease the incidence of complications in patients requiring tracheal reintubation [18].

Airway exchange catheters (AEC's) are thin, long, hollow tubes that are inserted into the trachea through the tracheal tube prior to extubation. They are blunt-ended, radio-opaque tubes made from semi-rigid thermostable polyurethane. They should not be mistaken for a bougie or an Aintree™ exchange catheter, which are also hollow and long, but serve different purposes. They have length markings on the external surface. They are manufactured by the Cook™ company and are available in various sizes (Table 20.1).

The AEC can be left in place for 2–72 h. The Cook™ AECs are only licensed for immediate tracheal tube exchange in most countries. Therefore, leaving an AEC in situ for retaining airway access following extubation, though widely practiced, is technically an off-label application [8]. Nevertheless, usually within an hour or so, one can clinically assess whether a reintubation will be required or not.

Precautions with the Use of an AEC [8]

(a) The AEC should be inserted to a depth of 20–22 cm with an oral ETT and a depth of 26–30 cm with a nasal ETT.
(b) The distal tip of the AEC should be above the carina/mid trachea at all times, otherwise it can lead to trauma and airway perforation.
(c) It can be left in place for 2–72 h.

Table 20.1 Airway exchange catheters

AEC size (Fr)	Length (cm)	Internal diameter of the catheter (mm)	Suitable size of tracheal tube for insertion (mm)
8	45	1.6	3 or larger
11	83	2.3	4 or larger
14	83	3.0	5 or larger
19	83	3.4	7 or larger

(d) It should be labelled carefully so that it is not mistaken for a nasogastric tube.
(e) Patients should be kept fasted when they have an AEC in place.
(f) Oxygen should be administered through a facemask and never through an AEC to avoid barotrauma.

Steps for Use of an AEC

1. When an extubation is planned, the lubricated AEC is inserted through the tracheal tube up to a predetermined depth. It should never be forced or advanced against resistance.
2. The oral cavity should be thoroughly suctioned.
3. The depth of the AEC should be noted and it should be taped on the forehead or cheek. It should be clearly labelled to avoid being mistaken for a nasogastric tube.
4. The patient should be in the recovery room or high dependency unit (HDU) in a supervised environment and should be kept fasted.
5. After the patient satisfies all the criteria for extubation, the tracheal tube can be removed, taking care that the AEC does not get dislodged or migrate.
6. Oxygen may be supplemented with a facemask. It should not be given through the AEC as cases of airway injury, barotrauma, pneumothorax, pneumomediastinum, etc. have been reported. [22–24]

Steps for Reintubation over an AEC

1. A smaller-sized tracheal tube with a soft, blunt bevelled tip is preferred for reintubation over an AEC. Alternatively, a Parker flex tube may also be used to avoid an arytenoid holdup.
2. A direct or videolaryngoscope may be used to retract the tongue and railroad the tracheal tube over the AEC [25].
3. The prior passage of an intermediate catheter (e.g. the Aintree catheter) over an 11- or 14-French AEC will facilitate the passage of a tracheal tube through the adult larynx by reducing the size discrepancy between the outer diameter of the AEC and the inner diameter of the tracheal tube [26].
4. Staged extubation sets use a guide wire placed through the AEC, which is left in the trachea after removal of the AEC. This is better tolerated by the patients due to the narrow diameter as compared to an AEC. For reintubation, the AEC needs to be reinserted in the trachea over the guidewire, before the tracheal tube is reinserted over it [17, 27]. However, the failures of reintubation are higher with smaller diameter guides and staged extubation sets [28, 29].
5. Following reintubation, the position of the tracheal tube should always be confirmed with capnography.

Complications such as failure to reintubate, accidental dislodgements, airway trauma, and pneumothorax have been reported with the use of AEC [30, 31].

5. *Extubation over a Flexible Bronchoscope or Video Endoscope*

In cases with longstanding neck masses or thyroid tumours where there is a risk of tracheomalacia or suspected airway collapse, a flexible bronchoscope or a video bronchoscope may be passed through the tracheal tube and extubation conducted while visualizing the trachea distal to the tip of the tracheal tube for dynamic airway collapse or oedema as it is withdrawn. This may be done either when the patient is fully awake or under deep inhalational anaesthesia with spontaneous breathing. If there is distal airway collapse, the tracheal tube is railroaded back into the trachea for a delayed extubation strategy or eventually a tracheostomy if this strategy fails. It is often prudent to wait for 48–72 h before extubation, till the oedema settles or fibrosis sets in and stabilizes the trachea enough to prevent airway collapse. Until such time, the tracheal tube serves as a stent to prevent collapse of the trachea. The patient should be closely monitored during this time, especially if not receiving mechanical ventilation.

6. *Cuff Leak Test*

This test is performed when airway oedema is suspected. This test is performed when the patient is on volume control mechanical ventilation. The set and expired tidal volume are noted on the ventilator when the ETT cuff is inflated. The cuff is deflated and the tidal volume leak is noted. If the leak is less than 10–25%, it suggests that there is airway oedema or collapsibility and maintenance of a patent airway following extubation is doubtful. In such cases, a delayed extubation strategy is suggested. Under normal circumstances, there should be a leak of more than 110–130 mL after the ETT cuff is deflated. Though not a foolproof test, in the presence of a leak, it may be safe to attempt an extubation, considering the other factors of extubation [3].

In a recent systematic review, the authors concluded that the absence of a cuff leak in an at-risk patient is associated with post-extubation stridor or need for re-intubation (High specificity), but the presence of a leak does not necessarily rule out the occurrence of stridor or need for re-intubation (Low sensitivity) [32]. The value of the cuff leak test is more for intensive care unit (ICU) patients rather than for extubation following an anaesthetic [9].

7. *Delayed Extubation*

Postponing extubation by a few hours to a few days may be appropriate if airway oedema or bleeding is anticipated. The airway oedema may settle in a few hours and make extubation relatively safer.

If there is a likelihood of redo surgery or a staged procedure within a few hours in a patient with a difficult reintubation, it may be prudent to leave the tracheal tube in place.

A delayed extubation strategy may be a safe alternative to tracheostomy in select cases of major intraoral surgeries in cancer patients. Extubation performed the following morning when expert help is available is a safe strategy, in case reintubation is required, in addition to providing time for airway oedema to settle and a secure airway in case a re-exploration in required soon after surgery [33].

8. *Elective Tracheostomy*

A tracheostomy may be performed upfront during surgery or following a failed extubation in an "at-risk" airway. Conditions in which an elective tracheostomy may be performed are when there is airway compromise due to major surgical excision of airway structures, bulky flaps, high chances of redo surgeries within a short time, facial trauma, etc. [33, 34] In resource-limited settings, due to the unavailability of trained help or advanced equipment to resecure the airway in case of a difficult intubation, performing a tracheostomy may also be a safer option. An elective tracheostomy may also be performed in cases where a patent airway cannot be maintained despite performing a delayed extubation.

9. *Measures to Reduce Airway Oedema*

Measures to reduce airway oedema are propped up position to improve venous drainage, nebulization with epinephrine and intravenous steroids for at least 12 h to reduce inflammatory oedema [35]. For patients in the ICU where the leak test is negative, but are otherwise ready for extubation, administering systemic steroids for at least 4 h before extubation is recommended. [36] Single-dose steroids are usually ineffective. Intravenously administered hydrocortisone or dexamethasone may be used to reduce inflammatory oedema. Steroids do not have any role in mechanical oedema following venous obstruction and dissection.

Prior to every extubation, the following two questions should be asked: (1) Is this an "at-risk" airway? (2) Is re-intubation going to be difficult? If the answer to either question is a "Yes," specific strategies for extubation of the "at-risk" airway outlined above should be followed. (Fig. 20.1) If the answer to both questions is a "Yes," it will be safer to perform extubation over an AEC or flexible bronchoscope, to be better prepared in case a reintubation is required.

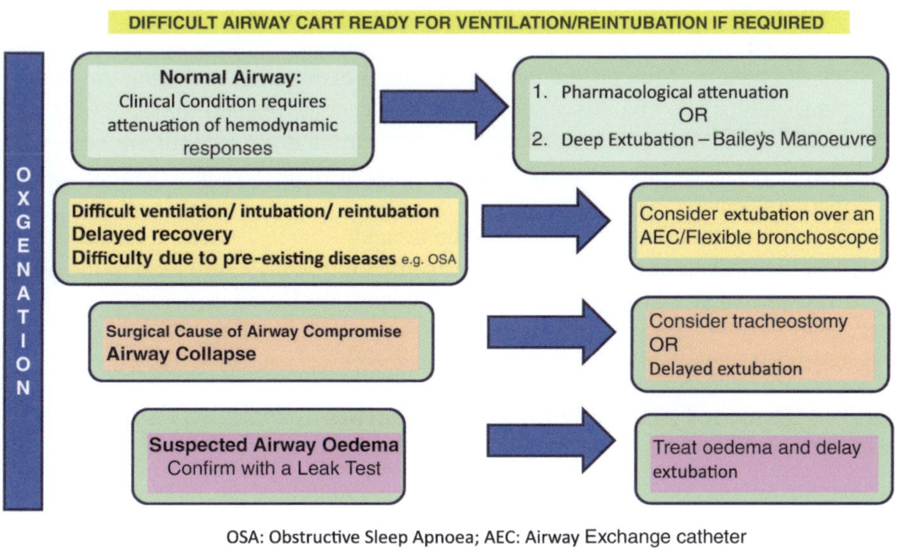

Fig. 20.1 Extubation of the at-risk airway. *OSA* obstructive sleep apnoea, *AEC* airway exchange catheter

20.6 Post-extubation Care

The patient should be placed in a monitored area soon after extubation

1. Oxygen supplementation during transfer and in the recovery room is mandatory.
2. Patients who have an airway in situ may not be able to express themselves and need counselling and reassurance. They may have some post-emergence delirium and should be restrained to avoid injuries and falls during transport and in the recovery room. A transport trolley and bed with side rails are mandatory.
3. Transfers should always be supervised by the accompanying anaesthesiologist with relevant monitoring in place.
4. Patients should preferably be transferred and nursed in the recovery room in a propped-up/head-up position unless contraindicated.
5. Basic levels of monitoring should be used during patient transfer. Advanced monitoring may be needed for high-risk patients.
6. Monitoring in the recovery room should include continuous ECG, pulse oximetry, NIBP, consciousness level, respiratory rate, pain score, and capnography.
7. Handover and communication should be detailed, clear, and well-documented. All healthcare providers should be aware of the airway plan and backup plan in case of extubation failure.
8. A calm environment and patient reassurance are helpful for patients with airway compromise, as anxiety may increase the work of breathing.
9. Along with the difficult airway cart, clip removers, wire cutters, etc. should be available in the recovery room.
10. A skilled anaesthesiologist who is aware of the airway plan should be immediately available should the need arise for a re-intubation or any other complications occur.
11. Adequate analgesia should be provided at all times.
12. All the details of the difficulties faced during extubation, including the airway plan, challenges, and concerns should be clearly explained to the patient and family and documented on an airway alert card and the anaesthesia notes and charts. This may be extremely helpful should the patient require another anaesthetic in future.
13. Airway oedema if suspected should be treated.
14. An airway examination should be performed following extubation in the event of suspected airway trauma or an unanticipated intubation difficulty if required.

20.7 Human Factors During Extubation

At extubation, the conditions are usually not as favourable as during tracheal intubation. The airway equipment may be packed away and monitoring may be inadequate. Skilled assistance may not be available [2]. In addition, various patient and operator factors may contribute to problems during extubation. These include but are not limited to communication difficulties, uncooperative patient, patient position, limited access to the airway, time pressure, and operator fatigue. It is important to be mindful of these human and other factors, which may increase the risk of complications during extubation [37, 38].

20.8 Extubation in the Intensive Care Unit

Extubation of critically ill patients is different from that in the operating room following a short duration of anaesthesia. These patients are often extubated after receiving days of mechanical ventilation. Disease resolution is required prior to extubation. It is important to evaluate whether the condition for which the patient was intubated and mechanically ventilated has resolved. One should distinguish between extubation failure and weaning failure. Airway oedema is quite common in these patients due to prolonged intubation. A leak test should be performed when airway oedema is suspected and should be addressed appropriately if present. It is important to keep in mind that these patients have a physiologically difficult airway due to their critical illness and may often have a poor response to oxygenation [39]. Accidental extubations are more common in this population than in the operating room and should be prevented.

20.9 Conclusion

It is important to remember that extubation is an elective procedure. Extubation failure has grave implications, with higher rates of death and brain damage than during other phases of anaesthesia. Hence, extubation should be planned carefully, with full preparation for reintubation in case of failure. Identify patients at risk for extubation, including risk for reintubation and use specific strategies, including the use of an AEC when in doubt. Most importantly, oxygenate the patient throughout the procedure.

Conflict of Interest Nil.

References

1. Kundra P, Shah AP, Ahmed SM et al. All India Difficult Airway Association 2025 guidelines for extubation of the "at-risk" airway. Indian J Anaesth. 2025;69(11):1187–207.
2. Difficult Airway Society Extubation Guidelines Group, Popat M, Mitchell V, et al. Difficult Airway Society guidelines for the management of tracheal extubation. Anaesthesia. 2012;67(3):318–40.

3. Cavallone LF, Vannucci A. Review article: extubation of the difficult airway and extubation failure. Anesth Analg. 2013;116(2):368–83.
4. Gómez-Ríos MÁ, Sastre JA, Onrubia-Fuertes X, et al. Spanish Society of Anesthesiology, Reanimation and Pain Therapy (SEDAR) Spanish Society of Emergency and Emergency Medicine (SEMES) and Spanish Society of Otolaryngology, Head and Neck Surgery (SEORL-CCC) guideline for difficult airway management. Part II. Rev Esp Anestesiol Reanim. 2024;71(3):207–47.
5. Barham NJ, Boomers OW, Sherry KM, Locke TJ. Myocardial ischaemia during tracheal extubation in patients after cardiac surgery: an observational study. Br J Anaesth. 1998;80:832–3.
6. Rose DK, Cohen MM, DeBoer DP. Cardiovascular events in the postanesthesia care unit: contribution of risk factors. Anesthesiology. 1996;84:772–81.
7. Leech P, Barker J, Fitch W. Proceedings: changes in intracranial pressure and systemic arterial pressure during the termination of anaesthesia. Br J Anaesth. 1974;46:315–6.
8. Law JA, Duggan LV, Asselin M, et al. Canadian Airway Focus Group updated consensus-based recommendations for management of the difficult airway: part 2. Planning and implementing safe management of the patient with an anticipated difficult airway. Can J Anaesth. 2021;68(9):1405–36.
9. Langeron O, Bourgain JL, Francon D, et al. Difficult intubation and extubation in adult anaesthesia. Anaesth Crit Care Pain Med. 2018;37(6):639–51.
10. Lumb AB, Greenhill SJ, Simpson MP, Stewart J. Lung recruitment and positive airway pressure before extubation does not improve oxygenation in the postanaesthesia care unit: a randomized clinical trial. Br J Anaesth. 2010;104:643–7.
11. Gómez-Ríos MÁ, Abad-Gurumeta A, Casans-Francés R, Esquinas AM. Safe extubation procedure of the difficult airway: "think twice, act wise". Minerva Anestesiol. 2020;86(8):802–4.
12. Tung A, Fergusson NA, Ng N, Hu V, Dormuth C, Griesdale DEG. Medications to reduce emergence coughing after general anaesthesia with tracheal intubation: a systematic review and network meta-analysis. Br J Anaesth. 2020. [published online ahead of print, 2020 Feb 22]. S0007-0912(20)30012-X.
13. Liu EH, Yih PS. Negative pressure pulmonary oedema caused by biting and endotracheal tube occlusion—a case for oropharyngeal airways. Singapore Med J. 1999;40(3):174–5.
14. Bennett SR, Grace D, Griffin SC. Cardiovascular changes with the laryngeal mask airway in cardiac anaesthesia. Br J Anaesth. 2004;92(6):885–7.
15. Ellard L, Brown DH, Wong DT. Extubation of a difficult airway after thyroidectomy: use of a flexible bronchoscope via the LMAClassic. Can J Anaesth. 2012;59(1):53–7.
16. Nair I, Bailey PM. Use of the laryngeal mask for airway maintenance following tracheal extubation. Anaesthesia. 1995;50(2):174–5.
17. Artime CA, Hagberg CA. Tracheal extubation. Respir Care. 2014;59(6):991–1005.
18. Mort TC. Continuous airway access for the difficult extubation: the efficacy of the airway exchange catheter. Anesth Analg. 2007;105:1357–62.
19. Hernandez G, Vaquero C, Colinas L, et al. Effect of postextubation high-flow nasal cannula vs noninvasive ventilation on reintubation and postextubation respiratory failure in high-risk patients: a randomized clinical trial. JAMA. 2016;316:1565–74.
20. Granton D, Chaudhuri D, Wang D, et al. High-flow nasal cannula compared with conventional oxygen therapy or noninvasive ventilation immediately postextubation: a systematic review and meta-analysis. Crit Care Med. 2020;48:e1129–36.
21. Hernandez G, Vaquero C, Gonzalez P, et al. Effect of postextubation high-flow nasal cannula vs conventional oxygen therapy on reintubation in low-risk patients: a randomized clinical trial. JAMA. 2016;315:1354–61.
22. Duggan LV, Law JA, Murphy MF. Brief review: supplementing oxygen through an airway exchange catheter: efficacy, complications, and recommendations. Can J Anaesth. 2011;58(6):560–8.
23. Baraka AS. Tension pneumothorax complicating jet ventilation via a cook airway exchange catheter. Anesthesiology. 1999;91:557–8.

24. Shehata IM, Hashim RM. Pneumomediastinum, pneumothorax, pneumoperitoneum, and subcutaneous emphysema complicating extubation of a difficult airway using an airway exchange catheter: is oxygen insufflation innocent?: a case report. A Pract. 2020;14(7):e01228.
25. Mort TC. Tracheal tube exchange: feasibility of continuous glottic viewing with advanced laryngoscopy assistance. Anesth Analg. 2009;108(4):1228–31.
26. Higgs A, Swampillai C, Dravid R, et al. Re-intubation over airway exchange catheters – mind the gap. Anaesthesia. 2010;65:859–60.
27. Sturgess DJ, Greenland KB, Senthuran S, Ajvadi FA, van Zundert A, Irwin MG. Tracheal extubation of the adult intensive care patient with a predicted difficult airway – a narrative review. Anaesthesia. 2017;72(2):248–61.
28. Corso RM, Sorbello M, Mecugni D, et al. Safety and efficacy of staged extubation set in patients with difficult airway: a prospective multicenter study. Minerva Anestesiol. 2020;86(8):827–34.
29. Furyk C, Walsh ML, Kaliaperumal I, Bentley S, Hattingh C. Assessment of the reliability of intubation and ease of use of the cook staged extubation set-an observational study. Anaesth Intensive Care. 2017;45(6):695–9.
30. McLean S, Lanam CR, Benedict W, Kirkpatrick N, Kheterpal S, Ramachandran SK. Airway exchange failure and complications with the use of the Cook Airway Exchange Catheter(R): a single center cohort study of 1177 patients. Anesth Analg. 2013;117:1325–7.
31. Parotto M, Cooper RM, Behringer EC. Extubation of the Challenging or Difficult Airway. Curr Anesthesiol Rep. 2020;10(4):334–40. https://doi.org/10.1007/s40140-020-00416-3. Epub 2020 Sep 4. PMID: 32901201; PMCID: PMC7471579.
32. Kuriyama A, Jackson JL, Kamei J. Performance of the cuff leak test in adults in predicting post-extubation airway complications: a systematic review and meta-analysis. Crit Care. 2020;24(1):640.
33. Myatra SN, Gupta S, D'Cruz AK, et al. Identification of patients for a delayed extubation strategy versus elective tracheostomy for postoperative airway management in major oral cancer surgery: a prospective observational study in seven hundred and twenty patients. Oral Oncol. 2021;121:105502.
34. Jacomet A, Tasman AJ. Airway management in facial trauma patients. Facial Plast Surg. 2015;31(4):319–24.
35. Kuriyama A, Umakoshi N, Sun R. Prophylactic corticosteroids for prevention of postextubation stridor and reintubation in adults: a systematic review and meta-analysis. Chest. 2017;151:1002–10.
36. Girard TD, Alhazzani W, Kress JP, et al. An Official American Thoracic Society/American College of Chest Physicians clinical practice guideline: liberation from mechanical ventilation in critically ill adults. Rehabilitation protocols, ventilator liberation protocols, and cuff leak tests. Am J Respir Crit Care Med. 2017;195(1):120–33.
37. Glavin RJ. Excellence in anesthesiology: the role of nontechnical skills. Anesthesiology. 2009;110:201–3.
38. Flin R, Crichton M. Safety at the sharp end. A guide to non-technical skills. Farnham: Ashgate Publishing Ltd; 2008.
39. Myatra SN, Divatia JV, Brewster DJ. The physiologically difficult airway: an emerging concept. Curr Opin Anaesthesiol. 2022;35(2):115–21.

Chapter 21
Airway Complications

Lauren C. Berkow

21.1 Introduction

Complications related to airway management can occur with any type of airway instrumentation or intervention. These complications can occur during or immediately after airway management, but sometimes present later and are more long-term. Complications can occur during the process of airway management (i.e., placement or removal of an airway device), but can also occur as a result of medications given to facilitate airway management. This chapter will cover direct mechanical or traumatic complications, as well as the physiological and hemodynamic complications that may occur. It will also briefly discuss some of the less common, more long-term complications that can occur after endotracheal intubation.

When difficulty is encountered during airway management, failed intubation or the need for a surgical airway may result. These topics and how to manage them are covered elsewhere in this book.

L. C. Berkow (✉)
Division of Neuroanesthesia, University of Florida College of Medicine, Gainesville, FL, USA
e-mail: lberkow@anest.ufl.edu

M. Á. Gómez-Ríos, A. van Zundert (eds.), *Evidence-based Guide to Difficult Airway Management*, https://doi.org/10.1007/978-3-032-30769-9_21

21.2 Short-Term/Acute Complications Associated with Airway Management

21.2.1 *Incidence*

Minor complications related to airway management are fairly common, while major complications are rarely reported. According to the American Society for Anesthesiologists (ASA) Closed Claims Program, 17% of reported claims were due to respiratory events associated with airway management, and 6% of claims reported direct airway injury [1]. The Fourth National Audit Project (NAP4), published in 2011 by the Royal College of Anesthetists and the Difficult Airway Society, collected airway-related complications over a one-year period. Major events, such as death, brain damage, or need for a surgical airway, were identified in 1 in 21,598 cases, with higher rates recorded outside the operating room setting [2]. A more recent study in the United Kingdom using similar methods found similar complication rates, with a higher incidence in patients with a predicted difficult airway (1 in 315) [3].

Both the ASA Closed Claims Program and the NAP4 report found that airway-related complications were higher during emergency airway management as well as when airway management was performed outside the operating room setting [1, 4, 5]. The incidence of airway-related complications both inside and outside the operating room was also found to be higher when a difficult intubation was encountered.

21.2.2 *Risk Factors*

Several risk factors increase the likelihood of complications related to airway management. Risk factors can be either patient-related (Table 21.1) or situation-related (Table 21.2), and often more than one of these types of risk factors play a role [1, 4, 5]. Patient factors may include congenital or acquired diseases that have been associated with difficult intubation (Table 21.3) [6]. Situational factors can also increase

Table 21.1 Risk factors for short-term airway complications: patient factors

Presence of risk factors for difficulty (see Table 21.3)
Coagulopathy
Obesity
Physiological difficulty
Increased oxygen demand
Decreased oxygen delivery
Acute or chronic respiratory insufficiency

Table 21.2 Risk factors for short-term airway complications: situational factors

Predicted or unpredicted difficult intubation
Emergent airway management
Intubation performed outside the operating room
Multiple intubation attempts
Poor planning for airway management
Reintubation after failed Eextubation

Table 21.3 Risk factors for difficulty with airway management

Congenital	Acquired
Down syndrome	Morbid obesity
Achondroplasia	Acromegaly
Micrognathia	Infections involving the airway
Mucopolysaccharidoses	Obstructive sleep apnea
Pierre Robin syndrome	Radiation to the head or neck
Goldenhar syndrome	Tumors involving the airway
Treacher Collins syndrome	Trauma or burns to the head or neck

the risk of complications. Poor airway assessment or lack of planning for difficulty or failure has been associated with an increase in complications [2]. Emergent airway management as well as airway management outside the operating room, where the needed personnel or equipment may not be immediately available, have also been associated with increased complication rates [5]. Multiple intubation attempts, difficult intubation, and failed extubation have also been associated with an increased risk of complications [4, 5, 7].

Patients may also present with a physiologically difficult airway, which increases their risk of hypoxia or hemodynamic instability during airway management. Critically ill patients often have increased oxygen demands, decreased oxygen delivery, or both, putting them at higher risk of desaturation and hemodynamic instability during airway management [8, 9]. Other patients that may present with a physiologically difficult airway include patients with acute respiratory insufficiency (due to coronavirus, pulmonary embolism, acute respiratory distress syndrome, or severe atelectasis), sepsis, or pregnancy [8, 9].

21.2.3 Emergent Airway Management

Emergent airway management has been associated with an increased risk of complications [2, 7, 10]. Major complications, including cardiac arrest, death, and hypoxic injury, are also higher with emergent airway management [10]. Most emergency airway management occurs outside the operating room, in the intensive care unit, procedural areas, or the emergency department.

Many factors contribute to this increased risk, including:

- Incomplete or inadequate airway assessment [1–3, 5, 10, 11].
- Inadequate preoxygenation due to lack of time or physiological factors that increase oxygen demand or decrease oxygen delivery [8, 12].
- Hemodynamic instability due to underlying medical or surgical conditions [8, 9].
- Increased incidence of airway edema (due to recent failed extubation, anaphylaxis, or other causes).

In addition, emergent airway management has been associated with an increased incidence of difficult intubation as well as the need for multiple intubation attempts, both of which are linked to higher rates of complications [2, 10, 12]. See Table 21.4 for a clinical scenario that illustrates these points.

Outside the operating room setting, experienced personnel and equipment to manage the airway may not be immediately available. Additional situational factors that may increase difficulty and complications include decreased access to the patient due to equipment or space constraints, higher noise levels and distractions, and the need for emergent intubation after hours (i.e., late at night or during weekend hours) [2, 12–16]. Standardization of airway equipment and personnel, including the creation of difficult airway carts and Airway Teams made available throughout the hospital, has been demonstrated to reduce the incidence of airway-related complications [13–15, 17–19]. (Grade B evidence) Simulation and teamwork training centered around emergent airway management have also been shown to decrease complication rates [14–16, 20, 21] (Grade C evidence).

Table 21.4 Clinical scenario

A 130 kg patient presents to the emergency department (ED) with severe respiratory distress. O_2 saturations are in the low 80 s, with BP 70/50. The team in the ED gives propofol and rocuronium for emergent intubation. Direct laryngoscopy is difficult, and a videolaryngoscope needs to be brought to the ED from another location before intubation is successful. During airway management, the patient becomes more hypoxic as well as hypotensive and bradycardic, requiring pressor support and aggressive bag mask ventilation
How could the management of this patient be improved and these complications prevented?
Patient related
Optimal preoxygenation and peri-oxygenation with high flow oxygen during intubation to reduce the hypoxia risk
Consideration of the use of other medications such as etomidate or ketamine as well as fluid and pressor resuscitation prior to administration to prevent hypotension
Systems related
Backup airway equipment such as videolaryngoscopy and flexible bronchoscopes immediately available in the ED prior to airway management
Team training and simulation for difficult airway patients
Airway Lead/Airway Team familiar with difficult airway guidelines and algorithms

21.2.4 *Physiological Complications*

Induction of anesthesia or the administration of medications to facilitate airway management, as well as the intubation procedure itself can result in a variety of physiological complications including hypoxia, hemodynamic instability, arrhythmias, cardiovascular collapse, and death [2, 10, 12].

21.2.4.1 Hypoxia

When sedation or general anesthesia is induced prior to airway management, the patient usually becomes apneic, requiring the airway manager to initiate ventilation, usually via a facemask. If mask ventilation is inadequate, hypoxia can occur. This can occur due to a variety of causes, including bronchospasm, laryngospasm, aspiration, airway obstruction, or esophageal intubation. Patients may also become hypoxic despite mask ventilation if oxygenation is inadequate. Hypoxia due to inadequate ventilation also causes hypercapnia, which can reduce pH and increase the risk of arrhythmia or neurological injury [8]. If untreated, hypoxia can lead to other complications such as hypotension, arrhythmias, brain damage, cardiac arrest, and death [10, 12].

Mort et al. studied airway-related complications in the ICU setting and found that over 70% of patients became hypoxic during airway management and 1 in 50 suffered a cardiac arrest [10]. The NAP4 report also found hypoxia to be a common theme in deaths due to airway management [2, 11].

Certain categories of patients are at higher risk of hypoxia during airway management [8]:

- Patients expected to desaturate more rapidly during a period of apnea due to increased oxygen demands: neonatal/pediatric patients, pregnant, obese, or hypermetabolic patients.
- Patients with decreased oxygen delivery or reserves: cardiovascular or pulmonary pathology (chronic obstructive pulmonary disease/emphysema, acute respiratory distress syndrome, congestive heart failure, pulmonary edema, severe asthma or bronchospasm, COVID infection, or low cardiac output states).

Good preoxygenation prior to airway management, as well as peri-oxygenation during airway management, can improve oxygenation and reduce the risk of hypoxia [8, 9, 12, 22–24] (Grade A evidence). Adequate preoxygenation can increase oxygen reserves and prolong safe apnea time. Delivery of oxygen both before and throughout airway management is recommended in the recently updated American Society of Anesthesiologists (ASA) Practice Guidelines for Management of the Difficult Airway as well as in the Difficult Airway Society guidelines for airway management in the critically ill patient, especially if difficulty is anticipated or if patients are at higher risk for hypoxia [25, 26] (Grade B evidence). Peri-oxygenation can be delivered via a variety of methods, including low or high-flow nasal cannula, nasal CPAP devices such as the SuperNO2VA (Vyaire Medical), or high-flow humidified nasal oxygen devices such as Optiflow (Fisher and Paykel) [27–29]. Many of these devices can be used during laryngoscopy in addition to preoxygenation to provide apneic oxygenation during airway management.

21.2.4.2 Hemodynamic Changes

Airway instrumentation, as well as the medications given to achieve intubating conditions, can cause changes in blood pressure, as well as heart rate and rhythm. Manipulation of the airway can trigger sympathetic and parasympathetic stimulation, with variable results [30, 31].

Hypotension is common both during and after intubation and occurs in over 50% of critically ill patients requiring airway management, especially if they have depressed cardiac function [8, 30]. If untreated, hypotension can progress to cardiac arrest. The causes of hypotension are multifactorial and include patient factors (critical illness, reduced cardiac function), effects of medications given to provide intubating conditions that produce vasodilation, as well as the effects of transitioning from spontaneous to positive pressure ventilation. The transition from spontaneous to positive pressure ventilation can trigger hypotension due to reduced venous return, even with minimal sedation, and can be more pronounced in the presence of hypovolemia. Postintubation hypotension can be difficult to predict or prevent in critically ill patients, so several guidelines suggest that the need for IV fluid boluses and vasopressors should be anticipated in these patients [9, 26, 31, 32] (Grade A evidence). Two recent large center trials, the INTUBE study and PREPARE study, both studied the use of vasopressors and fluid administration to reduce hemodynamic complications during airway management in the ICU setting and found that neither strategy reduced the incidence of cardiovascular instability [31, 32].

Sympathetic stimulation during airway instrumentation can trigger hypertension, tachycardia, or arrhythmias [30, 33]. Both laryngoscopy and endotracheal tube (ETT) placement can trigger this response. Several studies have demonstrated a reduced hyperdynamic response with the use of a videolaryngoscope or supraglottic airway (SGA) compared to direct laryngoscopy [34, 35] (Grade B evidence). Hypertension and tachycardia can lead to myocardial ischemia, cerebrovascular accidents, bleeding, or congestive heart failure, which can then lead to hypotension or cardiovascular collapse. This stimulation can be mitigated by providing adequate sedation and medications to blunt the sympathetic response prior to airway instrumentation, but should be dosed carefully to avoid hypotension [30, 33] (Grade B evidence).

21.2.4.3 Arrhythmias

Bradycardia can occur during airway management in conjunction with hypotension, and if unrecognized or untreated, can lead to cardiac arrest or death [36]. Bradycardia can be due to the vagal response to manipulation of the airway, especially in children who have higher vagal tone. The most common cause of bradycardia in both adults and children is hypoxia [10]. Treatment should include correction of hypoxia. Once hypoxia is corrected or ruled out, if bradycardia persists, anticholinergic medications such as glycopyrrolate or atropine should be administered, and other causes for the bradycardia should be investigated and treated [36]. Succinylcholine can also be a cause of bradycardia in children, as well as in adults who receive repeated doses.

More severe arrhythmias are less common but can occur during prolonged hypoxia and hypotension, especially in patients who are critically ill. Supraventricular tachycardia, ventricular tachycardia, ventricular fibrillation, and cardiac arrest can all occur and should be managed per advanced cardiac life support protocols (ACLS) [2, 10, 11, 30, 37].

Adequate fluid resuscitation when time allows and careful selection of medications can potentially reduce hemodynamic complications during airway management. Medications that are less likely to cause hypotension and myocardial depression, such as etomidate and ketamine, may be considered [37] (Grade B evidence). Adequate personnel and anticipation of the hemodynamic changes that can occur during airway management, especially in critically ill patients, are important for both prevention and management [2, 9, 11–14, 26, 30] (Grade A evidence). Some studies suggest that hemodynamic instability can still occur despite the use of fluid resuscitation and vasopressors [31, 33].

21.2.5 Sore Throat

Sore throat is a common complication after placement of an endotracheal tube or supraglottic airway. The incidence of sore throat varies in the literature between 14% and 60% [38–41]. Symptoms of sore throat vary widely, including pain, cough, dry throat, hoarseness, or trouble swallowing (dysphagia). Sore throat symptoms can be a result of injury or irritation to the uvula or oropharynx, pharyngitis, tracheitis, or laryngitis. These conditions can be caused by trauma (during laryngoscopy, airway device placement, or suctioning), or irritation or injury to mucosal structures from the airway device. Most symptoms are mild and short-lived, resolving within 24–48 h [38–40]. Severe or persistent symptoms should be evaluated by an otolaryngologist, as they may be due to a more severe laryngeal injury.

Several risk factors have been linked to the development of sore throat after airway management, including use of a larger ETT, higher cuff pressures, use of a nasogastric or double lumen tube, coughing during emergence, and tracheal intubation without the use of neuromuscular blockade [38–41].

Several strategies can be employed to reduce postoperative sore throat. Careful airway manipulation under ideal intubating conditions, use of an appropriately sized ETT or SGA, and avoidance of high cuff pressures have all been demonstrated to reduce sore throat incidence [41–43] (Grade B evidence). A cuff manometer can be used to monitor cuff pressures during surgery. ETT cuff pressures above 20 mm Hg and SGA cuff pressures above 60 mm Hg have been associated with a higher incidence of sore throat [42, 43]. Some newer ETTs and SGAs come with a built-in cuff manometer. Several studies have investigated whether the use of an ETT versus an SGA or specific types of SGA was associated with a reduced incidence of sore throat, but these studies were quite heterogeneous and presented inconclusive results [44] (Grade D evidence). Pharmacological agents can also be administered to reduce sore throat incidence, including IV or topical lidocaine or steroids, topical benzydamine, or lozenges, although the benefit of these medications is unclear [45, 46] (Grade C evidence).

21.2.6 Traumatic Complications

Traumatic injuries can occur both during induction and intubation as well as during extubation. Injuries to teeth are the most commonly reported injuries and a frequent source of patient complaints [1, 4, 47, 48]. Teeth can be cracked, dislodged, or avulsed, and can occur with any type of airway management or if patients bite down on an airway device or bite block. A dislodged tooth can potentially be aspirated into the trachea and require removal to avoid morbidity. Risk factors for dental injury include pre-existing poor dentition and difficult intubation [47]. Any teeth dislodged during airway management should be retrieved and placed in saline, and a dental consult is recommended postoperatively [47]. The use of protective devices such as mouthguards have not been shown to reduce the incidence of dental injury and may provide a false sense of security [48].

Other soft tissues inside the mouth and larynx can also be injured during laryngoscopy due to direct trauma from the laryngoscope blade. Injuries to the palate and tonsils have been reported during blind placement of the ETT during videolaryngoscopy [49]. These injuries can be mild or more severe, causing airway edema or obstruction. Risk factors for soft tissue injury include preexisting swelling, coagulopathy, prior neck radiation, and difficult intubation [50].

The vocal cords and arytenoids can also be injured during ETT or SGA placement. Arytenoid cartilage dislocation has been reported after intubation or extubation (if the cuff is not deflated prior to removal) and presents as hoarseness or a weak, breathy voice [51]. Vocal cord injuries can include lacerations, granulomas, or ulcers, and can also occur during either intubation or extubation. Most of these injuries heal over time, but may result in dysphonia [52]. Vocal cord paralysis can also occur after short- or long-term intubation and is further discussed in the section on long-term complications [52].

Other rare traumatic complications include temporomandibular joint dislocation, cervical spine injury in patients at risk (myelopathy, acute cervical spine injuries, severe cervical spine stenosis), and barotrauma or pneumothorax due to overinflation of the lung if very high positive pressures are delivered [53, 54].

21.2.7 Complications Associated with Nasal Intubation

Many of the complications described above that are associated with oral endotracheal intubation can also occur with nasotracheal intubation. Complications more specifically associated with nasotracheal intubation include bleeding within the nasal passages, nasal trauma, or sinus infection [1, 3, 4]. Since the nose is highly vascular, a risk of bleeding exists. This risk can be reduced by the use of topical vasoconstrictors such as oxymetazoline, cocaine, or phenylephrine, as well as the use of prewarmed and well-lubricated ETTs [55]. The nasal septum, turbinates, or adenoid tissues can be traumatized during nasal ETT placement, especially if a deviated septum is present or a larger ETT size is used. Nasal intubation has been associated with sinusitis due to an inflammatory response to the indwelling ETT and is more common with prolonged intubation [56]. If long-term intubation is planned, it is recommended to either use the oral route or to convert a nasal ETT to an oral ETT to reduce infection risk.

21.2.8 Aspiration

Induction of general anesthesia and administration of muscle relaxants result in the loss of airway reflexes and relaxation of the muscles of the esophagus. Aspiration of gastric contents into the trachea and lungs can occur during mask ventilation and placement of an airway device. Patients who are not adequately fasted, such as during emergency surgery, or patients with gastroesophageal reflux disease, bowel obstruction, pregnancy, or gastroparesis are at higher risk of aspiration during airway management [1–3, 11, 57]. Rapid securement of the airway, minimizing the need for mask ventilation during airway management, and use of a cuffed ETT can potentially reduce aspiration risk [25, 26, 57] (Grade B evidence). An SGA device does not fully protect against aspiration of stomach contents, so its use may increase the aspiration risk in patients with a full stomach. However, the reported incidence of aspiration during airway management with either an ETT or SGA is low [1–3, 11, 58].

21.2.9 Bronchospasm and Laryngospasm

Instrumentation of the airway can trigger bronchospasm, especially in patients with reactive airway disease (asthma, chronic obstructive pulmonary disease, smoking, or vaping). Prevention, as well as management of bronchospasm, can include the use of bronchodilators and ensuring an adequate depth of anesthesia during airway manipulation [8, 9, 59] (Grade A evidence). Laryngospasm can occur as a result of laryngeal stimulation from an airway device or secretions at any time during anesthesia. It is more common in children, and most often occurs during induction or emergence [60]. Laryngospasm can also progress to negative pressure pulmonary edema. Laryngospasm usually resolves with positive pressure ventilation but may also require the administration of muscle relaxants and reintubation of the airway [59–61].

21.2.10 Esophageal Intubation

Despite advanced airway techniques and the use of capnography, esophageal intubation still can occur, and if not recognized quickly, it can result in complications such as hypoxia, brain damage, and death [1–3, 11, 62, 63]. Esophageal intubation was the causative factor in 6% of airway complications reported by the NAP4 Project [2, 11]. The Project for Universal Management of Airways (PUMA), an international society of airway experts from many established airway societies, recently published consensus guidelines on preventing unrecognized esophageal intubation [62]. Use of end-tidal capnography to identify a sustained exhaled carbon dioxide waveform is recommended to confirm endotracheal intubation in order to avoid unrecognized esophageal intubation [13, 25, 26, 62, 63] (Grade A evidence). The lack of sustained carbon dioxide ("no trace, wrong place") should immediately prompt concern that the tube may not be in the trachea, and further assessment of the airway should be performed [62, 63] (Grade A evidence). The use of videolaryngoscopy has also been associated with reducing the incidence of unrecognized esophageal intubation [62, 63] (Grade B evidence). The presence of severe bronchospasm or cardiac arrest can be a confounding factor that may result in a lack of exhaled carbon dioxide despite the correct endotracheal placement of the tube [62, 63].

21.2.11 Unplanned Extubation

Unplanned extubation can occur in the operating room as well as in other locations where patients are intubated (the emergency department or intensive care unit). Unplanned extubation can occur as a result of external factors that result in a force that dislodges the tube, or as a result of "self-extubation" where the patient removes the tube prematurely [64]. Risk factors for unplanned or accidental extubation include lack of adequate securement of the tube, a change in patient position (turning or placing a patient prone), lack of sedation or restraints in the ICU setting, or lack of adequate staffing during manipulation of the ETT or change in position [64, 65]. Signs of accidental extubation may include loss of capnography, oxygen desaturation, a sudden leak around the endotracheal tube or in the ventilation system, or a decrease or loss of tidal volume. Unplanned extubation can result in hypoxia, hemodynamic instability, brain damage, and death, especially if it is unrecognized or if reintubation is delayed or difficult [64]. Strategies that can prevent unplanned extubation include adequate securement of the tube, use of end-tidal capnography, clear protocols for turning patients and weaning for extubation, and close monitoring of the tube during transport or any change in patient position [64, 65] (Grade B evidence).

21.3 Long-Term Complications Associated with Airway Management

Long-term or late complications can occur after longer periods of intubation or due to the presence of a tracheostomy. Most of these complications are quite rare and include vocal cord paralysis, laryngotracheal stenosis (subglottic stenosis), or structural changes to the trachea [66]. Stenosis is thought to be triggered by edema or tissue ischemia from the prolonged presence of the endotracheal tube, which leads to scarring and fibrosis. Symptoms can include dyspnea, stridor, or voice changes, and treatment may include stenting, dilatation, or tracheal resection in extreme cases [66]. Other structural changes can include tracheomalacia or fistula development (tracheoesophageal fistula or tracheoinnominate fistula), which may also require surgical repair [66].

21.3.1 Prevention/Summary

Airway-related complications can be prevented, or at least the incidence reduced, through a multifaceted strategy (Fig. 21.1). Standardization of equipment and personnel, the use of guidelines, algorithms, and cognitive aids, good airway assessment and planning, and the creation of airway plans and backup plans can all play a role in safer airway management [13, 14, 15, 25, 26] (Grade A evidence). Common messages of most published airway guidelines include improving the system, addressing human factors, and having the needed airway equipment available [25, 26]. The Difficult Airway Society created the concept of an "Airway Lead Network" in the United Kingdom, which has spread to other countries as well [67]. The

AIRWAY COMPLICATIONS

TYPES	RISK FACTORS	PREVENTION
Traumatic/Mechanical • Sore throat • Soft tissue injury • Dental damage • Vocal cord injury • Bleeding • Unplanned extubation • Unrecognized esophageal intubation	**Patient-Related** • Obesity • Physiological derangements – Increased oxygen demand – Decreased oxygen supply – Sepsis – Respiratory insufficiency • Coagulopathy	**Patient-Related** • Optimize oxygenation • Deliver oxygen throughout airway management • Perform a thorough airway assessment • Create multiple airway management plans • Anticipate hemodynamic changes
Physiological • Hypoxia • Hemodynamic instability – Hypotension – Hypertension – Arrhythmias • Aspiration • Bronchospasm • Laryngospasm	**Situational Factors** • Difficult intubation • Emergent airway management • Multiple intubation attempts • Intubation outside the OR (ED, ICU)	**Equipment-Related** • End-tidal capnography for all airway management in all locations • Standardize airway equipment • Have airway equipment immediately available
Long-Term • Subglottic stenosis • Tracheomalacia • Vocal cord paralysis • Fistulae – Tracheoesophageal – Tracheoinnominate	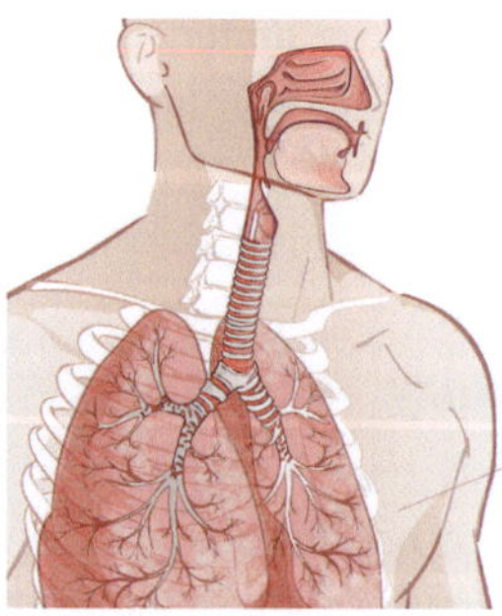	**Systems-Related** • Consider Airway Lead Network • Education – Guidelines – Algorithms – Simulation – Airway skills training • Teamwork and human factors training

Fig. 21.1 Airway complications

Airway Lead or Airway Team coordinates educational programs, adherence to guidelines, and standardization of equipment, addresses human factors, and performs audit analyses to identify gaps and improve practice [67, 68].

Highlights/Recommendations

1. Standardization of airway equipment throughout the hospital can reduce airway-related complications.
2. A complete airway assessment and prediction of difficulty with airway management should be performed on all patients when time permits.
3. Emergent airway management has been associated with an increased risk of complications as well as difficult intubation. These complications should be anticipated and the appropriate equipment to manage them should be available.
4. Patients requiring emergent intubation may have physiological disturbances that increase the risk of hypoxia and hemodynamic instability. These complications should be anticipated and the airway manager should be prepared to manage them.
5. Oxygen delivery throughout airway management (peri-oxygenation) can reduce the risk of hypoxia, especially in patients at higher risk of desaturation.
6. Postoperative sore throat is a common complication, and its risk can be reduced by the use of appropriately sized ETTs, careful airway manipulation under ideal conditions, and monitoring of cuff pressures.
7. Routine use of end-tidal capnography is recommended to confirm endotracheal intubation and to reduce the incidence of unrecognized esophageal intubation or unplanned extubation.
8. Long-term complications related to airway management are quite rare but can include vocal cord paralysis, tracheal stenosis, or the development of fistulae between the trachea and nearby structures.
9. The establishment of an Airway Lead or Airway Team in the hospital can address educational and equipment needs, as well as implement training related to airway skills, human factors, and teamwork.

References

1. Metzner J, Posner KL, Lam MS, Domino KB. Closed claims' analysis. Best Pract Res Clin Anaesthesiol. 2011;25(2):263–76. https://doi.org/10.1016/j.bpa.2011.02.007.
2. The Fourth National Audit Project of the Royal College of Anaesthetists and Difficult Airway Society (NAP4). Major complications of airway management in the United Kingdom: report and findings. https://www.nationalauditprojects.org.uk/downloads/NAP4%20Full%20Report.pdf. Accessed 25 Sept 2022.
3. Cumberworth A, Lewith H, Sud A, Jefferson H, Athanassoglou V, Pandit JJ. Major complications of airway management: a prospective multicentre observational study. Anaesthesia. 2022;77(6):640–8. https://doi.org/10.1111/anae.15668.
4. Domino KB, Posner KL, Caplan RA, Cheney FW. Airway injury during anesthesia: a closed claims analysis. Anesthesiology. 1999;91(6):1703–11. https://doi.org/10.1097/00000542-199912000-00023.

5. Joffe AM, Aziz MF, Posner KL, Duggan LV, Mincer SL, Domino KB. Management of difficult tracheal intubation: a closed claims analysis. Anesthesiology. 2019;131(4):818–29. https://doi.org/10.1097/ALN.0000000000002815.
6. Kim SO. Airway management. J Korea Med Ass. 2007;50(12):1048–56. https://doi.org/10.5124/jkma.2007.50.12.1048.
7. Marin J, Davison D, Pourmand A. Emergent endotracheal intubation associated cardiac arrest, risks, and emergency implications. J Anesth. 2019;33(3):454–62. https://doi.org/10.1007/s00540-019-02631-7.
8. Mosier JM, Joshi R, Hypes C, Pacheco G, Valenzuela T, Sakles JC. The physiologically difficult airway. West J Emerg Med. 2015;16(7):1109–17. https://doi.org/10.5811/westjem.2015.8.27467.
9. Kornas RL, Owyang CG, Sakles JC, Foley LJ, Mosier JM, Society for Airway Management's Special Projects Committee. Evaluation and management of the physiologically difficult airway: consensus recommendations from Society for Airway Management. Anesth Analg. 2021;132(2):395–405. https://doi.org/10.1213/ANE.0000000000005233.
10. Mort TC. The incidence and risk factors for cardiac arrest during emergency tracheal intubation: a justification for incorporating the ASA guidelines in the remote location. J Clin Anesth. 2004;16(7):508–16. https://doi.org/10.1016/j.jclinane.2004.01.007.
11. Cook TM, Woodall N, Harper J, Benger J, Fourth National Audit Project. Major complications of airway management in the UK: results of the Fourth National Audit Project of the Royal College of Anaesthetists and the Difficult Airway Society. Part 2: intensive care and emergency departments. Br J Anaesth. 2011;106(5):632–42. https://doi.org/10.1093/bja/aer059.
12. Mort TC. Preoxygenation in critically ill patients requiring emergency tracheal intubation. Crit Care Med. 2005;33(11):2672–5. https://doi.org/10.1097/01.ccm.0000187131.67594.9e.
13. Woodall N, Frerk C, Cook TM. Can we make airway management (even) safer?—lessons from national audit. Anaesthesia. 2011;66(suppl 2):27–33. https://doi.org/10.1111/j.1365-2044.2011.06931.x.
14. Mark LJ, Herzer KR, Cover R, Pandian V, Bhatti NI, Berkow LC, et al. Difficult Airway Response Team: a novel quality improvement program for managing hospital-wide airway emergencies. Anesth Analg. 2015;121(1):127–39. https://doi.org/10.1213/ANE.0000000000000691.
15. Berkow LC, Greenberg RS, Kan KH, Colantuoni E, Mark LJ, Flint PW, et al. Need for emergency surgical airway reduced by a comprehensive difficult airway program. Anesth Analg. 2009;109(6):1860–9. https://doi.org/10.1213/ane.0b013e3181b2531a.
16. Schnittker R, Marshall S, Horberry T, Young KL. Human factors enablers and barriers for successful airway management—an in-depth interview study. Anaesthesia. 2018;73(8):980–9. https://doi.org/10.1111/anae.14302.
17. Tsai AC, Krisciunas GP, Brook C, Basa K, Gonzalez M, Crimlisk J, et al. Comprehensive Emergency Airway Response Team (EART) training and education: impact on team effectiveness, personnel confidence, and protocol knowledge. Ann Otol Rhinol Laryngol. 2016;125(6):457–63. https://doi.org/10.1177/0003489415619178.
18. Showan AM, Sestito JA. Organization of personnel and resources for airway management in the hospital and office environment. Crit Care Clin. 2000;16(3):527–39. https://doi.org/10.1016/s0749-0704(05)70129-9.
19. Long L, Vanderhoff B, Smyke N, Shaffer LET, Solomon J, Steuer JD. Management of difficult airways using a hospital-wide "alpha team" approach. Am J Med Qual. 2010;25(4):297–304. https://doi.org/10.1177/1062860610366587.
20. Mehta N, Boynton C, Boss L, Morris H, Tatla T. Multidisciplinary difficult airway simulation training: two year evaluation and validation of a novel training approach at a District General Hospital based in the UK. Eur Arch Otorrinolaringol. 2013;270(1):211–7. https://doi.org/10.1007/s00405-012-2131-3.
21. DeMaria S Jr, Berman DJ, Goldberg A, Lin HM, Khelemsky Y, Levine AI. Team-based model for non-operating room airway management: validation using a simulation-based study. Br J Anaesth. 2016;117(1):103–8. https://doi.org/10.1093/bja/aew121.

22. Pavlov I, Medrano S, Weingart S. Apneic oxygenation reduces the incidence of hypoxemia during emergency intubation: a systematic review and meta-analysis. Am J Emerg Med. 2017;35(8):1184–9. https://doi.org/10.1016/j.ajem.2017.06.029.
23. Oliveira JE, Silva L, Cabrera D, Barrionuevo P, Johnson RL, Erwin PJ, Murad MH, et al. Effectiveness of apneic oxygenation during intubation: a systematic review and meta-analysis. Ann Emerg Med. 2017;70(4):483–94.e11. https://doi.org/10.1016/j.annemergmed.2017.05.001.
24. Binks MJ, Holyoak RS, Melhuish TM, Vlok R, Bond E, White LD. Apneic oxygenation during intubation in the emergency department and during retrieval: a systematic review and meta analysis. Am J Emerg Med. 2017;35(10):1542–6. https://doi.org/10.1016/j.ajem.2017.06.046.
25. Apfelbaum JL, Hagberg CA, Connis RT, Abdelmalak BB, Agarkar M, Dutton RP, et al. 2022 American Society of Anesthesiologists practice guidelines for management of the difficult airway. Anesthesiology. 2022;136(1):31–81. https://doi.org/10.1097/ALN.0000000000004002.
26. Higgs A, McGrath BA, Goddard C, Rangasami J, Suntharalingam G, Gale R, et al. DAS guidelines on the airway management of critically ill patients. Anaesthesia. 2018;73(8):1035–6. https://doi.org/10.1111/anae.14352.
27. Mitsuyama Y, Nakao S, Shimazaki J, Ogura H, Shimazu T. Effectiveness of high-flow nasal cannula for tracheal intubation in the emergency department. BMC Emerg Med. 2022;22(1):115. https://doi.org/10.1186/s12873-022-00674-w.
28. Guy L, Christensen R, Dodd B, Pelecanos A, Wyssusek K, Van Zundert A, et al. The effect of transnasal humidified rapid-insufflation ventilator exchange (THRIVE) versus nasal prongs on safe apnoea time in paralysed obese patients: a randomised controlled trial. Br J Anaesth. 2022;128(2):375–81. https://doi.org/10.1016/j.bja.2021.10.048.
29. Lodenius Å, Piehl J, Östlund A, Ullman J, Jonsson Fagerlund M. Transnasal humidified rapid-insufflation ventilatory exchange (THRIVE) vs. facemask breathing pre-oxygenation for rapid sequence induction in adults: a prospective randomised non-blinded clinical trial. Anaesthesia. 2018;73(5):564–71. https://doi.org/10.1111/anae.14215.
30. Mort TC. Complications of emergency tracheal intubation: hemodynamic alterations—part I. J Intensive Care Med. 2007;22(3):157–65. https://doi.org/10.1177/0885066607299525.
31. Russotto V, Tassistro E, Myatra SN, Parotto M, Antolini L, Bauer P, et al. Peri-intubation cardiovascular collapse in patients who are critically ill: insights from the INTUBE study. Am J Respir Crit Care Med. 2022;206(4):449–58. https://doi.org/10.1164/rccm.2021.
32. Janz DR, Casey JD, Semler MW, Russell DW, Dargin J, Vonderhaar DJ, et al. Effect of a fluid bolus on cardiovascular collapse among critically ill adults undergoing tracheal intubation (PrePARE): a randomised controlled trial. Lancet Respir Med. 2019;7(12):1039–47. https://doi.org/10.1016/S2213-2600(19)30246-2.
33. Hassan HG, el-Sharkawy TY, Renck H, Mansour G, Fouda A. Hemodynamic and catecholamine responses to laryngoscopy with vs. without endotracheal intubation. Acta Anaesthesiol Scand. 1991;35(5):442–7. https://doi.org/10.1111/j.1399-6576.1991.tb03325.x.
34. Maassen RL, Pieters BM, Maathuis B, Serroyen J, Marcus MA, Wouters P, et al. Endotracheal intubation using videolaryngoscopy causes less cardiovascular response compared to classic direct laryngoscopy, in cardiac patients according a standard hospital protocol. Acta Anaesthesiol Belg. 2012;63(4):181–6.
35. Wood ML, Forrest ET. The haemodynamic response to the insertion of the laryngeal mask airway: a comparison with laryngoscopy and tracheal intubation. Acta Anaesthesiol Scand. 1994;38(5):510–3. https://doi.org/10.1111/j.1399-6576.1994.tb03938.x.
36. Jones P, Dauger S, Peters MJ. Bradycardia during critical care intubation: mechanisms, significance and atropine. Arch Dis Child. 2012;97(2):139–44. https://doi.org/10.1136/adc.2010.210518.
37. Russotto V, Myatra SN, Laffey JG, Tassistro E, Antolini L, Bauer P, et al. Intubation practices and adverse peri-intubation events in critically ill patients from 29 countries. JAMA. 2021;325(12):1164–72. https://doi.org/10.1001/jama.2021.1727. Erratum in: JAMA. 2021;325(24)2507. https://doi.org/10.1001/jama.2021.9012.

38. Lee JY, Sim WS, Kim ES, Lee SM, Kim DK, Na YR, et al. Incidence and risk factors of postoperative sore throat after endotracheal intubation in Korean patients. J Int Med Res. 2017;45(2):744–52. https://doi.org/10.1177/0300060516687227.
39. El-Boghdadly K, Bailey CR, Wiles MD. Postoperative sore throat: a systematic review. Anaesthesia. 2016;71(6):706–17. https://doi.org/10.1111/anae.13438.
40. Levin PD, Chrysostomos C, Ibarra CA, Ledot S, Naito D, Weissman C, et al. Causes of sore throat after intubation: a prospective observational study of multiple anesthesia variables. Minerva Anestesiol. 2017;83(6):582–9. https://doi.org/10.23736/S0375-9393.17.11419-7.
41. Hu B, Bao R, Wang X, Liu S, Tao T, Xie Q, et al. The size of endotracheal tube and sore throat after surgery: a systematic review and meta-analysis. PLoS One. 2013;8(10):e74467. https://doi.org/10.1371/journal.pone.0074467.
42. Liu J, Zhang X, Gong W, Li S, Wang F, Fu S, et al. Correlations between controlled endotracheal tube cuff pressure and postprocedural complications: a multicenter study. Anesth Analg. 2010;111(5):1133–7. https://doi.org/10.1213/ANE.0b013e3181f2ecc7.
43. Seet E, Yousaf F, Gupta S, Subramanyam R, Wong DT, Chung F. Use of manometry for laryngeal mask airway reduces postoperative pharyngolaryngeal adverse events: a prospective, randomized trial. Anesthesiology. 2010;112(3):652–7. https://doi.org/10.1097/ALN.0b013e3181cf4346.
44. van Esch BF, Stegeman I, Smit AL. Comparison of laryngeal mask airway vs tracheal intubation: a systematic review on airway complications. J Clin Anesth. 2017;36:142–50. https://doi.org/10.1016/j.jclinane.2016.10.004.
45. Tanaka Y, Nakayama T, Nishimori M, Tsujimura Y, Kawaguchi M, Sato Y. Lidocaine for preventing postoperative sore throat. Cochrane Database Syst Rev. 2015;2015(7):CD004081. https://doi.org/10.1002/14651858.CD004081.pub3.
46. Sun L, Guo R, Sun L. Dexamethasone for preventing postoperative sore throat: a meta-analysis of randomized controlled trials. Ir J Med Sci. 2014;183(4):593–600. https://doi.org/10.1007/s11845-013-1057-0.
47. Newland MC, Ellis SJ, Peters KR, Simonson JA, Durham TM, Ullrich FA, Tinker JH. Dental injury associated with anesthesia: a report of 161,687 anesthetics given over 14 years. J Clin Anesth. 2007;19(5):339–45. https://doi.org/10.1016/j.jclinane.2007.02.007. PMID: 17869983
48. Skeie A, Schwartz O. Traumatic injuries of the teeth in connection with general anaesthesia and the effect of use of mouthguards. Endod Dent Traumatol. 1999;15(1):33–6. https://doi.org/10.1111/j.1600-9657.1999.tb00746.x.
49. Greer D, Marshall KE, Bevans S, Standlee A, McAdams P, Harsha W. Review of videolaryngoscopy pharyngeal wall injuries. Laryngoscope. 2017;127(2):349–53. https://doi.org/10.1002/lary.26134.
50. Loh KS, Irish JC. Traumatic complications of intubation and other airway management procedures. Anesthesiol Clin North Am. 2002;20(4):953–69. https://doi.org/10.1016/s0889-8537(02)00022-6.
51. Yamanaka H, Hayashi Y, Watanabe Y, Uematu H, Mashimo T. Prolonged hoarseness and arytenoid cartilage dislocation after tracheal intubation. Br J Anaesth. 2009;103(3):452–5. https://doi.org/10.1093/bja/aep169.
52. Colton House J, Noordzij JP, Murgia B, Langmore S. Laryngeal injury from prolonged intubation: a prospective analysis of contributing factors. Laryngoscope. 2011;121(3):596–600. https://doi.org/10.1002/lary.21403. Erratum in: Laryngoscope. 2020;130(9):2299. https://doi.org/10.1002/lary.28907.
53. Han I, Kim TK, Yoo JH, Park JH, Chung EY. Dislocation of the temporomandibular joint following general anesthesia. Korean J Anesthesiol. 2014;67(suppl):S113–4. https://doi.org/10.4097/kjae.2014.67.S.S113.
54. Epaud A, Levesque E, Clariot S. Dramatic cervical spine injury secondary to videolaryngoscopy in a patient suffering from ankylosing spondylitis. Anesthesiology. 2021;135(3):495–6. https://doi.org/10.1097/ALN.0000000000003866.

55. Kim YC, Lee SH, Noh GJ, Cho SY, Yeom JH, Shin WJ, et al. Thermosoftening treatment of the nasotracheal tube before intubation can reduce epistaxis and nasal damage. Anesth Analg. 2000;91(3):698–701. https://doi.org/10.1097/00000539-200009000-00038.
56. Stein M, Caplan ES. Nosocomial sinusitis: a unique subset of sinusitis. Curr Opin Infect Dis. 2005;18(2):147–50. https://doi.org/10.1097/01.qco.0000160904.56566.4a.
57. Smith C. Rapid-sequence intubation in adults: indications and concerns. Clin Pulm Med. 2001;8(3):147–65. https://doi.org/10.1097/00045413-200105000-00004.
58. Keller C, Brimacombe J, Bittersohl J, Lirk P, von Goedecke A. Aspiration and the laryngeal mask airway: three cases and a review of the literature. Br J Anaesth. 2004;93(4):579–82. https://doi.org/10.1093/bja/aeh228.
59. Bayable SD, Melesse DY, Lema GF, Ahmed SA. Perioperative management of patients with asthma during elective surgery: a systematic review. Ann Med Surg (Lond). 2021;70:102874. https://doi.org/10.1016/j.amsu.2021.102874.
60. Al-alami AA, Zestos MM, Baraka AS. Pediatric laryngospasm: prevention and treatment. Curr Opin Anaesthesiol. 2009;22(3):388–95. https://doi.org/10.1097/aco.0b013e32832972f3.
61. Larson CP Jr. Laryngospasm—the best treatment. Anesthesiology. 1998;89(5):1293–4.
62. Chrimes N, Higgs A, Hagberg CA, Baker PA, Cooper RM, Greif R, et al. Preventing unrecognised oesophageal intubation: a consensus guideline from the Project for Universal Management of Airways and international airway societies. Anaesthesia. 2022;77(12):1395–415. https://doi.org/10.1111/anae.15817.
63. Cook TM, Harrop-Griffiths AW, Whitaker DK, McNarry AF, Patel A, McGuire B. The 'no trace=wrong place' campaign. Br J Anaesth. 2019;122(4):e68–9. https://doi.org/10.1016/j.bja.2019.01.008.
64. Berkow L, Kanowitz A. Unplanned extubation in the perioperative environment. Anesth Patient Saf Found Newsl. 2022;37(1):14–6, 18.
65. McNett M, Kerber K. Unplanned extubations in the ICU: risk factors and strategies for reducing adverse events. J Clin Outcomes Manag. 2015;22(7):303–11.
66. Pacheco-Lopez PC, Berkow LC, Hillel AT, Akst LM. Complications of airway management. Respir Care. 2014;59(6):1006–21.
67. Baker PA, Behringer EC, Feinleib J, Foley LJ, Mosier J, Roth P, et al. Formation of an airway lead network: an essential patient safety initiative. Br J Anaesth. 2022;128(2):225–9. https://doi.org/10.1016/j.bja.2021.11.013.
68. Smith C, McNarry AF. Airway Leads and Airway Response Teams: improving delivery of safer airway management? Curr Anesthesiol Rep. 2020;10(4):370–7. https://doi.org/10.1007/s40140-020-00404-7.

Chapter 22
Airway Management in Morbid Obesity

Teresa López, Manuel A. Gómez-Ríos, and José Alfonso Sastre

Highlights

- Perform a screening for OSAHS using STOP-Bang in every obese patient. If the score is ≥4, the patient should be referred for polysomnography and CPAP treatment if necessary.
- Obesity is associated with greater difficulty in face mask ventilation, especially if it coexists with OSAHS.
- Globally, obese patients placed in the ramped position are no more difficult to intubate than lean patients.
- Preoxygenate obese patients in the head-up position and preferably with NIV techniques. Use apneic oxygenation during the apnea period.
- Rapid sequence induction is not routinely recommended for obese patients; however, its use is recommended in patients with associated risk factors or with previous bariatric surgery procedures.
- In obese patients, second-generation SAD should be reserved for highly selected patients undergoing short procedures and with continuous access to the airway.
- Videolaryngoscopes are superior to the Macintosh laryngoscope; therefore, they should be considered the technique of choice for intubation in obese patients.
- In obese patients, it is recommended to identify the cricothyroid membrane with ultrasonography and mark its position prior to anesthetic induction.

(continued)

T. López (✉) · J. A. Sastre
Department of Anesthesiology, Complejo Asistencial Universitario de Salamanca, Salamanca, Spain

M. A. Gómez-Ríos
Department of Anesthesia and Perioperative Medicine, Complejo Hospitalario Universitario de A Coruña, A Coruña, Spain

M. Á. Gómez-Ríos, A. van Zundert (eds.), *Evidence-based Guide to Difficult Airway Management*, https://doi.org/10.1007/978-3-032-30769-9_22

- Rocuronium is currently the neuromuscular relaxant of choice in obese patients. Sugammadex dosing should be based on adjusted body weight, and the dose of 16 mg/kg should be precalculated and immediately available.
- The use of CPAP/NIV in the postoperative period should be considered in obese patients, especially in patients previously using them for the treatment of OSAHS/OHS.

OSAHS: obstructive sleep apnea-hypopnea syndrome; **CPAP**: continuous positive airway pressure; **NIV**: noninvasive ventilation; **SAD**: supraglottic airway device; **OHS**: obesity-hypoventilation syndrome.

Table 22.1 Classification of obesity

Obesity class	Body mass index (BMI)
Overweight	25–29.9 kg/m^2
Obesity class 1	30–34.9 kg/m^2
Obesity class 2	35–39.9 kg/m^2
Obesity class 3	$\geq$ 40 kg/m^2

https://www.euro.who.int/en/health-topics/disease-prevention/nutrition/a-healthy-lifestyle/body-mass-index-bmi (Accessed on September 26, 2022) and the National Institutes of Health [United States Centers for Disease Control and Prevention. Defining adult overweight and obesity. https://www.cdc.gov/obesity/adult/defining.html (Accessed on September 26, 2022)]

22.1 Introduction

The prevalence of obesity has increased significantly in the last few decades worldwide. With increasing frequency, these patients undergo surgical procedures, either for the treatment of their obesity (bariatric surgery) or for the treatment of other elective or emergent surgical pathologies. The management of obese patients is a challenge for anesthesiologists, who may encounter difficulties in different aspects of the anesthetic procedure (vascular access, regional anesthesia, or airway control procedures). The management of the airway in these patients can be a source of significant morbidity and mortality and requires careful and meticulous planning and execution.

In adults, the World Health Organization [1] and the National Institutes of Health [2] have adopted a classification of obesity defined by the body mass index (BMI) (Table 22.1). The term morbid obesity is frequently used to define patients with a BMI $\geq$ 40 kg/m^2. The terms super obesity for cases with a BMI $\geq$ 50 kg/m^2 and super super obesity for those with a BMI $\geq$ 60 kg/m^2 are also used.

22.2 Anatomy and Physiology of the obese Patient

Patients suffering from obesity develop anatomical and physiological changes compared to the normal population. These changes can hinder airway management and reduce the safety threshold in these patients (Table 22.2).

Table 22.2 Anatomical and functional changes in the obese patient

	Changes	Anesthetic implications
Anatomical changes	Excessive soft tissue around the patient's face and cheeks	Difficult effective mask seal and bag-mask ventilation
	Large tongue	Difficult to displace it in the submental space for adequate exposure during laryngoscopy
	Increased adipose tissue deposition in the pharynx and hypopharynx	Narrowing of the airway and increased risk of airway obstruction
	Deposition of adipose tissue in the neck, shoulder, and back	Positioning the patient in the sniffing position for laryngoscopy requires specific adjustments
	Increased abdominal cavity contents	Increased intraabdominal pressure Increased incidence of hiatal hernia and gastroesophageal reflux disease Diminished TLC and VC
Functional changes	Reduced chest wall compliance	Diminished TLC and VC
	Reduced FRC	Faster desaturation during apnea
	Increased O_2 demand	
	Early airway closure	Resting room air hypoxemia
	Microatelectasis	
	Decreased ventilation of the relatively well-perfused lung bases and ventilation-perfusion mismatch	
	Increased CO_2 production	Increased hypercapnia during apnea
	Larger gastric volumes	Neumonitis in case of bronchial aspiration
	Lower gastric pH	

TLC total lung capacity, *VC* vital capacity, *FRC* functional residual capacity

22.3 Preanesthetic Evaluation

In the preanesthetic consultation of the obese patient, it is mandatory to rule out the presence of obstructive sleep apnea-hypopnea syndrome (OSAHS), which can greatly influence the anesthetic induction, extubation, and postoperative recovery. Its prevalence rate is approximately 70% in patients undergoing bariatric surgery [3], but it may be underdiagnosed. The STOP-Bang questionnaire (Table 22.3) [4] is the best validated screening tool in obese patients [5]. It is easy to calculate, takes only a few minutes to perform and has shown a good correlation with the severity of postoperative apneas. For the obese patients, a STOP-Bang score of 0–3 indicates a low risk of OSAHS, a STOP-Bang score of 4–5 suggests an intermediate risk and a STOP-Bang score of 6–8 indicates a high risk situation [6]. The STOP-Bang score may be used as an effective predictor of difficult airway in obese patients; in different studies, those with diagnosed OSAHS or with a STOP-Bang score ≥ 3 have significantly higher frequency of difficult mask ventilation (both before and after muscle relaxation), and more difficulty in laryngoscopy and intubation [7–10] (grade of recommendation B). However, another study has shown that OSAHS is not a risk factor for difficult intubation in morbidly obese patients when the ramped position is used [11], so this position has been recommended for preoxygenation and intubation. Patients with suspected undiagnosed OSAHS who do not require urgent surgery should be referred to a physician specializing in sleep disorders to perform a polysomnography [5] and start treatment with nocturnal continuous positive airway pressure (CPAP) in severe cases or in those with significant associated cardiovascular comorbidity [12].

Moreover, it is important to have a high index of suspicion to detect a possible obesity-hypoventilation syndrome (OHS). Its diagnosis is based on the presence

Table 22.3 STOP-Bang questionnaire

Snoring	Do you snore loudly (loud enough to be heard through closed doors)?
Tired	Do you often feel tired, fatigued or sleepy during the daytime?
Observed	Has anyone observed you stop breathing during your sleep?
Blood **p**ressure	Do you have or are you being treated for high blood pressure?
BMI	BMI more than 35 kg/m^2?
Age	Age over 50 years old?
Neck circumference	Neck circumference > 40 cm?
Gender	Male?

Chung F, Subramanyam R, Liao P, Sasaki E, Shapiro C, Sun Y. High STOP-Bang score indicates a high probability of obstructive sleep apnoea. Br J Anaesth 2012;108(5):768–775. https://doi.org/10.1093/bja/aes022

of obesity, sleep-disordered breathing, and awake daytime hypercapnia in the absence of other causes for hypoventilation [13]. The prevalence of OHS increases in parallel with the increase in BMI, reaching 30.4% in subjects with BMI ≥ 40 kg/m^2 [14]. The American Thoracic Society recommends obtaining an arterial blood gas in severely obese patients with signs and symptoms of OHS if they have a serum bicarbonate >27 mEq/L, which cannot be explained by another cause [15]. If the diagnosis of OHS is confirmed, CPAP is the first-line treatment, followed by noninvasive ventilation (NIV) with two levels of pressure (BiPAP) in case of failure [12].

Finally, obesity may be associated with chronic obstructive pulmonary disease (COPD) and asthma. In addition, obesity by itself can generate an obstructive syndrome [12]. It is therefore necessary to assess the existence of these pathologies and establish the appropriate treatment to minimize the risk of perioperative bronchospasm.

In obese patients, as in any other patient, the airway must be exhaustively examined, regardless of the procedure and the anesthetic technique used. This exam includes the evaluation of the face and cheeks, the presence of a beard, the degree of mouth opening, Mallampati scoring, thyromental distance, mandibular movement, range of movement of the neck, and neck circumference. The exploration should be directed systematically to detect clinical indicators of difficult mask ventilation and difficult tracheal intubation. It is widely accepted that there is no single clinical indicator of a difficult airway and that the presence of several of these indicators increases the possibilities of difficulty.

1. *Facemask ventilation:* According to various studies, obesity is an independent predictor of difficult mask ventilation [16–18]. Additionally, snoring and OSAHS are also considered independent predictors; therefore, the coexistence of both factors indicates a high probability of difficult mask ventilation [16]. Neck circumference, Mallampati classification grade III–IV, limited mandibular protrusion, and male gender are independent predictors for difficult mask ventilation in this population [19]. A high BMI is also a risk factor for difficult mask ventilation combined with difficult laryngoscopy [20]. However, obesity is not a predictor of impossible mask ventilation, but OSAHS is [21].
2. *Intubation:* Historically, obese patients have been considered more difficult to intubate than normal-weight patients; we now know that this does not always correspond to reality [18, 22–31]. In fact, a reduction in BMI is associated with a significant decrease in Mallampati score, but there is no significant decrease in laryngoscopy grade [32]. Indeed, the isolated BMI does not take into account the patient's percentage of lean mass, nor the distribution of body fat. However, there are some features in these patients that are associated with greater laryngoscopy or intubation difficulty, such as increased neck circumference [22, 27, 30, 33–38], short thyromental distance [35, 39, 40], high neck circumference to thyromental distance ratio [41, 42], high Mallampati score [11, 23, 34, 35, 37, 39, 41–43], high upper lip bite test [40, 44], and high waist and chest circumferences [37].

3. *Supraglottic airway devices (SADs):* The literature on predictors of SADs insertion and ventilation failure in obese patients is less extensive than that for face mask ventilation and intubation. In one study, BMI has been identified as a risk factor for failure of SADs [45], but this association has not been found in other subsequent studies [46, 47].

Recently, there has been increasing interest in advanced techniques, such as neck X-rays and ultrasounds, to predict difficult intubations. However, no clear radiographic or sonographic parameters have been validated for predicting a difficult airway. In obese patients, fat pads around the neck and deposited anterior to the trachea might lower submandibular space compliance and might limit optimal head extension; more than 15 ultrasonographic measured parameters have been used in prospective studies [48], like the soft tissue thickness measured anterior to the epiglottis, tracheal wall, vocal cords commissure, and hyoid bone. Other advanced imaging modalities, such as computerized tomography or magnetic resonance imaging, may be employed, but their use is usually restricted to airway assessment in complex head and neck pathologies.

22.4 Approach to Airway Management

22.4.1 Positioning

Proper positioning of the obese patient is the first step in facilitating intubation. Unlike lean patients, who are placed in the sniffing position (head extended and neck flexed) (Fig. 22.1), obese patients should be placed in the ramped position (Fig. 22.2). To do this, the patient's head and shoulders must be raised above the horizontal plane until the external auditory meatus is aligned with the sternal notch; this can be achieved using blankets or specialized instruments designed for this purpose. The ramped position allows alignment of the oral, pharyngeal, and laryngeal axes in the obese patient, improving glottic exposure with respect to the sniffing position [49, 50] (grade of recommendation A). Additionally, the ramped

Fig. 22.1 Supine position

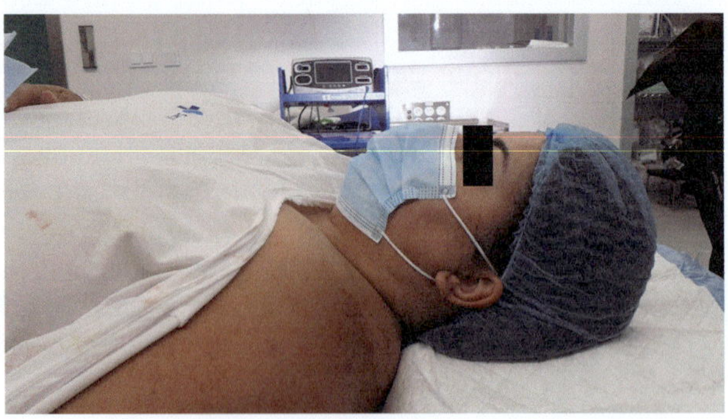

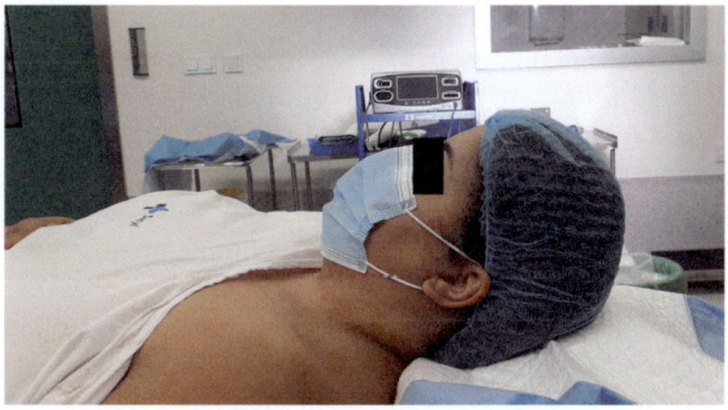

Fig. 22.2 Ramped position

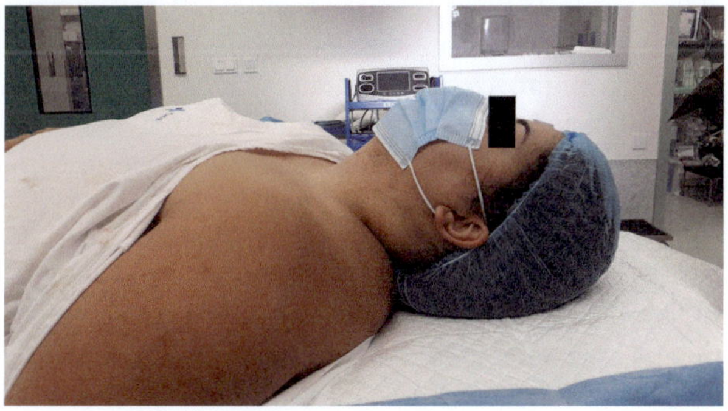

Fig. 22.3 Modified ramped position

position improves lung mechanics and minimizes the impact of obesity on respiratory function, favoring preoxygenation and maximizing the safe apnea time [5].

According to some authors, the position achieved by reconfiguring the operating room table by flexing it at the trunk-thigh hinge and raising the back (trunk) portion of the table is equivalent to the ramped position for the purpose of direct laryngoscopy and intubation [51] (grade of recommendation A).

A modified ramped position has recently been described for obese women (Fig. 22.3); in this position, the shoulders remain elevated, and the head hyperextended using a special pillow to bring the breasts away from the laryngoscope. Compared to the conventional ramped position, the modified ramped position provides better intubating conditions, improves the laryngeal view, and eliminates the need for repositioning of obese females during insertion of the laryngoscope [52] (grade of recommendation A).

22.4.2 Preoxygenation

Preoxygenation in obese patients is especially important, since desaturation after the onset of apnea occurs significantly faster than in lean patients, due to smaller functional residual capacity (FRC) and higher oxygen consumption [53, 54]. To increase the effectiveness of preoxygenation and safe apnea time, different strategies have been described.

As in the case of intubation, the position of the patient is decisive to optimize preoxygenation. The decrease in FRC in the obese patient is exacerbated by the supine position, as the diaphragm is displaced cranially. Therefore, preoxygenation in the head-up position would increase FRC and can significantly extend the tolerance to apnea [55–57] (grade of recommendation A).

Preoxygenation in spontaneous ventilation with a facemask is followed by rapid desaturation after induction in obese patients, despite a high inspired oxygen fraction (less than 1 min in case of very severe obesity) [12]. For conventional preoxygenation, tidal volume and eight vital capacity breathing techniques are equivalent [58]. The application of CPAP during preoxygenation decreases the formation of atelectasis [59], improves oxygenation [59, 60], and prolongs the time of safe apnea [60] without increasing the volume of gastric gas [61] (grade of recommendation A). NIV improves end-expiratory lung volume [62] and arterial oxygenation [62–66], achieving higher EtO_2 more rapidly [63, 66], albeit modestly increasing gastric distention [63] (grade of recommendation A).

On the other hand, in obese patients, apneic oxygenation techniques are of special interest, since they significantly delay desaturation once apnea has begun. Thus, the simple administration of conventional oxygen therapy through nasal cannulas [67, 68], an intraoral tube [69], or a nasopharyngeal catheter [70] can significantly increase the safe apnea time if the upper airway remains patent (grade of recommendation A). Buccal oxygenation with an oral 3.5 mm Ring, Adair and Elwyn (RAE) tube provides safe apnea times modestly higher than the nasal cannulas, being a reliable alternative that can be used in situations where nasal oxygenation is contraindicated or not feasible [71].

In recent years, the use of high flow nasal oxygenation (HFNO) as an alternative or complement to conventional preoxygenation has been investigated. According to two recent meta-analyses, compared with conventional oxygen therapy or NIV, the use of HFNO may be associated with a longer safe apnea time without a beneficial impact on the risk of hypoxemia, oxygenation, and CO_2 elimination in patients with obesity [72, 73] (grade of recommendation A). Regarding side effects, compared to conventional preoxygenation and facemask ventilation during apnea, the use of HFNO results in significantly less gastric insufflation [74].

22.4.3 Risk of Bronchial Aspiration

Obese patients have usually been considered to have a higher risk of bronchial aspiration, due to the higher intra-abdominal pressure and greater frequency of gastroesophageal reflux and hiatus hernia [75]. In addition, obesity is a risk factor for the development of diabetes mellitus, which can also increase the possibility of aspiration if there is autonomic neuropathy (gastroparesis).

Obese patients have a higher risk of aspiration than lean patients in accordance with the Roberts and Shirley criteria (gastric volume > 25 mL and pH < 2.5) [76], but the risk is equalized with the administration of ranitidine and metoclopramide [77]. However, it has been found that obesity is associated with a faster transit of both solids and liquids through the stomach [78]. In fact, the guidelines of the European Society of Anaesthesiology and the American Society of Anesthesiologists do not consider obesity to be a risk factor of aspiration and recommend that obese patients who are without gastroparesis or symptomatic gastroesophageal reflux follow the same fasting guidelines as patients of normal weight [79, 80]. Similarly, rapid sequence induction is not routinely recommended for obese patients who adhere to fasting guidelines and have no associated risk factors [81] (grade of recommendation D).

On the other hand, bariatric surgery procedures can induce pathophysiological changes that increase the risk of bronchial aspiration. Patients with an adjustable gastric band are at high risk of pulmonary inhalation during the induction of general anesthesia due to a disorder of esophageal motility and dilation above the band [12]; the dilatation may persist following band deflation. Sleeve gastrectomy decreases the pressure of the lower esophageal sphincter and increases the inefficiency of esophageal motility, with increased acid reflux [82]. A significant increase in aspiration cases has been reported after both procedures [83]. Also, the Roux-en-Y gastric bypass can affect esophageal motility [82]. Therefore, in all these obese patients, it seems reasonable to perform a rapid sequence induction and secure the airway by endotracheal intubation (grade of recommendation B).

22.4.4 *Selection of the Airway Control Device*

Different studies have shown that the use of second-generation SADs is safe in obese patients [84–87]. In any case, it seems prudent to reserve SADs for highly selected patients undergoing short procedures and with continuous access to the airway; in these cases, a Plan B should always be available for intubation in the event of airway device failure [5]. Second-generation SADs with a high success rate of fiberoptic-guided intubation through SADs are preferred [87, 88] (grade of recommendation B).

Tracheal diameters reduce slightly with increasing BMI [89]; therefore, the size of the endotracheal tube or the SAD should be selected based on ideal weight.

22.4.5 *Airway Management*

Major complications in airway management in the United Kingdom were extensively studied in the fourth National Audit Project of the Royal College of Anaesthetists and the Difficult Airway Society [90]. In the group of obese patients, a higher frequency of anesthesia-related events was observed, and this was attributed to several facts:

1. Often, there was a lack of recognition and planning for potential airway problems.
2. As a result of the reduced safe apnea time, when airway complications occurred, they occurred rapidly with a potentially catastrophic outcome.
3. Rescue airway techniques such as SADs and emergency cricothyroidotomy had an increased failure rate.
4. Adverse events occurred more frequently in obese patients when the anesthesiologist was inexperienced.

For all these reasons, careful planning of the airway approach in these patients is essential, establishing an initial plan and rescue strategies that must be implemented immediately in the event of failure of the primary plan, and that must be known by the entire team. Likewise, the presence of personnel experienced in the management of these patients is a fundamental requirement.

Taking into account the higher frequency of facemask ventilation difficulties in obese patients, if intubation problems are also anticipated, intubation should be performed with the patient awake, either with a fiberoptic bronchoscope or a videolaryngoscope [91]. It is important to optimize topical anesthesia in these patients, as sedation can precipitate airway obstruction, especially in those with OSAHS [5].

In case of intubation of an anesthetized patient, it has been suggested to use a SAD to maintain oxygenation in the interval between the onset of apnea and endotracheal intubation, given the ease of insertion [92] and the better oxygenation achieved with these devices compared to facemask ventilation [93] (grade of recommendation A). There is an ongoing debate about whether videolaryngoscopes are the first choice in this type of patients, compared to conventional laryngoscopes [94]. According to two recent meta-analyses, videolaryngoscopes are superior to the Macintosh laryngoscope in relation to success rate, intubation time, and glottic visualization [95, 96] (grade of recommendation A). Videolaryngoscopes with a tracheal tube guide channel are superior to the Macintosh laryngoscope for all outcomes, while videolaryngoscopes without a tracheal tube guide channel are superior to the Macintosh laryngoscope for all outcomes except for intubation time. A high rate of success in intubation has also been documented with video-intubating laryngeal masks, which minimize apnea time and desaturation in these patients [97–99] (grade of recommendation B).

In case of "can't-intubate-can't-oxigenate" (CICO) situation, the first rescue option should always be a SAD. However, it should be noted that the probability of ventilation failure with these devices is greater if facemask ventilation and intubation are difficult [100–102]; thereby, if after a maximum of three attempts to insert a SAD, effective ventilation is not achieved, an emergency front-of-neck access (FONA) should be performed without delay [103].

The FONA is a challenge for the anesthesiologist, since it is a procedure that is performed infrequently and usually on an emergent basis. The difficulty in the obese patient is even greater, since the accuracy in locating the cricothyroid membrane by palpation may be reduced due to the accumulation of fat in the anterior cervical region; in fact, increased neck circumference is significantly associated with inaccuracy in identifying the cricothyroid membrane [104]. It has been found that the ultrasound-guided approach offered a significantly higher success rate in the identification of the cricothyroid membrane than the palpation technique, and although it requires a longer time, the difference is not statistically significant [105] (grade of recommendation B); the transverse technique is faster than the longitudinal technique [106]. It is therefore recommended, in obese patients and other patients in whom difficulty in managing the airway is anticipated, that the cricothyroid membrane be identified with ultrasonography and marked with the patient in an extended-neck position prior to anesthetic induction (grade of recommendation D). In this way, if the initial airway management plan fails and it is necessary to proceed to a FONA, the patient can be returned to the extended-neck position, and the marking of the cricothyroid membrane will again be correct [107].

22.5 Airway Management Pharmacology

Obesity has significant effects on the metabolism and pharmacokinetic profiles of most anesthetic agents. For many of them, dosing to total body weight is rarely appropriate and increases the risk of relative overdose. Lipid-soluble drugs have a larger volume of distribution and are metabolized faster in patients who are obese. The effects of opioids can also be altered and patients with OSAHS are especially sensitive to them. When possible, anesthetic medications should be titrated to effect with incremental doses. Suggested starting doses for obese patients are shown in Table 22.4, and relative terms for describing patients' weight are shown in Table 22.5 [5].

Highly lipid-soluble halogenated agents can be associated with delayed awakening in obese patients. There is evidence of faster postoperative recovery after desflurane than after sevoflurane, isoflurane, or propofol anesthesia [108–110], although the huge impact on the environment prevents us from using desflurane in the anesthesia practice.

Table 22.4 Suggested initial dosing for anesthetic drugs for healthy obese adults

Lean body weight	Adjusted body weight	Total body weight
Propofol (induction) Thiopental Fentanyl Morphine Rocuronium Atracurium Vecuronium Paracetamol Bupivacaine Lidocaine	Propofol (infusion) Antibiotics Low molecular weight heparin Alfentanil Neostigmine (maximum 5 mg) Sugammadex	Succinylcholine

Modified from Nightingale CE, Margarson MP, Shearer E, Redman JW, Lucas DN, Cousins JM, et al. Peri-operative management of the obese surgical patient 2015: Association of Anaesthetists of Great Britain and Ireland Society for Obesity and Bariatric Anaesthesia. Anaesthesia. 2015;70:859–876. https://doi.org/10.1111/anae.13101

Table 22.5 Terms for describing patients' weight

Total body weight (TBW)	The actual weight of the patient
Ideal body weight (IBW)	What the patient should weigh with a normal ratio of lean to fat mass IBW (kg) = height (cm)—100 (men) IBW (kg) = height (cm)—105 (women)
Lean body weight (LBW)	The patient's weight excluding fat. Many of the formulae for calculating lean body weight are complex. Regardless of total body weight, lean body weight rarely exceeds 100 kg in men and 70 kg in women
Adjusted body weight (ABW)	Takes into account the fact that obese patients have increased lean body mass and an increased volume of distribution for drugs. It is calculated by adding 40% of the excess weight to the IBW ABW (kg) = IBW (kg) + 0.4 [TBW (kg) − IBW (kg)]

Modified from Nightingale CE, Margarson MP, Shearer E, Redman JW, Lucas DN, Cousins JM, et al. Peri-operative management of the obese surgical patient 2015: Association of Anaesthetists of Great Britain and Ireland Society for Obesity and Bariatric Anaesthesia. Anaesthesia. 2015;70:859–876. https://doi.org/10.1111/anae.13101

In patients at high-risk of hypoxemia during induction, such as the obese patient, the use of succinylcholine is not recommended, because the fasciculations increase oxygen consumption, decrease safe apnea time, and prolong the recovery of oxygen saturation [111, 112] (grade of recommendation A); moreover, its effect is unlikely to wear off before hypoxemia occurs [113, 114]. On the other hand, different studies have shown that neuromuscular transmission and spontaneous ventilation recover more quickly with the rocuronium-sugammadex combination than with succinylcholine [115, 116]; hence, rocuronium is currently considered the neuromuscular relaxant of choice in obese patients [5] (grade of recommendation A). The sugammadex dose of 16 mg/kg should be precalculated and immediately available in all cases [117]. Sugammadex dosing should be based on adjusted body weight, with reversal times similar to total body weight doses, but significantly shorter than those achieved with ideal body weight doses [118] (grade of recommendation A). Although recovery of neuromuscular transmission is rapid with sugammadex, profound desaturation may occur before return of spontaneous ventilation, especially in obese patients, so the clinical management of the CICO situation should focus primarily on restoration of airway patency, oxygenation, and ventilation consistent with the practice guidelines for management of the difficult airway [119].

22.6 Emergence from Anaesthesia

Obese patients are at higher risk of perioperative complications (mainly associated with the respiratory function) and problems during extubation, as shown in NAP4 [90]. Therefore, extubation must be planned as meticulously as intubation. The patient should be extubated as soon as possible, awake and in the sitting position, when neuromuscular transmission and airway reflexes have fully recovered [5, 12]. Insertion of a nasopharyngeal airway before awakening in patients with OSAHS may mitigate the upper airway obstruction that commonly occurs after extubation [5]. Oxygen supplementation should be administered to all patients until they are able to maintain baseline oxygen saturation in ambient air [12].

Postoperative pulmonary considerations are similar to those of the intraoperative phase: keeping the lung open and preventing atelectasis. It has been shown that there is more atelectasis and a reduction in lung volumes post-extubation in obese patients than in lean patients [120]. Short-term respiratory physiotherapy promotes more rapid recovery of postoperative lung function in the obese during the first 24 h [121] (grade of recommendation A). The rationale for the postoperative use of NIV is an increased FRC, improved lung compliance, ventilation, and oxygenation, and decreased upper airway obstruction and work of breathing. It should be started once the patient is awake, following commands, and breathing spontaneously [122]; early initiation of short-term NIV promotes more rapid recovery of postoperative lung function and oxygenation, and the effect lasts 24 h after discontinuation [123] (grade of recommendation A). Although the use of NIV is associated with a lower frequency of respiratory complications, it has not been shown to reduce the frequency of reintubation and unplanned Intensive Care Unit (ICU) admissions [65]. Subjects with OHS (with or without OSAHS) are more likely to develop postoperative respiratory and heart failure and prolonged intubation time compared with patients with OSAHS alone [124]; therefore, it is imperative that after extubation, these patients be immediately transitioned to the NIV strategy used to treat their underlying OSAHS/OHS. Initially, the use of NIV was not widely accepted for obese patients following gastrointestinal surgery because of concerns that pressurized air may inflate the stomach and proximal intestine, resulting in anastomotic disruption. However, various studies have shown that NIV is safe and does not increase these types of complications [125–128] (grade of recommendation A).

The role of HFNO in the postoperative period of obese patients is controversial. In a study, prophylactic extubation onto HFNO following cardiac surgery did not improve atelectasis, oxygenation, respiratory rate, or dyspnea or reduce the need for escalation of respiratory support when compared to standard oxygen therapy [129]. However, in a later study, the use of continuous HFNO compared with intermittent NIV did not result in a worse rate of treatment failure among obese cardiothoracic surgery subjects [130]. In fact, in recent guidelines, it is suggested to use HFNO to prevent respiratory failure in the immediate postoperative period in high-risk and/or obese patients undergoing cardiac or thoracic surgery [131]. On the other hand, HFNO has been shown to reduce postoperative hypoxemia and atelectasis in morbidly obese patients undergoing bariatric surgery compared to conventional oxygen therapy [132].

Recommendations

Recommendation	Grade of recommendation
The STOP-bang score is an effective predictor of difficult airway in obese patients; those with diagnosed OSAHS or with a STOP-bang score ≥ 3 have a significantly higher frequency of difficult mask ventilation and more difficulty in laryngoscopy and intubation	B
The ramped position allows the alignment of the oral, pharyngeal, and laryngeal axes in the obese patient, improving glottic exposure concerning the sniffing position	A
The position achieved by reconfiguring the operating room table by flexing it at the trunk-thigh hinge and raising the back (trunk) portion of the table is equivalent to the ramped position for the purpose of direct laryngoscopy and intubation	A
Compared to the conventional ramped position, the modified ramped position in females provides better intubating conditions, improves the laryngeal view, and eliminates the need for repositioning during insertion of the laryngoscope	A
Preoxygenation in the head-up position increases FRC and can significantly extend the tolerance to apnea	A
The application of CPAP during preoxygenation decreases the formation of atelectasis, improves oxygenation, and prolongs the time of safe apnea without increasing the volume of gastric gas	A
NIV for preoxygenation improves end-expiratory lung volume and arterial oxygenation, achieving higher EtO_2 more rapidly, albeit modestly increasing gastric distention	A
The administration of conventional oxygen therapy during apnea through nasal cannulas, an intraoral tube, or a nasopharyngeal catheter can significantly increase the safe apnea time if the upper airway remains patent	A
Compared with conventional oxygen therapy or NIV, the use of HFNO may be associated with a longer safe apnea time without a beneficial impact on the risk of hypoxemia, oxygenation, and CO_2 elimination in patients with obesity	A
Rapid sequence induction is not routinely recommended for obese patients who adhere to fasting guidelines and have no associated risk factors	D
In patients with adjustable gastric band and sleeve gastrectomy, the risk of bronchial aspiration is increased, so it is reasonable to perform a rapid sequence induction and secure the airway by endotracheal intubation	B
Second-generation SADs with a high success rate of fiberoptic-guided intubation through them is preferred	B
SADs can be used to maintain oxygenation in the interval between the onset of apnea and endotracheal intubation, given the ease of insertion and the better oxygenation achieved with these devices compared to face mask ventilation	A

Recommendation	Grade of recommendation
Videolaryngoscopes are superior to the Macintosh laryngoscope in success rate, intubation time, and glottic visualization; therefore, they are the devices of first choice for intubation in the obese patient	A
A high rate of success in intubation has been documented with video intubating laryngeal masks, which minimize apnea time and desaturation in these patients	B
The ultrasound-guided approach offered a significantly higher success rate in the identification of the cricothyroid membrane than the palpation technique, and although it requires a longer time, the difference is not statistically significant	B
It is recommended, in obese patients and other patients in whom difficulty in managing the airway is anticipated, that the cricothyroid membrane be identified with ultrasonography and marked with the patient in an extended-neck position prior to anesthetic induction	D
There is evidence of faster postoperative recovery after desflurane than after sevoflurane, isoflurane, or propofol anesthesia in obese patients, so desflurane can be considered the maintenance agent of choice in these patients. However, due to desflurane's environmental impact, desflurane is no longer used in many countries	A
In patients at high-risk of hypoxemia during induction, such as the obese patient, the use of succinylcholine is not recommended, because the fasciculations increase oxygen consumption, decrease safe apnea time, and prolong the recovery of oxygen saturation	A
Neuromuscular transmission and spontaneous ventilation recover more quickly with the rocuronium-sugammadex combination than with succinylcholine; hence, rocuronium is currently considered the neuromuscular relaxant of choice in obese patients	A
Sugammadex dosing should be based on adjusted body weight, with reversal times similar to total body weight doses, but significantly shorter than those achieved with ideal body weight doses	A
Short-term respiratory physiotherapy promotes more rapid recovery of postoperative lung function in the obese during the first 24 h	A
Early initiation of short-term NIV after extubation promotes more rapid recovery of postoperative lung function and oxygenation, and the effect lasts 24 h after discontinuation	A
NIV is safe and does not increase anastomotic disruption after gastrointestinal surgery	A

OSAHS: obstructive sleep apnea-hypopnea syndrome; **FRC**: functional residual capacity; **CPAP**: continuous positive airway pressure; **NIV**: noninvasive ventilation; **HFNO**: high flow nasal oxygenation; **SAD**: supraglottic airway device.

References

1. https://www.euro.who.int/en/health-topics/disease-prevention/nutrition/a-healthy-lifestyle/body-mass-index-bmi. Accessed on 26 Sept 2022.
2. United States Centers for Disease Control and Prevention. Defining adult overweight and obesity. https://www.cdc.gov/obesity/adult/defining.html. Accessed on 26 Sept 2022.
3. Frey W, Pilcher J. Obstructive sleep-related breathing disorders in patients evaluated for bariatric surgery. Obes Surg. 2003;13:676–83. https://doi.org/10.1381/096089203322509228.
4. Chung F, Yegneswaran B, Liao P, Chung SA, Vairavanathan S, Islam S, et al. STOP Questionnaire. Anesthesiology. 2008;108:812–21. https://doi.org/10.1097/aln.0b013e31816d83e4.
5. Nightingale CE, Margarson MP, Shearer E, Redman JW, Lucas DN, Cousins JM, et al. Perioperative management of the obese surgical patient 2015: association of anaesthetists of Great Britain and Ireland society for obesity and bariatric. Anaesthesia. 2015;70:859–76. https://doi.org/10.1111/anae.13101.
6. Chung F, Yang Y, Liao P. Predictive performance of the STOP-bang score for identifying obstructive sleep apnea in obese patients. Obes Surg. 2013;23:2050–7. https://doi.org/10.1007/s11695-013-1006-z.
7. Toshniwal G, McKelvey GM, Wang H. STOP-bang and prediction of difficult airway in obese patients. J Clin Anesth. 2014;26:360–7. https://doi.org/10.1016/j.jclinane.2014.01.010.
8. Khan MN, Ahmed A. Accuracy of STOP-bang questionnaire in predicting difficult mask ventilation: an observational study. Cureus. 2021;13:e15955. https://doi.org/10.7759/cureus.15955.
9. Seet E, Chung F, Wang CY, Tam S, Kumar CM, Ubeynarayana CU, et al. Association of obstructive sleep apnea with difficult intubation: prospective multicenter observational cohort study. Anesth Analg. 2021;133:196–204. https://doi.org/10.1213/ANE.0000000000005479.
10. Nagappa M, Wong DT, Cozowicz C, Ramachandran SK, Memtsoudis SG, Chung F. Is obstructive sleep apnea associated with difficult airway? Evidence from a systematic review and meta-analysis of prospective and retrospective cohort studies. PLoS One. 2018;13:e0204904. https://doi.org/10.1371/journal.pone.0204904.
11. Neligan PJ, Porter S, Max B, Malhotra G, Greenblatt EP, Ochroch EA. Obstructive sleep apnea is not a risk factor for difficult intubation in morbidly obese patients. Anesth Analg. 2009;109:1182–6. https://doi.org/10.1213/ane.0b013e3181b12a0c.
12. De Jong A, Rollé A, Souche FR, Yengui O, Verzilli D, Chanques G, et al. How can I manage anaesthesia in obese patients? Anaesth Crit Care Pain Med. 2020;39:229–38. https://doi.org/10.1016/j.accpm.2019.12.009.
13. Mokhlesi B, Tulaimat A, Faibussowitsch I, Wang Y, Evans A. Obesity hypoventilation syndrome: prevalence and predictors in patients with obstructive sleep apnea. Sleep Breath. 2007;11:117–24. https://doi.org/10.1007/s11325-006-0092-8.
14. Macavei VM, Spurling KJ, Loft J, Makker HK. Diagnostic predictors of obesity-hypoventilation syndrome in patients suspected of having sleep disordered breathing. J Clin Sleep Med. 2013;9:879–84. https://doi.org/10.5664/jcsm.2986.
15. Mokhlesi B, Masa JF, Afshar M, Balachandran JS, Brozek JL, Dweik RA, et al. Evaluation and management of obesity hypoventilation syndrome an official American Thoracic Society clinical practice guideline. Am J Respir Crit Care Med 2019;200:E6-E24. doi:https://doi.org/10.1164/rccm.201905-1071ST.
16. Langeron O, Masso E, Huraux C, Guggiari M, Bianchi A, Coriat P, et al. Prediction of difficult mask ventilation. Anesthesiology. 2000;92:1229–36. https://doi.org/10.1097/00000542-200005000-00009.
17. Kheterpal S, Han R, Tremper KK, Shanks A, Tait AR, O'Reilly M, et al. Incidence and predictors of difficult and impossible mask ventilation. Anesthesiology. 2006;105:885–91. https://doi.org/10.1097/00000542-200611000-00007.

18. Moon TS, Fox PE, Somasundaram A, Minhajuddin A, Gonzales MX, Pak TJ, et al. The influence of morbid obesity on difficult intubation and difficult mask ventilation. J Anesth. 2019;33:96–102. https://doi.org/10.1007/s00540-018-2592-7.
19. Leoni A, Arlati S, Ghisi D, Verwej M, Lugani D, Ghisi P, et al. Difficult mask ventilation in obese patients: analysis of predictive factors. Minerva Anestesiol. 2014;80:149–57.
20. Kheterpal S, Healy D, Aziz MF, Shanks AM, Freundlich RE, Linton F, et al. Incidence, predictors, and outcome of difficult mask ventilation combined with difficult laryngoscopy: a report from the multicenter perioperative outcomes group. Anesthesiology. 2013;119:1360–9. https://doi.org/10.1097/ALN.0000435832.39353.20.
21. Kheterpal S, Martin L, Shanks AM, Tremper KK. Prediction and outcomes of impossible mask ventilation: a review of 50.000 anesthetics. Anesthesiology. 2009;110:891–7. https://doi.org/10.1097/ALN.0b013e31819b5b87.
22. Brodsky JB, Lemmens HJM, Brock-Utne JG, Vierra M, Saidman LJ. Morbid obesity and tracheal intubation. Anesth Analg. 2002;94:732–6. https://doi.org/10.1097/00000539-200203000-00047.
23. Ezri T, Medalion B, Weisenberg M, Szmuk P, Warters RD, Charuzi I. Increased body mass index per se is not a predictor of difficult laryngoscopy. Can J Anesth. 2003;50:179–83. https://doi.org/10.1007/BF03017853.
24. Lundstrøm LH, Møller AM, Rosenstock C, Astrup G, Wetterslev J. High body mass index is a weak predictor for difficult and failed tracheal intubation. Anesthesiology. 2009;110:266–74. https://doi.org/10.1097/ALN.0b013e318194cac8.
25. Sheff SR, May MC, Carlisle SE, Kallies KJ, Mathiason MA, Kothari SN. Predictors of a difficult intubation in the bariatric patient: does preoperative body mass index matter? Surg Obes Relat Dis. 2013;9:344–9. https://doi.org/10.1016/j.soard.2012.02.004.
26. Dohrn N, Sommer T, Bisgaard J, Rønholm E, Larsen JF. Difficult tracheal intubation in obese gastric bypass patients. Obes Surg. 2016;26:2640–7. https://doi.org/10.1007/s11695-016-2141-0.
27. Hashim MM, Ismail MA, Esmat AM, Adeel S. Difficult tracheal intubation in bariatric surgery patients, a myth or reality? Br J Anaesth. 2016;116:557–8. https://doi.org/10.1093/bja/aew039.
28. Saasouh W, Laffey K, Turan A, Avitsian R, Zura A, You J, et al. Degree of obesity is not associated with more than one intubation attempt: a large centre experience. Br J Anaesth. 2018;120:1110–6. https://doi.org/10.1016/j.bja.2018.01.019.
29. Wang T, Sun S, Huang S. The association of body mass index with difficult tracheal intubation management by direct laryngoscopy: a meta-analysis. BMC Anesthesiol. 2018;18:1–13. https://doi.org/10.1186/s12871-018-0534-4.
30. Raju Vegesna AR, Al-Anee KN, Bashah MMM, Faraj JH. Airway management in bariatric surgery patients, our experience in Qatar: a prospective observational cohort study. Qatar Med J. 2020;2020:1–12. https://doi.org/10.5339/qmj.2020.2.
31. Mahmoud M, Hasanin AM, Mostafa M, Alhamade F, Abdelhamid B, Elsherbeeny M. Evaluation of super-obesity and super-super-obesity as risk factors for difficult intubation in patients undergoing bariatric surgery. Surg Obes Relat Dis. 2021;17:1279–85. https://doi.org/10.1016/j.soard.2021.03.028.
32. Shimonov M, Schechter P, Boaz M, Waintrob R, Ezri T. Does body mass index reduction by bariatric surgery affect laryngoscopy difficulty during subsequent anesthesia? Obes Surg. 2017;27:737–9. https://doi.org/10.1007/s11695-016-2355-1.
33. Iyer US, Koh KF, Chia NCH, Macachor J, Cheng A. Perioperative risk factors in obese patients for bariatric surgery: a Singapore experience. Singapore Med J. 2011;52:94–9.
34. Juvin P, Lavaut E, Dupont H, Lefevre P, Demetriou M, Dumoulin JL, et al. Difficult tracheal intubation is more common in obese than in lean patients. Anesth Analg. 2003;97:595–600. https://doi.org/10.1213/01.ANE.0000072547.75928.B0.

35. Gonzalez H, Minville V, Delanoue K, Mazerolles M, Concina D, Fourcade O. The importance of increased neck circumference to intubation difficulties in obese patients. Anesth Analg. 2008;106:1132–6. https://doi.org/10.1213/ane.0b013e3181679659.
36. Riad W, Vaez MN, Raveendran R, Tam AD, Quereshy FA, Chung F, et al. Neck circumference as a predictor of difficult intubation and difficult mask ventilation in morbidly obese patients. Eur J Anaesthesiol. 2016;33:244–9. https://doi.org/10.1097/EJA.0000000000000324.
37. Emik E, Gümüs-Özcan F, Demirgan S, Selcan A. Evaluation of the correlation between preoperative airway assessment tests, anthropometric measurements, and endotracheal intubation difficulty in obesity class III patients undergoing bariatric surgery. Medicine (Baltimore). 2021;100:e27188. https://doi.org/10.1097/MD.0000000000027188.
38. Sinha A, Jayaraman L, Punhani D. Predictors of difficult airway in the obese are closely related to safe apnea time! J Anaesthesiol Clin Pharmacol. 2020;36:25–30. https://doi.org/10.4103/joacp.JOACP_164_19.
39. Ahmed A, Zaky M, El-Mekawy N, Ollaek M, Sami W, Mohamed D. Evaluation of thyromental height test in prediction of difficult airway in obese surgical patients: an observational study. Indian J Anaesth. 2021;65:880–5. https://doi.org/10.4103/ija.IJA.
40. Kheirabadi D, Honarmand A, Rasouli M, Safavi M, Maracy M. Comparison of airway assessment tests for prediction of difficult intubation in obese patients: importance of thyromental height and upper lip bite test. Minerva Anestesiol. 2022;88:114–20. https://doi.org/10.23736/S0375-9393.21.15764-5.
41. Kim WH, Ahn HJ, Lee CJ, Shin BS, Ko JS, Choi SJ, et al. Neck circumference to thyromental distance ratio: a new predictor of difficult intubation in obese patients. Br J Anaesth. 2011;106:743–8. https://doi.org/10.1093/bja/aer024.
42. Siriussawakul A, Rattana-arpa S, Jirachaipitak S, Chatsiriphattana A, Nimmannit A, Wong-in N. The performance of the neck circumference for a difficult laryngoscopy in obese patients. J Med Assoc Thail. 2016;99:484–90. https://doi.org/10.1016/j.ijoa.2017.01.011.
43. Özdilek A, Beyoglu CA, Erbabacan ŞE, Ekici B, Altındaş F, Vehid S, et al. Correlation of neck circumference with difficult mask ventilation and difficult laryngoscopy in morbidly obese patients: an observational study. Obes Surg. 2018;28:2860–7. https://doi.org/10.1007/s11695-018-3263-3.
44. Richa F, Chalhoub V, Gebrayel WB, El-Hage C, El Jamal P, Yazbeck P. Upper lip bite test versus modified Mallampati classification in predicting difficult laryngoscopy and/or intubation among morbidly obese patients. J Clin Anesth. 2020;63:109761. https://doi.org/10.1016/j.jclinane.2020.109761.
45. Ramachandran SK, Mathis MR, Tremper KK, Shanks AM, Kheterpal S. Predictors and clinical outcomes from failed laryngeal mask airway unique™: a study of 15.795 patients. Anesthesiology. 2012;116:1217–26. https://doi.org/10.1097/ALN.0b013e318255e6ab.
46. Theiler L, Gutzmann M, Kleine-Brueggeney M, Urwyler N, Kaempfen B, Greif R. I-gel™ supraglottic airway in clinical practice: a prospective observational multicentre study. Br J Anaesth. 2012;109:990–5. https://doi.org/10.1093/bja/aes309.
47. Saito T, Liu W, Chew STH, Ti LK. Incidence of and risk factors for difficult ventilation via a supraglottic airway device in a population of 14.480 patients from South-East Asia. Anaesthesia. 2015;70:1079–83. https://doi.org/10.1111/anae.13153.
48. Petrişor C, Trancă S, Szabo R, Simon R, Prie A, Bodolea C. Clinical versus ultrasound measurements of hyomental distance ratio for the prediction of difficult airway in patients with and without morbid obesity. Diagnostics. 2020;10:1–9. https://doi.org/10.3390/diagnostics10030140.
49. Collins JS, Lemmens HJM, Brodsky JB, Brock-Utne JG, Levitan RM. Laryngoscopy and morbid obesity: a comparison of the "sniff" and "ramped" positions. Obes Surg. 2004;14:1171–5. https://doi.org/10.1381/0960892042386869.
50. Lebowitz PW, Shay H, Straker T, Rubin D, Bodner S. Shoulder and head elevation improves laryngoscopic view for tracheal intubation in nonobese as well as obese individuals. J Clin Anesth. 2012;24:104–8. https://doi.org/10.1016/j.jclinane.2011.06.015.

51. Rao SL, Kunselman AR, Schuler HG, Desharnais S. Laryngoscopy and tracheal intubation in the head-elevated position in obese patients: a randomized, controlled, equivalence trial. Anesth Analg. 2008;107:1912–8. https://doi.org/10.1213/ane.0b013e31818556ed.
52. Hasanin A, Tarek H, MMA M, Arafa A, Safina AG, Elsherbiny MH, et al. Modified-ramped position: a new position for intubation of obese females: a randomized controlled pilot study. BMC Anesthesiol. 2020;20:1–7. https://doi.org/10.1186/s12871-020-01070-2.
53. Berthoud MC, Peacock JE, Reilly CS. Effectiveness of preoxygenation in morbidly obese patients. Br J Anaesth. 1991;67:464–6. https://doi.org/10.1093/bja/67.4.464.
54. Jense HG, Dubin SA, Silverstein PI, O'Leary-Escolas U. Effect of obesity on safe duration of apnea in anesthetized humans. Anesth Analg. 1991;72:89–93. https://doi.org/10.1213/00000539-199101000-00016.
55. Altermatt FR, Muñoz HR, Delfino AE, Cortínez LI. Pre-oxygenation in the obese patient: effects of position on tolerance to apnoea. Br J Anaesth. 2005;95:706–9. https://doi.org/10.1093/bja/aei231.
56. Dixon BJ, Dixon JB, Carden JR, Burn AJ, Schachter LM, Playfair JM, et al. Preoxygenation is more effective in the 25° head-up position than in the supine position in severely obese patients: a randomized controlled study. Anesthesiology. 2005;102:1110–5. https://doi.org/10.1097/00000542-200506000-00009.
57. Couture EJ, Provencher S, Somma J, Lellouche F, Marceau S, Bussières JS. Effect of position and positive pressure ventilation on functional residual capacity in morbidly obese patients: a randomized trial. Can J Anesth. 2018;65:522–8. https://doi.org/10.1007/s12630-018-1050-1.
58. Rapaport S, Joannes-Boyau O, Bazin R, Janvier G. Comparison of eight deep breaths and tidal volume breathing preoxygenation techniques in morbid obese patients. Ann Fr Anesth Reanim. 2004;23:1155–9. https://doi.org/10.1016/j.annfar.2004.10.012.
59. Coussa M, Proietti S, Schnyder P, Frascarolo P, Suter M, Spahn DR, et al. Prevention of atelectasis formation during the induction of general anesthesia in morbidly obese patients. Anesth Analg. 2004;98:1491–5. https://doi.org/10.1213/01.ANE.0000111743.61132.99.
60. Gander S, Frascarolo P, Suter M, Spahn DR, Magnusson L. Positive end-expiratory pressure during induction of general anesthesia increases duration of nonhypoxic apnea in morbidly obese patients. Anesth Analg. 2005;100:580–4. https://doi.org/10.1213/01.ANE.0000143339.40385.1B.
61. Cressey D, Berthoud M, Reilly C. Effectiveness of continuous positive airway pressure to enhance pre-oxygenation in morbidly obese women. Anaesthesia. 2001;56:680–4. https://doi.org/10.1046/j.1365-2044.2001.01374-3.x.
62. Futier E, Constantin JM, Pelosi P, Chanques G, Massone A, Petit A, et al. Noninvasive ventilation and alveolar recruitment maneuver improve respiratory function during and after intubation of morbidly obese patients: a randomized controlled study. Anesthesiology. 2011;114:1354–63. https://doi.org/10.1097/ALN.0b013e31821811ba.
63. Delay JM, Sebbane M, Jung B, Nocca D, Verzilli D, Pouzeratte Y, et al. The effectiveness of noninvasive positive pressure ventilation to enhance preoxygenation in morbidly obese patients: a randomized controlled study. Anesth Analg. 2008;107:1707–13. https://doi.org/10.1213/ane.0b013e318183909b.
64. Harbut P, Gozdzik W, Stjernfält E, Marsk R, Hesselvik JF. Continuous positive airway pressure/pressure support pre-oxygenation of morbidly obese patients. Acta Anaesthesiol Scand. 2014;58:675–80. https://doi.org/10.1111/aas.12317.
65. Carron M, Zarantonello F, Tellaroli P, Ori C. Perioperative noninvasive ventilation in obese patients: a qualitative review and meta-analysis. Surg Obes Relat Dis. 2016;12:681–91. https://doi.org/10.1016/j.soard.2015.12.013.
66. Chiang TL, Tam KW, Chen JT, Wong CS, Yeh CT, Huang TY, et al. Non-invasive ventilation for preoxygenation before general anesthesia: a systematic review and meta-analysis of randomized controlled trials. BMC Anesthesiol. 2022;22:1–14. https://doi.org/10.1186/s12871-022-01842-y.

67. Ramachandran SK, Cosnowski A, Shanks A, Turner CR. Apneic oxygenation during prolonged laryngoscopy in obese patients: a randomized, controlled trial of nasal oxygen administration. J Clin Anesth. 2010;22:164–8. https://doi.org/10.1016/j.jclinane.2009.05.006.
68. Moon TS, Tai K, Kim A, Gonzales MX, Lu R, Pak T, et al. Apneic oxygenation during prolonged laryngoscopy in obese patients: a randomized, double-blinded, controlled trial of nasal cannula oxygen administration. Obes Surg. 2019;29:3992–9. https://doi.org/10.1007/s11695-019-04077-y.
69. Heard A, Toner AJ, Evans JR, Aranda Palacios AM, Lauer S. Apneic oxygenation during prolonged laryngoscopy in obese patients: a randomized, controlled trial of buccal RAE tube oxygen administration. Anesth Analg. 2017;124:1162–7. https://doi.org/10.1213/ANE.0000000000001564.
70. Baraka AS, Taha SK, Siddik-Sayyid SM, Kanazi GE, El-Khatib MF, Dagher CM, et al. Supplementation of pre-oxygenation in morbidly obese patients using nasopharyngeal oxygen insufflation. Anaesthesia. 2007;62:769–73. https://doi.org/10.1111/j.1365-2044.2007.05104.x.
71. Mohanty R, George L, George S, Babu M. Apnoeic oxygenation during simulated difficult intubation in obese patients: comparison of buccal ring, Adair and Elwyn tube versus nasal cannula: a prospective randomized controlled trial. Anesth Essays Res. 2021;15:408–12. https://doi.org/10.4103/aer.aer_114_21.
72. Hung KC, Ko CC, Chang PC, Wang KF, Teng IC, Lin CH, et al. Efficacy of high-flow nasal oxygenation against peri- and post-procedural hypoxemia in patients with obesity: a meta-analysis of randomized controlled trials. Sci Rep. 2022;12:1–11. https://doi.org/10.1038/s41598-022-10396-5.
73. Bright MR, Harley WA, Velli G, Zahir SF, Eley V. High-flow nasal cannula for apneic oxygenation in obese patients for elective surgery: a systematic review and meta-analysis. Anesth Analg. 2022;00:1–11. https://doi.org/10.1213/ANE.0000000000006304.
74. Jiang W, Shi L, Zhao Q, Zhang W, Xu M, Wang W, et al. Ultrasound assessment of gastric insufflation in obese patients receiving transnasal humidified rapid-insufflation ventilatory exchange during general anesthesia induction. Nan Fang Yi Ke Da Xue Xue Bao 2020;30;40:1543–1549. doi:https://doi.org/10.12122/j.issn.1673-4254.2020.11.
75. Asai T. Who is at increased risk of pulmonary aspiration? Br J Anaesth. 2004;93:497–500. https://doi.org/10.1093/bja/aeh234.
76. Roberts R, Shirley M. Reducing the risk of acid aspiration during cesarean section. Anesth Analg. 1974;53:859–68. https://doi.org/10.1213/00000539-197453060-00010.
77. Mahajan V, Hashmi J, Singh R, Samra T, Aneja S. Comparative evaluation of gastric pH and volume in morbidly obese and lean patients undergoing elective surgery and effect of aspiration prophylaxis. J Clin Anesth. 2015;27:396–400. https://doi.org/10.1016/j.jclinane.2015.03.004.
78. Lu C, An X, Yu Y, Jiao L, Canarutto D, Li G, et al. Pooled analysis of gastric emptying in patients with obesity: implications for oral absorption projection. Clin Ther. 2021;43:1768–88. https://doi.org/10.1016/j.clinthera.2021.08.006.
79. Smit I, Kranke P, Murat I, Smith A, O'Sullivan G, Søreide E, et al. Perioperative fasting in adults and children: guidelines from the European Society of Anaesthesiology. Eur J Anesth. 2011;l28:556–69. https://doi.org/10.1097/EJA.0b013e3283495ba1.
80. American Society of Anesthesiologists Committee. Practice guidelines for preoperative fasting and the use of pharmacologic agents to reduce the risk of pulmonary aspiration: application to healthy patients undergoing elective procedures: an updated report. Anesthesiology. 2011;114:495–511. https://doi.org/10.1097/ALN.0b013e3181fcbfd9.
81. Brodsky J. Patients with obesity need not routinely undergo rapid sequence anesthetic induction. Bariatr Times. 2018;15:8–10.
82. Jaruvongvanich V, Matar R, Ravi K, Murad MH, Vantanasiri K, Wongjarupong N, et al. Esophageal pathophysiologic changes and adenocarcinoma after bariatric surgery: a systematic review and meta-analysis. Clin Transl Gastroenterol. 2020;11:e00225. https://doi.org/10.14309/ctg.0000000000000225.

83. Jean J, Compère V, Fourdrinier V, Marguerite C, Auquit-Auckbur I, Milliez PY, et al. The risk of pulmonary aspiration in patients after weight loss due to bariatric surgery. Anesth Analg. 2008;107:1257–9. https://doi.org/10.1213/ane.0b013e31817f1563.
84. Prabha R, Raman R, Khan MP, Kaushal D, Siddiqui AK, Abbas H. Comparison of I-gel for general anesthesia in obese and nonobese patients. Saudi J Anaesth. 2018;12:529–34. https://doi.org/10.4103/sja.SJA_79_18.
85. Shariffuddin II, Chaw SH, Ng LW, Lim CH, Fitry M, Abidin Z, et al. Clinical performance of the LMA protector™ airway in moderately obese patients. BMC Anesthesiol. 2020;20:1–8. https://doi.org/10.1186/s12871-020-01100-z.
86. Tian Y, Wu XY, Li L, Ma L, Li YF. A clinical trial evaluating the laryngeal mask airway-supreme in obese children during general anesthesia. Arch Med Sci. 2017;13:183–90. https://doi.org/10.5114/aoms.2017.64719.
87. Moser B, Keller C, Audigé L, Dave MH, Bruppacher HR. Fiberoptic intubation of severely obese patients through supraglottic airway: a prospective, randomized trial of the Ambu® AuraGain™ laryngeal mask vs the i-gel™ airway. Acta Anaesthesiol Scand. 2019;63:187–94. https://doi.org/10.1111/aas.13242.
88. Mendonca C, Tourville CC, Jefferson H, Nowicka A, Patteril M, Athanassoglou V. Fibreoptic-guided tracheal intubation through i-gel and LMA protector TM supraglottic airway devices—a randomised comparison. Anaesthesia. 2019;74:203–10. https://doi.org/10.1111/anae.14475.
89. D'Anza B, Knight J, Greene J. Does body mass index predict tracheal airway size? Laryngoscope. 2015;125:1093–7. https://doi.org/10.1002/lary.24943.
90. Cook T, Woodall N, Frerk C, Project FNA. Major complications of airway management in the UK: results of the fourth National Audit Project of the Royal College of Anaesthetists and the difficult airway society. Part 1: Anaesthesia. Br J Anaesth. 2011;106:617–31. https://doi.org/10.1093/bja/aer058.
91. Moore AR, Schricker T, Court O. Awake videolaryngoscopy-assisted tracheal intubation of the morbidly obese. Anaesthesia. 2012;67:232–5. https://doi.org/10.1111/j.1365-2044.2011.06979.x.
92. Abdi W, Dhonneur G, Amathieu R, Adhoum A, Kamoun W, Slavov V, et al. LMA supreme versus facemask ventilation performed by novices: a comparative study in morbidly obese patients showing difficult ventilation predictors. Randomized Control Trial. Obes Surg. 2009;19:1624–30. https://doi.org/10.1007/s11695-009-9953-0.
93. Sinha A, Jayaraman L, Punhani D, Panigrahi B. ProSeal laryngeal mask airway improves oxygenation when used as a conduit prior to laryngoscope guided intubation in bariatric patients. Indian J Anaesth. 2013;57:25–30. https://doi.org/10.4103/0019-5049.108557.
94. King MR, Jagannathan N. Should videolaryngoscopy be the standard of care for routine tracheal intubation in obese adults? J Clin Anesth. 2018;45:33–4. https://doi.org/10.1016/j.jclinane.2017.12.006.
95. Hoshijima H, Denawa Y, Tominaga A, Nakamura C, Shiga T, Nagasaka H. Videolaryngoscope versus Macintosh laryngoscope for tracheal intubation in adults with obesity: a systematic review and meta-analysis. J Clin Anesth. 2018;44:69–75. https://doi.org/10.1016/j.jclinane.2017.11.008.
96. Carron M, Linassi F, Ieppariello G. Videolaryngoscopy versus direct laryngoscopy for patients with obesity requiring tracheal intubation: a meta-analysis. Obes Surg. 2021;31:3327–9. https://doi.org/10.1007/s11695-021-05357-2.
97. Dhonneur G, Ndoko SK, Yavchitz A, Foucrier A, Fessenmeyer C, Polliand C, et al. Tracheal intubation of morbidly obese patients: LMA CTrach TM vs direct laryngoscopy. Br J Anaesth. 2006;97:742–5. https://doi.org/10.1093/bja/ael219.
98. Gaszynski T. Totaltrack video intubating laryngeal mask in super-obese patients—series of cases. Ther Clin Risk Manag. 2016;12:335–8. https://doi.org/10.2147/TCRM.S95695.
99. Gómez-Ríos M, Casans-Francés R, Freire-Vila E, Sastre JA, López T, Garzón JC. A prospective evaluation of the Totaltrack video laryngeal mask in paralyzed, anesthetized obese patients. J Clin Anesth. 2020;61:109688. https://doi.org/10.1016/j.jclinane.2019.109688.

100. Thomsen JLD, Nørskov AK, Rosenstock CV. Supraglottic airway devices in difficult airway management: a retrospective cohort study of 658104 general anaesthetics registered in the Danish Anaesthesia database. Anaesthesia. 2019;74:151–7. https://doi.org/10.1111/anae.14443.
101. Saito T, Asai T, Taguchi A, Sophia CTH, Liu W, Thinn KK, et al. Prediction of failed facemask ventilation: new scoring system for difficult airway. J Anesth. 2020;34:367–72. https://doi.org/10.1007/s00540-020-02761-3.
102. Saito T, Asai T, Taguchi A, Sophia CTH, Liu W, Thinn KK, et al. Correlation between failed facemask ventilation, failed ventilation through a supraglottic airway and difficult tracheal intubation in unexpected difficult airways: an observational study. J Clin Anesth. 2020;60:34–5. https://doi.org/10.1016/j.jclinane.2019.08.024.
103. Frerk C, Mitchell VS, McNarry AF, Mendonca C, Bhagrath R, Patel A, et al. Difficult Airway Society 2015 guidelines for management of unanticipated difficult intubation in adults. Br J Anaesth. 2015;115:827–48.
104. You-Ten KE, Desai D, Postonogova T, Siddiqui N. Accuracy of conventional digital palpation and ultrasound of the cricothyroid membrane in obese women in labour. Anaesthesia. 2015;70:1230–4. https://doi.org/10.1111/anae.13167.
105. Hung KC, Chen IW, Lin CM, Sun CK. Comparison between ultrasound-guided and digital palpation techniques for identification of the cricothyroid membrane: a meta-analysis. Br J Anaesth. 2021;126:e9–e11. https://doi.org/10.1016/j.bja.2020.08.012.
106. Kristensen MS, Teoh WH, Rudolph SS, Hesselfeldt R, Børglum J, Tvede MF. A randomised cross-over comparison of the transverse and longitudinal techniques for ultrasound-guided identification of the cricothyroid membrane in morbidly obese subjects. Anaesthesia. 2016;71:675–83. https://doi.org/10.1111/anae.13465.
107. Kristensen MS, Teoh WH. Ultrasound identification of the cricothyroid membrane: the new standard in preparing for front-of-neck airway access. Br J Anaesth. 2021;126:22–7. https://doi.org/10.1016/j.bja.2020.10.004.
108. McKay RE, Malhotra A, Cakmakkaya OS, Hall KT, McKay WR, Apfel CC. Effect of increased body mass index and anaesthetic duration on recovery of protective airway reflexes after sevoflurane vs desflurane. Br J Anaesth. 2010;104:175–82. https://doi.org/10.1093/bja/aep374.
109. Strum EM, Szenohradszki J, Kaufman WA, Anthone GJ, Manz IL, Lumb PD. Emergence and recovery characteristics of desflurane versus sevoflurane in morbidly obese adult surgical patients: a prospective, randomized study. Anesth Analg. 2004;99:1848–53. https://doi.org/10.1213/01.ANE.0000136472.01079.95.
110. Liu FL, Cherng YG, Chen SY, Su YH, Huang SY, Lo PH, et al. Postoperative recovery after anesthesia in morbidly obese patients: a systematic review and meta-analysis of randomized controlled trials. Can J Anesth. 2015;62:907–17. https://doi.org/10.1007/s12630-015-0405-0.
111. Taha SK, El-Khatib MF, Baraka AS, Haidar YA, Abdallah FW, Zbeidy RA, et al. Effect of suxamethonium vs rocuronium on onset of oxygen desaturation during apnoea following rapid sequence induction. Anaesthesia. 2010;65:358–61. https://doi.org/10.1111/j.1365-2044.2010.06243.x.
112. Tang L, Li S, Huang S, Ma H, Wang Z. Desaturation following rapid sequence induction using succinylcholine vs. rocuronium in overweight patients. Acta Anaesthesiol Scand. 2011;55:203–8. https://doi.org/10.1111/j.1399-6576.2010.02365.x.
113. Benumof J, Dagg R, Benumof R. Critical hemoglobin desaturation will occur before return to an unparalyzed state following 1 mg/kg intravenous succinylcholine. Anesthesiology. 1997;87:979–82. https://doi.org/10.1097/00000542-199710000-00034.
114. Heier T, Feiner JR, Lin J, Brown R, Caldwell JE. Hemoglobin desaturation after succinylcholine-induced apnea. Anesthesiology. 2001;94:754–9. https://doi.org/10.1097/00000542-200105000-00011.
115. Lee C, Jahr J, Candiotti K, Warriner B, Zornow M, M N. Reversal of profound neuromuscular block by sugammadex administered three minutes after: a comparison with spontaneous

recovery from succinylcholine. Anesthesiology. 2009;110:1020–5. https://doi.org/10.1097/ALN.0b013e31819dabb0.

116. Sørensen MK, Bretlau C, Gätke MR, Sørensen AM, Rasmussen LS. Rapid sequence induction and intubation with rocuronium-sugammadex compared with succinylcholine: a randomized trial. Br J Anaesth. 2012;108:682–9. https://doi.org/10.1093/bja/aer503.
117. Bisschops MMA, Holleman C, Huitink JM. Can sugammadex save a patient in a simulated "cannot intubate, cannot ventilate" situation? Anaesthesia. 2010;65:936–41. https://doi.org/10.1111/j.1365-2044.2010.06455.x.
118. Liao JQ, Shih D, Lin TY, Lee M, Lu CW. Appropriate dosing of sugammadex for reversal of rocuronium/vecuronium-induced muscle relaxation in morbidly obese patients: a meta-analysis of randomized controlled trials. J Int Med Res. 2022;50:1–12. https://doi.org/10.1177/03000605221116760.
119. Naguib M, Brewer L, Lapierre C, Kopman AF, Johnson KB. The myth of rescue reversal in "can't intubate, can't ventilate" scenarios. Anesth Analg. 2016;123:82–92. https://doi.org/10.1213/ANE.0000000000001347.
120. Eichenberger AS, Proietti S, Wicky S, Frascarolo P, Suter M, Spahn DR, et al. Morbid obesity and postoperative pulmonary atelectasis: an underestimated problem. Anesth Analg. 2002;95:1788–92. https://doi.org/10.1097/00000539-200212000-00060.
121. Zoremba M, Dette F, Gerlach L, Wolf U, Wulf H. Short-term respiratory physical therapy treatment in the PACU and influence on postoperative lung function in obese adults. Obes Surg. 2009;19:1346–54. https://doi.org/10.1007/s11695-009-9922-7.
122. Imber DAE, Pirrone M, Zhang C, Fisher DF, Kacmarek RM, Berra L. Respiratory management of perioperative obese patients. Respir Care. 2016;61:1681–92. https://doi.org/10.4187/respcare.04732.
123. Zoremba M, Kalmus G, Begemann D, Eberhart L, Zoremba N, Wulf H, et al. Short term non-invasive ventilation post-surgery improves arterial blood-gases in obese subjects compared to supplemental oxygen delivery—a randomized controlled trial. BMC Anesthesiol. 2011;11:10. https://doi.org/10.1186/1471-2253-11-10.
124. Kaw R, Bhateja P, Paz Y, Hernandez AV, Ramaswamy A, Deshpande A, Aboussouan L. Postoperative complications in patients with unrecognized obesity hypoventilation syndrome undergoing elective noncardiac surgery. Chest. 2016;149:84–91. https://doi.org/10.1378/chest.14-3216.
125. de Raaff CAL, Kalff MC, Coblijn UK, de Vries CEE, de Vries N, Bonjer HJ, et al. Influence of continuous positive airway pressure on postoperative leakage in bariatric surgery. Surg Obes Relat Dis. 2018;14:186–90. https://doi.org/10.1016/j.soard.2017.10.017.
126. Reijers SNH, Nijland LMG, Bosschieter PFN, de Raaff CAL, Ravesloot MJL, van Veen RN, et al. The effect of postoperative CPAP use on anastomotic and staple line leakage after bariatric surgery. Sleep Breath. 2021;25:1037–43. https://doi.org/10.1007/s11325-020-02199-7.
127. Das F, Emk S, Án A, Fmr V. Noninvasive positive pressure ventilation for acute respiratory failure following upper abdominal surgery. Cochrane Database Syst Rev. 2015:CD009134. https://doi.org/10.1002/14651858.CD009134.
128. Tong S, Gower J, Morgan A, Gadbois K, Wisbach G. Noninvasive positive pressure ventilation in the immediate post-bariatric surgery care of patients with obstructive sleep apnea: a systematic review. Surg Obes Relat Dis. 2017;13:1227–33. https://doi.org/10.1016/j.soard.2017.02.009.
129. Corley A, Bull T, Spooner AJ, Barnett AG, Fraser JF. Direct extubation onto high-flow nasal cannulae post-cardiac surgery versus standard treatment in patients with a BMI ≥30: a randomised controlled trial. Intensive Care Med. 2015;41:887–94. https://doi.org/10.1007/s00134-015-3765-6.
130. Stéphan F, Bérard L, Rézaiguia-Delclaux S, Amaru P. High-flow nasal cannula therapy versus intermittent noninvasive ventilation in obese subjects after cardiothoracic surgery. Respir Care. 2017;62:1193–202. https://doi.org/10.4187/respcare.05473.

131. Rochwerg B, Einav S, Chaudhuri D, Mancebo J, Mauri T, Helviz Y, et al. The role for high flow nasal cannula as a respiratory support strategy in adults: a clinical practice guideline. Intensive Care Med. 2020;46:2226–37. https://doi.org/10.1007/s00134-020-06312-y.
132. Ferrando C, Puig J, Serralta F, Carrizo J, Pozo N, Arocas B, et al. High-flow nasal cannula oxygenation reduces postoperative hypoxemia in morbidly obese patients: a randomized controlled trial. Minerva Anestesiol. 2019;85:1062–70. https://doi.org/10.23736/S0375-9393.19.13364-0.

Chapter 23
Obstetric Airway Management

Sonia Vaida, Luis Gaitini, Mostafa Somri, and Jansie Prozesky

Airway management in the obstetric patient continues to be a major predicament for the anesthesiologist. Despite improved preoperative airway assessment and preparedness, better simulation training, and the availability of advanced airway technology, airway difficulties in obstetric patients can cause minor to devastating maternal and neonatal complications.

Cesarean deliveries (CDs) are rarely performed under general anesthesia and studying the management of the obstetric difficult airway by enrolling pregnant patients in prospective, randomized, controlled trials raises serious ethical and practical concerns. Therefore, there is a limited number of comparative, prospective, randomized studies on the obstetric airway in general and particularly the difficult airway. The evidence is based largely on observational and retrospective studies, case series, and case reports.

23.1 Incidence of Difficult and Failed Intubation

The reported incidence of difficult and failed intubation varies largely in the obstetric anesthesia literature, depending on the criteria used to define the airway event.

In the most recent large multicenter (45 institutions) retrospective, observational cohort study that included 14,437 patients undergoing CD under general anesthesia,

S. Vaida (✉) · J. Prozesky
Department of Anesthesiology, Penn State College of Medicine, Penn State Milton S. Hershey Medical Center, Hershey, PA, USA
e-mail: svaida@pennstatehealth.psu.edu; jprozesky@pennstatehealth.psu.edu

L. Gaitini · M. Somri
Department of Anesthesiology, Bnai-Zion Medical Center, Haifa, Israel
e-mail: Mostafa.somri@b-zion.org.il

M. Á. Gómez-Ríos, A. van Zundert (eds.), *Evidence-based Guide to Difficult Airway Management*, https://doi.org/10.1007/978-3-032-30769-9_23

difficult intubation was found in 1:49 cases, corresponding to 2.03% of patients. Failed intubation occurred in 1:808, corresponding to 0.12% of patients. Reported complications following difficult airway cases were: pharyngeal injury, aspiration, dental injury, and cardiac arrest. Risk factors for difficult intubation included increased body mass index (BMI), Mallampati score III or IV, small hyoid-to-mentum distance, limited jaw protrusion, limited mouth opening, and cervical spine limitations [1].

23.2 Factors Contributing to Obstetric Airway Challenges

23.2.1 Physiologic Changes in Pregnancy Affecting Airway Management

Airway changes start as early as the second trimester, progress during pregnancy, and persist in the post-partum period for at least 48 h after delivery [2]. Fluid retention during pregnancy leads to airway edema. Valsalva maneuvers, fluid, and oxytocin administration during labor and delivery, as well as reduction of plasma colloid osmotic pressure in preeclamptic patients, can further exacerbate fluid retention, resulting in worsening airway edema [2–4].

Kodali et al. [2] showed that during labor, there is a further decrease in oral volume as well as pharyngeal area and volume, leading to a progressive increase in the Mallampati score.

Laryngeal edema causing airway narrowing may prevent the passage of a standard-size endotracheal tube (ETT), despite adequate laryngoscopic vocal cord visualization. Therefore, a smaller size ETT is preferred for intubating the trachea (e.g., 6.5 mm internal diameter ETT).

Nasal intubation is best avoided, given the increased risk of severe epistaxis due to significant mucosal vascular engorgement and tissue friability during pregnancy.

Breast enlargement may interfere with the insertion of the laryngoscope blade, and therefore, a short-handled laryngoscope is preferred.

Increased oxygen consumption and reduced functional residual capacity during pregnancy increase the risk of hypoxemia even after very brief periods of apnea during induction of general anesthesia or extubation.

23.2.2 Emergency Situation

General anesthesia is mostly performed in the stressful environment of an emergent/urgent CD. Concerns for fetal well-being may hinder proper airway evaluation, preoxygenation, and correct patient positioning, resulting in suboptimal conditions for intubation [5].

23.2.3 Lack of Experience with the Obstetric Airway

With the widespread use of neuraxial anesthesia, the administration of general anesthesia for CD is steadily declining. According to the data from the National Anesthesiology Clinical Outcomes Registry (NACOR), in the United States, general anesthesia is administered in 5.8% of cases. The majority of cases requiring general anesthesia are emergency procedures [6]. Nowadays, trainees have significantly less exposure to airway management in obstetric patients. Therefore, acquiring and retaining these vital skills requires frequent simulation training [7].

23.3 Planning for the Obstetric Airway

23.3.1 Airway Evaluation

Every patient presenting to the labor and delivery unit should be examined by an anesthesiologist, including a comprehensive airway evaluation, regardless of the type of anesthesia to be administered, if any. Due to the progressive changes during labor, including exacerbation of airway edema, it is highly recommended to reevaluate the airway right before induction of general anesthesia, in addition to the initial pre-labor/early labor evaluation.

Ultrasonography of the anterior neck is gaining popularity as a non-invasive, point-of-care tool to evaluate the airway in obstetric patients. Ultrasound airway parameters, such as soft tissue thickness at the level of the hyoid bone, epiglottis, and vocal cords, can predict difficult airways in pregnant patients [3, 8, 9]. Identifying the cricothyroid membrane (CTM), by palpation is challenging, especially in patients with intangible anatomical landmarks on the front of the neck, during stressful conditions of an airway emergency. Gadd et al. reported a linear relationship between the CTM depth and neck circumference in normal-weight and obese pregnant patients [10]. Ultrasonography can reliably guide the preemptive location of the CTM to expedite front-of-neck access if necessary [11].

23.3.2 Equipment

A difficult airway cart customized to institutional standards should be available and checked at least once daily. In addition to the standardized equipment, the difficult airway cart must include a short-handled laryngoscope designed to address pregnancy-related anatomical changes, such as increased breast size and weight gain.

23.3.2.1 Videolaryngoscopes

Videolaryngoscopes (VLs) offer a better safety profile and the clear advantage of improved glottic visualization, higher first-attempt endotracheal intubation rate as well as decreased risk of hypoxemia and failed intubation rate in the general population [12]. (Grade A evidence) A few comparative studies have recently been added to numerous reports of successful use of VLs for initial intubation in obstetric patients with normal or predicted difficult airways or as rescue devices after failed direct laryngoscopy [12–14].

A mixed-methods systematic review and meta-analysis including four randomized controlled studies (428 patients), 35 case reports/case series, and nine observational studies compared videolaryngoscopy and direct laryngoscopy for endotracheal intubation in obstetrics. The authors reported better glottic visualization with videolaryngoscopy but no difference in first-attempt success rate or time to complete endotracheal intubation [14] (Grade A).

There are many different VL models, with different designs, characteristics, and clinical advantages. Blajic et al. prospectively compared the C-MAC (a MacIntosh-type blade VL), King Vision (a channeled VL), and direct laryngoscopy. The time to successfully intubate the trachea was similar for all three devices. While the C-MAC was the easiest to insert, the King Vision VL was found to offer the highest rate of grade 1 laryngoscopic view. Based on their findings, the authors recommend VLs as primary intubation devices for obstetric patients undergoing CD [15] (Grade A).

To date, there are no short-handled VLs specifically designed for obstetric patients. However, the McGrath Series 5 and King Vision VL have obstetric airway-friendly features. The McGrath Series 5 laryngoscope has an adjustable blade length, and the King Vision VL has the advantage of allowing the laryngoscope blade to be inserted separately and then, once positioned in the oropharynx, the monitor to be attached.

23.3.2.2 Supraglottic Airway Devices

SADs have a very well-established role in obstetric airway management as rescue devices after attempts at intubation failed [1, 4, 16] (Grade A, B). The continued development and improvements of SADs (laryngeal mask airways and non-laryngeal mask airways) have resulted in safer airway devices.

Second-generation SADs (e.g., LMA Supreme, i-gel, etc.) with a gastric drain should be used preferentially as they offer an improved oropharyngeal seal and better protection against regurgitation and pulmonary aspiration of gastric contents.

SADs should be used early in the algorithm of difficult airways to avoid hypoxemia and airway trauma caused by multiple attempts at intubation. Cricoid pressure should be transiently released to facilitate the successful placement of SADs [17] (Grade A, B).

Some studies looked into the use of SADs as primary airway devices in fasted patients with normal weight and airway anatomy [18–21]. A recent meta-analysis by White et al. included 14 studies to compare SADs to endotracheal intubation in patients undergoing elective CD. The authors found no difference in the first-attempt success rate and major adverse event rates but concluded that "the analysis remains underpowered and therefore inconclusive." [22].

23.3.3 Patient Positioning

Optimizing patients' head/neck position before induction of general anesthesia significantly improves intubation conditions. Head-up position to 25–30 degrees can prolong safe apnea time by increasing the functional residual capacity [23], improve glottic visualization during laryngoscopy [4] and minimize the risk of pulmonary aspiration of gastric contents (Grade A, B). The "ramped up" position further improves intubation conditions, especially in overweight parturients. This position can be achieved by placing pillows, blankets, or commercially available devices under the upper body, in order to align the level of the external auditory meatus to the sternal notch.

23.3.4 Preoxygenation

Pregnant patients tend to desaturate quickly, even after brief periods of apnea, due to increased oxygen consumption and decreased functional residual capacity. Preoxygenation before induction of general anesthesia, using low-flow or high-flow nasal oxygen, as well as mask oxygenation or gentle mask ventilation, prolongs the period of apnea [4, 24, 25] (Grade A, D).

The optimal preoxygenation technique to significantly reduce hypoxemia during the induction of general anesthesia in the parturient is yet to be determined.

In emergencies such as fetal distress, eight deep breaths with 100% oxygen are recommended before rapid sequence induction of general anesthesia [26].

23.4 Management of Difficult Airway

The Obstetric Anesthetists' Association and Difficult Airway Society in the United Kingdom have developed evidence-based guidelines for the management of difficult and failed tracheal intubation to facilitate the decision-making process for obstetric patients [4]. These comprehensive guidelines are based on a systematic approach to address all aspects of airway management in obstetrics including steps to "optimize a safe general anesthetic technique in the obstetric patient," "management after declaring failed tracheal intubation," "management of the "can't intubate-can't-oxygenate" (CICO), situation," "emergency front-of-neck airway access

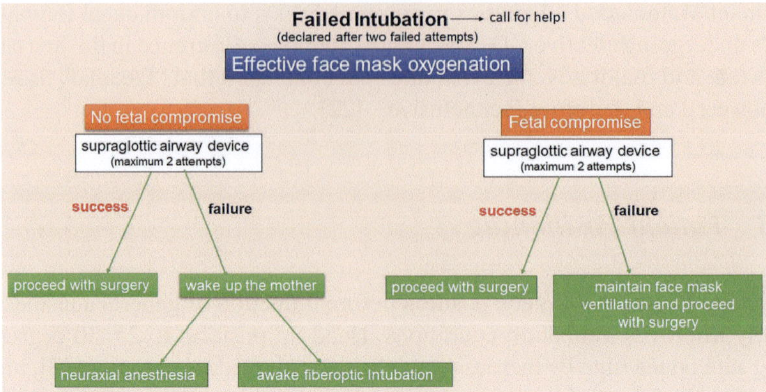

Fig. 23.1 Failed intubation: effective face mask oxygenation

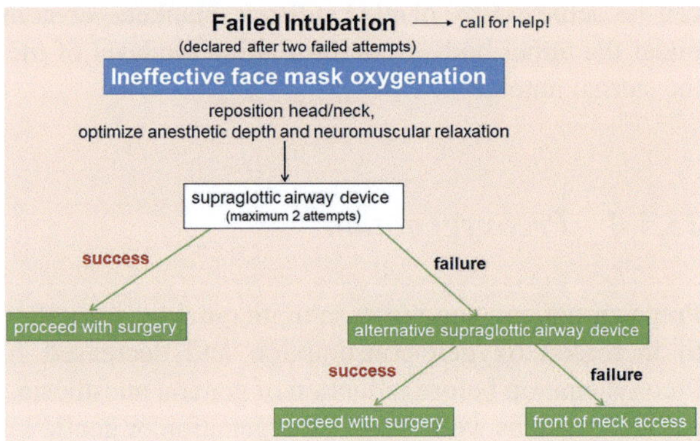

Fig. 23.2 Failed intubation: ineffective face mask oxygenation

(FONA)." The authors offer guidance to decide whether to awaken the mother or proceed with general anesthesia after failed intubation if the airway is efficiently secured with an SAD or adequate face mask ventilation [4]. We recommend adapting these guidelines to graphically friendly, succinct algorithms specific to each institution, based on local resources and equipment, while considering the presence or absence of fetal distress (Figs. 23.1, and 23.2).

23.4.1 Predicted Difficult Airway

When examining the airway, one should consider multiple aspects of airway management, including difficulty with face mask ventilation, endotracheal intubation, SAD placement and ventilation, and FONA. The location of the cricothyroid membrane should be identified and marked to facilitate FONA, should that become necessary.

The anesthetic approach in these cases should be guided by the urgency of delivery.

23.4.1.1 Neuraxial Anesthesia

Placing a "prophylactic" epidural catheter in early labor is recommended for a possible extension of labor epidural analgesia to surgical anesthesia for CD, should this be indicated. However, the reported incidence of failure to convert an existing satisfactory labor epidural analgesic to epidural anesthesia for CD varies between 1.7% and 19.8% [27, 28]. Predictors of failure to convert epidural analgesia to surgical anesthesia include young age, greater urgency of the CD, multiple epidural boluses administered by the clinician, etc. [29, 30].

Therefore, a contingency plan should be in place to address possible complications of neuraxial anesthesia necessitating airway manipulation, such as failure to provide surgical anesthesia, high neuraxial block, or total spinal, resulting in respiratory arrest, local anesthetic toxicity, and be fully prepared to administer general anesthesia. Maternal hemodynamic instability caused by post-partum hemorrhage may also prompt airway manipulation with conversion to GA [31].

Good communication with the obstetric team to anticipate CD in a patient with a labor epidural will allow for adequate planning for safe conversion to adequate surgical anesthesia.

Spinal anesthesia is the preferred method for surgical delivery with catheter techniques (such as combined spinal epidural or continuous spinal), providing the additional flexibility of supplementation of the block.

23.4.1.2 Awake Fiberoptic-Aided Intubation

Awake fiberoptic-aided intubation with a flexible bronchoscope is the safest technique for securing the airway in cases of a predicted difficult airway. However, the procedure may be time-consuming, and it requires special technical skills, experience, and continued practice. Psychological preparation of the parturient, including a detailed explanation of the technique, is essential.

The risk of causing bleeding is increased when the nasal route is used in a pregnant patient with an engorged and highly vascular nasal mucosa, and, therefore, the oral route is preferred. In addition to prophylaxis for pulmonary aspiration, an antisialagogue (e.g., glycopyrrolate 0.2 mg IV) should be administered before the procedure to control secretions and increase the effectiveness of topical anesthetics.

Airway topicalization with selective nerve blocks or direct application of local anesthetics may blunt airway reflexes. Attention must be paid to the total dose of local anesthetics in topical anesthesia, considering the increased mucosal vascularization and sensitivity of peripheral nerves to local anesthetics during pregnancy.

More recently, videolaryngoscopy for awake intubation was added to the airway techniques armamentarium. A systematic review and meta-analysis of videolaryngoscopy compared with fiberoptic bronchoscopy for awake tracheal intubation in the general population analyzed eight studies including 429 patients. The authors reported comparable success rates and safety with a shorter intubation time with videolaryngoscopy [32] (Grade A).

When providing conscious sedation for "awake" intubation one should consider the increased risk of pulmonary aspiration of gastric contents in a pregnant patient, as well as the effects of placental transfer of sedatives, possibly resulting in neonatal sedative effects or respiratory depression.

Remifentanil, an ultra-short-acting phenylpiperidine opioid, can be used for maternal sedation to decrease anxiety and improve patient cooperation during awake intubation. It crosses the placenta, but it is rapidly hydrolyzed by nonspecific plasma and tissue esterase [33].

Dexmedetomidine, a selective α-2 agonist, has also been successfully administered in obstetric patients to provide sympatholysis, sedation, anxiolysis, and analgesia [34].

23.4.2 Unpredicted Difficult Airway

Management of the unanticipated difficult tracheal intubation must concentrate on the maintenance of oxygenation while preventing upper airway trauma. The number of intubation attempts should be limited to two. Repeated attempts at intubation increase the risk of hypoxia and aspiration. Atraumatic manipulation of the airway is crucial, as every intubation attempt may increase airway edema and the risk of bleeding.

Call for skilled help should be initiated very early in the process and failed intubation must be declared after two failed intubation attempts. It is very important to inform the obstetricians and the entire operating room team of a difficult airway emergency.

If the first attempt at intubation fails, the second intubation attempt conditions must be optimized to increase the chances of success in securing the airway.

- The most experienced/qualified anesthesiologist should perform the second intubation attempt and immediately assume the leadership role to coordinate team efforts.
- Demand silence in the operating room to facilitate clear communication with team members.
- The head and neck should be checked for correct positioning.
- If necessary, additional induction agents or neuromuscular blocking agents should be administered.
- Cricoid pressure should be released and external laryngeal manipulation should be optimally performed to improve glottic visualization.
- An alternative laryngoscope type or size should be used, with a preference for videolaryngoscopy.

In obstetric patients, videolaryngoscopy is superior to conventional laryngoscopy in terms of glottic visualization [14]; however, it can cause significant pharyngeal trauma, mainly if a rigid stylet is required to facilitate intubation [35]. The increased upper airway tissue friability seen in obstetric patients might make them more prone to this complication.

If the second intubation attempt fails, an SAD should be inserted. Among numerous available SADs, the choice should be made based on availability and expertise, with preference to the second-generation SAD. Given the increased risk of regurgitation and pulmonary aspiration of gastric contents, the stomach should be drained through the second-generation SADs dedicated channel.

Regardless of what type of SADs are used, it is crucial to choose the correct size and ensure optimal positioning. SADs are mostly inserted blindly, often resulting in malpositioning. Malpositioning of an SAD can be corrected by applying a jaw lift, reinserting the device using a railroading technique (bougie, orogastric tube), or laryngoscopically facilitated repositioning [36].

Mushambi et al., recommend a maximum of two attempts at SAD placements [4]. Alternative SADs may provide adequate oxygenation and ventilation in circumstances where the first-choice SAD fails.

A properly functioning SDA may be left in place until the completion of the CD. The decision to leave a SAD in place or proceed to an exchange with an ETT should be based on the adequacy of oxygenation and ventilation and the expected length of the surgical procedure. If possible, the exchange procedure should be postponed after delivery of the newborn (Grade 4) [16]. There are several techniques to facilitate endotracheal intubation through a SAD, including blind intubation or facilitation by light wands, optical stylets, or a fiberoptic bronchoscope [37]. Exchanging the SAD with an ETT may be challenging, but removing the SAD before attempting endotracheal intubation can lead to a life-threatening CICO situation.

If the SAD fails to provide adequate oxygenation and ventilation, the decision-making process should be further guided by the urgency of delivery, the effectiveness of face mask ventilation, and the well-being of the fetus.

23.4.2.1 Effective Mask Ventilation

If accurate oxygenation can be properly maintained through face mask ventilation and there is no fetal compromise, the mother should be awakened. After re-evaluating the urgency of the CD, a decision needs to be made on whether to proceed with awake intubation or neuraxial anesthesia.

In case of fetal distress, continued face mask ventilation should be considered to allow prompt fetal delivery. The optimal attempt at conventional mask ventilation should be a two-person effort.

23.4.2.2 Ineffective Mask Ventilation

Failure to maintain oxygenation at this stage becomes a life-threatening CICO situation, prompting FONA [4]. According to Kinsella, the incidence of FONA after failed intubation in obstetric patients is 1:60 [38]. The Difficult Airway Society guidelines for the management of unanticipated difficult intubation, published in 2015, recommend scalpel cricothyroidotomy as the “fastest and most reliable method of securing the airway in the emergency setting” [39].

23.5 Extubation

Tracheal extubation in pregnant patients is performed when the patient is awake and following commands, to avoid aspiration. Adverse airway events may be common during this time, as preexisting pregnancy-related laryngeal edema can exacerbate after intubation. A strategy for safe extubation should be formulated immediately after intubation.

Airway exchange catheters are well tolerated in awake patients as long as carinal irritation is avoided and can be used for staged extubation in patients with difficult intubation and/or expected difficult extubation.

After extubation, close follow-up of the patient and good communication with post-anesthesia unit (PACU) staff is crucial.

23.6 Conclusions

Emergency CD often requires general anesthesia in a highly stressful environment, further complicated by the complexity of airway management of these patients.

Failed intubation must be declared after two unsuccessful attempts to intubate the trachea with direct or videolaryngoscopy, keeping in mind that adequate oxygenation takes priority over endotracheal intubation in difficult airway situations. Development and implementation of an airway management strategy requires frequent simulation-based training with institutionally available advanced airway equipment.

Recommendations	Evidence level
Adequate difficult airway equipment should be available in every obstetric unit.	D
Administration of high-flow nasal oxygenation before induction of general anesthesia in the parturient decreases the risk of hypoxemia after brief periods of apnea.	A
Low-flow nasal oxygen administration, face mask oxygenation, or gentle face mask ventilation are efficient preoxygenation alternative techniques.	D
Head-up position before induction of general anesthesia improves intubation conditions.	A
Videolaryngoscopy has gained popularity as the primary intubating device in obstetric patients.	A, B
Supraglottic airway devices should be used as rescue devices, early in the difficult airway algorithm.	B
Cricoid pressure should be temporarily released during the insertion of a Supraglottic Airway Device.	A, B
Upper airway ultrasonography measurements have predictive value in detecting difficult airways.	A, C
Identifying and marking the cricothyroid membrane before induction of general anesthesia can help expedite the front-of-neck access in a cannot-intubate/cannot-oxygenate situation.	C, D

References

1. Reale SC, Bauer ME, Klumpner TT, Aziz MF, Fields KG, Hurwitz R, Saad M, Kheterpal S, Bateman BT, Multicenter Perioperative Outcomes Group Collaborators. Frequency and risk factors for difficult intubation in women undergoing general anesthesia for cesarean delivery: a multicenter retrospective cohort analysis. Anesthesiology. 2022;136:697–708.
2. Kodali BS, Chandrasekhar S, Bulich LN, Topulos GP, Datta S. Airway changes during labor and delivery. Anesthesiology. 2008;108:357–62.
3. Ahuja P, Jain D, Bhardwaj N, Jain K, Gainder S, Kang M. Airway changes following labor and delivery in preeclamptic parturients: a prospective case control study. Airway changes following labor and delivery in preeclamptic parturients: a prospective case control study. Int J Obstet Anesth. 2018;33:17–22.
4. Mushambi MC, Kinsella SM, Popat M, Swales H, Ramaswamy KK, Winton AL, Quinn AC, Obstetric Anaesthetists' Association, Difficult Airway Society. Obstetric Anaesthetists' Association and Difficult Airway Society guidelines for the management of difficult and failed tracheal intubation in obstetrics. Anaesthesia. 2015;70(11):1286–306.
5. Rucklidge M, Hinton C. Difficult and failed intubation in obstetrics. Continuing Educ Anaesthesia Crit Care Pain. 2012;12(2):86–91.

6. Juang J, Gabriel RA, Dutton RP, Palanisamy A, Urman RD. Choice of anesthesia for cesarean delivery: an analysis of the national anesthesia clinical outcomes registry. Anesth Analg. 2017;124:1914–7.
7. Mushambi M, Jaladi S. Airway management and training in obstetric anaesthesia. Curr Opin Anaesthesiol. 2016;29(3):261–7.
8. Carsetti A, Sorbello M, Adrario E, Donati A, Falcetta S. Airway ultrasound as predictor of difficult direct laryngoscopy: a systematic review and meta-analysis. Anesth Analg. 2022;134(4):740–50.
9. Vajanthri SY, Mohammed S, Kumar M, Chhabra S, Bhatia P, Kamal M, Paliwa B. Evaluation of ultrasound airway assessment parameters in pregnant patients and their comparison with that of non-pregnant women: a prospective cohort study. Int J Obstet Anesth. 2023; Online ahead of print
10. Gadd K, Wills K, Harle R, Terblanche N. Relationship between severe obesity and depth to the cricothyroid membrane in third-trimester non-labouring parturients: a prospective observational study. Br J Anaesth. 2018;20(5):1033–9.
11. Lavelle A, Drew T, Fennessy P, McCaul C, Shannon J. Accuracy of cricothyroid membrane identification using ultrasound and palpation techniques in obese obstetric patients: an observational study. Int J Obstet Anesth. 2021;48:103205.
12. Hansel J, Rogers AM, Lewis SR, Cook TM, Smith AF. Videolaryngoscopy versus direct laryngoscopy for adults undergoing tracheal intubation: a Cochrane systematic review and meta-analysis update. Br J Anaesth. 2022;129(4):612–23.
13. Aziz MF, Kim D, Mako J, Hand K, Brambrink AM. A retrospective study of the performance of video laryngoscopy in an obstetric unit. Anesth Analg. 2012;115(4):904–6.
14. Howle R, Onwochei D, Harrison SL, Desai N. Comparison of videolaryngoscopy and direct laryngoscopy for tracheal intubation in obstetrics: a mixed-methods systematic review and meta-analysis. Can J Anaesth. 2021;68(4):546–65.
15. Blajic I, Hodzovic I, Lucovnik M, Mekis D, Novak-Jankovic V, Stopar Pintaric T. A randomized comparison of C-MAC™ and king vision® videolaryngoscopes with direct laryngoscopy in 180 obstetric patients. Int J Obstet Anesth. 2019;39:35–41.
16. Mhyre JM, Healy D. The unanticipated difficult intubation in obstetrics. Anesth Analg. 2011;112(3):648–52.
17. Li CW, Xue FS, Xu YC, Liu Y, Mao P, Liu KP, Yang QY, Zhang GH, Sun HT. Cricoid pressure impedes insertion of, and ventilation through, the ProSeal laryngeal mask airway in anesthetized, paralyzed patients. Anesth Analg. 2007;104(5):1195–8.
18. Panneer M, Babu S, Murugaiyan P. Comparison of I-gel versus endotracheal tube in patients undergoing elective cesarean section: a prospective randomized control study. Anesth Essays Res. 2017;11:930–3.
19. Saini S, Ahuja S, Guleria K. To evaluate the use of ProSeal laryngeal mask airway in patients undergoing elective lower segment cesarean section under general anesthesia: a prospective randomized controlled study. J Obstet Anaesth Crit Care. 2016;6:11.
20. Yao WY, Li SY, Yuan YJ, et al. Comparison of supreme laryngeal mask airway versus endotracheal intubation for airway management during general anesthesia for cesarean section: a randomized controlled trial. BMC Anesthesiol. 2019;19:123.
21. Han TH, Brimacombe J, Lee EJ, Yang HS. The laryngeal mask airway is effective (and probably safe) in selected healthy parturients for elective cesarean section: a prospective study of 1067 cases. Can J Anaesth 2001;48:9 (11) 1117–1121.
22. White LD, Thang C, Hodsdon A, Melhuish TM, Barron FA, Godsall MG, Vlok R. Comparison of Supraglottic airway devices with endotracheal intubation in low-risk patients for cesarean delivery: systematic review and meta-analysis. Anesth Analg. 2020;131(4):1092–101.
23. Hignett R, Fernando R, McGlennan A, McDonald S, Stewart A, Columb M, Adamou T, Dilworth P. A randomized crossover study to determine the effect of a 30°head-up versus a supine position on the functional residual capacity of term parturients. Anesth Analg. 2011;113(5):1098.

24. Wong CA, Mushambi M. Peri-intubation oxygenation for Caesarean delivery: is there an optimal technique? Br J Anaesth. 2022;129(4):468–71.
25. Zhou S, Zhou Y, Cao X, Ni X, Du W, Xu Z, Liu Z. The efficacy of high flow nasal oxygenation for maintaining maternal oxygenation during rapid sequence induction in pregnancy: a prospective randomised clinical trial. Eur J Anaesthesiol. 2021;38(10):1052–8.
26. Chiron B, Laffon M, Ferrandiere M, Pittet JF, Marret H, Mercier C. Standard preoxygenation technique versus two rapid techniques in pregnant patients. Int J Obstet Anesth. 2004;13(1):11.
27. Paech MJ, Godkin R, Webster S. Complications of obstetric epidural analgesia and anaesthesia: a prospective analysis of 10 995 cases. Int J Obstet Anesth. 1998;7:5–11.
28. Orbach-Zinger S, Friedman L, Avramovich A, Ilgiaeva N, Orvieto R, Sulkes J, Eidelman LA. Risk factors for failure to extend labor epidural analgesia to epidural anesthesia for cesarean section. Acta Anaesthesiol Scand. 2006;50:793–7.
29. Grap SM, Patel GR, Huang J, Vaida SJ. Risk factors for labor epidural conversion failure requiring general anesthesia for cesarean delivery. J Anaesthesiol Clin Pharmacol. 2022;38(1):118–23.
30. Bauer ME, Kountanis JA, Tsen LC, Greenfield ML, Mhyre JM. Risk factors for failed conversion of labor epidural analgesia to cesarean delivery anesthesia: a systematic review and metaanalysis of observational trials. Int J Obstet Anesth. 2012;21:294–309.
31. Patel S, Wali A. Airway management of the obstetric patient. Curr Anesthesiol Rep. 2020;10:350–60.
32. Alhomary M, Ramadan E, Curran E, Walsh SR. Videolaryngoscopy vs. fibreoptic bronchoscopy for awake tracheal intubation: a systematic review and meta-analysis. Anaesthesia. 2018;73:1151–61.
33. Machata AM, Gonano C, Holzer A, et al. Awake nasotracheal fiberoptic intubation: patient comfort, intubating conditions, and hemodynamic stability during conscious sedation with remifentanil. Anesth Analg. 2003;97:904–8.
34. Sng BL, Dabas R, Sia AT. Intravenous dexmedetomidine use in obstetric anaesthesia: a weapon in our armoury? Int J Obstet Anesth. 2018 Nov;36:1–2.
35. Pham Q, Lentner M, Hu A. Soft palate injuries during orotracheal intubation with the videolaryngoscope. Ann Otol Rhinol Laryngol. 2017;126(2):132–7.
36. Van Zundert AA, Kumar CM, Van Zundert TC. Malpositioning of supraglottic airway devices: preventive and corrective strategies. Br J Anaesth. 2016 May;116(5):579–82.
37. Timmermann A. Supraglottic airways in difficult airway management: successes, failures, use and misuse. Anaesthesia. 2011;66(Suppl 2):45–56. (pt wxcahnge la partea cu diff airway
38. Kinsella SM, Winton AL, Mushambi MC, Ramaswamy K, Swales H, Quinn AC, Popat M. Failed tracheal intubation during obstetric general anaesthesia: a literature review. Int J Obstet Anesth. 2015 Nov;24(4):356–74.
39. Frerk C, Mitchell VS, McNarry AF, Mendonca C, Bhagrath R, Patel A, O'Sullivan EP, Woodall NM, Ahmad I, Difficult Airway Society Intubation Guidelines Working Group. Difficult Airway Society 2015 guidelines for management of unanticipated difficult intubation in adults. Br J Anaesth. 2015;115(6):827–48.

Chapter 24
Paediatric Airway Management

Chloe Heath, Neil Hauser, and Britta S. von Ungern-Sternberg

24.1 Introduction

Paediatric patients represent a diverse group of patients from extremely premature neonates to large adult-sized adolescents. The expert management of paediatric airways, in both theatre and in outside areas, is particularly important as perioperative respiratory adverse events are the most common cause of mortality and morbidity in children without cardiac malformations. Airway incidents in children are a frequent problem in paediatric anaesthesia, contributing significantly to mortality and morbidity statistics. Human factors and unfamiliarity with the nuances of paediatric airways are recognised as variables contributing to adverse outcomes in airway management.

A difficult paediatric airway, although rare in terms of predictability, is potentially one of the most challenging situations a clinician may face. A poor tolerance of even short periods of apnoea with limited ability to adequately pre-oxygenate, a propensity for upper airway obstruction, and the exponential effect of oedema on

C. Heath (✉)
Department of Anaesthesia and Pain Medicine, Perth Children's Hospital, Perth, WA, Australia

Perioperative Medicine Team, Perioperative Care Program, Kids Institute, Perth, WA, Australia

N. Hauser · B. S. von Ungern-Sternberg
Department of Anaesthesia and Pain Medicine, Perth Children's Hospital, Perth, WA, Australia

Perioperative Medicine Team, Perioperative Care Program, Kids Institute, Perth, WA, Australia

Division of Emergency Medicine, Anaesthesia and Pain Medicine, Medical School, The University of Western Australia, Perth, WA, Australia
e-mail: Neil.Hauser@health.wa.gov.au

M. Á. Gómez-Ríos, A. van Zundert (eds.), *Evidence-based Guide to Difficult Airway Management*, https://doi.org/10.1007/978-3-032-30769-9_24

airway resistance all contribute to a potentially stressful clinical situation with the chance of a rapid deterioration in patient status. Fortunately, difficult paediatric airways remain a relatively rare event. Unfortunately, the complications associated with managing a difficult paediatric airway are common and occur in 20% of children, with 3% suffering severe complications including cardiac arrest [1].

Recognising the anatomical and physiological differences between paediatric, particularly neonatal, and adult airways can help clinicians to plan for and hopefully avoid the adverse events that may occur during intubation attempts in paediatric patients. An underlying theme in the literature on the management of paediatric airways is to keep it simple, adhere to familiar techniques, and have a plan to respond to clinical changes, remembering that the simplest technique of effective bag and mask ventilation is more likely to save the life of the littlest patients and not the newest airway gadget [2].

24.2 Anatomical and Physiological Airway Differences in Paediatric Patients

24.2.1 Anatomical Differences

Anatomical and physiological differences exist between paediatric and adult patients. These differences are generally most pronounced in patients under 1 year of age. This is also reflected in the increased rate of adverse airway events reported in infants compared with older children. Age-related anatomical and physiological differences are a consequence of normal paediatric development. These developmental changes necessitate experience with a range of techniques to ensure safe airway management through the spectrum of premature neonatal to adolescent airways. Each of these stages presents a range of airway challenges that will be encountered by clinicians managing these young patients. Table 24.1 lists the commonly-cited anatomical differences noted with paediatric airways [3]. These differences in airway anatomy combine to increase the risk of technical difficulties when managing infant airways.

Infants have a predisposition to upper airway obstruction because of reduced muscular tone and increased tissue laxity. Patency of the upper airway improves gradually over the first 8 weeks of life with increases in both tissue and muscle tone. Growth of the mandible and maxilla contributes further to improved airway patency as their size increases relative to that of the tongue. This reduces the impact of difficulty with laryngoscopy due to the tongue's relatively large size at birth. Early in life, the larynx is higher in the neck to allow the infant to breathe during feeding. This cephalad position in the neck means that a straight blade is frequently more useful during laryngoscopy in infants. At the same time, control of the epiglottis is more challenging in this age group due to its angle over the laryngeal inlet, its shape and floppiness, adding further difficulty to performing laryngoscopy.

Table 24.1 Commonly cited anatomical differences encountered in paediatric airways

Paediatric airways	Consequence of anatomical differences
Relatively large tongue compared to oral cavity	Potentially difficult laryngoscopy due to the challenge of displacing the tongue
Prominent occiput (especially in neonates and infants)	Requires a head ring/shoulder roll to position the head correctly
Large head relative to body size	Alignment of oral, pharyngeal, and tracheal axis is challenging
Large and floppy epiglottis that is more cephalad and anterior	Potentially more difficult to obtain a satisfactory view of the vocal cords
Relatively narrow nasal passages and delicate, highly vascular nasal mucosa in neonates and infants	Nasal instrumentation may be difficult and carries an increased risk of mucosal trauma and epistaxis; appropriately sized equipment and a gentle technique should be used
Floor of mouth is softer and more compressible	Ensure correct positioning of fingers during mask ventilation to avoid compression anatomical structures
Until puberty, the cricoid ring forms the narrowest portion of the airway	The size of the cricoid ring determines ETT size, increased risk of airway swelling
Soft compliant trachea	With obstruction of the upper airway, there is a greater risk of extra-thoracic tracheal collapse

Adapted from BvUS & C. Sims 2nd ed. [2, 3]

Due to the shape of the larynx in infants, the choice of the endotracheal tube (ETT) size* is important to limit the risk of airway tissue trauma and thus reduce the risk of oedema, which will in turn increase the airway resistance. The classic description of an infant airway is "funnel-shaped" with the inlet tapering towards the circular cricoid ring when the vocal cords are widely abducted. More recent MRI studies have suggested that the narrowest part is indeed the subglottic region. The subglottic region is relatively pliable and easily accommodates the passing of an ETT. The insertion of an incorrectly sized ETT in an infant predisposes to post-extubation stridor and subglottic stenosis because of oedema, mucosal ischaemia, and scarring. This may further be exacerbated by the over-inflation of an ETT cuff. As such, it is important when selecting a cuffed ETT in paediatric patients to use a high-volume low-pressure cuff, or micro cuff. In addition, the cuff pressure should be checked at both inflation and intermittently thereafter, once the ETT has been placed, to ensure a pressure of less than 20 cmH_2O. This will limit the risk of pressure necrosis associated with over-inflation of ETT cuffs.

***ETT Size**

Uncuffed ETT size for child over 2 years: Age/4 + 4 = ETT size (inside diameter mm), with a cuffed ETT a ½ size smaller.

Cuffed ETT size for a child over 2 years: Age/4 + 3.5 = ETT size (inside diameter mm).

A cuffed ETT in general is preferred, even in children under 2 years of age, provided an appropriately sized cuff and ETT have been selected and the cuff pressure is measured to avoid excessive pressure on the tracheal mucosa.

Table 24.2 Physiological differences and the consequences associated with airway management

Paediatric physiology	Consequences of physiological differences
Higher rate of oxygen consumption	Greater metabolic demand and need for supplementary oxygen during airway manipulation
Reduced function residual capacity	Limited oxygen reserves with more rapid reduction of oxygen stores and less margin for apnoea
Reduced pulmonary compliance	Predisposition to small airway closure with subsequent accelerated hypoxaemia
Soft compliant ribcage	Indrawing of the chest with upper airway obstruction, with further airway closure and hypoxaemia
Obligate nasal breather	Copes poorly with any nasal congestion/obstruction

24.2.2 *Physiological Differences*

Physiological differences in paediatric patients have the potential to add further challenges to airway management. A proportionately higher rate of oxygen consumption, together with a relatively reduced functional residual capacity (FRC) and frequent inability to pre-oxygenate, combine to result in a reduced tolerance of apnoeic periods. Consequently, accelerated rates of desaturation during airway management can occur. The FRC is the oxygen reservoir for all patients and paediatric patients have low absolute FRC values. In infancy, FRC values are as low as 80 mL (17–25 mL/kg), with FRC values increasing to 3000 mL (30–35 mL/kg) by adulthood. Additionally, the relative reduction in pulmonary compliance seen in younger paediatric patients, together with a predisposition for small airway closure, adds to the propensity of atelectasis and accelerated rates of desaturation. Table 24.2 illustrates commonly cited physiological differences and their consequences.

The anatomical and physiological differences noted above and in Tables 24.1 and 24.2 are more marked in neonates. This reflects the age-related time required for structures to develop, illustrating the importance of developmental respiratory physiology knowledge. At birth, the lung is underdeveloped, with alveolar multiplication and maturation continuing until 8 years of age [4]. This under-development is exacerbated in premature infants due to inadequate surfactant production prior to 34 weeks of gestation.

24.3 Pre-operative Airway Assessment and Specific Syndromes

The ability to assess a paediatric airway pre-operatively is largely dependent on the age and developmental status of the patient. Co-operative older children and adolescents may be assessed with the same tools used to assess an adult airway. Infants, younger children, and uncooperative children are largely assessed by observation and reference to previous anaesthetic and airway records if available. Table 24.3

Table 24.3 Anatomical structures to observe on assessment of the paediatric airway

Mouth opening and size of the mouth	Functional and/or anatomical limitation reducing mouth opening
Abnormal tongue size	Age-related relative size or associated with mucopolysaccharide diseases
Abnormal neck position or limited range of neck movement	Consider the potential for undiagnosed atlanto-axial instability in trisomy 21 patients Reduced range of motion with Goldenhar
Position and size of mandible	Note the presence of micro/retrognathia
Mid-face anomalies associated with syndromes	Difficulties associated with the insertion of the laryngoscope and subsequent laryngoscopy

details the anatomical structures that should be examined during an airway assessment. In paediatric patients, the unanticipated difficult airway is a small proportion of the difficult airway population when compared to adults [5]. Difficult paediatric airways are generally predictable, with syndromal or abnormal facies evident on examination. This allows for appropriate planning and preparation, including necessary equipment and experienced personnel, including surgical support from Ear, Nose and Throat (ENT) specialists.

The approach to any paediatric airway can be determined by a pragmatic classification described below [6].

1. Normal airway—a patient without a history, sign, or symptom of a difficult airway.
2. Impaired normal airway—includes disease states that affect airway management, e.g. respiratory tract infections and resultant upper airway obstruction and rapid desaturation.
3. Abnormal or difficult airway. Much like adults, difficult paediatric airways may then further be divided into:

    3.1. Difficulty with bag-mask ventilation (BMV)
    3.2. Difficulty with laryngoscopy
    3.3. Difficulty with supraglottic airway device (SAD) insertion or any combination of the three.

4. A fourth definition may also be included in paediatrics due to their limited cardiorespiratory reserve to include patients with abnormalities that result in difficult airway management with traditional approaches [7, 8].

A useful strategy in paediatric patients of any age is to observe for and note any malformations, deformations, or disruptions as these may increase airway complexity [9]. Malformations include any abnormal tissue development, e.g. cleft lip and palate or microcephaly [9]. Deformations occur in normal tissues that have been exposed to abnormal forces, e.g. Robin sequence [9]. Disruptions occur when normal tissue is broken down, e.g. hemifacial microsomia and other facial clefts [8]. Table 24.4 presents syndromes that are known difficult airway associations [3].

Table 24.4 Facial syndromes associated with a difficult airway

Anatomical airway variances of concern	Anatomical variance associated with airway management difficulty	Predicted progression with increasing age and growth of the patient
Apert syndrome	Anomalies of the mid-face and mandibular hypoplasia	Airway management progressively becomes more difficult
Hunter and hurlers syndromes	Mucopolysaccharide deposition in the tissues of the airway—tongue and larynx particularly affected	Airway management progressively becomes more difficult
Robin sequence	Mandibular hypoplasia (micrognathia)	Improves with patient's growth
Goldenhar (hemifacial microsomia)	Potentially reduced cervical spine range of motion as a result of vertebral abnormalities, asymmetrical mandibular size	Airway management potentially becomes more difficult with increasing age
Treacher Collins	Reduced mouth size and associated mandibular hypoplasia The larynx is funnel-shaped	Airway management progressively becomes more difficult Potential issues with advancing ETT

Adapted from BvUS & C. Sims 2nd ed. [3]

The presence of retrognathia or micrognathia is one of the most important features to note. If a small mandible is present on examination, there is less space between the tongue and the soft palate, increasing the risk of upper airway obstruction. There is also less space to compress the tongue on laryngoscopy, thus reducing the view of the vocal cords obtainable during direct laryngoscopy and intubation [3].

24.4 Approach to Airway Management

24.4.1 General Considerations

Regular practice, continuing medical education, and simulation training are all essential for practitioners involved in difficult airway management [6]. The paediatric airway may be classified as difficult, as described above, due to (1) an abnormal airway or (2) an impaired otherwise normal airway [10]. All anticipated difficult airway management should involve early referral to a specialist paediatric centre with careful planning and multidisciplinary input, ideally with ENT involvement. Whilst clinical urgency can impact the extent of planning, local expertise and resources should always be considered.

Prior to the administration of sedative agents, a clear airway management plan, including consideration for potential complications and their management must be established and agreed upon [6, 11]. All equipment and medications required to establish a safe paediatric airway and manage potential complications must be prepared in advance for immediate use. Ideally, a designated difficult airway trolley is available, and at a minimum, equipment should include: ETT's and supraglottic airway devices, a variety of laryngoscope blades, a videolaryngoscope, stylets, forceps, facemasks, airway adjuncts, a self-inflating ventilation bag and T-piece, suction, an oxygen source, and vascular access equipment [5, 6, 12].

24.4.2 Airway Algorithms, Guidelines, and Cognitive Aids

Paediatric airway algorithms were historically drafted by adapting those from adult practice. However, the adaptation of adult algorithms to guide paediatric airway practice is inappropriate given the anatomical, physiological, and neurodevelopmental differences between adults and children [6]. In more recent times, The Difficult Airway Society has published a paediatric specific guideline, and The American Society of Anaesthesiologists (ASA) in consultation with the Society for Paediatric Anaesthesia (SPA) & the Paediatric Difficult Intubation (PeDI) Collaborative have published an algorithm for the management of the difficult paediatric airway [11, 13]. A group of paediatric airway experts has also published a Framework Approach for the management of the paediatric airway [6]. Similar to the Vortex approach, the Framework Approach is a concept-based cognitive aid. Concept-based cognitive aids are more likely to become a natural component of situational awareness and reduce the risk of task fixation [14, 15]. Continual reassessment and appropriate redirection of focus, including working through all optimisation steps to achieve safe oxygenation, is essential in airway management [14].

24.4.3 The Framework Approach

24.4.3.1 Principles

The authors of this approach aimed to produce a universally accepted framework that could be implemented in any clinical environment. To achieve this, the authors acknowledged the need for a simple, intuitive, and forward-only algorithm. In addition, the authors created an "open-box" approach to account for the ever-evolving development of new equipment and techniques. The "open-box" recognises the need to incorporate local expertise, opinion, resources (such as equipment), and facilities at different sites [6].

In the context of the difficult paediatric airway in a patient undergoing sedation or anaesthesia, the first decision point is the appropriateness of proceeding with patient management at the specific institution. This decision should be based on available local facilities and expertise (Fig. 24.1) [6].

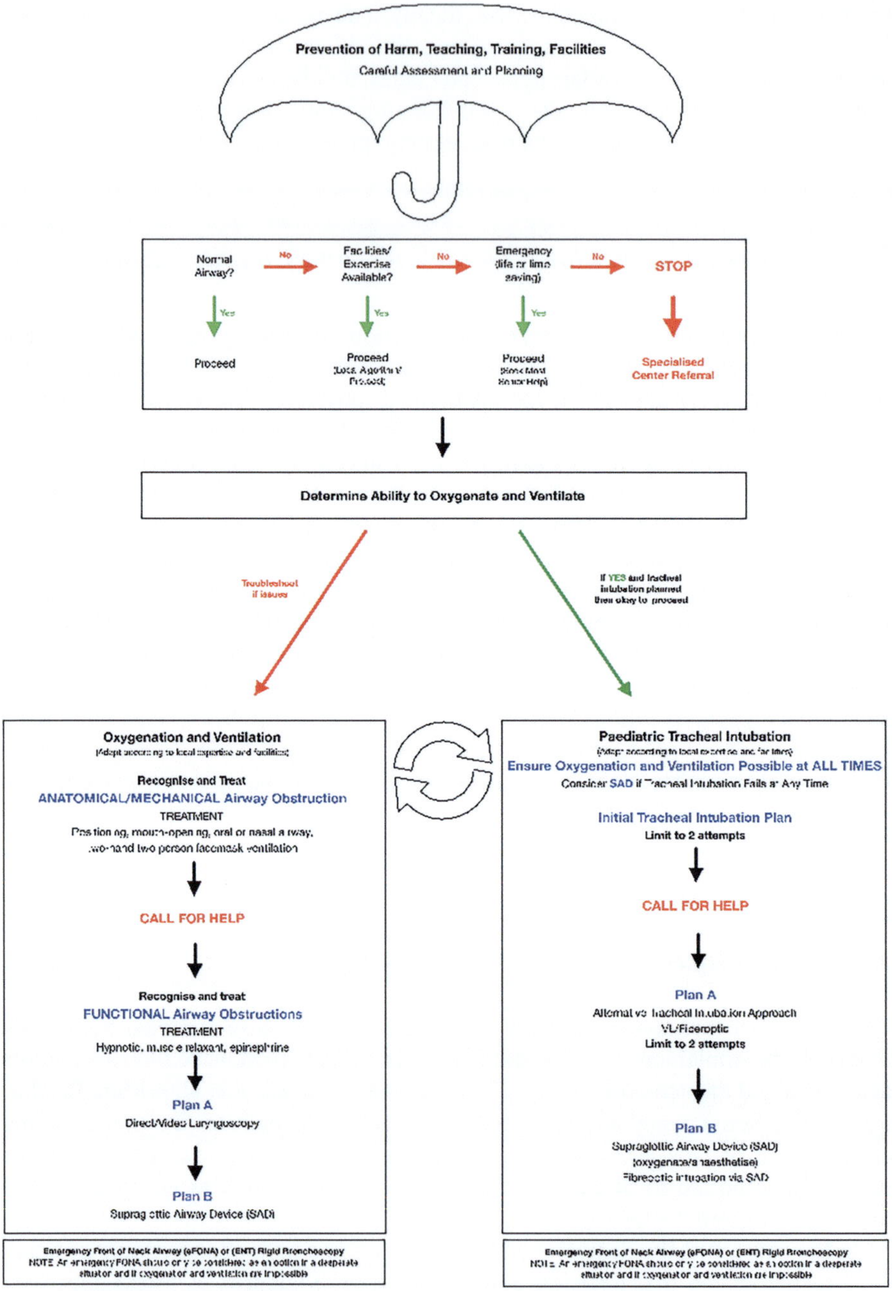

Fig. 24.1 The framework approach. (Adapted from Engelhardt et al. [6])

24.4.3.2 Clear Separation of Airway Problems

If the decision is made to proceed with airway management, the framework approach has two pathways (Fig. 24.1):

1. Oxygenation and ventilation.
2. Tracheal intubation.

Safe oxygenation (and ventilation) must be the priority in airway management. The overarching goal of the framework approach is the prevention of perioperative hypoxia rather than the insertion of an ETT [6].

If prior to tracheal intubation, oxygenation (and ventilation) is problematic, the practitioner will troubleshoot oxygenation and ventilation (Fig. 24.1). If oxygenation is safe peri-intubation, the practitioner can proceed with tracheal intubation (Fig. 24.1). Difficult airway management is a dynamic process, and the framework approach allows movement between the two pathways if oxygenation (and ventilation) is inadequate at any time during attempted tracheal intubation. Oxygenation and effective ventilation (facemask) must always be prioritised over tracheal intubation [6, 16].

Note the framework approach emphasises:

1. Practice should be adapted to local expertise and facilities.
2. Prevention (of avoidable harm), teaching, training, and resource utilisation are at the core of safe airway management.
3. Help should be sought early.

Like the vortex approach in adults, three basic techniques to restore oxygenation and ventilation are covered: face mask ventilation, supraglottic airway insertion, and tracheal intubation [14].

Oxygenation and Ventilation

The first step after encountering difficulties is to prevent, recognise, and treat airway obstruction with skills and medications, respectively. In the context of airway management, it is imperative that the clinician recognises and treats airway obstruction by distinguishing between mechanical and functional airway obstruction (Table 24.5). Once these have been considered and optimally treated, the clinician moves to plan A (tracheal intubation). With failure to intubate, plan B is insertion of a supraglottic airway device [6].

Tracheal Intubation

In the context of the difficult paediatric airway, there is no one best technique for tracheal intubation. All approaches to the management of a difficult airway require unique consideration and careful planning. The priority remains oxygenation and

Table 24.5 Causes and treatment of airway obstruction during anaesthesia

Anatomical/mechanical airway obstruction		**Treatment**
Inadequate head position	→	Reposition, re-open
Large adenoids/tonsils/obesity	→	Oropharyngeal, nasopharyngeal airway
Difficult facemask technique	→	Two-hand, two-person technique
Blood, foreign body, secretions	→	Suction, removal
Alveolar collapse	→	Alveolar recruitment manoeuvre
Gastric hyperinflation	→	Decompression by orogastric tube
Functional airway obstruction		**Treatment**
Inadequate depth of anaesthesia	→	Deepen anaesthesia
Laryngospasm	→	Propofol, muscle relaxation
Opioid-induced muscle rigidity +/− vocal cord closure	→	Muscle relaxation
Bronchospasm	→	Epinephrine, bronchodilators

Adapted from Engelhardt et al. [6]

avoidance of airway trauma [6]. Whilst the framework approach is not specifically designed for difficult airway management, the same principles still apply. Following two attempts of the initial intubation plan, an alternative technique should be pursued with a further limit of two attempts before moving to consider abandonment or feasibility of using a supraglottic airway in the context of the planned surgery or fibreoptic intubation via the supraglottic airway if not already attempted [1, 6, 17]. Specific equipment and airway techniques to manage the difficult airway are discussed in further detail in the remainder of the chapter.

24.4.3.3 Conclusion

The open-box design of the framework approach ensures that local expertise and protocols are factored into airway management. This approach to airway management is universally applicable, easily adapted to diverse clinical situations, and provides a tool for use in both training and during critical clinical airway management scenarios [6, 14]. Combined with teaching, training, and regular practice, the framework approach provides a paediatric-specific, intuitive, and time-critical approach to airway management that can help to reduce airway-related morbidity and mortality [6].

24.5 Equipment and Techniques to Manage the Difficult Airway

In paediatric anaesthesia practice, respiratory events are the most common cause of adverse events. Infants and neonates are at the highest risk [18]. Over 20% of adverse events are due to intubation-related factors, including ETT and supraglottic device use, endobronchial intubation, dislodged airway devices, and equipment failure [18]. Suitable equipment aligning with national and international standards, as well as a dedicated difficult paediatric airway trolley, must be available for the safe management of paediatric airways [6].

24.5.1 Oxygenation

Hypoxia is frequently associated with bradycardia, which is the most common warning sign of impending cardiac arrest in children (54%) [18]. Clinicians, however, must consider that oxygen as a drug is not without risk, particularly in premature babies and neonates. Preterm neonates (gestational age <37 weeks) are most at risk of negative outcomes due to oxidative stress, possibly related to oxygen free radical formation [18, 19]. Oxygen, like any other drug, must be titrated to ensure the dose correlates with the needs of the patient to achieve optimal physiological status [18].

24.5.1.1 Bag-Mask Oxygenation and Ventilation

Bag-mask oxygenation via a T-piece or anaesthesia circuit is a core skill for all airway practitioners and is the default technique for safe oxygenation in airway management. Dysmorphic features such as micrognathia and distorted anatomy can create difficulties in achieving an adequate seal in children. Difficult airways may require airway manoeuvres such as jaw thrust, chin lift, and head tilt in addition to adjuncts such as oral and nasopharyngeal airways or, in some instances, a two-operator technique.

24.5.1.2 Preoxygenation

Preoxygenation is essential in patients with difficult airways. Children, and in particular neonates, have short apnoea times prior to desaturation due to the anatomical and physiological differences discussed previously. Preoxygenation is recommended by current airway management guidelines to increase safe apnoea time for laryngoscopy and tracheal intubation [18, 20–22]. In children, preoxygenation often occurs in combination with gas induction of anaesthesia. The un-cooperative child creates challenges with preoxygenation and this must be considered in the airway management plan, especially in the presence of a difficult airway [18]. The importance of continuing oxygenation during tracheal intubation is emphasised in this context.

24.5.1.3 Oxygenation During Tracheal Intubation

Maintaining oxygenation during attempted intubation has physiological advantages. The benefit of increased time to desaturation can translate to less airway trauma if the practitioner does not feel rushed and this may limit multiple attempts at securing the airway [18]. Trauma to the airway through instrumentation and multiple attempts can increase the grade of airway difficulty through the accumulation of blood and secretions, airway oedema and potential airway obstruction [1, 18]. Repeated attempts at tracheal intubation may render a paediatric airway impossible to intubate or lead to an inability to oxygenate and ventilate the patient [16, 17]. This is of particular relevance in children and, most importantly, neonates due to the small lumen diameter of the trachea [18]. The PeDI-Collaborative is a multicentre international group of anaesthesiologists dedicated to assessing, understanding, and improving the outcomes of children with Difficult Direct Laryngoscopy (DDL). The group recommends routine use of oxygen during attempts at tracheal intubation in difficult airway patients [23]. This aligns with the 2022 ASA guidelines for difficult airway management [13]. These recommendations are on the basis that available evidence demonstrates that supplemental oxygen prolongs apnoea time and results in less adverse events [24, 25].

Various techniques for oxygenation during tracheal intubation are described. Those suggested by PeDI-Collaborative for difficult airway management are outlined. These techniques can be applied to both the apnoeic and spontaneously breathing child.

Nasal Oxygenation

Nasal oxygenation techniques require strict attention to the maintenance of airway patency for effectiveness. Patient positioning is key [18].

1. *Low Flow Nasal Cannula*

Nasal cannulae are placed during preoxygenation or pre-laryngoscopy, with flow being established during laryngoscopy and tracheal intubation. Limitations include the potential to affect the mask seal and thus oxygenation if placed during induction. Flow rates of 1–2 L/kg/min have been safely used in small children [26]. In the recently published OPTIMISE study, all patients received supplemental oxygen (1 L/kg/min low flow nasal cannula) during laryngoscopy until the correct tracheal tube position was confirmed. This study, which compared direct and video laryngoscopy in infants, suggested that the addition of supplemental oxygen during laryngoscopy may improve first pass success due to an increase in safe apnoea time [25].

2. *Nasal High Flow (NHF)*

This technique involves the delivery of oxygen at flow rates exceeding that of the patient's own inspiratory effort via the administration of oxygen and air warmed to body temperature at >99% relative humidity [18, 27]. In addition to providing a reliable fractional inspired oxygen, this technique also decreases the work of breathing and provides a small degree of continual positive airway pressure (4–6 cm H20) [18, 28]. In the paediatric population, this can avoid the need for tracheal intubation through the provision of respiratory support to maintain oxygenation in patient groups such as premature neonates, infants with bronchiolitis, critically unwell patients requiring transport, and patients with post-extubation stridor [27].

Specific to paediatric anaesthesia, NHF is still relatively novel compared with other clinical areas such as intensive care. However, in the context of difficult paediatric airway management in anaesthesia practice, applications include preoxygenation, oxygenation during tracheal intubation, and oxygenation for tubeless anesthesia [6]. Nasal High Flow oxygen has been shown to double the expected time to desaturation below 90% in apnoeic well children [28, 29]. Of note, unlike the adult literature, there is no evidence in the paediatric population that NHF provides partial carbon dioxide clearance in apnoeic patients. Age and physical status of the patient will dictate the suitability and success of apnoeic oxygenation [18]. The absence of ventilation and a steady increase in carbon dioxide, with the potential for adverse effects caused by respiratory acidosis, such as cardiac arrhythmias and vasodilation, is a pertinent consideration when assessing the suitability of the technique, and transcutaneous monitoring of carbon dioxide is recommended [18, 28, 30]. Furthermore, complications in children have been documented, e.g. abdominal distension, barotrauma, pneumothoraces, and pneumomediastinum [27]. To mitigate these risks, NHF requires airway patency, adequate leak around the nares (cannula <50% nare diameter), and no concurrent face mask ventilation [18]. Weight-based flow rates as suggested by Humphreys et al. are shown in Table 24.6 [29].

Pharyngeal Oxygenation

1. *Tracheal Tube or Modified Nasal Trumpet* via *Nare Connected to Anaesthesia Circuit*

Either a modified nasal trumpet or an appropriately sized uncuffed tracheal tube can be placed in the external portion of the nasal airway. The anaesthesia circuit is then connected to this to deliver oxygen while intubation is attempted [23, 31].

Table 24.6 Nasal high flow rates

Weight (kg)	Flow rate
0–12	2 L/kg/min
13–15	30 L/min
16–30	35 L/min
31–50	40 L/min
>50	50 L/min

Table adapted from Humphreys et al. [29]

2. *Tracheal Tube (Oral RAE) in the Corner of the Mouth*

The anaesthesia circuit can be connected to a pharyngeally placed oral RAE tracheal tube to deliver oxygen while intubation is attempted.

3. *Supraglottic Airway with Bronchoscopic Adaptor*

This method of oxygenation during attempted intubation is applicable only to intubation techniques via the supraglottic airway (see hybrid techniques below).

24.5.2 Endotracheal Intubation

Within the paediatric population, infants have the highest incidence of difficult laryngoscopy (4.7%), compared to less than 1% in the older child. Overall, difficult laryngoscopy is rare in children compared to adults, with a reported incidence of 1.37% versus 9% [18, 32].

24.5.2.1 Techniques for the Management of a Difficult Paediatric Airway

A variety of tools and techniques are available for managing difficult paediatric airways. Patient and staff factors, including operator-dependent expertise and preference, will further guide the chosen technique. At the start, all clinicians must consider the need for an awake versus sedated or asleep approach to intubation in the difficult airway [33].

An awake approach to airway management is ideal in those with anticipated difficult ventilation. For example, this would include patients with severely limited mouth opening, blocked upper airway, or poor access to the oral cavity. In these patients, ventilation via the natural airway with adjuncts or a supraglottic device may not be possible, and therefore, rescue ventilation techniques are precluded. However, in paediatrics, awake approaches to airway management are commonly precluded, with practicalities dependent on both the age and developmental maturity of the patient. The availability of drugs such as dexmedetomidine and ketamine has broadened the feasibility of sedated approaches to airway management in the difficult paediatric airway [34]. In patients with no anticipated ventilation difficulties, an approach to tracheal intubation under general anaesthesia can be pursued [9, 31].

Regarding spontaneous versus controlled ventilation (with or without neuromuscular blockade), the PeDI registry has published results that show a higher incidence of non-severe complications in the management of difficult paediatric airways with spontaneously ventilated children. The key factor associated with these complications was airway reactivity during attempted airway manipulation [9, 35]. Adequate depth of anaesthesia prior to airway manipulation is crucial.

Video Laryngoscopes

Videolaryngoscopes are either standard (non-angulated) or non-standard (angulated) [26]. The most commonly encountered videolaryngoscopes are the GlideScope and the Storz C-MAC (SVL). The GlideScope is a hyper-angulated 60° blade available from neonate to adult sizes. The Storz C-MAC is available in Miller and MAC blade configurations (standard) from neonate to adult sizes and the hyper angulated (60°) D-blade is available down to a size 2 MAC equivalent.

Standard blades do not require the use of a stylet for ETT insertion. Other advantages include placement of the blade either into the vallecula or in front of the epiglottis to lift the epiglottis, ability to perform direct laryngoscopy, and the ability to perform a retromolar approach to create more intraoral space [36, 37].

Non-standard hyper-angulated blades are designed to improve visualisation, particularly for an anterior glottis [24]. Use of a stylet is routine with hyper-angulated blades, although techniques vary depending on the utilised blade regarding how the stylet should be curved and whether it is inserted congruently with the blade or from the corner of the mouth [36, 38, 39]. Hyper-angulated videolaryngoscope blades, compared to non-angulated blades, can introduce more difficulty in converting an adequate view to a successful intubation [36]. This is referred to as the view tube discrepancy and troubleshooting this issue is as per adult practice.

Two recent randomised controlled trials, the VISI trial and OPTIMISE trial, compared the success rate of first-attempt tracheal intubation between videolaryngoscopy (standard blade) and direct laryngoscopy in infants (<12 months and δ52 weeks postmenstrual age, respectively) without known or anticipated difficult airways [25, 40]. In the OPTIMISE trial, all laryngoscopy attempts were combined with the additional intervention of low flow nasal oxygen (1 L/kg/min) [25]. Both trials found videolaryngoscopy with a standard blade improves first-attempt tracheal intubation success rate, particularly in small infants δ6.5 kg [25, 40].

Specific to paediatric difficult airways, data from the PeDI Registry also shows superiority favouring video laryngoscopy in both visualisation and intubation in children with difficult airways [36]. Case series looking at the efficacy of the SVL in paediatric difficult airways have also shown high success when compared with direct laryngoscopy [36, 41, 42]. Regarding glottic views, studies have shown consistent superiority of the SVL compared to direct laryngoscopy in a range of groups (manikin, normal paediatric airway, and difficult paediatric airway) [36, 42–47].

Evidence to guide the choice of videolaryngoscope blade is limited. A recent observational study assessed the efficacy of standard and non-standard blades to perform tracheal intubation in paediatric patients from the Difficult Intubation Registry. Success rates of initial and eventual tracheal intubation by weight stratification were measured. In infants weighing <5 kg, videolaryngoscopy with standard blades was associated with a significantly greater success rate than videolaryngoscopy with non-standard blades [48]. Other studies comparing different videolaryngoscopes are limited, generally have small numbers, and were conducted on simulated patients (manikins) or children with normal airways [36]. Furthermore, specific to infants and neonates, experience is limited and therefore evidence is lacking.

Table 24.7 Flexible bronchoscopes sizes for paediatric practice with correlation of ETT sizes

	Olympus		Karl Storz		Verathon	
	ETT	OD (mm)	ETT	OD (mm)	ETT	OD (mm)
Neonate/infant	2.5 3.0	2.2 2.8	3.5 3.0 3.5	3.1 2.8 3.0		
Paediatric	4.0 4.5	3.8 4.1	4.0 4.5	3.7 4.0		
Teen	5.5	5.1	5.5 6.0	5.2 5.5	6.0 6.5	5.0 5.8

Adapted from Stein et al. [24]

Flexible Bronchoscopy

Flexible bronchoscopy is the gold standard for the management of difficult paediatric airways in patients with limited mouth opening [26]. Data generated by the PeDI-Registry has shown the highest first attempt success using flexible bronchoscopy compared with other techniques, particularly in infants [26, 49]. Notably, in older children with normal mouth opening, intubation success rates are comparable between videolaryngoscopy and flexible bronchoscopy [26]. Table 24.7 details flexible bronchoscope sizes and correlating ETT sizes for paediatric practice.

Oxygenation techniques during flexible bronchoscopic intubation align with adult practice, including nasal oxygenation (low flow or NHF), pharyngeal oxygenation via an (oral) ETT placed in the opposite nare or an inverted Hudson mask over the mouth [18, 50]. Oxygenation and a degree of ventilation can also be achieved through the use of a paediatric endoscopy face mask during oral or nasal flexible bronchoscopy. Insufflation of oxygen via the bronchoscope working channel is not recommended due to the risk of barotrauma [18].

Complete airway obstruction during induction of anaesthesia, whether intravenous or inhalational, is of particular concern in the difficult airway. However, unlike adult practice, the option for awake flexible bronchoscopic intubation in the difficult paediatric airway is rarely an option. Awake intubation with local anaesthetic and sedation may be tolerated in select older children [18]. Hybrid awake techniques have also been described as discussed below.

Optical Stylets

Optical stylets can be used in the management of difficult paediatric airways, both as stand-alone intubation devices and adjuncts to direct or videolaryngoscopy [18]. Advantages include usefulness in patients with limited mouth opening and the ability to watch the tracheal tube advance into the glottis [51]. The Bonfils and Shikani are the two most commonly used devices.

Table 24.8 Optical stylet sizes for paediatric practice with correlation of ETT sizes

	Paediatric		Teen	
	OD (mm)	ETT	OD (mm)	ETT
Karl Storz	Bambrink 2.0 Bonfils 3.5	2.5 4.0	Bonfils 5.0 C-Mac 5.5	4.0 4.5
Clarus (Shikani)	Shikani 2.4	3.0	Shikani 5.1	5.5
MP multiview stylet scope	Stylet Scope 2.5 Stylet Scope 3.5	3.0 4.0	Stylet scope 5.0	5.5
UE video stylet	Small	3.0	Large	5.5

Adapted from Stein et al. [24]

Evidence around their utility in paediatric practice is limited with varied results regarding its efficiency [51–56]. Furthermore, proficiency in the use of optical stylets takes time, making unfamiliarity with the device a major limitation [51, 57]. Table 24.8 presents the sizes of types of optical stylets available.

Hybrid Techniques

Hybrid techniques have the advantage of combining the benefits and minimizing the pitfalls of isolated techniques [24].

1. *Intubation via Supraglottic Airway (SGA) Device*

Studies in children, including those with difficult airways, have demonstrated the effective use of SGAs as conduits for tracheal intubation [58–61]. This technique has been described in both awake and anesthetised patients following insertion of the SGA. One study comparing this technique to videolaryngoscopy showed higher first-attempt success, through the SGA, in anaesthetised infants with difficult airways [49].

A range of SGA devices are suitable as tracheal intubation conduits for paediatric patients with difficult airways (see Table 24.9) [62]. The air-Q uniquely has a detachable 15-mm adaptor compared with other SGAs, which may be advantageous.

Significant advantages of this technique include the ability to maintain continuous oxygenation and ventilation during intubation via a triple port adapter connected to the supraglottic device and the option of using the SGA as the primary airway if intubation is not possible [49, 58, 61, 63]. An important consideration with this technique is not to dislodge the tracheal tube when the SGA device is removed. Advancing the bronchoscope beyond the tracheal tube during removal of the SGA is advised. An alternate option is to leave the SGA in situ if safe to do so.

A muscle relaxant may facilitate easier tracheal tube placement by preventing coughing, laryngospasm, and vocal cord closure around the scope [31]. When using spontaneous ventilation, it is important to maintain an adequate depth of anaesthesia [64]. If airway reactivity is noted, neuromuscular blockade should be considered [26].

Table 24.9 Suggested maximum cuffed endotracheal tube sizes for supraglottic airways

	Neonate/infant		Paediatric		Teen	
	Size	ETT	Size	ETT	Size	ETT
LMA unique	1 1.5	3.0[a] 3.5[a]	2 2.5 3	4.0[a] 5.0[a] 6.0	4 5	6.0 7.0
Air-Q intubating laryngeal airway	0.5 1.0	4.0 4.5	1.5 2.0 2.5	5.5 6.0 6.5	3.5 4.5	7.5 8.5
i-gel supraglottic airway	1.0 1.5	3.0[a] 4.0[a]	2 2.5 3	5.0[a] 5.0[a] 6.0	4 5	7.0 8.0
Ambu AuraGain laryngeal mask	1.0 1.5	3.0[a] 3.5[a]	2 2.5 3	4.5[a] 5.0[a] 6.0	4 5 6	6.0 7.0 7.5

Adapted from Stein et al. [24]
Note the size of the LMA is weight-dependent and varies across devices
[a]Not recommended to put the pilot balloon through the SAD conduit

2. *Intubation Combining a Videolaryngoscope with Flexible Bronchoscope*

This technique has several advantages. Compared to either technique alone, visualisation is improved with the ability to visualise both the insertion of the tube into both the glottis and confirmation of tracheal placement [26, 65]. Furthermore, manoeuvrability of the fibreoptic bronchoscope is improved as the videolaryngoscope displaces soft tissue [26]. The disadvantage of this technique is the requirement for two experienced clinicians. The PeDI Registry found a 79% success rate in children (0.5 to 310 months) in a case series of 71 children [35, 65].

3. *Intubation Combining a Non-angulated Videolaryngoscope with Optical Stylet*

With this technique, the videolaryngoscope is initially used to perform laryngoscopy and assess airway grade. The video stylet acts as the ETT rigid stylet and, compared to the use of optical stylets in isolation, passage of the ETT into the larynx is visualised. If neither a direct nor videolaryngoscopy view is obtained, the video stylet becomes the primary method of intubation [24].

Rigid Bronchoscope

Rigid bronchoscopes are recommended by the Difficult Airway Society in the management of obstructed paediatric airways prior to front of neck access (FONA) [11]. Rigid bronchoscopes can deliver 100% oxygen, splint open an obstructed airway, facilitate the removal of foreign bodies, and facilitate insertion of a tracheal tube [18]. However, the use of rigid bronchoscopes requires proficiency, which highlights the urgent need for the multi-disciplinary management and the early involvement of ENT colleagues in the management of the paediatric difficult airway.

24.5.3 Supraglottic Airway Devices (SGAs)

SGAs. Particularly second-generation SGAs, may prevent the need for tracheal intubation in children with a difficult airway, are an excellent airway device for rescuing difficult ventilation, and an excellent conduit for fibreoptic intubation [26, 66].

24.5.4 Emergency Front of Neck Access

Elective FONA contingency planning may be considered as part of the airway management plan in children with known difficult airways [6]. In an emergency, FONA is likely to be futile in a child and should only ever be attempted in a cannot intubate cannot oxygenate scenario as a last resort when all other means of relieving mechanical and functional airway obstruction are exhausted [67, 68]. Of the anticipated and unanticipated difficult airways from the PeDI registry, FONA was attempted in 2% of cases [1]. In paediatric practice, there is no evidence to guide the choice of cannula or scalpel technique for front of neck access, with the majority of successful cases being performed by a surgeon through surgical tracheotomy [69–71]. A consideration in infants and neonates is that the smallest neonatal ETT diameter is larger than the average neonatal cricothyroid membrane [72]. A surgical approach may not be feasible in some patients [24].

24.5.4.1 Needle Cricothyroidotomy Ventilation

In the case of cannula FONA, ventilation can be either flow-regulated or pressure-regulated. Barotrauma and surgical emphysema are significant risks, especially in the context of small lung volumes and obstructed airways [18]. Such devices are relatively contraindicated in neonates and infants with upper airway obstruction. Expert panels have advised the cautious use of the Manujet in children. The lowest driving pressure should always be the starting pressure and titrated up based on chest movement with the goal of restoring oxygenation. Respiratory rate should be dictated by the time required for full chest recoil [11, 18]. Use of these devices must be complimented by efforts to achieve a patent upper airway and paralysis of the patient to eliminate laryngospasm [18]. The Rapid O_2 insufflator is a flow-regulated volume ventilation device. Recommendation for use is: flow of 1 L/min/year of age with I:E ratio of 1:4 at a rate of 12 bpm [18].

The Ventrain is another device on the market to enable effective oxygenation and ventilation via a small-bore cannula. This is a flow-regulated oxygenation ventilation device. The Ventrain limits high intrathoracic pressures with the capability for expiratory ventilation assistance via suction with proximal airway obstruction [18, 26]. This has advantages over the above techniques that depend on passive exhalation [24].

24.5.5 Ultrasound

As in adult practice, ultrasound has utility in paediatric airway management to:

- Aid in diagnosing vocal cord dysfunction.
- Assessment of airway anatomy (sizing).
- Assessment of appropriate endotracheal and tracheostomy tube sizing.
- Confirming oesophageal versus tracheal intubation.
- Assessment of the cricothyroid membrane for emergency airway access.
- Assessment of tracheal rings for US-guided tracheostomy [73].

24.5.6 Neuromuscular Blocking Agents (NMBA)

The use of neuromuscular blocking agents in difficult airway management must be guided by the clinical situation. In general, the recommendation is to avoid NBMs in certain patient groups, such as those with mucopolysaccharidosis, head and neck radiation, and airway masses, given the risk of worsening ventilation [26]. However, NMBAs can facilitate the safe management of difficult airways in some clinical situations.

The PeDI registry published results to show that a higher incidence of non-severe complications in the management of difficult paediatric airways was associated with spontaneously ventilated children compared to controlled ventilation (with or without neuromuscular blocker). The key factor associated with these complications was airway reactivity during attempted airway manipulation [26, 35]. Of note, muscle relaxants should always be used in the "cannot intubate cannot oxygenate" situation before any FONA attempt.

24.5.7 Difficult Airway Trolley

Difficult airway trolleys should be available in locations where all routine paediatric airway management is performed [5]. In paediatric appropriate sizing and models, equipment should fall under the categories of (1) basic airway devices and medications, (2) intubating SGAs and ETTs, (3) optical stylets, bougies, and tube exchange catheters, (4) videolaryngoscopes, (5) flexible bronchoscope, and (6) front of neck airway equipment [5].

24.5.8 Extubation

While the underlying anatomical, physiological, and surgical considerations will differ with each patient, all the same general considerations (timing, place, personnel) for extubation should be applied to the paediatric patient. The preparation in terms of personnel and equipment should be the same as that for intubation.

References

1. Fiadjoe JE, Nishisaki A, Jagannathan N, et al. Airway management complications in children with difficult tracheal intubation from the Pediatric Difficult Intubation (PeDI) registry: a prospective cohort analysis. Lancet Respir Med. 2016;4(1):37–48.
2. von Ungern-Sternberg BS, Engelhardt T. Life is really simple, but we insist on making it complicated (Confucius). Paediatr Anaesth. 2020;30(3):203.
3. Sims C, Weber D, Johnson C. A guide to pediatric anesthesia. 2nd ed. Cham: Springer; 2020. p. 77–115.
4. Feldman JM. Optimal ventilation of the anesthetized pediatric patient. Anesth Analg. 2015;120(1):165–75.
5. Murray DJ, Massy-Westropp C, Narayana-Reddy K, Marsh J. Description and function of a difficult airway service. Paediatr Anaesth. 2020;30(3):375–82.
6. Engelhardt T, Fiadjoe JE, Weiss M, et al. A framework for the management of the pediatric airway. Paediatr Anaesth. 2019;29(10):985–92.
7. Nykiel-Bailey SM, McAllister JD, Schrock CR, Molter DW, Marsh JK, Murray DJ. Difficult airway consultation service for children: steps to implement and preliminary results. Paediatr Anaesth. 2015;25(4):363–71.
8. von Ungern-Sternberg BS. Rare events can be fatal and must not be ignored; how much needs to happen before we act? Paediatr Anaesth. 2015;25(4):332–3.
9. Garcia-Marcinkiewicz AG, Stricker PA. Craniofacial surgery and specific airway problems. Paediatr Anaesth. 2020;30(3):296–303.
10. Engelhardt T, Weiss M. A child with a difficult airway: what do I do next? Curr Opin Anaesthesiol. 2012;25(3):326–32.
11. Black AE, Flynn PE, Smith HL, Thomas ML, Wilkinson KA. Development of a guideline for the management of the unanticipated difficult airway in pediatric practice. Paediatr Anaesth. 2015;25(4):346–62.
12. Engelhardt T, Machotta A. Universal algorithms and approaches to airway management. In: Narasimhan J, Fiadjoe JE, editors. Management of the difficult pediatric airway. Cambridge University Press; 2019.
13. Apfelbaum JL, Hagberg CA, Connis RT, et al. 2022 American Society of Anesthesiologists Practice guidelines for management of the difficult airway. Anesthesiology. 2022;136(1):31–81.
14. Frykholm P. Visual aids for pediatric airway management. Paediatr Anaesth. 2020;30(3):371–4.
15. Chrimes N. The vortex: a universal 'high-acuity implementation tool' for emergency airway management. Br J Anaesth. 2016;117(Suppl 1):i20–7.
16. Weiss M, Engelhardt T. Proposal for the management of the unexpected difficult pediatric airway. Paediatr Anaesth. 2010;20(5):454–64.
17. Engelhardt T, Virag K, Veyckemans F, Habre W. Airway management in paediatric anaesthesia in Europe-insights from APRICOT (Anaesthesia Practice In Children Observational Trial): a prospective multicentre observational study in 261 hospitals in Europe. Br J Anaesth. 2018;121(1):66–75.
18. Baker P. Oxygenation techniques for children with difficult airways. In: Narasimhan J, Fiadjoe JE, editors. Management of the difficult pediatric airway. Cambridge University Press; 2019.
19. The International Liaison Committee on Resuscitation. The International Liaison Committee on Resuscitation (ILCOR) consensus on science with treatment recommendations for pediatric and neonatal patients: pediatric basic and advanced life support. Pediatrics. 2006;117(5):e955–77.

20. Apfelbaum JL, Hagberg CA, Caplan RA, et al. Practice guidelines for management of the difficult airway: an updated report by the American Society of Anesthesiologists Task Force on Management of the Difficult Airway. Anesthesiology. 2013;118(2):251–70.
21. Frerk C, Mitchell VS, McNarry AF, et al. Difficult Airway Society 2015 guidelines for management of unanticipated difficult intubation in adults. Br J Anaesth. 2015;115(6):827–48.
22. Law JA, Broemling N, Cooper RM, et al. The difficult airway with recommendations for management—part 2—the anticipated difficult airway. Can J Anaesth. 2013;60(11):1119–38.
23. Pediatric Difficult Intubation (PeDI) Registry. https://www.pediregistry.org/. Accessed 22 Jan 2023.
24. Stein ML, Park RS, Kovatsis PG. Emerging trends, techniques, and equipment for airway management in pediatric patients. Paediatr Anaesth. 2020;30(3):269–79.
25. Riva T, Engelhardt T, Basciani R, et al. Direct versus video laryngoscopy with standard blades for neonatal and infant tracheal intubation with supplemental oxygen: a multicentre, non-inferiority, randomised controlled trial. Lancet Child Adolesc Health. 2022;7(2):101–11.
26. Fiadjoe J, Nishisaki A. Normal and difficult airways in children: "What's new" – current evidence. Paediatr Anaesth. 2020;30(3):257–63.
27. Hutchings FA, Hilliard TN, Davis PJ. Heated humidified high-flow nasal cannula therapy in children. Arch Dis Child. 2015;100(6):571–5.
28. Humphreys S, Schibler A. Nasal high-flow oxygen in pediatric anesthesia and airway management. Paediatr Anaesth. 2020;30(3):339–46.
29. Humphreys S, Lee-Archer P, Reyne G, Long D, Williams T, Schibler A. Transnasal humidified rapid-insufflation ventilatory exchange (THRIVE) in children: a randomized controlled trial. Br J Anaesth. 2017;118(2):232–8.
30. Humphreys S, Schibler A, von Ungern-Sternberg BS. Carbon dioxide monitoring in children—a narrative review of physiology, value, and pitfalls in clinical practice. Paediatr Anaesth. 2021;31(8):839–45.
31. Stricker P, Kovatis PG. Flexible bronchoscopic techniques: nasal and oral approaches. In: Narasimhan J, Fiadjoe JE, editors. Management of the difficult pediatric airway. Cambridge University Press; 2019.
32. Heinrich S, Birkholz T, Ihmsen H, Irouschek A, Ackermann A, Schmidt J. Incidence and predictors of difficult laryngoscopy in 11,219 pediatric anesthesia procedures. Paediatr Anaesth. 2012;22(8):729–36.
33. Sequera-Ramos L, Laverriere EK, Garcia-Marcinkiewicz AG, Zhang B, Kovatsis PG, Fiadjoe JE. Sedation versus general anesthesia for tracheal intubation in children with difficult airways: a cohort study from the Pediatric Difficult Intubation Registry. Anesthesiology. 2022;137(4):418–33.
34. Buck ML. Dexmedetomidine use in pediatric intensive care and procedural sedation. J Pediatr Pharmacol Ther. 2010;15(1):17–29.
35. Garcia-Marcinkiewicz AG, Adams HD, Gurnaney H, et al. A retrospective analysis of neuromuscular blocking drug use and ventilation technique on complications in the Pediatric Difficult Intubation Registry using propensity score matching. Anesth Analg. 2020;131(2):469–79.
36. Hunyady AI, Peyton J, Lee S, Par R. Video laryngoscopy equipment and techniques. In: Management of the difficult pediatric airway. Cambridge University Press; 2019.
37. Holm-Knudsen R. The difficult pediatric airway—a review of new devices for indirect laryngoscopy in children younger than two years of age. Paediatr Anaesth. 2011;21(2):98–103.
38. Fiadjoe JE, Gurnaney H, Dalesio N, et al. A prospective randomized equivalence trial of the GlideScope Cobalt® video laryngoscope to traditional direct laryngoscopy in neonates and infants. Anesthesiology. 2012;116(3):622–8.
39. Levitan RM, Heitz JW, Sweeney M, Cooper RM. The complexities of tracheal intubation with direct laryngoscopy and alternative intubation devices. Ann Emerg Med. 2011;57(3):240–7.
40. Garcia-Marcinkiewicz AG, Kovatsis PG, Hunyady AI, et al. First-attempt success rate of video laryngoscopy in small infants (VISI): a multicentre, randomised controlled trial. Lancet. 2020;396(10266):1905–13.

41. Wald SH, Keyes M, Brown A. Pediatric video laryngoscope rescue for a difficult neonatal intubation. Paediatr Anaesth. 2008;18(8):790–2.
42. Hackell RS, Held LD, Stricker PA, Fiadjoe JE. Management of the difficult infant airway with the Storz Video Laryngoscope: a case series. Anesth Analg. 2009;109(3):763–6.
43. Sun Y, Lu Y, Huang Y, Jiang H. Pediatric video laryngoscope versus direct laryngoscope: a meta-analysis of randomized controlled trials. Paediatr Anaesth. 2014;24(10):1056–65.
44. Vadi MG, Roddy KJ, Ghazal EA, Um M, Neiheisel AJ, Applegate RL 2nd. Comparison of the GlideScope Cobalt® and Storz DCI® video laryngoscopes in children younger than 2 years of age during manual in-line stabilization: a randomized trainee evaluation study. Pediatr Emerg Care. 2017;33(7):467–73.
45. Vlatten A, Aucoin S, Litz S, Macmanus B, Soder C. A comparison of the STORZ video laryngoscope and standard direct laryngoscopy for intubation in the Pediatric airway—a randomized clinical trial. Paediatr Anaesth. 2009;19(11):1102–7.
46. Fiadjoe JE, Stricker PA, Hackell RS, et al. The efficacy of the Storz Miller 1 video laryngoscope in a simulated infant difficult intubation. Anesth Analg. 2009;108(6):1783–6.
47. Saracoglu KT, Eti Z, Kavas AD, Umuroglu T. Straight video blades are advantageous than curved blades in simulated pediatric difficult intubation. Paediatr Anaesth. 2014;24(3):297–302.
48. Peyton J, Park R, Staffa SJ, et al. A comparison of videolaryngoscopy using standard blades or non-standard blades in children in the Paediatric Difficult Intubation Registry. Br J Anaesth. 2021;126(1):331–9.
49. Burjek NE, Nishisaki A, Fiadjoe JE, et al. Videolaryngoscopy versus fiber-optic intubation through a supraglottic airway in children with a difficult airway: an analysis from the Multicenter Pediatric Difficult Intubation Registry. Anesthesiology. 2017;127(3):432–40.
50. Holm-Knudsen R, Eriksen K, Rasmussen LS. Using a nasopharyngeal airway during fiberoptic intubation in small children with a difficult airway. Paediatr Anaesth. 2005;15(10):839–45.
51. Subramanyam R, Mahmoud M. Optical stylet and light-guided equipment and techniques. In: Narasimhan J, Fiadjoe JE, editors. Management of the difficult pediatric airway. Cambridge University Press; 2019.
52. Bein B, Wortmann F, Meybohm P, Steinfath M, Scholz J, Dörges V. Evaluation of the pediatric Bonfils fiberscope for elective endotracheal intubation. Paediatr Anaesth. 2008;18(11):1040–4.
53. Aucoin S, Vlatten A, Hackmann T. Difficult airway management with the Bonfils fiberscope in a child with Hurler syndrome. Paediatr Anaesth. 2009;19(4):421–2.
54. Vlatten A, Aucoin S, Litz S, MacManus B, Soder C. A comparison of Bonfils fiberscope-assisted laryngoscopy and standard direct laryngoscopy in simulated difficult pediatric intubation: a manikin study. Paediatr Anaesth. 2010;20(6):559–65.
55. Shikani AH. New "seeing" stylet-scope and method for the management of the difficult airway. Otolaryngol Head Neck Surg. 1999;120(1):113–6.
56. Kaufmann J, Laschat M, Engelhardt T, Hellmich M, Wappler F. Tracheal intubation with the Bonfils fiberscope in the difficult pediatric airway: a comparison with fiberoptic intubation. Paediatr Anaesth. 2015;25(4):372–8.
57. Gravenstein D, Liem EB, Bjoraker DG. Alternative management techniques for the difficult airway: optical stylets. Curr Opin Anaesthesiol. 2004;17(6):495–8.
58. Jagannathan N, Sequera-Ramos L, Sohn L, Wallis B, Shertzer A, Schaldenbrand K. Elective use of supraglottic airway devices for primary airway management in children with difficult airways. Br J Anaesth. 2014;112(4):742–8.
59. Jagannathan N, Sohn LE, Sawardekar A, et al. A randomized trial comparing the Ambu® Aura-i ™ with the air-Q™ intubating laryngeal airway as conduits for tracheal intubation in children. Paediatr Anaesth. 2012;22(12):1197–204.
60. Jagannathan N, Kho MF, Kozlowski RJ, Sohn LE, Siddiqui A, Wong DT. Retrospective audit of the air-Q intubating laryngeal airway as a conduit for tracheal intubation in pediatric patients with a difficult airway. Paediatr Anaesth. 2011;21(4):422–7.
61. Huang AS, Sarver A, Widing A, Hajduk J, Jagannathan N. The design of the perfect pediatric supraglottic airway device. Paediatr Anaesth. 2020;30(3):280–7.

62. Huang AS, Hajduk J, Jagannathan N. Advances in supraglottic airway devices for the management of difficult airways in children. Expert Rev Med Devices. 2016;13(2):157–69.
63. Kovatsis PG. Continuous ventilation during flexible fiberscopic-assisted intubation via supraglottic airways. Paediatr Anaesth. 2016;26(4):457–8.
64. Abelson D. Laryngospasm notch pressure ('Larson's maneuver') may have a role in laryngospasm management in children: highlighting a so far unproven technique. Paediatr Anaesth. 2015;25(11):1175–6.
65. Olomu PN, Hsu G, Lockman JL. Hybrid approaches to the difficult pediatric airway. In: Narasimhan J, Fiadjoe JE, editors. Management of the difficult pediatric airway. Cambridge University Press; 2019.
66. Sharma B, Sood J, Sahai C, Kumra VP. Troubleshooting ProSeal LMA. Indian J Anaesth. 2009;53(4):414–24.
67. Okada Y, Ishii W, Sato N, Kotani H, Iiduka R. Management of pediatric 'cannot intubate, cannot oxygenate'. Acute Med Surg. 2017;4(4):462–6.
68. Koers L, Janjatovic D, Stevens MF, Preckel B. The emergency paediatric surgical airway: a systematic review. Eur J Anaesthesiol. 2018;35(8):558–65.
69. Prunty SL, Aranda-Palacios A, Heard AM, et al. The 'can't intubate can't oxygenate' scenario in pediatric anesthesia: a comparison of the Melker cricothyroidotomy kit with a scalpel bougie technique. Paediatr Anaesth. 2015;25(4):400–4.
70. Stacey J, Heard AM, Chapman G, et al. The 'can't intubate can't oxygenate' scenario in pediatric anesthesia: a comparison of different devices for needle cricothyroidotomy. Paediatr Anaesth. 2012;22(12):1155–8.
71. Prunty SL, Heard AM, Chapman G, Challen A, Vijayasekaran S, von Ungern-Sternberg BS. "Cannot intubate, cannot oxygenate": a novel 2-operator technique for cannula tracheotomy in an infant animal model-a feasibility study. Paediatr Anaesth. 2021;31(12):1298–303.
72. Overmann KM, Boyd SD, Zhang Y, Kerrey BT. Apneic oxygenation to prevent oxyhemoglobin desaturation during rapid sequence intubation in a pediatric emergency department. Am J Emerg Med. 2019;37(8):1416–21.
73. Daniel SJ, Bertolizio G, McHugh T. Airway ultrasound: point of care in children-the time is now. Paediatr Anaesth. 2020;30(3):347–52.

Chapter 25
Prehospital and Trauma Airway Management

Christopher Choi, Tony Garcia, Siddharth Dave, and Kunal Karamchandani

Highlights

- Prehospital airway management involves ensuring airway patency and adequate oxygenation/ventilation.
- Endotracheal intubation in the prehospital setting should be considered when the rescue airway is inadequate based on the team's expertise.
- Trauma airway management requires addressing anatomical, physiological, and logistical challenges.
- Time permitting, trauma airway assessment should include looking for anatomic as well as physiologic difficulties using POCUS.
- Pre-oxygenation, as well as hemodynamic optimization, should be considered in patients with a physiologically difficult airway.

Airway management in trauma patients begins from the time of first responder arrival and continues until a definitive airway can be secured and maintained. The priorities for airway management differ between the prehospital and hospital settings, likely due to alterations in the circumstances, equipment, and personnel. Despite being one of the most performed procedures, airway management in these settings continues to be associated with significant morbidity and mortality. While the overarching goal of prehospital airway management is to provide an open airway allowing oxygenation and ventilation with rapid transport to a trauma center,

C. Choi · T. Garcia · S. Dave · K. Karamchandani (✉)
Division of Critical Care Medicine, Department of Anesthesiology and Pain Management, University of Texas Southwestern Medical Center, Dallas, TX, USA
e-mail: Christopher.Choi@UTSouthwestern.edu; Tony.Garcia@UTSouthwestern.edu; Siddharth.Dave@UTSouthwestern.edu; Kunal.Karamchandani@UTSouthwestern.edu

M. Á. Gómez-Ríos, A. van Zundert (eds.), *Evidence-based Guide to Difficult Airway Management*, https://doi.org/10.1007/978-3-032-30769-9_25

airway management for trauma patients in the hospital is focused on establishing and/or maintaining a definitive airway. Providers involved with airway management in the prehospital and trauma settings often encounter anatomic, physiologic, or logistical challenges either by themselves or in combination.

25.1 Prehospital Airway Management

Airway management is one of the most important components of prehospital care in an adult trauma patient, as the inability to maintain a patent airway may lead to rapid deterioration and death. Establishing a definitive airway is not always the priority, and instead, the focus is on instituting and maintaining an open airway, allowing oxygenation and ventilation, while protecting from gross aspiration. Airway management in the prehospital setting is inherently difficult, both due to the circumstances and patient-related challenges. There is never an opportunity to perform any sort of pre-procedural examination, assessment, or management of the patient and their airway often occurs simultaneously. Hence, the process should be simplified as much as possible, and the initial set of questions should include: Is the airway open? Is the oxygen saturation adequate? Is the patient able to ventilate? If the answer to all these questions is "yes," then the only treatment necessary is supplemental oxygen, and the patient should be transferred to the nearest trauma center at the earliest so that definitive care can be instituted [1]. If the answer to any of these questions is "no," then the prehospital airway management should begin with BLS (basic life support) airway maneuvers. These maneuvers may include a jaw thrust, oropharyngeal airway (OPA), or nasopharyngeal airway (NPA) insertion in the absence of any contraindications (conscious, intact gag reflex, basilar skull fracture, etc.). If the airway is not patent after such maneuvers, then bag-valve-mask (BVM) ventilation should be initiated. If successful, based on available resources and the time to the nearest trauma center, either BVM ventilation should be continued, or advanced airway management (rescue airway placement or tracheal intubation) should be considered. Since BVM is best performed with two providers, one maintaining a mask seal and the other providing manual ventilation, this may not be possible in all situations, and advanced airway management may be preferred. In cases of hemodynamic instability, patients must be resuscitated prior to placement of an advanced airway to reduce the risk of cardiovascular collapse, including peri-intubation arrest.

25.1.1 Rescue Airway

The rescue airway (alternative airway or blind insertion airway device) is an important addition to the prehospital airway management armamentarium. If BVM ventilation is not effective, then a rescue airway is a logical next step in prehospital airway management. Extra-glottic devices (EGDs) have traditionally been utilized as "rescue" airways in the event of an inability to place an endotracheal tube. These include supraglottic and retroglottic devices. The supraglottic devices sit above the glottis opening, whereas retroglottic devices sit behind the glottis and have two inflatable balloons. One balloon sits in the pharynx while the other sits in the esophagus (air passes through openings in between the two balloons when both are inflated). While traditionally considered rescue devices, EGDs have been elevated in priority and can be used as a primary airway in certain situations [2]. Studies evaluating the use of rescue devices in the prehospital setting, both for trauma activations and out-of-hospital cardiac arrests (OHCA), have shown conflicting results. A meta-analysis comparing patient outcomes with endotracheal intubation (ETI) versus supraglottic airway (SGA) placement in patients with OHCA in the prehospital setting revealed that patients who receive ETI were more likely to obtain ROSC, survive to hospital admission, and survive neurologically intact when compared to SGA [3]. On the other hand, a meta-analysis reviewing prehospital airway management demonstrated a higher frequency of ROSC in adults with SGA versus ETI, but overall revealed no evidence of a difference in survival between the use of BVM, SGA, and ETI for adults/mixed ages and pediatric patients with cardiac arrest [4]. Similarly, prehospital ETI in trauma patients was not shown to be associated with improved outcomes, with most evidence leaning towards harm [5]. Insertion of rescue airways does not require the level of experience or expertise of an orotracheal intubation [6, 7]. However, providers must keep in mind that the rescue airway is not a definitive airway, does not prevent aspiration, and may be prone to inappropriate insertion and potential gastric insufflation. Reassuringly, the risk of clinically significant aspiration with EGDs seems low [8]. Nevertheless, providers should minimize peak inspiratory pressures on the ventilator and/or avoid aggressive manual bag ventilation. In the absence of clear evidence, the decision to continue with a rescue airway or to insert an advanced airway should be made on a case-by-case basis, keeping the providers' experience and the distance to the nearest healthcare facility in mind.

25.1.2 Endotracheal Intubation

In cases where BVM ventilation is inadequate, rescue airways are not available or ineffective, prehospital ETI may be necessary. However, ETI is a low-frequency, high-liability skill, and depending on the emergency medical system (EMS), paramedics may not have sufficient attempts to remain proficient in definitive airway management [9]. Also, recent data would suggest that there may not be a mortality benefit with ETI over other methods of airway management [4], and its role during OHCA has been questioned [10]. Similarly, there are conflicting reports on outcomes in trauma patients having prehospital ETI. A review of prehospital intubations at a trauma system demonstrated no survival benefit and increased prehospital time [11], while improved survival of severely injured patients who had prehospital intubation *without any delay in transport* was reported by another center [12]. Currently, basic and advanced airway management (including tracheal intubation) remain a part of the National EMS Education Standards and the National EMS Scope of Practice Model [13, 14]. However, initial paramedic training continues to suffer from a lack of access to live human patient clinical opportunities for airway management learning [15, 16]. In light of these factors and the conflicting evidence, prehospital ETI should be reserved for situations with clear indications for definitive airway management when appropriate experience and expertise are available and transfer time is not impacted. Figure 25.1 describes an algorithmic approach to airway management in the prehospital setting.

25.2 Trauma Airway Management in the Hospital Setting

The initial step of the primary survey in the evaluation of a trauma patient is airway assessment. Airway assessment should entail ensuring patency of the airway to confirm adequate oxygenation and ventilation, or the presence of a secure airway with

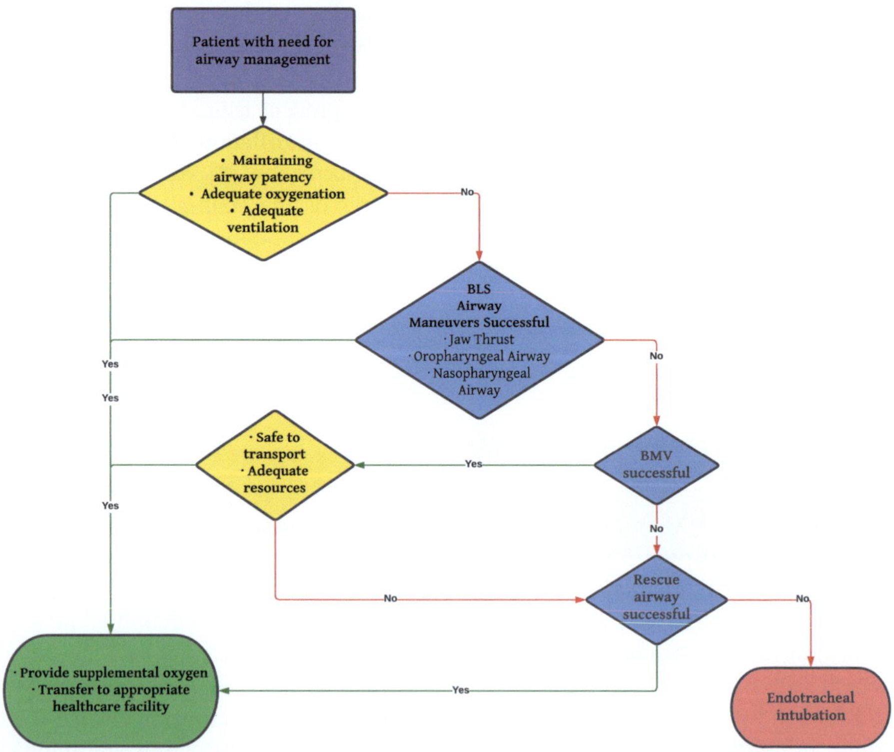

Fig. 25.1 Flowchart depicting prehospital airway management BLS, basic life support; BMV, bag-mask ventilation

a cuffed tube placed in the trachea [17]. While prehospital airway management may have provided temporary patency of the airway, as described earlier, the assessment of airway adequacy by trained trauma airway personnel should occur immediately upon hospital arrival.

25.2.1 Indications for Airway Management

While the airway, breathing, circulation (ABC) have become ubiquitous with trauma resuscitation over the years, the decision to intubate a trauma patient is often more complicated. Many patients with traumatic injuries are often able to maintain their native airway well enough to oxygenate and ventilate adequately. Practice management guidelines by the Eastern Association for the Surgery of Trauma (EAST) guide indications for early tracheal intubation in trauma patients [18]. Since delayed intubation in moderately to severely injured patients is associated with increased morbidity and worse outcomes, intubation should be undertaken without delay in high-risk patients [19]. Trauma assessment can then continue once a secure airway is established. The indications for intubation in the trauma setting, based on the EAST practice management guidelines [18] and the ATLS course manual (tenth edition) [17], are listed in Table 25.1.

Airway obstruction is a common indication for intubation in patients with trauma and can be caused by direct trauma of the head and neck, burns, gastric contents, or aspiration of foreign objects. Visual inspection of the airway and the ability of a patient to phonate can point towards airway patency. Inability to maintain adequate arterial oxygen saturation is another indication for tracheal intubation, and hypoxemia in trauma patients can lead to worse outcomes [20]. Similarly, inability to

Table 25.1 Indications for securing the airway in a trauma patient

ATLS	EAST
Need for ventilation or oxygenation Inadequate respiratory efforts Hypoxia, hypercarbia, cyanosis Combativeness Apnea	Hypoventilation
Acute neuro deterioration (GCS $\leq$ 8)	Persistent hypoxemia
Need for airway protection Severe maxillofacial fractures Laryngeal or tracheal injury Inhalation injury/facial burns TBI (unconscious/combative)	Cognitive impairment (GCS $\leq$ 8)
	Hemorrhagic shock/cardiac arrest
	Airway obstruction
	Major inhalation injury/facial burns

ATLS advanced trauma life support, *EAST* Eastern Association for the Surgery of Trauma, *GCS* Glasgow coma scale

maintain adequate ventilation is an indication for urgent tracheal intubation irrespective of the arterial oxygen saturation. While supplemental oxygen administration can potentially maintain oxygenation, it may mask hypoventilation, thus highlighting the importance of monitoring ventilation and CO_2 clearance in these patients. Acute neurological deterioration is an indication for intubation as it may lead to airway obstruction and/or hypoxemia and hypoventilation. The Glasgow Coma Scale (GCS) score should be obtained as part of the primary survey, with scores of 8 or less being an indication for intubation [18]. The utility of using only the GCS score as an indication for securing the airway has recently been questioned, with some evidence that intubation can be safely deferred in patients with GCS scores between 6 and 8 [21]. However, there remains a risk of hypoxemia as well as hypoventilation-induced hypercarbia in many of these patients. With a concern for severe brain injury and raised intracranial pressure in patients with a low GCS score, episodes of hypoxemia and hypercarbia may not be well tolerated. Hence, patients with low GCS should be closely monitored with a low threshold for tracheal intubation. Other than a depressed GCS score, agitation may also prove to be a discretionary indication, as in many instances, a patient's agitation may be related to alterations in respiratory function and potential head injury. Hemorrhagic shock with hemodynamic instability is another indication for tracheal intubation. These patients tend to have a "physiologically difficult airway" and are at high risk of hemodynamic collapse and cardiac arrest during the peri-intubation period and upon initiation of positive pressure ventilation [22]. Such patients will likely need emergent surgical intervention necessitating an airway and are also more likely to receive large volume resuscitation, which may worsen their respiratory status. Therefore, it may be better to establish the airway early in relatively controlled conditions. However, in certain cases, such as suspected cardiac tamponade, it may be reasonable to proceed to the operating room and perform intubation with the ability to emergently intervene surgically in the event of hemodynamic collapse after intubation. Other indications for early intubation in trauma are related to specific injuries. With airway injuries, a definitive airway is frequently needed and should be established early as ongoing edema, hematoma formation, or tissue disruption can rapidly progress to airway obstruction [23]. Similarly, with acute cervical spine injuries, patients with lesions above C5 might require early intubation. Although patients with lower cervical injuries may initially have adequate ventilation, these patients will eventually require intubation and can have life-threatening ventilatory compromise if intubation is delayed [24].

25.2.2 Airway Assessment

Time permitting, airway assessment should be performed prior to initiating the procedure to identify an anatomically difficult airway and prepare accordingly. Many of the commonly used methods for assessing the airway before elective intubation are not feasible in this setting, where the patient may be uncooperative, agitated,

Table 25.2 MOANS and LEMON difficult airway predictors

MOANS	LEMON[a]
M = Suboptimal **M**ask seal (i.e., bushy beards, lower facial disruption)	L = Look externally (facial trauma, large incisors, beard or moustache, and large tongue)
O = **O**besity or **O**bstruction (i.e., foreign body, pregnancy, angioedema)	E = Evaluate with 3-3-2 rule (incisor distance <3 fingerbreadths, hyoid/mental distance <3 fingerbreadths, thyroid-to-mouth distance <2 fingerbreadths)
A = **A**ge > 55 years	M = Mallampati score (Mallampati score ≥3)
N = **N**o teeth	O = Obstruction (presence of any condition that could cause an obstructed airway)
S = **S**tiff lungs (i.e., ARDS, pulmonary edema)	N = Neck mobility (limited neck mobility)

[a]The score, with a maximum of 10 points, was calculated by assigning 1 point for each of the LEMON criteria

unstable, or delirious [25]. Various scoring systems have been used in the trauma setting to rapidly identify patients likely to have an anatomically difficult airway. MOANS (Table 25.2) may help identify difficult mask ventilation, and LEMON (Table 25.2) can predict difficult laryngoscopy and intubation (Table 25.2) [26]. The HEAVEN criteria (hypoxemia, extremes of size, anatomic challenges, vomit/blood/fluid, exsanguination, neck mobility) incorporate physiological data with anatomical challenges to take into account the physiologically difficult airway and have been proposed as a more relevant airway assessment tool in the emergency setting [27]. Each of the criteria is associated with lower intubation success, and the total number of criteria is inversely proportional to first attempt success, overall intubation success, and first attempt success without desaturation. It does not require the patient to be awake or cooperative and applies to a laryngoscopic view with either direct or videolaryngoscopy [28]. The MACOCHA score (Mallampati score III or IV, sleep Apnea syndrome, decreased cervical mobility, mouth opening <3 cm, Coma defined by a Glasgow score < 8, severe Hypoxemia, and if the practitioner is not an anesthetist), that combines anatomic, physiologic, and operator characteristics may help predict first pass success in critically ill trauma patients [29].

When patients are at the end of their physiologic reserve, as is often the case during trauma intubations, the process of intubation can tip the patient into complete hemodynamic collapse and cardiac arrest. The incidence of hemodynamic collapse associated with ETI in critically ill patients is estimated to be around 40% [30]. There are several explanations for this. First, each commonly used induction drug can lead to hypotension by itself. Second, the apnea caused by the induction of anesthesia pauses any respiratory compensation for metabolic acidosis if present, and ETI also ameliorates the hypoxia/hypercarbia-associated sympathetic drive. Finally, the shift from negative to positive pressure ventilation can reduce venous preload as well as increase afterload on the right ventricle (RV). All these factors can lead to hemodynamic compromise and cardiac arrest in this at-risk population. Therefore, it is prudent to first or, at least, concomitantly address major physiological disturbances prior to and/or during the process of ETI. Point-of-care ultrasound (POCUS) may be helpful in these scenarios to identify underlying physiologic perturbations and optimize patients prior to ETI, as well as tailor the process to avoid patient harm related to the procedure [31]. While the use of fluid bolus prior to ETI in critically ill patients is not beneficial [32], the trauma patient might benefit from resuscitation prior to ETI since massive exsanguination is common in trauma patients. The use of empiric vasopressors/inotropes in this setting is not evidence-based and should be avoided unless deemed medically necessary, and should be directed by POCUS exam. The shock index (heart rate/systolic blood pressure) can also provide some objective risk stratification, with a cut-off of approximately 0.8 or higher for predicting the risk of post-intubation hypotension and a cut-off of approximately 0.9 or higher for predicting the risk of post-intubation cardiac arrest [33].

25.2.3 Airway Management

Airway management in the trauma setting is marred by anatomic, physiologic, and situational challenges. Preoxygenation before induction of anesthesia for the procedure is difficult due to time constraints as well as patient agitation/lack of cooperation. These patients are at risk for rapid desaturation during intubation in the absence of adequate preoxygenation, and hence, all efforts should be made to pre-oxygenate with noninvasive ventilation and/or high-flow nasal oxygen (HFNO), especially in patients with moderate-severe hypoxemia [25] (Grade A). Apneic oxygenation with HFNO or nasal cannula should also be considered in these patients as it can decrease the incidence of desaturation (Grade A). Bag mask and positive end-expiratory pressure ventilation may be used for apneic patients at low risk of aspiration [34]. In a hypoxic agitated patient, wherein preoxygenation is either ineffective or difficult to apply, a delayed sequence intubation with a sedating dose of ketamine to allow for adequate preoxygenation induction can be performed [35]. Management of the anatomically difficult airway has been greatly improved over the past two decades with the multitude of devices available on the market for both ventilation and laryngoscopy. First-pass success is now more widely achieved, which is critical given that repeated attempts at intubation are independently associated with adverse events [36]. However, factors such as operator expertise, time pressure, and the patient's underlying physiologic state still present a challenge, even more so in the critically ill patient, where there is little margin for error. Rapid sequence induction (RSI) is routinely utilized to minimize aspiration risk and is recommended by EAST as the tracheal intubation procedure of choice for trauma patients [18]. RSI helps facilitate rapid unconsciousness and paralysis, leading to immediate airway management while reducing the amount of time and risk of aspiration. However, RSI may not always be appropriate. In the patient with a suspected difficult airway, one should proceed with caution, as a cannot ventilate/cannot intubate situation in these patients may be detrimental.

The EAST recommends succinylcholine as the muscle relaxant of choice for RSI due to its rapid onset; however, many contraindications exist and limit its use. With the ready availability of sugammadex, non-depolarizing muscle relaxants such as rocuronium and vecuronium may also be considered for RSI (Grade C evidence). No specific induction agent has been recommended by trauma guidelines, but recent evidence suggests that the use of propofol as an induction agent for ETI in critically ill patients may be independently associated with hemodynamic collapse and poor outcomes. Hence, propofol should be avoided in the trauma setting [37] (Grade B evidence). Etomidate is perhaps the most commonly used induction agent for emergency intubations in emergency departments in North America [38]. However, the potential of adrenal suppression, even with a single dose, in critically ill patients remains a concern. Ketamine is a close second and has been used in the unstable trauma population due to its preservation of heart rate and blood pressure [39]. Direct head-to-head comparisons between ketamine and etomidate as induction agents for TI have yielded mixed results, and the choice and dose of an induction agent for RSI should be carefully selected and tailored to the individual patient as dictated by hemodynamic conditions and setting.

The selection of the laryngoscopy technique for tracheal intubation in trauma patients is determined mostly by local practices. In trauma centers with anesthesiologists as primary responders for airway management, direct laryngoscopy has been used successfully with a 99% success rate [40]. In places where trauma airways are managed by emergency medicine physicians, video laryngoscopy (VL) is used predominantly with good success rates [41]. Systematic reviews and meta-analyses show no overall difference between the two techniques, and the preference of one over the other is often related to a provider's comfort and experience with the device [25].

25.2.4 Difficult Airway in Trauma

Many factors may make intubation in the trauma setting difficult. These patients could have an anatomically or physiologically, or logistically difficult airway or a combination of two or all three. With traumatic injuries and potential full stomach situations, there may be significant airway soiling with blood and vomitus, making intubation conditions difficult [42]. When active regurgitation is present and significant, the suction-assisted laryngoscopy airway decontamination (SALAD) technique can be employed. It involves decontamination of the oral airway using the Ducanto suction catheter (a large-bore, multiport, "always on," softer- plastic suction device that is anatomically shaped like a patient's airway, making it easy to position and work with other complementary devices used to clear a patient's airway) while simultaneously preserving VL [43] (Fig. 25.2).

Spinal fractures and the risk of spinal cord injury are a major concern in trauma patients, specifically those suffering from blunt trauma. For patients with suspected cervical spine injuries (CSI), the possibility of secondary injury during tracheal

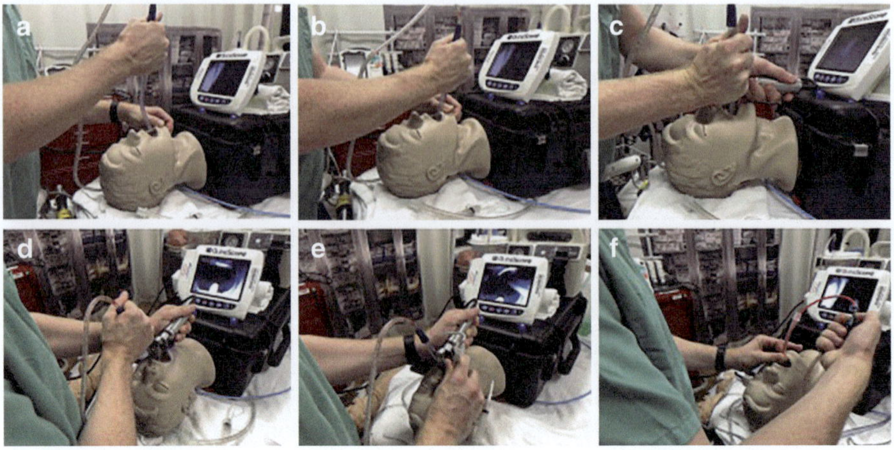

Fig. 25.2 The SALAD technique. (**a**) The rigid suction catheter (RSC) is gripped overhand. (**b**) The RSC displaces the structures of the upper airway. (**c**) The airway is continuously suctioned as the laryngoscope blade is positioned. (**d**) The RSC is withdrawn and repositioned to the left of the laryngoscope blade and seated in the *hypopharynx* in order to provide continuous suction. (**e**) The endotracheal tube is delivered through the *vocal cords*. (**f**) The endotracheal tube is suctioned prior to ventilation. (Reproduced with permission from Root et al. [44])

intubation is real. The management of suspected cervical spine injury includes immobilization with a hard cervical collar, and although the evidence supporting neck immobilization to stabilize the spinal column and prevent further severity of injury is not robust [45], it has become standard-of-care until CSI is ruled out. However, cervical collars alone do not seem to provide satisfactory motion reduction, and therefore, carefully removing the collar and applying manual in-line stabilization (MILS) seems to be the best approach for intubation in patients with suspected CSI. During routine tracheal intubation, the neck is manipulated to align the oropharyngeal, pharyngeal, and laryngeal axes to improve the glottic view. In patients with suspected CSI, this manipulation is not recommended. This can also make glottic visualization more difficult with DL, thus making the argument to use other adjuvants such as tracheal tube introducer/bougie or VL to improve the first pass success.

Early airway control is critical in the patient with traumatic brain injury (TBI). As previously mentioned, a GCS < 8 is a strong indication for tracheal intubation. If intubation is deemed necessary, it is important to determine if the patient is exhibiting clinical signs of increased ICP and if there is any imaging available. A quick bedside POCUS exam to measure the optic nerve sheath diameter can provide some helpful objective data, as a diameter > 5 mm is associated with an ICP >20 mm Hg [46]. In this population, extra care must be taken to reduce the sympathetic response to laryngoscopy. The cerebral autoregulation curve is disrupted in TBI, so even a small increase in blood pressure can result in a significant change in ICP.

Facial and neck trauma leads to specific concerns due to the potential for airway injury or compromise. When maxillofacial injuries are present, providers should recognize that preoxygenation may be difficult since obtaining a good seal with a bag-valve-mask device can be challenging. If high-impact force was involved (>50 times the force of gravity), pan-facial fractures may be present, which can lead to airway compromise [47]. If there are many varied injuries, a submental intubation or tracheostomy may be the safest initial choice for airway management. Retrograde intubation is relatively contraindicated, as the guidewire may not have a clear path cephalad into the oral/nasal cavity. There may also be significant bleeding, which can worsen during the intubation process. Trismus can be present, but this usually resolves with neuromuscular blockade. Of note, swelling at the temporomandibular joints suggests the presence of condylar fractures, which can create a mechanical obstruction limiting mouth opening [48].

Primary airway trauma is uncommon, with a reported incidence of <1%. However, when present, mortality is high, with airway injury being a major cause of early death in trauma [23]. Clinical signs of significant laryngotracheal injury include dysphagia, hoarseness, stridor, upper airway bleeding, subcutaneous emphysema, expanding hematoma, or obvious disruption of the larynx or trachea [48]. Radiographic evaluation with CT is often necessary but not always possible unless the airway is secured. Of note, some patients with blunt trauma to the neck may initially seem stable but develop airway compromise over the next few hours; therefore, frequent exams are prudent. Laryngeal injuries may be worsened by cricoid pressure, rigid laryngoscopy, intubating stylets, blind techniques, and even by the endotracheal tube itself [49]. Specifically, blind placement of an endotracheal tube or bougie distal to the epiglottis can create a false tract that can distort anatomy even further. The safest way to secure an airway is to place an endotracheal tube under direct visualization. If the patient is cooperative, awake fiberoptic intubation or awake tracheostomy is ideal. Spontaneous breathing can be preserved with an inhalational induction, although this process is slow and not safe with all clinical specialties. If RSI is chosen, it is important to avoid cricoid pressure since it can displace fractures of the laryngotracheal complex [50]. Laryngoscopy (video or direct) can be utilized in this scenario to find the glottic opening. However, we recommend passing a fiberoptic scope through the glottis first, prior to "railroading" the endotracheal tube carefully into the intact portion of the trachea. Positive pressure ventilation should be avoided/minimized throughout the intubation. If lower tracheal or bronchus damage is suspected, a double-lumen tube or a deep-positioned single-lumen tube can be used to isolate and ventilate the intact side.

Important Recommendations

- Anticipate and prepare for anatomic, physiologic, and/or logistical challenges with prehospital and trauma airway management.
- Ensure airway patency as well as adequate oxygenation and ventilation during prehospital airway management.
- Endotracheal intubation during the prehospital setting should be reserved for rescue airway failure and should not delay transfer to a healthcare facility.
- Time permitting, trauma airway management should include airway assessment.
- Every attempt should be made to optimize hemodynamics prior to tracheal intubation to avoid peri-intubation hemodynamic collapse.
- A stepwise strategy for airway management with backup plans should be implemented.
- Anticipate a soiled airway in the case of facial/neck trauma and prepare accordingly.

Clinical Situation

Patient is a previously healthy 25 y/o male who presents to the emergency department via emergency medical services after a motor vehicle collision. His Glasgow coma score is 8, and you are called to the bedside for endotracheal intubation. Vitals are notable for tachycardia (heart rate, 110 b/min) and hypotension (noninvasive blood pressure, 90/55 mm Hg). He is otherwise breathing comfortably with oxygen saturation of 97% on 2 L/min nasal cannula. Airway exam reveals a Mallampati score of 1, thyromental distance >3 cm, and interincisor gap >3 fingerbreadths without any signs of neck trauma. The cervical immobilization collar is in place.

"How to Do"
This is a classic example of a physiologically difficult airway

1. Since there is no urgent need to secure the airway, you should try to optimize the patient's hemodynamics.
2. Utilize point-of-care ultrasound (POCUS) to guide your peri-intubation hemodynamic optimization and management. In this case, POCUS determined that the patient was hypovolemic with inspiratory collapse of the inferior vena cava (IVC) and a "kissing ventricle" sign.
3. Administer a fluid bolus prior to tracheal intubation and reassess fluid status via POCUS.

(continued)

4. Carefully titrate induction medications. In this case, etomidate or ketamine, accompanied by succinylcholine or rocuronium for rapid sequence induction, would be appropriate.
5. Carefully remove cervical collar and have a trained operator provide manual in-line stabilization during laryngoscopy.

References

1. McMullan J, Rodriquez D, Hart KW, Lindsell CJ, Vonderschmidt K, Wayne B, et al. Prevalence of prehospital hypoxemia and oxygen use in trauma patients. Mil Med. 2013;178(10):1121–5.
2. Lyng JW, Baldino KT, Braude D, Fritz C, March JA, Peterson TD, et al. Prehospital supraglottic airways: an NAEMSP position statement and resource document. Prehosp Emerg Care. 2022;26(sup1):32–41.
3. Benoit JL, Gerecht RB, Steuerwald MT, McMullan JT. Endotracheal intubation versus supraglottic airway placement in out-of-hospital cardiac arrest: a meta-analysis. Resuscitation. 2015;93:20–6.
4. Carney N, Totten AM, Cheney T, Jungbauer R, Neth MR, Weeks C, et al. Prehospital airway management: a systematic review. Prehosp Emerg Care. 2022;26(5):716–27.
5. Fevang E, Perkins Z, Lockey D, Jeppesen E, Lossius HM. A systematic review and meta-analysis comparing mortality in pre-hospital tracheal intubation to emergency department intubation in trauma patients. Crit Care. 2017;21(1):192.
6. Middleton PM, Simpson PM, Thomas RE, Bendall JC. Higher insertion success with the i-gel supraglottic airway in out-of-hospital cardiac arrest: a randomised controlled trial. Resuscitation. 2014;85(7):893–7.
7. Russi CS, Miller L, Hartley MJ. A comparison of the king-LT to endotracheal intubation and Combitube in a simulated difficult airway. Prehosp Emerg Care. 2008;12(1):35–41.
8. Steuerwald MT, Robinson BR, Hanseman DJ, Makley A, Pritts TA. Prehospital airway technique does not influence incidence of ventilator-associated pneumonia in trauma patients. J Trauma Acute Care Surg. 2016;80(2):283–8.
9. Pepe PE, Roppolo LP, Fowler RL. Prehospital endotracheal intubation: elemental or detrimental? Crit Care. 2015;19(1):121.
10. Wang HE, Benger JR. Endotracheal intubation during out-of-hospital cardiac arrest: new insights from recent clinical trials. J Am Coll Emerg Physicians Open. 2020;1(1):24–9.
11. Stockinger ZT, McSwain NE Jr. Prehospital endotracheal intubation for trauma does not improve survival over bag-valve-mask ventilation. J Trauma. 2004;56(3):531–6.
12. Meizoso JP, Valle EJ, Allen CJ, Ray JJ, Jouria JM, Teisch LF, et al. Decreased mortality after prehospital interventions in severely injured trauma patients. J Trauma Acute Care Surg. 2015;79(2):227–31.
13. Administration NHTS. National emergency medical services education standards: ems.gov; 2021. Available from: https://www.ems.gov/assets/EMS_Education-Standards_2021_FNL.pdf
14. Officials NAoSE. National EMS scope of practice model 2019 (Report No. DOT HS 812-666). Washington, DC: National Highway Traffic Safety Administration; 2019. Available from: https://www.ems.gov/assets/National_EMS_Scope_of_Practice_Model_2019.pdf
15. Johnston BD, Seitz SR, Wang HE. Limited opportunities for paramedic student endotracheal intubation training in the operating room. Acad Emerg Med. 2006;13(10):1051–5.
16. Wang HE, Seitz SR, Hostler D, Yealy DM. Defining the learning curve for paramedic student endotracheal intubation. Prehosp Emerg Care. 2005;9(2):156–62.

17. Galvagno SM Jr, Nahmias JT, Young DA. Advanced Trauma Life Support® update 2019: management and applications for adults and special populations. Anesthesiol Clin. 2019;37(1):13–32.
18. Mayglothling J, Duane TM, Gibbs M, McCunn M, Legome E, Eastman AL, et al. Emergency tracheal intubation immediately following traumatic injury: an Eastern Association for the Surgery of Trauma practice management guideline. J Trauma Acute Care Surg. 2012;73(5 Suppl 4):S333–40.
19. Miraflor E, Chuang K, Miranda MA, Dryden W, Yeung L, Strumwasser A, et al. Timing is everything: delayed intubation is associated with increased mortality in initially stable trauma patients. J Surg Res. 2011;170(2):286–90.
20. Davis DP, Dunford JV, Poste JC, Ochs M, Holbrook T, Fortlage D, et al. The impact of hypoxia and hyperventilation on outcome after paramedic rapid sequence intubation of severely head-injured patients. J Trauma. 2004;57(1):1–8; discussion -10.
21. Hatchimonji JS, Dumas RP, Kaufman EJ, Scantling D, Stoecker JB, Holena DN. Questioning dogma: does a GCS of 8 require intubation? Eur J Trauma Emerg Surg. 2021;47(6):2073–9.
22. Mosier JM, Joshi R, Hypes C, Pacheco G, Valenzuela T, Sakles JC. The physiologically difficult airway. West J Emerg Med. 2015;16(7):1109–17.
23. Kummer C, Netto FS, Rizoli S, Yee D. A review of traumatic airway injuries: potential implications for airway assessment and management. Injury. 2007;38(1):27–33.
24. Hassid VJ, Schinco MA, Tepas JJ, Griffen MM, Murphy TL, Frykberg ER, et al. Definitive establishment of airway control is critical for optimal outcome in lower cervical spinal cord injury. J Trauma. 2008;65(6):1328–32.
25. Karamchandani K, Wheelwright J, Yang AL, Westphal ND, Khanna AK, Myatra SN. Emergency airway management outside the operating room: current evidence and management strategies. Anesth Analg. 2021;133(3):648–62.
26. Hagiwara Y, Watase H, Okamoto H, Goto T, Hasegawa K, Japanese Emergency Medicine Network Investigators. Prospective validation of the modified LEMON criteria to predict difficult intubation in the ED. Am J Emerg Med. 2015;33(10):1492–6.
27. Kuzmack E, Inglis T, Olvera D, Wolfe A, Seng K, Davis D. A novel difficult-airway prediction tool for emergency airway management: validation of the HEAVEN criteria in a large air medical cohort. J Emerg Med. 2018;54(4):395–401.
28. Nausheen F, Niknafs NP, MacLean DJ, Olvera DJ, Wolfe AC Jr, Pennington TW, et al. The HEAVEN criteria predict laryngoscopic view and intubation success for both direct and video laryngoscopy: a cohort analysis. Scand J Trauma Resusc Emerg Med. 2019;27(1):50.
29. De Jong A, Molinari N, Terzi N, Mongardon N, Arnal JM, Guitton C, et al. Early identification of patients at risk for difficult intubation in the intensive care unit: development and validation of the MACOCHA score in a multicenter cohort study. Am J Respir Crit Care Med. 2013;187(8):832–9.
30. Russotto V, Myatra SN, Laffey JG, Tassistro E, Antolini L, Bauer P, et al. Intubation practices and adverse peri-intubation events in critically ill patients from 29 countries. JAMA. 2021;325(12):1164–72.
31. Khorsand S, Chin J, Rice J, Bughrara N, Myatra SN, Karamchandani K. Role of point-of-care ultrasound in emergency airway management outside the operating room. Anesth Analg. 2023;137:124.
32. Russell DW, Casey JD, Gibbs KW, Ghamande S, Dargin JM, Vonderhaar DJ, et al. Effect of fluid bolus Administration on cardiovascular collapse among critically ill patients undergoing tracheal intubation: a randomized clinical trial. JAMA. 2022;328(3):270–9.
33. Althunayyan SM. Shock index as a predictor of post-intubation hypotension and cardiac arrest; a review of the current evidence. Bull Emerg Trauma. 2019;7(1):21–7.
34. Casey JD, Janz DR, Russell DW, Vonderhaar DJ, Joffe AM, Dischert KM, et al. Bag-mask ventilation during tracheal intubation of critically ill adults. N Engl J Med. 2019;380(9):811–21.
35. Weingart SD, Trueger NS, Wong N, Scofi J, Singh N, Rudolph SS. Delayed sequence intubation: a prospective observational study. Ann Emerg Med. 2015;65(4):349–55.

36. Hasegawa K, Shigemitsu K, Hagiwara Y, Chiba T, Watase H, Brown CA 3rd, et al. Association between repeated intubation attempts and adverse events in emergency departments: an analysis of a multicenter prospective observational study. Ann Emerg Med. 2012;60(6):749–54 e2.
37. Russotto V, Tassistro E, Myatra SN, Parotto M, Antolini L, Bauer P, et al. Peri-intubation cardiovascular collapse in patients who are critically ill: insights from the INTUBE study. Am J Respir Crit Care Med. 2022;206(4):449–58.
38. Brown CA 3rd, Bair AE, Pallin DJ, Walls RM, NEAR III Investigators. Techniques, success, and adverse events of emergency department adult intubations. Ann Emerg Med. 2015;65(4):363–70 e1.
39. Baekgaard JS, Eskesen TG, Sillesen M, Rasmussen LS, Steinmetz J. Ketamine as a rapid sequence induction agent in the trauma population: a systematic review. Anesth Analg. 2019;128(3):504–10.
40. Stephens CT, Kahntroff S, Dutton RP. The success of emergency endotracheal intubation in trauma patients: a 10-year experience at a major adult trauma referral center. Anesth Analg. 2009;109(3):866–72.
41. Michailidou M, O'Keeffe T, Mosier JM, Friese RS, Joseph B, Rhee P, et al. A comparison of video laryngoscopy to direct laryngoscopy for the emergency intubation of trauma patients. World J Surg. 2015;39(3):782–8.
42. Sakles JC, Corn GJ, Hollinger P, Arcaris B, Patanwala AE, Mosier JM. The impact of a soiled airway on intubation success in the emergency department when using the GlideScope or the direct laryngoscope. Acad Emerg Med. 2017;24(5):628–36.
43. DuCanto J, Serrano KD, Thompson RJ. Novel airway training tool that simulates vomiting: suction-assisted laryngoscopy assisted decontamination (SALAD) system. West J Emerg Med. 2017;18(1):117–20.
44. Root CW, Mitchell OJL, Brown R, Evers CB, Boyle J, Griffin C, West FM, et al. Suction Assisted Laryngoscopy and Airway Decontamination (SALAD): a technique for improved emergency airway management. Resusc Plus. 2020;1–2:100005.
45. Kwan I, Bunn F, Roberts I. Spinal immobilisation for trauma patients. Cochrane Database Syst Rev. 2001;2001(2):CD002803.
46. Maissan IM, Dirven PJ, Haitsma IK, Hoeks SE, Gommers D, Stolker RJ. Ultrasonographic measured optic nerve sheath diameter as an accurate and quick monitor for changes in intracranial pressure. J Neurosurg. 2015;123(3):743–7.
47. Saini S, Singhal S, Prakash S. Airway management in maxillofacial trauma. J Anaesthesiol Clin Pharmacol. 2021;37(3):319–27.
48. Kovacs G, Sowers N. Airway management in trauma. Emerg Med Clin North Am. 2018;36(1):61–84.
49. Jain U, McCunn M, Smith CE, Pittet JF. Management of the traumatized airway. Anesthesiology. 2016;124(1):199–206.
50. Shilston J, Evans DL, Simons A, Evans DA. Initial management of blunt and penetrating neck trauma. BJA Educ. 2021;21(9):329–35.

Chapter 26
Airway Management in Critical Care

Andy Higgs

Highlights

- Airway management in critically ill patients has higher morbidity and mortality compared to the operating room setting, with ICU patients experiencing more avoidable airway-related complications.
- The MACOCHA score is a validated tool for assessing difficult airways in critical care and predicting intubation difficulty.
- Recent advancements, including videolaryngoscopy, preoxygenation strategies, and structured airway rescue plans, have improved intubation outcomes.
- Rapid Sequence Induction (RSI) techniques are evolving, integrating apnoeic oxygenation and prophylactic mask ventilation to reduce hypoxia-related complications.
- Haemodynamic instability is a major concern, occurring in over 42% of intubations, necessitating pre-intubation cardiovascular optimization.
- The use of cognitive aids, checklists, and team-based approaches enhances patient safety and improves first-pass success rates.
- COVID-19 airway management requires specific protocols to reduce aerosolization risk while ensuring rapid and safe intubation.

A. Higgs (✉)
Intensive Care Medicine & Anaesthesia, Warrington Teaching Hospitals, Cheshire, UK
e-mail: andyhiggs@doctors.org.uk

M. Á. Gómez-Ríos, A. van Zundert (eds.), *Evidence-based Guide to Difficult Airway Management*, https://doi.org/10.1007/978-3-032-30769-9_26

26.1 Introduction

Outcomes of airway management are discernibly poorer in critically ill patients than in the Operating Room, especially in the ICU. The UK's 4th National Audit Project of the RCoA showed that compared to these other settings, the ICU saw the most potentially avoidable airway mortality [1]. More than a decade later, the international INTUBE study conducted in 27 countries described haemodynamic instability in >42% of intubations, severe hypoxaemia in approximately 10%, and cardiac arrest in more than 3%. Nearly 90% of patients needed increased or new cardiovascular support [2].

There are multiple reasons for this. It is important to understand that a majority of airway-related deaths and near-misses occur in patients who have already had their airway secured; most involve tube obstruction or partial/complete displacement [3]. Displacements often occur during intercurrent interventions like patient turns, proning, nasogastric tube insertion or uncontrolled patient movement during waking, weaning, sedation holds or simply agitation incidents whilst airway operators are not immediately present. The duration of intubation may be days or weeks, during which time the airway swells due to prolonged instrumentation or generalized whole-body oedema. ICU patients with V/Q abnormalities are dependent on high concentrations of inspired oxygen and PEEP; they are often haemodynamically unstable. Basic airway monitors such as waveform capnography are inconsistently used: only about 25% of intubations in the INTUBE dataset used this modality [2].

Urgency and the traditional lack of specific airway guidelines focussed on the critically ill may result in poor planning. Patients in the ICU are usually intubated for airway protection or for physiological support. This means abandoning intubation in the face of difficulty is not an option. Overall, these patients have a greater need for more urgent intubation whilst at the same time being far more vulnerable to the complications of difficult or prolonged intubation attempts [1].

Recently, such developments as a proper appreciation of the importance of Human Factors in airway management mortality and morbidity, specific algorithms and training in critical care airway manoeuvres, videolaryngoscopy, and a clearer understanding of when and how to perform airway rescue in patients with severe physiological abnormalities, such as high oxygen requirements and PEEP dependency, have shown discernible improvements in outcomes [4].

26.2 Airway Evaluation

The most well-validated technique to assess the airway in the critically ill is the MACOCHA score. This consists of seven variables: high (3 or 4) Mallampati score (which can be performed in the supine position [5]), obstructive sleep apnoea, reduced range of neck extension, mouth opening <3 cm, coma, severe hypoxaemia ($SpO_2 < 80\%$), and airway operator with less than 2 years anaesthesia training [6]. A score of ≥ 3 predicts complicated airway management. Other major risk factors include age >75 years, hypotension, no preoxygenation, and even simple obesity [7].

26.3 Approach to Intubation: RSI

To enhance team performance and clinical outcomes, an agreed and rehearsed strategy is vital. In response to the clear evidence of high airway risk in critically ill adults identified in the NAP4 audit, the Difficult Airway Society (Fig. 26.1) devised such an approach [4], as have other organizations [8, 9].

Critically ill patients are at risk of pulmonary aspiration, and overall, this caused 50% of deaths reported in NAP4. 'Rapid Sequence Induction—Intubation' was first described by Safar in 1970 and has continually evolved since [10]. Most operators agree that RSI is indicated in ICU and ED patients, but there is little agreement about what RSI is in the third decade of the twenty-first century.

Recently, the PUMA collaboration has attempted to clarify the inchoate nature of RSI and defines it as 'a technique to minimize the risk of pulmonary aspiration by minimizing the time interval between drug-induced loss of intrinsic airway reflexes and restoration of airway protection with a cuffed tube' [11]. PUMA resolves RSI into three domains: essential, recommended, and optional (see Fig. 26.2).

A detailed discussion of this approach is beyond the remit of this chapter, but, specific to critical care, essential per-oxygenation components include preoxygenation, apnoeic oxygenation between laryngoscopy attempts if mask ventilation is not used and rescue mask ventilation if the oxygen saturation falls below an agreed level. Mask ventilation before and between intubation attempts has traditionally been contraindicated in RSI because of the risk of causing aspiration, but the actual incidence is low [12], and Casey et al. demonstrated that mask ventilation incorporating 5–10 cm H_2O PEEP between induction and laryngoscopy significantly reduced peri-intubation oxygen desaturation in critically ill adults. Such prophylactic mask ventilation also gives an early indication of whether rescue oxygenation will be possible if airway management fails. There was no increased incidence of aspiration, although the study was not powered sufficiently to confirm this [13]. Mask ventilation peak inspiratory pressure should be kept below 20 cm H_2O.

The vexed question of cricoid pressure (CP) remains controversial, with a much-quoted, if under-powered, study claiming non-inferiority when avoiding CP in anaesthesia [14]. CP is optional in the PUMA approach, leaving it for local decision-making, but if CP is used it must be applied by a trained practitioner who should confirm, prior to induction, with the airway operator that it will be removed if difficulty in (1) mask ventilation, (2) laryngoscopy, (3) passage of the tracheal tube, (4) insertion of an SGA or (5) active vomiting occurs. CP reduces gastric insufflation when mask ventilation is used. Apply 10 N awake, increasing to 30 N after loss of consciousness [4]. Left para-tracheal pressure may protect against gastric insufflation to a greater degree than CP, with a non-inferior laryngeal view [15]. Gastric ultrasound is sensitive and specific to identify gastric residue, but it takes time and training [16].

An existing nasogastric tube should be aspirated prior to induction. A 20° head-up position is recommended to facilitate preoxygenation, laryngoscopy, and reduce passive regurgitation.

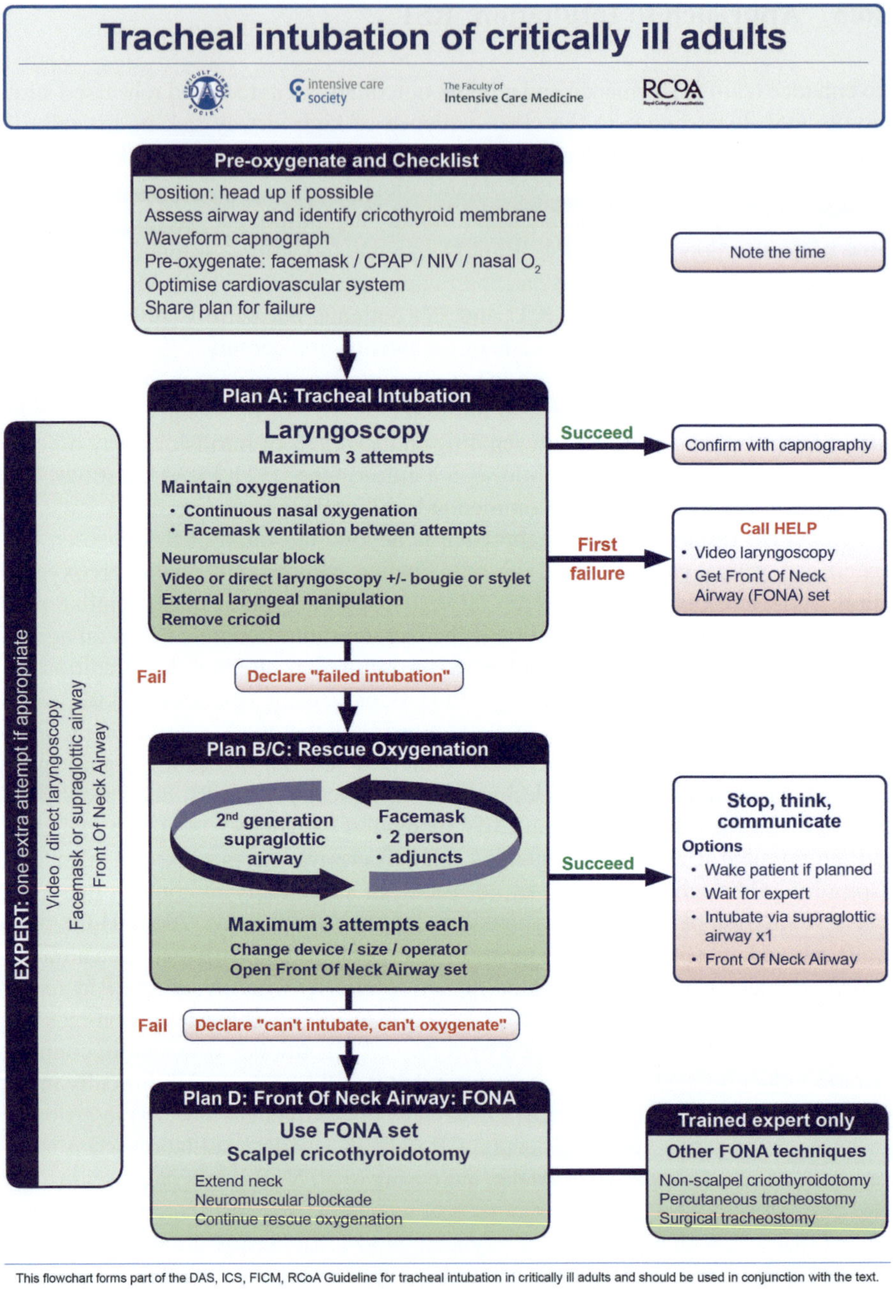

Fig. 26.1 DAS critically ill adult algorithm

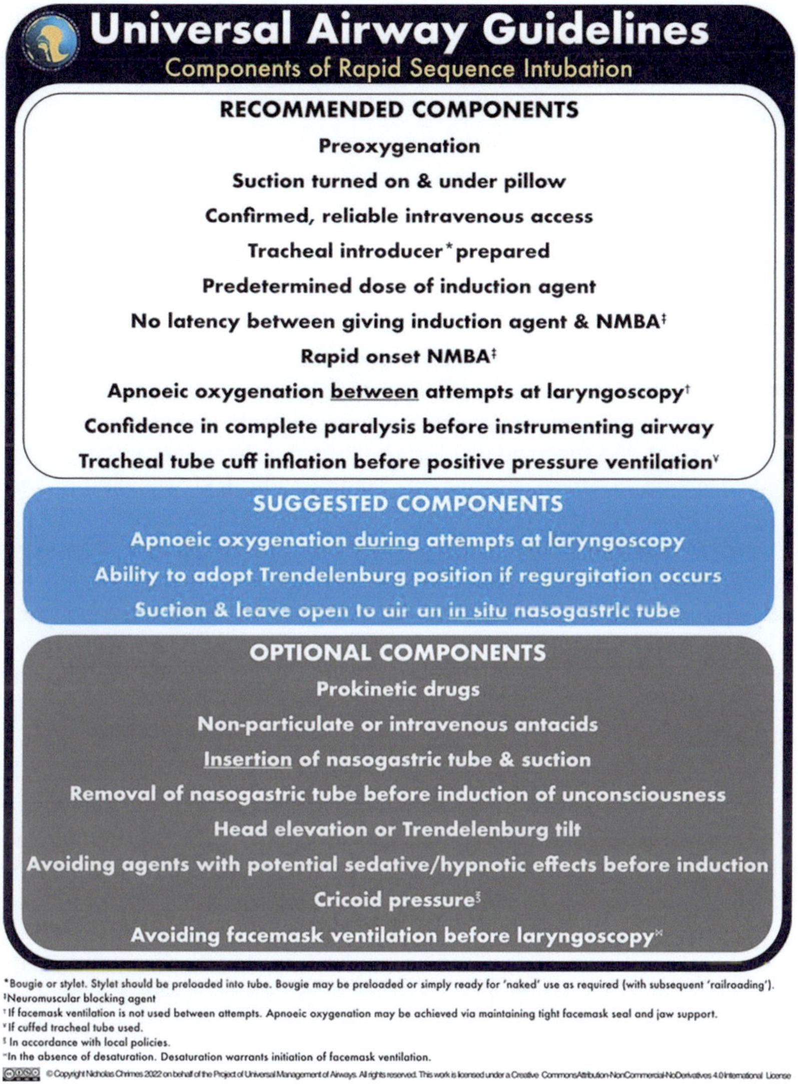

Fig. 26.2 PUMA rapid sequence intubation

26.3.1 RSI Drugs

The induction agent should be selected according to operator experience and cardiovascular profile (see haemodynamic management). The intubation profile of induction drugs is largely irrelevant when NMBAs are used. Use of muscle relaxants is associated with greater success and fewer complications [17]. Traditionally, succinylcholine is the muscle relaxant of choice, but rocuronium (1.2 mg/kg) produces equally good intubating conditions with fewer side effects [18]. Critically ill patients are at especially high risk of hyperkalaemic cardiac arrest with succinylcholine, and it may be best simply to avoid this agent in case it is administered in error. See Plan D for discussion of sugammadex use.

In summary, an RSI consisting of preoxygenation, pre-determined dose of induction agent immediately followed by rapid-onset NMBA, together with apnoeic oxygenation +/or mask ventilation with CPAP and videolaryngoscopy (see below) should be used.

26.3.2 *Performance of Intubation (RSI)*

26.3.2.1 Peroxygenation

Peri-intubation desaturation is the second most common complication of attempted tracheal intubation in ICU patients [2]. Peroxygenation refers to maintaining alveolar oxygenation during efforts to achieve intubation; it includes preoxygenation (before induction) and manoeuvres during intubation including nasal oxygen and intermittent gentle facemask ventilation. Traditionally, RSI was confined to face mask preoxygenation, but now includes using standard facemask, CPAP, NIV, HFNO, prophylactic or rescue facemask ventilation. Possible use of prophylactic veno-venous ECMO is not discussed in this chapter.

The literature examining this topic is regarded as conflicting, but can be rationalized when set in a physiological context of what the issues and therapeutic goals are. Essentially, critically ill patients present a spectrum of patients with varying degrees of V/Q mismatch. At the severe end of this distribution, FRC is severely impaired (usually the indication for intubation), and so it is imperative that as much of the FRC as possible is recruited. This is done with non-invasive ventilation, including PEEP [19, 20], using an anaesthesia-type facemask in the semi-recumbent position (25–30° upright) [21]. This should be performed for 3–4 minutes or until end-tidal oxygen is at least 85%. The pressure-support element of NIV recruits alveoli and the PEEP stabilizes this; it also minimizes the absorption atelectasis consequent on using 100% oxygen. Positioning the patient correctly optimizes this recruitment. Trendelenburg can be used provided haemodynamic stability is maintained [22]. Clearly, known impediments to oxygenation, such as pneumothoraces and pulmonary collapse amenable to physical therapy, should be corrected as is possible prior to induction.

Formal NIV was only used in 11% of the INTUBE intubations, probably because it can be time-consuming and cumbersome to set up, and concerns regarding gastric insufflation or even cardiovascular compromise [2]. A technique widely used in the UK, Australia, and New Zealand is manual pressure-supported breaths (with PEEP) using a Waters circuit. This is advantageous compared to the same technique using a self-inflating bag because the latter doesn't permit detection of a leak at the interface and also adds to the work of breathing in spontaneously breathing patients [4].

However, alveolar de-recruitment occurs immediately after the facemask is removed to pass the tube. During these efforts, apnoeic oxygenation can be used. This relies on the phenomenon whereby less CO_2 is excreted by diffusion into the alveoli than oxygen is extracted, consequent on the differing solubilities and metabolism of these two gases. This generates a negative intra-pulmonary pressure of $-20cmH_2O$, provided the airway is kept open to the atmosphere [23]. Its success is aided by high (60–70 L/min) flow rates, optimal airway opening, and humidification. This technique can be combined with NIV [24] using the Optiflow Switch™ device; the latter ensures that the gas inflow to the nasal canulae stops when a set pressure is detected under the face mask, thereby preventing high intra-thoracic pressures. In only moderately sick patients, HFNO may be of use [25].

The PREVENT trial [26] compared intermittent face mask ventilation to controls during RSIs and confirmed that the safe apnoeic period is extended using this technique; $SpO_2 < 80\%$ was very significantly reduced (10.3 vs 22.8%). While not powered to detect pulmonary aspiration, higher rates of this complication were not seen (3.2%), so confirming the contemporary practice of many operators who routinely apply low-pressure facemask breaths between loss of consciousness and full muscle relaxation [4]. This technique is probably superior to HFNO alone [27].

As alluded to above, there is a linear relationship between SpO_2 at induction and lowest SpO_2 during intubation [28]; the worse the V/Q mismatch, the less effective HFNO is, and so mask recruitment with NIV becomes more important, certainly when the PaO_2/FiO_2 [P/F]is <200. The FLORALI-2 study demonstrated 24% of patients preoxygenated with NIV developed a $SpO_2 < 80\%$. This compares to 35% preoxygenated with HFNO [25].

It should be emphasized that a decisive factor in avoiding peri-intubation desaturation is achieving first pass success with minimal procedural duration.

26.4 Plan A: Laryngoscopy

First pass success (FPS) in ICU is about 80% [2], and First Pass Failure is associated with worse mortality and peri-procedural complications [29]. Until recently, the optimal laryngoscope technique has been a matter of controversy in the literature, but multiple international guidelines now recommend routine use of VL. RCTs are often quite small, exclude Difficult Intubation patients, employ different blades and airway adjuncts, involve disparate groups of operators in different clinical settings, but it may be that RCTs and the consequent meta-analyses are the wrong tools to evaluate low-rate complications; intubation registries could yield more useful data [30, 31].

A 2022 Cochrane Collaboration review demonstrated reduced complications in ICU airway management across most domains, including reduced risk ratios against MacIntosh DL [32] (Table 26.1):

Some studies have suggested higher complication rates and worse outcomes when VL is used, but these have suffered from methodological problems, including adjunct use such as bougies or stylets being used in only 20% of cases, and only 20% were well-practiced operators [33], but Prekker et al. demonstrated improved outcomes using VL [34].

While it is now clear that adjuncts such as bougies or equally successful stylets are crucial to manipulate the tube into the airway [35, 36], and that training with a device is vital. Sufficient training may be needed in excess of 75 intubations using hyper-angulated VLs [37] and at least 15 uses with MAC VLs [38].

Table 26.1 Risk ratios of VL vs DL

Blade	Failed intubation	Hypoxaemia	FPS	View (grade 3/4)	Oesophageal intubation
MAC-VL	**0.41** (0.26–0.65)	**0.72** (0.42–0.99)	**1.05** (1.02–1.09)	**0.38** (0.29–0.48)	**0.51** (0.22–1.21)
HA-VL	**0.51** (0.34–0.76)	0.49 (0.22–1.11)	**1.03** (1.00–1.05)	**0.15** (0.10–0.24)	**0.39** (0.18–0.81)

Bold: Sig. From Hansel et al. [32]

A common criticism of VL use is that operators need to maintain DL skills, but traditional skills can easily be maintained by using MAC VL to achieve a direct view of the larynx and restricting use of the video image to when an indirect view is strictly necessary. Sakles has demonstrated that upper airway secretions and airway soiling do not reduce the utility of VL [39]. VL, especially with a screen visible to the entire team, also improves teamwork.

It is clear that the same airway equipment should be used throughout hospitals, such that wherever operators are called to intubate patients, whether in the ICU, ED, general wards, or the OR, they are able to use the same devices in all locations so that familiarity gain can be realized [4]. Adequate training is needed to avoid the predictable situation in which a good view can be attained, but passing the tube is difficult and time-consuming: in critically ill patients, this leads to desaturation and increased complications. Purchasing decisions should reflect the needs of the most junior operators, who may need to use devices alone in an emergency, rather than the idiosyncratic individual preferences of influential senior members of the department [1].

VL requires the use of adjuncts such as a stylet or bougie to enable passage of the tube using an indirect view. Stylets may cause rare, but severe complications. The STYLETTO study demonstrated stylet utility and occasional laryngeal, mediastinal and oesophageal trauma [40]. Bougies are certainly as successful [41].

It is important that the tube inserted is of sufficient size to accommodate adult bronchoscopes.

The number of times the airway should be instrumented is a matter of considerable debate. Multiple attempts are associated with poorer airway and patient mortality/morbidity outcomes, but cannot be said to cause these as multiple attempts is a surrogate for difficult airway management. However, it is obvious that attempts should be limited as much as possible because airway instrumentation is undeniably injurious, and the law of diminishing returns applies—serial attempts are sequentially less likely to succeed. The commonest approach is to confine initial attempts to three times with material improvements in technique (different device type/size, different operator, ensuring muscle relaxation, etc.) to achieve a best effort. A fourth attempt is permitted by a new operator (an 'expert'), who can reasonably be expected to be more successful than earlier personnel. This 3 + 1 approach is advocated by the Difficult Airway Society [4], Canadian Airway Focus Group [30], and in original studies, which show that the vast majority of patients are successfully intubated within 4 attempts and that limiting clinicians to fewer efforts would, in the critically ill, necessarily require a high rate of neck rescue [42, 43].

26.5 Confirmation of Endotracheal Tube Position

Unrecognized oesophageal intubation is especially hazardous in critically ill patients because their tolerance of no alveolar ventilation is extremely poor and continues to cause avoidable mortality in the ICU. This issue was recently addressed by a guideline endorsed by almost all the main airway special interest societies in the world [31].

Routine VL is advocated, and the operator and assistant are encouraged to verbalize the laryngeal view obtained. When any tube is placed into the airway, its position must be confirmed by eliciting 'sustained exhaled CO_2' using waveform capnography [31]. Again, it is good practice for both the operator and the trained assistant to verbalize whether Sustained Exhaled CO_2 is present. Indeed, alternative techniques to confirm CO_2 are not acceptable if it is feasible to use waveform capnography. Clinical examination cannot be used to exclude OI [44].

Sustained exhaled CO_2 is defined by four criteria:

1. Amplitude rises during exhalation and falls during inspiration.
2. Consistent or increasing amplitude over at least seven breaths.
3. Peak amplitude more than 1 kPa (7.5 mm Hg) above baseline.
4. Reading is clinically appropriate [31].

Failure to meet these criteria does not itself define oesophageal intubation, but means that the likelihood of OI has exceeded an unacceptably high threshold risk and should usually prompt immediate removal of the tube and mask oxygenation. Only if it is clear that removing the tube would be dangerous (clear risk that mask oxygenation will fail, or significant aspiration cannot be avoided), should the tube be left in situ as concurrent measures to immediately exclude OI using VL and one additional method (usually bronchoscopy) is performed. However, if oxygen desaturation occurs in the absence of sustained exhaled CO_2, immediate removal of the tube is mandated in all circumstances [31] (see Fig. 26.3).

If sustained exhaled CO_2 is absent, alongside the above measures, a rapid 'Quick Check' should be performed to exclude technical problems with the tube or circuit and patient confounders such as cardiac arrest/bronchospasm. Note that in the presence of good quality chest compressions, low levels of CO_2 below Sustained Exhaled CO2 criteria should not be assumed to be caused by insufficient cardiac output [1].

Specific to the critically ill, it is sometimes the case that the exhaled CO_2 level remains low even when tracheal position and tube patency has been formally and correctly confirmed, e.g., massive PE. Only in these (rare) cases can the tube be left in situ (as long as VL and bronchoscopic views confirm tracheal placement) as attempts to raise the cardiac output and pulmonary blood flow are instituted [31].

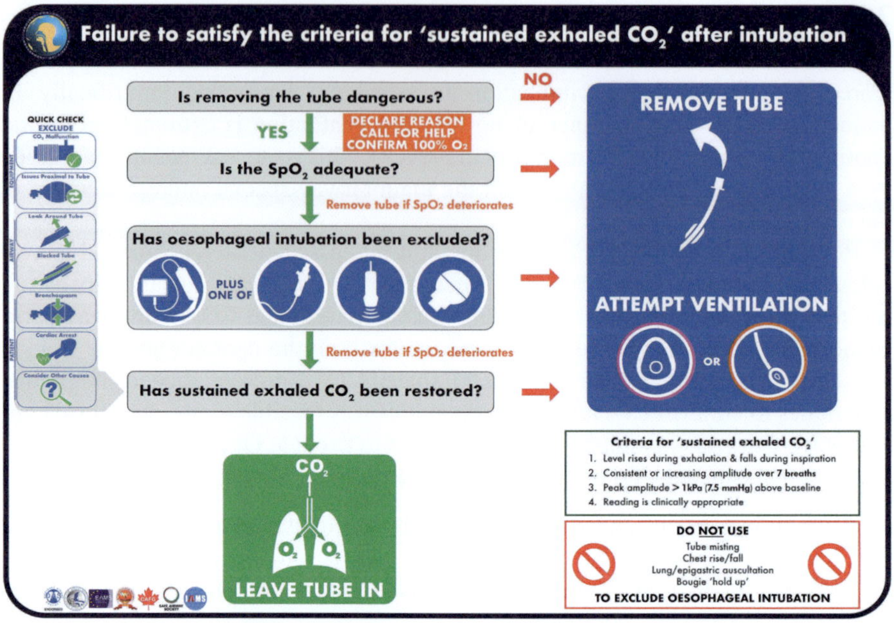

Fig. 26.3 PUMA preventing unrecognized oesophageal intubation

26.6 Failed Laryngoscopy: Plans B and C

Tracheal intubation, rather than other forms of airway management, is supremely important in the ICU, but intubation does fail, and rescue oxygenation using an SGA or face mask must be deployed. Profound hypoxaemia and cardiac arrest are common complications in the critically ill [45]. Traditionally, re-oxygenation with these two types of devices is conceptualized as two distinct phases (SGA oxygenation is Plan B, and a final attempt at FM oxygenation is Plan C in the traditional DAS approach) of management, but in reality, these two approaches merge into an alternating cycle of attempts using an SGA and then using an FM. This realization is best described in the VORTEX approach, in which serial attempts must differ in order to achieve an optimal attempt, or best effort, is achieved within three attempts [46].

The objective is successful alveolar oxygenation, indicated by an adequate waveform capnography trace and stable or improving peripheral oxygen saturation. According to the VORTEX Approach, this is the Green Zone. Failure is said to be entering into the Vortex. These principles were adopted by the DAS critical care guideline in 2018 [4].

Confirmed alveolar oxygen delivery using face mask or SGA after laryngoscopy/intubation has failed affords the team the opportunity to 'Stop, Think and Communicate'. This is essentially an airway 'time out' during which the team can consider the options and/or call rapidly available help. The options are: (1) Wait for an expert operator who can attend promptly, (2) intubate through an SGA (single attempt), (3) allow the patient to emerge from sedation and reverse neuromuscular blockade ('waking the patient'), and (4) proceed to perform an emergency front of neck airway [4] (see Fig. 26.1).

In the critically ill, second-generation SGAs are preferred because they possess better airway seals, which facilitate higher ventilation pressures and improved protection against aspiration of regurgitated material, together with gastric drainage ports [47]. As the tip of SGA devices dwells in the hypopharynx, their use necessitates the release of cricoid pressure [48], if the latter is used. NG tubes need not be removed in order to place an SGA.

Intubation via an SGA can be practiced in manikins and can be done either by loading a small tube over a flexible intubating laryngoscope and passing both through an SGA which has been placed to oxygenate the patient's lungs after failed intubation, or using a specialized airway exchange catheter (AEC) such as an Aintree Intubation Catheter. The latter is a short (57 cm) AEC, which fits snuggly over a flexible intubation scope. This combination is then passed through the rescue SGA. This allows the Aintree Catheter to be placed into the trachea under direct vision—an important safety feature. The flexible scope and SGA are then removed, leaving only the AIC in the trachea, and a >/= 7.0 mm tracheal tube is then railroaded over the AIC into the airway. If the initial FOS/AIC combination is passed through a bronchoscopic catheter mount, ventilation with 100% oxygen via the rescue SGA is possible during the intubation sequence [49]. NAP4 called for the immediate availability of flexible scopes in emergency locations and this has been widely achieved, consequent on the advent of disposable devices.

'Waking' the patient is only considered if the patient was conscious prior to the intubation attempt. As many ICU patients cannot achieve an adequate conscious level and adequate spontaneous respiration after a failed intubation attempt, which may also have traumatized the airway, this option rarely exists in the ICU, except when intubation is performed to enable diagnostic interventions such as ERCP. Whether awakening the patient is potentially possible should be agreed by the team before induction.

Rescue face mask oxygenation represents the final stage before eFONA is performed. In the critically ill, it should be done using full muscle relaxation and CPAP up to 20 cm H_2O [50].

At any point in the intubation strategy, an 'expert operator' might attend who may perform one attempt at any or all of the 3 upper airway techniques (tube, SGA, and FM), proceed to eFONA, or merely supervise other members of the team.

26.7 Plan D: Neck Rescue

When attempts to secure adequate gas exchange using one of the three upper airway approaches (tracheal tube, SGA, facemask) fail, the airway needs to be salvaged by 'Neck Rescue', a term which means the same as eFONA, but is more intuitive for inexperienced assistants and non-English speakers to understand in an emergency [51].

26.7.1 General Remarks

Neck rescue is more difficult in the critically ill because patients are on beds rather than firm operating tables, lighting is sub-optimal, trained assistance is often absent, and it is required out-of-hours and more often performed by junior staff. Life-threatening hypoxaemia supervenes much more rapidly, as does haemodynamic collapse. Aspiration of gastric contents is common [1].

It is important to bear in mind that before any rescue attempt is made, the operator should ensure the frequently overlooked precaution of confirming SGA oxygenation has been tried [52] and that neuromuscular blockade is adequate. Even during efforts to gain sub-glottic access, oxygenation attempts using an SGA or face mask should continue because, early on in most CICO situations, it is often possible to at least partially, if inadequately, supply the lungs with some oxygen. This may delay hypoxaemic cardiac arrest. The operator should also quickly exclude other causes of apparent CICO, such as a blocked device/circuit, or even excessive cricoid pressure (see Fig. 26.4).

26.7.2 Priming for Neck Rescue

A primary cause of death and major morbidity in failed airway management is delay in recognizing and executing neck rescue. This is due to both logistical and psychological reasons: operators lack the situational awareness to perceive their evolving failure and don't ensure necessary equipment is immediately available when they do eventually realize this need. A crucial technique in mitigating these failures is 'priming' for neck rescue [53]. In essence, this refers to building into the airway algorithm easily recognized events which should, when they occur, automatically trigger pre-defined actions which smooth the transition cognitively and logistically to timely sub-glottic access (see Fig. 26.1). These events are described (Table 26.2):

It is important to understand that there is no SpO_2 which mandates neck rescue. If optimal 'best' efforts at all three upper airway approaches (tube, SGA, face mask) have failed, then even if the SpO_2 is 100%, nothing is to be gained by delaying immediate sub-glottic access if lethal hypoxaemia is to be avoided.

Sugammadex is usually non-applicable in ICU or ED CICO events. If the indication for intubation is respiratory failure, then simply reversing neuro-muscular blockade but not the respiratory depressant effects of induction agents is unwise. Often, the upper airway has been traumatized by repeated intubation efforts, meaning that when neuro-muscular tone recovers, any marginal airway patency is lost entirely. Later attempts at neck rescue are hindered by a lack of paralysis [54].

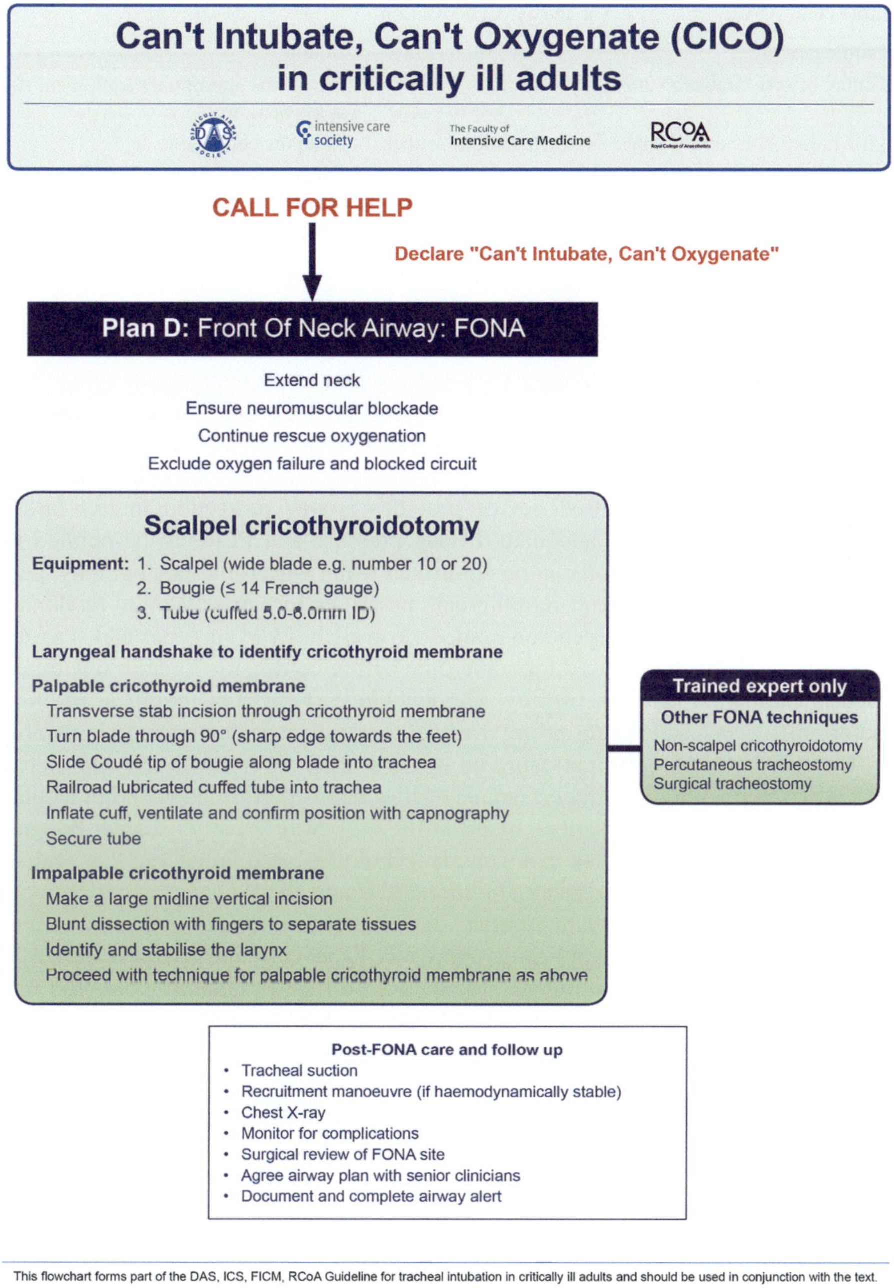

Fig. 26.4 DAS critically ill adult neck rescue algorithm

Table 26.2 Airway strategy event and associated action

Priming event	Action
Failure of first intubation attempt	Ensure the appropriate equipment is at the bedside
First failure of a second upper airway technique (either SGA or face mask oxygenation)	Open the equipment
Failure of best efforts at all three upper airway techniques	Declare 'CICO' loudly and clearly; perform neck rescue

26.7.3 Optimal Technique for Neck Rescue

The best technique is still debated [55], but a settled view may be emerging. The facets of an ideal technique include: rapidly performed, easily learned on manikins, uses simple equipment which is universally available on the ICU, simple method of oxygenation via the device, applicable to non-obese and obese patients with anatomy which is unclear, cuffed device provides airway protection in non-fasted patients and which allows adequate driving pressure and PEEP to be applied in hypoxic individuals, position can be confirmed using waveform capnography, permits exhalation to avoid high intrathoracic pressures in hypovolaemia, facilitates pulmonary toilet, doesn't depend on immediate availability of surgeons and is a reliable airway which can be used for some time before conversion to definitive trans-tracheal intubation or tracheostomy. The technique should not require using fine motor skills, which deteriorate during stressful situations at heart rates >115 bpm [56].

These criteria are only met using an open, scalpel approach to the sub-glottis (cricothyroid membrane). Precise details of how this is performed vary, but a commonly used technique is described by the Difficult Airway Society: 'scalpel-bougie-tube' [4]. NAP4 demonstrated that cannula techniques often failed, but that scalpel techniques were universally successful in the ICU and ED [1].

Whilst several different techniques are described, it is wisest to restrict oneself to one pre-rehearsed, widely applicable approach. Especially one which is useful in obese patents, in whom anatomical structures are difficult to identify, but who disproportionately require such interventions: A midline incision through the skin and subcutaneous tissues, block retraction of the pre-tracheal musculature followed by a single, horizontal stab incision using a 10 or 20 scalpel blade, insertion of a bougie to the level of the clavicles and railroading a 6.0 mm cuffed tracheal tube [4].

More complications accrue from the delayed performance of neck rescue rather than from the procedure itself. Using such a technique is very successful, even in extremely challenging circumstances such as the battlefield (67–85% success) [57] and the London HEMS team describe 100% success rates [58].

Regular, deliberate training is beneficial and reduces reaction times to the performance of neck rescue when it is indicated [59]. Annual practice by intensivists is mandated in some jurisdictions [8].

Unfortunately, emergency sub-glottic access is rarely performed and failure does occur. Evidence suggests that 'scalpel-bougie-tube' should be tried first and that if this initial attempt fails, then a second attempt using this same technique is best [60]. However, Intensivists are well-versed in percutaneous tracheostomy, and it is well-recognized that this can be used as an emergency approach in many patients. The recent INTUBE study described four emergency neck rescue events: one used scalpel cricothyroidotomy, one surgical tracheostomy and two were rescued using percutaneous tracheostomy [2]. Suitable patients include those in whom an initial cricothyroidotomy has failed, those with inaccessible cricothyroid membranes, or patients who have recently had an existing tracheostomy removed [4].

26.7.4 Post-rescue management

After the neck rescue has been performed, check for Sustained Exhaled CO_2 using waveform capnography. Perform a bronchoscopy and CXR to exclude endobronchial intubation and other complications. Once stabilized, conversion to a tracheal tube or, more usually, a tracheostomy is required. Maintain a low index of suspicion for pharyngo-oesophageal trauma [4].

26.8 Post-intubation Recruitment Manoeuvre

As long as cardiovascular stability is maintained, preserving lung volumes using an immediate post-intubation RM (applying 40 cmH_2O for 30 s) has been shown to sustain better PaO2 for up to 30 min post-intubation [61].

26.8.1 Delayed Sequence Induction

Some agitated patients cannot tolerate formal face mask preoxygenation. A common mitigation strategy is to administer small (0.25-0.5 mg/kg) boluses of ketamine as procedural sedation (to a total of 2 mg/kg). This is referred to as Delayed Sequence Induction, DSI [62, 63]. Ketamine best preserves spontaneous respiration, airway tone, and reflexes, together with cardiovascular stability and amnesia-analgesia. When the patient is sedated with preserved spontaneous breathing and airway reflexes, preoxygenation and optimal positioning are performed.

26.8.2 Awake Tracheal Intubation

If anatomical difficulty is anticipated which is thought unamenable to hyper-angulated VL, awake intubation (ATI) is an option provided the patient (1) is cooperative, (2) agrees, (3) does not have raised intracranial pressure or (4) PEEP-dependence, (5) the operator is competent to perform awake intubation in difficult circumstances, and (6) there is time to do it. One reason given for using awake techniques in the critically ill is that a patient may not tolerate the apnoea entailed in traditional RSI, with the traditional injunction to avoid mask ventilation before laryngoscopy; the PREVENT trial nullifies this concern to a significant extent [13]. When ATI is used, it smooths the transition to spontaneous modes of respiratory support and helps maintain haemodynamic stability [64].

26.8.3 Double Set-Up

In patients in whom ATI would usually be considered as intubation under anaesthesia is hazardous, but in whom contraindications to ATI exist, the wisest course is often to use a 'double set-up' technique. In essence, this simply refers to performing an RSI after fully preparing the patient, equipment, and the team for an emergency front-of-neck airway, should airway management fail [65].

26.9 Haemodynamic Management

Cardiovascular instability is the single most common major systemic complication of intubation in the critically ill [2, 45]. The INTUBE study data described haemodynamic instability in 42.6% of patients and cardiac arrest in 3.1%. Defined as SBP ≤65 mmHg at least once and/or ≤ 90 mmHg for ≥30 min despite 500–1000 mL fluid bolus and/or new pharmacological support [43], risk factors include age >75, high SOFA score, hypoxaemia, no preoxygenation, and cardiovascular indication for critical care [7, 66]. Haemodynamic instability is independently associated with ICU mortality, even when corrected for severity of illness [2, 7, 67, 68].

26.9.1 Pre-intubation Assessment and Monitoring

The cardiovascular status of these patients should be assessed fully before induction. Occult hypovolaemia is common in sepsis, peripherally oedematous, and perioperative patients. Increasingly, right ventricular failure is noted to be present [69]. Pre-induction bedside echocardiography is a useful technique which should be available in the modern ICU/ED. Any existing conditions should be ameliorated prior to induction as time, equipment, skills, and pathology allow.

Because of the rapid and dramatic manifestation of CVS instability, it is wisest to secure invasive arterial monitoring prior to intubation if at all possible [4]. Even if urgency means this is not possible, certainly a member of the team should be nominated to pay close attention to the BP and HR and instructed to inform the team leader of pre-defined levels of haemodynamic perturbation, in real time, so that the need for clinical response is realized and actioned promptly. The Team Leader should consider empowering an appropriately trained team member to administer pre-defined boluses of pressor or inotrope, should pre-agreed levels of hypotension occur, even without waiting for explicit instructions to do so. Communication is vital [4].

26.9.2 Vascular Access and Fluid Management

Reliable IV or IO access is crucial. A traditional technique to mitigate cardiovascular collapse is fluid bolus administration. However, in several studies, a 500 mL crystalloid bolus [70, 71] has been shown to have no demonstrable benefit. In the absence of overt hypovolaemia, a likely better approach is close monitoring, prompt diagnosis, and either pre-emptive pressor bolus or infusion pre-induction (inotrope if cardiac failure). An ongoing (FLUVA) trial (ClinicalTrials.gov identifier: NCT05318066) is comparing pre-induction fluid bolus against pre-induction pressor.

Vasopressors are used in published intubation bundles claiming improved outcomes [72], but the ideal agent is still debated. Infusions of the likely most appropriate pressors should be prepared before induction. Clearly, haemorrhagic shock should be treated as far as possible pre-intubation.

26.9.3 Selection of the Induction Agent

The much-vexed question of which induction agent to use has received recent attention. The most common drug used in Europe is propofol. This drug needs more aggressive dosing-reductions in critically sick patients than other agents and is increasingly eschewed in favour of ketamine, etomidate, or midazolam [4].

Post-hoc analysis of the INTUBE dataset [68] demonstrated propofol was independently associated with hypotension and, in turn, with higher mortality. In the past, there has been concern regarding etomidate's potential to inhibit 11 B-hydroxylase, but this is not generally regarded as a current issue [73, 74]. In the past, Ketamine has been avoided in patients with raised ICP, but its ability to maintain MAP obviates this, and it is increasingly used in trauma protocols [75].

In a recent direct head-to-head comparison of etomidate and ketamine, ketamine caused slightly more post-induction hypotension (25% vs 17%), but etomidate was associated with a significantly higher 7-day mortality, if only a non-significantly increased 1-month mortality [76].

26.9.4 Awake Tracheal Intubation: A Selective Alternative

Awake intubation can be used to avoid the cardiac depressant and/or vasodilatory effects of induction doses of sedatives. This takes time, skill, and compliant patients without raised ICP or dependency on NIV.

26.10 Human Factors Including Checklists

A full consideration of Human factors in airway management is beyond the remit of this chapter, but post-hoc analysis of the NAP4 dataset showed that HFs played a part in nearly all of the cases in this national audit. Training for the entire multidisciplinary team (MDT) on whichever pieces of equipment they may be called upon to use during real-world, in-house simulation is key. Staffing should ensure that individuals trained in intubation, together with airway assistants and runners familiar with all relevant policies and equipment, are available.

26.10.1 Use of Checklists

The use of checklists remains subject to discussion. Procedural checklists have been shown to improve compliance when several steps are required to perform complex invasive tasks [77]. This includes airway management. Indeed, Jaber showed that an intubation protocol reduced life-threatening complications from 34% to 21% compared to the earlier controls [72]. Corl used a modified version of this checklist and saw FPS increase 16% and a 13% reduction in all complications [78] but Janz conducted a randomized controlled checklist study in which there were no steps which optimized the patient, in which operators had a high level of prior airway expertise and use of checklists was common across several procedures already, and failed to demonstrate any impact [79], as did a meta-analysis including 3260 patients [80].

However, there is an increasing acceptance that checklist use is appropriate and likely to be useful when they lead to pre-intubation physiological optimization and/or when teams are relatively inexperienced in out-of-theatre airway management [81]. The DAS approach is to use a checklist that aims to optimally prepare the patient, the equipment, and the airway team and to best prepare for difficulty [4]. This is conducted prior to intubation during preoxygenation and is used to confirm not only logistical optimization, but to ensure all team members acknowledge each other and understand the airway strategy, together with everyone's role in it. They are empowered to speak up when they think errors of omission or commission have occurred or, simply, when they have concerns about any aspect of the procedure (see Fig. 26.5).

26.10.2 Role of the 'Time-Keeper'

A potentially powerful feature of checklists is to appoint a 'time-keeper' who measures preoxygenation and how much time has elapsed since the onset of apnoea. This is vital as appreciation of time is lost when operators are distracted by demanding tasks such that they fail to progress through the steps in algorithms in a timely fashion. This can mean that oxygen stored in the FRC is consumed before a reliably patent airway has been achieved.

26.10.3 Use of Cognitive Aids

Cognitive aids are aide-mémoires which are designed to be used in real-time to help unload the operator's cognitive burden. The entire team must be familiar with these prior to their introduction into clinical practice [46].

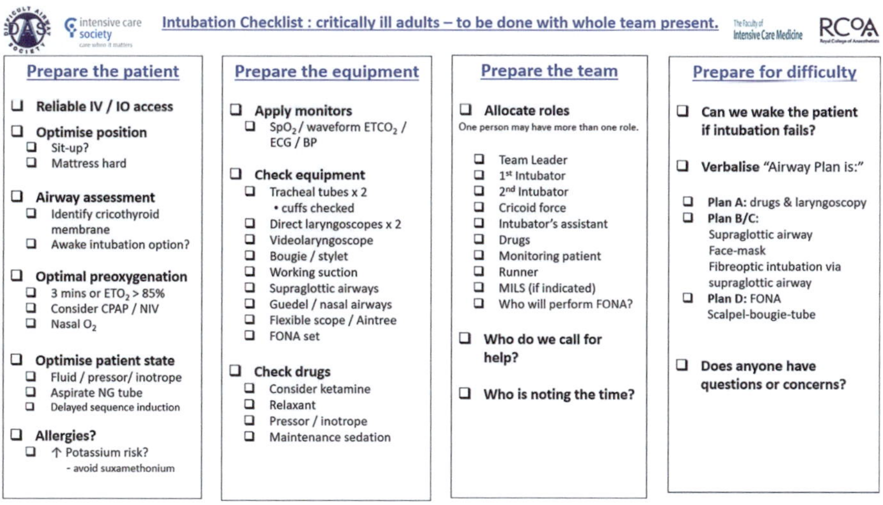

Intubation Checklist : critically ill adults – to be done with whole team present.

Prepare the patient

- ❑ **Reliable IV / IO access**
- ❑ **Optimise position**
  - ❑ Sit-up?
  - ❑ Mattress hard
- ❑ **Airway assessment**
  - ❑ Identify cricothyroid membrane
  - ❑ Awake intubation option?
- ❑ **Optimal preoxygenation**
  - ❑ 3 mins or ETO_2 > 85%
  - ❑ Consider CPAP / NIV
  - ❑ Nasal O_2
- ❑ **Optimise patient state**
  - ❑ Fluid / pressor/ inotrope
  - ❑ Aspirate NG tube
  - ❑ Delayed sequence induction
- ❑ **Allergies?**
  - ❑ ↑ Potassium risk?
    - avoid suxamethonium

Prepare the equipment

- ❑ **Apply monitors**
  - ❑ SpO_2 / waveform $ETCO_2$ / ECG / BP
- ❑ **Check equipment**
  - ❑ Tracheal tubes x 2
    - • cuffs checked
  - ❑ Direct laryngoscopes x 2
  - ❑ Videolaryngoscope
  - ❑ Bougie / stylet
  - ❑ Working suction
  - ❑ Supraglottic airways
  - ❑ Guedel / nasal airways
  - ❑ Flexible scope / Aintree
  - ❑ FONA set
- ❑ **Check drugs**
  - ❑ Consider ketamine
  - ❑ Relaxant
  - ❑ Pressor / inotrope
  - ❑ Maintenance sedation

Prepare the team

- ❑ **Allocate roles**

One person may have more than one role.

  - ❑ Team Leader
  - ❑ 1st Intubator
  - ❑ 2nd Intubator
  - ❑ Cricoid force
  - ❑ Intubator's assistant
  - ❑ Drugs
  - ❑ Monitoring patient
  - ❑ Runner
  - ❑ MILS (if indicated)
  - ❑ Who will perform FONA?
- ❑ **Who do we call for help?**
- ❑ **Who is noting the time?**

Prepare for difficulty

- ❑ **Can we wake the patient if intubation fails?**
- ❑ **Verbalise** "Airway Plan is:"
  - ❑ **Plan A:** drugs & laryngoscopy
  - ❑ **Plan B/C:** Supraglottic airway, Face-mask, Fibreoptic intubation via supraglottic airway
  - ❑ **Plan D:** FONA, Scalpel-bougie-tube
- ❑ **Does anyone have questions or concerns?**

Fig. 26.5 DAS critically ill adult intubation checklist

26.10.4 *Care of the Intubated Patient*

Departmental Leaders must ensure that complications are minimized by considering the following general points. All staff, including members of the MDT, should receive regular in-house simulation training, and when new devices are introduced, the most junior members of the team are trained to use them before applying them in real-life.

It is important that the airway history of each patient in the ICU is recorded and that unit handovers highlight patients with known difficult airways and those with risk factors. Attending consultants should confirm that an appropriate plan for intubation (or extubation) is discussed and understood at each shift change. This should anticipate using only devices and techniques with which the staff are familiar.

Videolaryngoscopes with which the staff are experienced should be immediately available. Bed - head signs should alert staff to patients known or suspected to be problematic. NAP4 led to instructions for the immediate availability of flexible intubation scopes (to intubate or simply inspect problematic airways) in the UK, and this is now a standard of care in the developed world, and, indeed, wherever feasible. Airway devices should be common throughout the hospital (OR, ED, ICU, wards) so that operators maximize their familiarity with key pieces of equipment and are not faced with unfamiliar equipment in emergency situations.

Decisions to intubate (or extubate) potentially difficult patients should be made during daytime hours if possible so that adequately trained members of the MDT are immediately available [4].

26.10.4.1 Post-intubation Phase and Complication Prevention

In critical care practice, the post-intubation phase is associated with the highest risks of complications [1]. Thomas showed that 80% of incidents relate to partial or total displacement of a tracheal tube (including tracheostomies) or complete or partial obstruction [3]. All staff must be able to diagnose and manage these complications. Specifically, these measures should be followed:

- The depth of the tube should be recorded on the chart and checked at every shift change and whenever clinical deterioration occurs.
- Cuff pressure is optimal at 20–25 cm H_2O, or 30 if necessary [82].
- Apparent cuff leak should be assumed to be partial extubation until proven otherwise [83].
- Not using capnography was associated with >70% of ICU airway events in NAP4. Bedside staff must be trained in its basic interpretation [3].
- Respiratory deterioration, especially 'red flags', mandates immediate examination of the tube and breathing circuit, especially following patient movement or procedures (Table 26.3).

Table 26.3 Intubated patient airway red flags

1. Absence or change in capnograph waveform with ventilation
2. Absence or change of chest wall movement with ventilation
3. Increasing airway pressure
4. Reducing tidal volume
5. Inability to pass a suction catheter through the endotracheal tube
6. Obvious air leak
7. Vocalization with a cuffed tube in place and inflated
8. Apparent deflation or need for regular re-inflation of the pilot balloon
9. Discrepancy between actual and recorded tube insertion depth
10. Surgical emphysema

Adapted from McGrath BA. National Tracheostomy Safety Project [4, 84]

26.11 COVID-19 Patients

COVID-19 is a novel B-coronavirus (SARS-CoV-2) which emerged in Wuhan, China in late 2019. It can cause a severe acute viral pneumonitis, fibrosis, cardiomyopathy, and pericarditis complicated by multiple organ failure [85]. It is spread by infected respiratory aerosols <5 microns in diameter (which spread over 6–7 m and remain in the air for prolonged periods) and larger droplets over short (1–2 m) distances, particularly in poorly ventilated spaces. It is especially liable to be infectious in the period 2 days before symptoms begin to 9 days after their onset. Patients classically present to critical care after the first week [86].

This caused particular concern amongst airway managers when it was first described because it is highly contagious and the related SARS epidemic in 2003–4 claimed the lives of a disproportionately high number of Health Care Workers, especially those involved in airway procedures [87]. However, it is now clear that vaccination, using enhanced aerosol Personal Protective Equipment including (0.3 μm particle Filtering Face Piece/FFP3-N95) fit-tested mask, eye protection, full fluid-repellent gown, elbow-length gloves, and appropriate clinical care has resulted in anaesthesia and critical care staff suffering a lower incidence of COVID-19 than other patient-facing HCWs, the three to four times higher risk of COVID-19 seen in patient-facing HCWs notwithstanding [88].

Alarming levels of concern for personal safety were a consequence of poor understanding by the scientific community regarding its mode of transmission, namely aerosols. These are generated by increased flow rates in the lower airways and the consequent increased shear stress at the air-mucous membrane interface. It was initially believed that almost all airway interventions were aerosol-generating procedures (AGPs), but it is now clear that the most prolific AGPs are coughing and sneezing, together with shouting and dyspnoeic breathing. Tracheal intubation,

SGA insertion and removal (without coughing), face mask ventilation, extubation without coughing, HFNO, and NIV are no more aerosol-generating than regular respiration [89]. Overall, dyspnoeic, coughing COVID-19-positive patients should be regarded as contagious, and an appropriate intubation technique is required to avoid exposure to an infection-level viral load.

However, airway management in COVID-19 patients remains more challenging due to:

- Inability to assess the airway because of NIV helmets/masks.
- Fewer staff.
- Limited equipment availability and PPE.
- Fear of infection complicates otherwise straightforward interventions.

26.11.1 Intubation Strategy in COVID-19 Patients

An approach using techniques with which the team is well-versed is crucial. Indeed, novel approaches are likely to lead to more human errors and should be avoided. Novel equipment like 'intubation boxes' adds complexity, impedes difficult airway manipulation, and may increase local viral load and should be avoided [90]. An appropriate technique includes a 'modified' RSI performed after a pre-procedural team briefing using a dedicated COVID-19 checklist. This is of particular importance since communication is extremely difficult when understandably anxious staff wear enhanced PPE.

Intubation should only be performed when absolutely necessary and should be performed by experienced staff in a well-ventilated (>12 air changes/hour) room. A COVID-specific algorithm should be followed [86, 91].

Meticulous preoxygenation with the use of PEEP is followed by videolaryngoscopy. The latter can increase the distance between the operator's face and the patient's airway; it also increases FPS, which is advantageous as these patients desaturate abruptly during apnoea. Post-induction bag-valve-mask ventilation maintains PEEP, extending the safe apnoeic period [26]. A two-handed vice-grip 'VE technique' is indicated. The cuff should be inflated about 5 cm H_2O above peak airway pressure.

If intubation fails, a second-generation SGA, which permits higher seal pressures, is best, but even these higher airway pressures may be insufficient to maintain a safe oxygen saturation. Rapid recourse to an open EFONA using a cuffed tracheal tube is required. Cannula oxygen insufflation techniques cannot be expected to maintain safe oxygen levels and will generate aerosols [86].

The viral filter should be inserted as close to the patient as possible and circuit disconnections should be minimized using a push-and-twist technique and the tube clamped during planned or inadvertent disconnections. In-line suction is mandated. All equipment should be promptly and carefully disposed of to avoid contamination [86, 91].

Recommendations

1. Use the MACOCHA Score to assess whether severe complications are likely to arise during intubation in critically ill adults [LoE: B].
2. Use a pre-intubation checklist which facilitates physiological optimization and sharing of the mental model regarding the procedure within the airway team [LoE: D].
3. Use a rapid sequence intubation technique [LoE: D].
4. Maintain SpO_2 during intubation attempts using thorough preoxygenation with NIV or HFNO, together with intermittent facemask ventilation between attempts [LoE: B].
5. Optimize the cardiovascular system as far as possible prior to attempting intubation, but be ready to deploy vasopressor support early [LoE: D].
6. Use videolaryngoscopy as a routine [LoE: B].
7. Exclude unrecognized oesophageal intubation by confirming Sustained Exhaled CO_2 using waveform capnography [LoE: D].
8. When intubation attempts are failing, remember priming techniques to prepare for neck rescue, and should the latter become necessary, use an open (surgical) cricothyroidotomy technique [LoE: D].

References

1. Cook TM, Woodall N, Harper J, Benger J, Fourth National Audit Project. Major complications of airway management in the UK: results of the Fourth National Audit Project of the Royal College of Anaesthetists and the Difficult Airway Society. Part 2: intensive care and emergency departments. Br J Anaesth. 2011;106:632–42.
2. Russotto V, Myatra SN, Laffey JG, et al. Intubation practices and adverse peri-intubation events in critically ill patients from 29 countries. JAMA. 2021;325:1164–72.
3. Thomas AN, McGrath BA. Patient safety incidents associated with airway devices in critical care: a review of reports to the UK national patient safety agency. Anaesthesia. 2009;64:358–65.
4. Higgs A, McGrath BA, Goddard C, et al. Guidelines for the management of tracheal intubation in critically ill adults. Br J Anaesth. 2018;120:323–52.
5. Bindra A, Prabhakar H, Singh GP, et al. Is the modified Mallampati test performed in supine position a reliable predictor of difficult tracheal intubation? J Anesth. 2010;24:482–5. https://doi.org/10.1007/s00540-010-0905-6.
6. De Jong A, Molinari N, Terzi N, et al. Early identification of patients at risk for difficult intubation in the intensive care unit: development and validation of the MACOCHA score in a multi-center cohort study. Am J Respir Crit Care Med. 2013;187:832–9.
7. De Jong A, Rolle A, Molinari N, et al. Cardiac arrest and mortality related to intubation procedure in critically ill adult patients: a multicenter cohort study. Crit Care Med. 2018;46:532–9.
8. Quintard H, l'Her E, Pottecher J, Adnet F, Constantin JM, De Jong A, Diemunsch P, Fesseau R, Freynet A, Girault C, Guitton C, Hamonic Y, Maury E, Mekontso-Dessap A, Michel F, Nolent P, Perbet S, Prat G, Roquilly A, Tazarourte K, Terzi N, Thille AW, Alves M, Gayat E, Donetti L. Intubation and extubation of the ICU patient. Anaesth Crit Care Pain Med. 2017;36:327–41.
9. Myatra SN, Ahmed SM, Kundra P, Garg R, Ramkumar V, Patwa A, Shah A, Raveendra US, Shetty SR, Doctor JR, Pawar DK, Ramesh S, Das S, Divatia JV. Republication: all India diffi-

cult airway association 2016 guidelines for tracheal intubation in the intensive care unit. Indian J Crit Care Med. 2017;21:146–53.
10. Stept WJ, Safar P. Rapid induction/intubation for prevention of gastric-content aspiration. Anesth Analg. 1970;49:633–6.
11. Project for the Universal Management of Airways Group. Universal Principles for Rapid Sequence Intubation. 2019. Available from https://www.universalairway.org. Accessed 3 Jan 2023.
12. Driver BE, Klein LR, Schick AL, Prekker ME, Reardon RF, Miner JR. The occurrence of aspiration pneumonia after emergency endotracheal intubation. Am J Emerg Med. 2018;36:193–6.
13. Casey JD, et al. Bag-mask ventilation during tracheal intubation of critically ill adults. NEJM. 2019;380(9):811–21.
14. Birenbaum A, Hajage D, Roche S. Effect of cricoid pressure compared with a sham procedure in the rapid sequence induction of anesthesia. The IRIS randomized clinical trial. JAMA Surg. 2019;154(1):9–17. https://doi.org/10.1001/jamasurg.2018.3577.
15. Dongwook W, Hyerim K, Chang J, et al. Effect of paratracheal pressure on the glottic view during direct laryngoscopy: a randomized double-blind, noninferiority trial. Anesth Analg. 2021;133:491–9.
16. Kruisselbrink R, Gharapetian A, Chaparro LE, et al. Diagnostic accuracy of point-of-care gastric ultrasound. Anesth Analg. 2019;128:89–95.
17. Heuer JF, Barwing TA, Barwing J, et al. Incidence of difficult intubation in intensive care patients: analysis of contributing factors. Anaesth Intensive Care. 2012;40:120–7.
18. Welch JL, Seupaul RA. Update: does rocuronium create better intubating conditions than succinylcholine for rapid sequence intubation. Ann Emerg Med. 2017;69:e55–6.
19. Baillard C, Fosse JP, Sebbane M, et al. Non-invasive ventilation improves preoxygenation before intubation of hypoxic patients. Am J Respir Crit Care Med. 2006;174:171–7.
20. Baillard C, Prat G, Jung B, et al. Effect of preoxygenation using non-invasive ventilation before intubation on subsequent organ failures in hypoxaemic patients: a randomised clinical trial. Br J Anaesth. 2018;120:361–7.
21. Dixon BJ, Dixon JB, Carden JR, Burn AJ, Schachter LM, Playfair JM, Laurie CP, O'Brien PE. Preoxygenation is more effective in the 25 degrees head-up position than in the supine position in severely obese patients: a randomized controlled study. Anesthesiology. 2005;102:1110–5.
22. Mosier JM, Hypes CD, Sakles JC. Understanding preoxygenation and apnoeic oxygenation during intubation in the critically ill. Intensive Care Med. 2017;43:226–8.
23. De Jong A, Rolle A, Ducros L, Aarab Y, Monet C, Jaber S. Clinical applications of high-flow nasal cannula in the operating room high flow nasal cannula. Cham: Springer; 2021. p. 101–8.
24. Jaber S, Monnin M, Girard M, et al. Apnoeic oxygenation via high-flow nasal cannula oxygen combined with non-invasive ventilation preoxygenation for intubation in hypoxaemic patients in the intensive care unit: the single-centre, blinded, randomised controlled OPTINIV trial. Intensive Care Med. 2016;42:1877–87.
25. Frat JP, Ricard JD, Quenot JP, et al. Non-invasive ventilation versus high-flow nasal cannula oxygen therapy with apnoeic oxygenation for preoxygenation before intubation of patients with acute hypoxaemic respiratory failure: a randomised, multicentre, open-label trial. Lancet Respir Med. 2019;7:303–12.
26. Casey JD, Janz DR, Russell DW, et al. Bag-mask ventilation during tracheal intubation of critically ill adults. N Engl J Med. 2019;380:811–21.
27. Vaughan EM, Seitz KP, Janz DR, et al. Bag-mask ventilation versus apnoeic oxygenation during tracheal intubation in critically ill adults: a secondary analysis of 2 randomized trials. J Intensive Care Med. 2022;37:899–907.
28. McKown AC, Casey JD, Russell DW, et al. Risk factors for and prediction of hypoxemia during tracheal intubation of critically ill adults. Ann Am Thorac Soc. 2018;15:1320–7.
29. De Jong A, Rolle A, Pensier J, Capdevila M, Jaber S. First-attempt success is associated with fewer complications related to intubation in the intensive care unit. Intensive Care Med. 2020;46:1278–80.

30. Law JA, Duggan LV, Asselin M. Canadian Airway Focus Group updated consensus-based recommendations for management of the difficult airway: part 2. Planning and implementing safe management of the patient with an anticipated difficult airway. Can J Anesth. 2021;68:1405–36. https://doi.org/10.1007/s12630-021-02008-z.
31. Chrimes N, Higgs A, Hagberg CA, et al. Prevention of unrecognised oesophageal intubation: consensus guideline—from the project for universal management of airways and international airway societies. Anaesthesia. 2022;77(12):1395–415.
32. Hansel J, Rogers AM, Lewis SR, et al. pub3Videolaryngoscopy versus direct laryngoscopy for adults undergoing tracheal intubation. Cochrane database systemic Review. 2022;4(4):CD011136. https://doi.org/10.1002/14651858.CD011136.
33. Lascarrou JB, Boisrame-Helms J, Bailly A, et al. Video laryngoscopy vs direct laryngoscopy on successful first-pass orotracheal intubation among ICU patients: a randomized clinical trial. JAMA. 317:483–93.
34. Prekker ME, Driver BE, Trent SA, et al. Video versus direct laryngoscopy for tracheal intubation of critically ill adults. N Engl J Med. 2023;389:418.
35. Jaber S, Rolle A, Godet T, et al. Effect of the use of an endotracheal tube and stylet versus an endotracheal tube alone on first attempt intubation success: a multicentre, randomised clinical trial in 999 patients. Intensive Care Med. 2021;47:653–64.
36. Driver BE, Semler MW, Self WH, et al. Effect of use of a Bougie vs endotracheal tube with stylet on successful intubation on the first attempt among critically ill patients undergoing tracheal intubation: a randomized clinical trial. JAMA. 2021;326:2488–97.
37. Aziz MF, Abrons RO, Cattano D. First-attempt intubation success of video laryngoscopy in patients with anticipated difficult direct laryngoscopy: a multicenter randomized controlled trial comparing the C-MAC D-blade versus the glidescope in a mixed provider and diverse patient population. Anesth Analg. 2016;122:740–50.
38. Amalric M, Larcher R, Brunot V. Impact of videolaryngoscopy expertise on first-attempt intubation success in critically ill patients. Crit Care Med. 2020;48:889–96.
39. Sakles JC, Corn GJ, Hollinger P, et al. The impact of a soiled airway on intubation success in the emergency department when using the Glidescope or the direct laryngoscope. Acad Emerg Med. 2017;24(5):628–36.
40. Jaber S, Rollé A, Godet T, et al. Effect of the use of an endotracheal tube and stylet versus an endotracheal tube alone on first-attempt intubation success: a multicentre, randomised clinical trial in 999 patients. Intensive Care Med. 2021;47:653–64.
41. Driver BE, Semler MW, Self WH, et al. Effect of use of a bougie vs endotracheal tube with stylet on successful intubation on the first attempt among critically ill patients undergoing tracheal intubation: a randomized clinical trial. JAMA. 2021;326:2488–97.
42. Sakles JC, Douglas MJK, Hypes CD, et al. Management of patients with predicted difficult airways in an academic emergency department. J Emerg Med. 2017;53(2):163–71. https://doi.org/10.1016/j.jemermed.2017.04.003. Epub 2017 Jun 9.
43. Jaber S, Amraoui J, Lefrant JY, et al. Clinical practice and risk factors for immediate complications of endotracheal intubation in the intensive care unit: a prospective, multi-centre study. Critical Care Med. 2006;34:2355–61.
44. Hansel J, Law JA, Chrimes N, Higgs A, Cook TM. Clinical tests for confirming tracheal intubation or excluding oesophageal intubation: a diagnostic test accuracy systematic review and meta-analysis. Anaesthesia. 2023. https://doi.org/10.1111/anae.16059.
45. Mort TC. The incidence and risk factors for cardiac arrest during emergency tracheal intubation: a justification for incorporating the ASA guidelines in the remote location. J Clin Anesth. 2004;16:508–16.
46. http://vortexapproach.org/: Supplementary Fig. 1. Accessed 21 Jan 2023.
47. Cook TM, Kelly FE. Time to abandon the 'vintage' laryngeal mask airway and adopt second-generation supraglottic airway devices as first choice. Br J Anaesth. 2015;115:497–9.
48. Cook TM. The cricoid debated balancing risks and benefits. Anaesthesia. 2016;71:721–2.

49. Berkow LC, Schwartz JM, Kan K, Corridore M, Heitmiller ES. Use of the laryngeal mask airway-Aintree intubating catheter-fiberoptic bronchoscope technique for difficult intubation. J Clin Anesth. 2011;23:534–9.
50. Ramachandran SK, Kheterpal S. Difficult mask ventilation: does it matter? Anaesthesia. 2011;66:40–4.
51. Chrimes N, Higgs A, Law JA, et al. Project for universal management of airways—part 1: concept and methods. Anaesthesia. 2020;75:1671–82. https://doi.org/10.1111/anae.15269.
52. Rosenstock CV, Nørskov AK, Wetterslev J, Lundstrøm LH. Emergency surgical airway management in Denmark: a cohort study of 452 461 patients registered in the Danish Anaesthesia Database. Br J Anaesth. 2016;117(S1):i75–82.
53. Chrimes N. The vortex: a universal 'high-acuity implementation tool' for emergency airway management. Br J Anaesth. 2016;117:i20–7.
54. Curtis RP. Persistent 'can't intubate, can't oxygenate' crisis despite reversal of rocuronium with sugammadex: the importance of timing. Anaesth Intensive Care. 2012;40:722.
55. Baker PA, O'Sullivan EP, Kristensen MS, Lockey D. The great airway debate: is the scalpel mightier than the cannula? Br J Anaesth. 2016;117(S1):i17–9. https://doi.org/10.1093/bja/aew219.
56. Siddle BK. Sharpening the warrior's edge: the psychology and science of training. Millstadt: PPCT Management Systems Inc.; 1995.
57. Mabry RL. An analysis of battlefield cricothyrotomy in Iraq and Afghanistan. J Spec Oper Med. 2012;12:17–23.
58. Lockey D, Crewdson K, Weaver A, Davies G. Observational study of the success rates of intubation and failed intubation airway rescue techniques in 7256 attempted intubations of trauma patients by pre-hospital physicians. Br J Anaesth. 2014;113:220–5.
59. Wong DT, Prabhu AJ, Coloma M, et al. What is the minimum training required for successful cricothyroidotomy? A study in mannequins. Anesthesiology. 2003;98:349–53.
60. Duggan LV, Lockhart SL, Cook TM, O'Sullivan EP, Dare T, Baker PA. The Airway App: exploring the role of smartphone technology to capture emergency front-of-neck airway experiences internationally. Anaesthesia. 2018;73(6):703–10.
61. Constantin JM, Godet T, Jabaudon M, Bazin JE, Futier E. Recruitment maneuvers in acute respiratory distress syndrome. Ann Transl Med. 2017;5:290.
62. Weingart SD, Trueger NS, Wong N, et al. Delayed sequence intubation: a prospective observational study. Ann Emerg Med. 2015;65:349–55.
63. Bandyopadhyay A, Kumar P, Jafra A, et al. Peri-intubation hypoxia after delayed versus rapid sequence intubation in critically injured patients on arrival to trauma triage: a randomized controlled trial. Anesth Analg. 2023;136(5):913–9. https://doi.org/10.1213/ANE.0000000000006171.
64. Mosier JM, Sakles JC, Law JA, et al. Tracheal intubation in the critically ill. Where we came from and where we should go. Am J Respir Crit Care Med. 2020;201:775–88. https://doi.org/10.1164/rccm.201908-1636CI.
65. Law JA, Duggan LV, Asselin M, Baker P. Canadian Airway Focus Group updated consensus-based recommendations for management of the difficult airway: part 1. Difficult airway management encountered in an unconscious patient. Can J Anesth/J Can Anesth. 2021;68:1373–404.
66. Perbet S, De Jong A, Delmas J, et al. Incidence of and risk factors for severe cardiovascular collapse after endotracheal intubation in the ICU: a multi center observational study. Crit Care. 2015;19:257.
67. Heffner AC, Swords DS, Nussbaum ML, Kline JA, Jones AE. Predictors of the complication of postintubation hypotension during emergency airway management. J Crit Care. 2012;27:587–93.
68. Russotto V, Tassistro E, Myatra SN, et al. Peri-intubation cardiovascular collapse in patients who are critically ill: insights from the INTUBE study. Am J Respir Crit Care Med. 2022;206:449–58.

69. Al-Saadi MA, Heidari B, Donahue KR, Shipman EM, Kinariwala KN, Masud FN. Pre-existing right ventricular dysfunction as an independent risk factor for post intubation cardiac arrest and hemodynamic instability in critically ill patients: a retrospective observational study. J Intensive Care Med. 2023;38:169–78.
70. Janz DR, Casey JD, Semler MW, et al. Effect of a fluid bolus on cardiovascular collapse among critically ill adults undergoing tracheal intubation (PrePARE): a randomised controlled trial. Lancet Respir Med. 2019;7:1039–47.
71. Russell DW, Casey JD, Gibbs KW, et al. Effect of fluid bolus administration on cardiovascular collapse among critically ill patients undergoing tracheal intubation: a randomized clinical trial PREPARE-II. JAMA. 2022;328:270–9.
72. Jaber S, Jung B, Corne P, et al. An intervention to decrease complications related to endotracheal intubation in the intensive care unit: a prospective, multiple-center study. Intensive Care Med. 2010;36:248–55.
73. Katz J, Greenberg S. Etomidate is NOT a first-line induction agent in critically ill patients: primum non nocere-above all, do no harm. Crit Care Med. 2018;46:1495–6. https://doi.org/10.1097/CCM.0000000000003291.
74. Lynde GC, Jabaley CS. Etomidate is a first-line induction agent in critically ill patients. Crit Care Med. 2018;46:1492–4. https://doi.org/10.1097/CCM.0000000000003290.
75. Ballow SL, Kaups KL, Anderson S, et al. A standardized rapid sequence intubation protocol facilitates airway management in critically injured patients. J Trauma Acute Care Surg. 2012;73:1401–5. https://doi.org/10.1097/TA.0b013e318270dcf5.
76. Matchett G, Gasanova I, Riccio CA, et al. Etomidate versus ketamine for emergency endotracheal intubation: a randomized clinical trial. Intensive Care Med. 2022;48:78–91.
77. Arriaga AF, Bader AM, Wong JM, et al. Simulation-based trial of surgical-crisis checklists. N Engl J Med. 2013;368:246–53.
78. Corl KA, Dado C, Agarwal A, et al. A modified Montpellier protocol for intubating intensive care unit patients is associated with an increase in first-pass intubation success and fewer complications. J Crit Care. 2018;44:191–5.
79. Janz DR, Semler MW, Joffe AM, et al. A multicenter randomized trial of a checklist for endotracheal intubation of critically ill adults. Chest. 2018;153:816–24.
80. Turner JS, Bucca AW, Propst SL, et al. Association of checklist use in endotracheal intubation with clinically important outcomes: a systematic review and meta-analysis. JAMA Netw Open. 2020;3:e209278.
81. De Jong A, Jaber S. Do not throw the intubation checklist out with the bath water! Chest. 2018;153:771–3.
82. Rello J, Soñora R, Jubert P, Artigas A, Rué M, Vallés J. Pneumonia in intubated patients: role of respiratory airway care. Am J Respir Crit Care Med. 1996;154:111–5.
83. Kearl RA, Hooper RG. Massive airway leaks: an analysis of the role of endotracheal tubes. Crit Care Med. 1993;21:518–21.
84. McGrath BA, Bates L, Atkinson D, Moore JA. Multidisciplinary guidelines for the management of tracheostomy and laryngectomy airway emergencies. Anaesthesia. 2012;67:1025–41.
85. Public Health England. COVID-19: infection prevention and control guidance. 2020. https://www.gov.uk/government/publications/wuhan-novel-coronavirus-infection-prevention-andcontrol/wuhan-novel-coronavirus-wn-cov-infection-preventionand-control-guidance#mobile-healthcare-equipment. Accessed 15 Jan 2023.
86. Cook TM, El-Boghdadly K, McGuire B, McNarry AF, Patel A, Higgs A. Consensus guidelines for managing the airway in patients with COVID-19. Anaesthesia. 2020;75:785–99. https://doi.org/10.1111/anae.15054.
87. Loeb M, McGeer A, Henry B, et al. SARS among critical care nurses, Toronto. Emerg Infect Dis. 2004;10:251–5.
88. Shields A, Faustini SE, Perez-Toledo M, et al. SARS-CoV-2 seroprevalence and asymptomatic viral carriage in healthcare workers: a cross-sectional study. Thorax. 2020;75(12):1089–94. https://doi.org/10.1136/thoraxjnl-2020-215414.

89. Chui J, Hui D, Chan M. How should aerosol generating procedures be defined? BMJ. 2022;378:e065903.
90. Kearsley R. Intubation boxes for managing the airway in patients with COVID-19. Anaesthesia. 2020;75(7):969. https://doi.org/10.1111/anae.15081.
91. Brewster DJ, Chrimes NC, Do T, et al. Consensus statement. Safe Airway Society principles of airway management & tracheal intubation specific to the COVID19 adult patient group. Med J Aust. 2020;212(10):472–81. https://doi.org/10.5694/mja2.50598.

Chapter 27
Airway Management During Cardiopulmonary Resuscitation

Basma Mohamed and Lauren C. Berkow

27.1 Introduction

Airway management during cardiopulmonary resuscitation has been updated in the most recent guidelines and has been the focus of multiple studies in out-of-hospital cardiac arrest (OHCA). The incidence of OHCA is 76.5 per 100,000 in the United States, with 10.6% of patients surviving and 8.2% recovering with good functional status [1, 2]. Adequate oxygenation and ventilation are essential to prevent further secondary injury to the organs from hypoxia. Airway management during cardiac arrest usually starts with a basic maneuver, such as opening the airway using head tilt-chin lift and bag-mask ventilation. Studies and the American Heart Association guidelines reviewed the impact of different airway management strategies on survival to hospital discharge and neurological outcomes. In this chapter, we review the recent literature and the most recent guidelines regarding updates in airway management during cardiopulmonary resuscitation for adults, pediatrics, and neonates, as well as patients in unique situations, such as trauma and pregnant patients.

B. Mohamed (✉)
Department of Anesthesiology, Duke University School of Medicine, Durham, NC, USA
e-mail: basma.mohamed@duke.edu

L. C. Berkow
Division of Neuroanesthesia, University of Florida College of Medicine, Gainesville, FL, USA
e-mail: lberkow@anest.ufl.edu

M. Á. Gómez-Ríos, A. van Zundert (eds.), *Evidence-based Guide to Difficult Airway Management*, https://doi.org/10.1007/978-3-032-30769-9_27

27.2 Airway Management During Cardiopulmonary Resuscitation (CPR) Guidelines

The American Heart Association guidelines emphasize the importance of focusing on circulation and hemodynamic status before proceeding with airway management and breathing. Similar to airway management during cardiopulmonary resuscitation, airway management for hemodynamically unstable patients should prioritize hemodynamic stability and circulation optimization before airway management. Airway management will impact the physiological responses during and after tracheal intubation. The changes from spontaneous to positive pressure ventilation may increase intrathoracic pressure and decrease venous return, resulting in lower cardiac output and peri-intubation cardiac arrest [3, 4]. Airway management during CPR provides adequate oxygenation and ventilation and prevents hypoxia-related injury. The goal is to improve overall and neurological survival.

The use of an advanced airway strategy has been the focus of recent guidelines (since 2019). Per the most recent (2025) American Heart Association (AHA) guidelines, either bag-mask ventilation or an advanced airway strategy may be considered during CPR for an adult patient with cardiac arrest in any setting (in-hospital or out-of-hospital cardiac arrest) based on the situation and the skillset of the first responders (Grade B evidence) [5, 6]. The decision-making will be based on multiple factors, including the possibility of interrupting chest compression, a malpositioned device, or the possible success rate of first-pass placement of an advanced airway. Providers should weigh the risk of proceeding with an advanced airway versus the potential benefits. Placement of an advanced airway can be delayed until two rounds of chest compressions are completed, assuming bag-mask ventilation is adequate. The 2025 guidelines also emphasize the use of rescue breathing at ten breaths per minute (or one breath every 6 s) before an advanced airway is placed (Grade B evidence) and while using an advanced airway device (Grade C evidence) or a compression-to-ventilation ratio of 30:2 (Grade B evidence). Clinicians and first responders to patients with cardiac arrest should receive the appropriate training and master one airway management technique and one backup technique. [5] Table 27.1 summarizes the updated recommendations from the AHA guidelines regarding airway management during cardiopulmonary resuscitation.

27.2.1 Airway Management During Out-of-Hospital Cardiac Arrest (OHCA)

Airway management is a critical procedure in out-of-hospital cardiac arrest (OHCA). Emergency medical services medical directors and clinicians must attend to the process of airway management, not only through evaluating the success of first-pass intubation but also through monitoring the physiological consequences of airway management, as well as preparation and teamwork related to the success of

Table 27.1 Updated airway management during adult cardiac arrest per the American Heart Association Guidelines

Grade of evidence	Recommendations for adult cardiac arrest patient
C	For lay rescuers trained in CPR and ventilation, or healthcare professionals, it is reasonable to start rescue breaths in addition to chest compressions
C	Healthcare providers should use the head tilt-chin lift maneuver to open the airway when no cervical spine injury is suspected
C	The use of an airway adjunct may be reasonable in patients with no cough or gag reflex
C	In patients with suspected skull base fracture or coagulopathy, an oropharyngeal airway is preferred
C	Routine use of cricoid pressure is not recommended
C	If cervical spine injury is suspected, healthcare providers should open the airway using the jaw thrust
C	In head and neck trauma, opening the airway can be performed using head tilt-chin lift if one cannot open the airway using jaw thrust
C	In head and neck trauma, lay rescuers should not use immobilization devices, as this may cause more harm
C	Ventilation to a visible chest rise (around 500–600 ml tidal volume) is reasonable
C	Rescue breaths should be delivered over 1 s
C	Avoid excessive ventilation (too many breaths or too large a volume) during CPR
C	In adults with spontaneous circulation who need support for ventilation, give rescue breaths at 1 breath every 6 s (or 10 breaths per minute)
B	Before placement of an advanced airway, CPR should be performed in cycles of 30 compressions to 2 breaths
C	If an advanced airway is in place, deliver 1 breath every 6 s or 10 breaths per minute
C	It is reasonable to delay ventilation for witnessed shockable OHCA
B	Either bag-mask ventilation or an advanced airway strategy may be considered during CPR for adult cardiac arrest in any setting, depending on the situation and skill set of the provider
B	If an advanced airway is used, a supraglottic airway can be used for adults with OHCA in settings with low tracheal intubation success rates or minimal training for endotracheal tube placement
B	If an advanced airway is used, either a supraglottic airway or endotracheal intubation can be used for adults with OHCA in settings with high tracheal intubation success rates or optimal training for endotracheal tube placement
B	If an advanced airway is used in the in-hospital setting by expert providers trained in these procedures, either a supraglottic airway or an endotracheal tube placement can be used
B	If advanced airway placement will interrupt chest compressions, providers may consider deferring insertion of the airway until the patient fails to respond to initial CPR and defibrillation attempts or obtains ROSC
C	Continuous waveform capnography is recommended in addition to clinical assessment as the most reliable method of confirming and monitoring correct placement of an endotracheal tube

Sources: Kleinman ME, Buick JE, Huber N, Idris AH, Levy M, Morgan SG, et al. Part 7: Adult Basic Life Support: 2025 American Heart Association Guidelines for Cardiopulmonary Resuscitation and Emergency Cardiovascular Care. Circulation. 2025 Oct 21;152(16_suppl_2):S448-S478.6. Wigginton JG, Agarwal S, Bartos JA, Coute RA, Drennan IR, Haamid A,et al. Part 9: Adult Advanced Life Support: 2025 American Heart Association Guidelines for Cardiopulmonary Resuscitation and Emergency Cardiovascular Care. Circulation. 2025 Oct 21;152(16_suppl_2):S538-S577

airway management in the pre-hospital setting, without compromising perfusion, oxygenation, and neurological outcomes. Considerations related to airway management in OHCA include: [4–6]

1. Prioritize treating hypoxemia over placing an advanced airway device. Addressing hypoxemia includes other measures to improve oxygenation, including bag-mask ventilation or passive oxygen insufflation.
2. Anticipation and management of the physiological consequences of airway management, including worsening hemodynamic status after initiating positive pressure ventilation.
3. Anticipating the difficulty of placing an advanced airway device should prompt clinicians to plan for alternative oxygenation and ventilation methods.
4. Practicing evidence-based methods of confirming advanced airway device placement. Waveform capnography is the most reliable method to confirm the initial and ongoing monitoring and function of an advanced airway device. It is now a class I recommendation (Grade C evidence) from the American Heart Association [5, 6].
5. Optimizing ventilation and oxygenation after advanced airway management should focus on the goals of care for the patient after the return of spontaneous circulation (ROSC).

   (a) The ventilation goal usually is normocapnia, while mainly in the OHCA setting, and after obtaining ROSC, many healthcare providers tend to hyperventilate, which might be beneficial in traumatic brain injury patients, but may not be beneficial in hypotensive patients, with the results of decreased preload and worsening of hemodynamic status after ROSC.
   (b) Deliver supplemental oxygen to maintain $SPO_2 > 94\%$.
   (c) While often utilized in the intensive care unit, protective lung ventilation may not be a preferred strategy for OHCA.

27.3 Airway Management Techniques and Devices During CPR

Airway management in clinical practice is a stepwise approach based on the availability of resources and the stage of resuscitation.

27.3.1 Rescue Breathing

Rescue breathing using bag-mask ventilation (BMV) is a practical technique to use for airway management in advanced life support. It is a fast way to improve and maintain oxygenation with minimal interruption of chest compressions. The most recent guidelines recommend using either BMV or an advanced airway during CPR for adult cardiac arrest in any setting based on the provider's clinical skills and the situation where the arrest occurs (Grade B evidence) [5, 6]. It has been shown that either technique's outcomes depend on the clinical provider's skills and experience. As a result, the appropriate decision regarding the choice of airway management will depend on the patient's condition and the clinical skills of the airway management provider. As this is the first technique used for airway management during CPR, optimization of the technique is essential to ensure appropriate oxygenation and improved survival [5–7]. Measures to optimize bag-mask ventilation include:

1. Maintain an open airway and appropriate facemask seal in addition to the need for jaw thrust and head tilt.
2. Maintain a patent airway using an oropharyngeal or nasopharyngeal airway.
3. A visible chest rise is needed to confirm adequate tidal volume and the appropriate technique.
4. Deliver adequate tidal volumes at the lowest pressure to minimize gastric insufflation, regurgitation, and aspiration.
5. Bag-mask ventilation should be synchronized with chest compressions in a compression-to-ventilation ratio of 30:2. Once ROSC is obtained, rescue breaths should continue at the same rate.
6. A modified 2-rescuer CPR technique* is preferred as it prevents unintentional desynchrony between BMV ventilation and chest compression.

   *During the modified 2-rescuer CPR technique, the first rescuer performs chest compressions and thereafter squeezes the BVM resuscitator bag during the ventilatory pause, while the second rescuer creates a two-handed mask-face seal. [8].

One of the disadvantages of BMV is aspiration. However, data on the incidence of aspiration in patients receiving BMV only compared to those with an advanced airway are conflicting. In addition, aspiration may occur during CPR, even in the setting of advanced airway placement. Aspiration may occur despite the advanced airway placement, as this might occur at the time of the cardiac arrest before any intervention, or may also occur as a result of increased gastric pressure that occurs during CPR. [9–11].

27.3.2 Advanced Airway Management

Placement of an advanced airway may result in interruption of chest compressions, malpositioning of the airway device, or physiological consequences related to positive pressure ventilation and hyperventilation. Therefore, the choice of proceeding with advanced airway management or continuing with bag-mask ventilation should take into account the risks and benefits of an advanced airway technique, as well as the clinical skills of the provider. The 2025 AHA guidelines highlight the following recommendations when choosing an advanced airway technique (see Fig. 27.1):

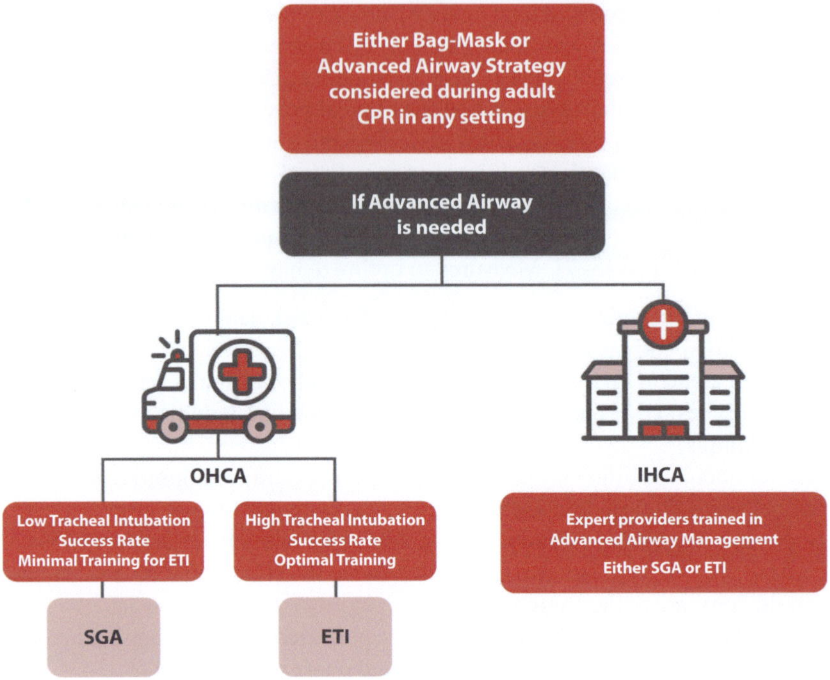

Fig. 27.1 Schematic representation of ACLS recommendations for use of advanced airways during CPR. (Reprinted with permission from Circulation. 2025;152(suppl 2):S538–S577. ©2025 American Heart Association, Inc.)

1. If the decision is made to proceed with an advanced airway, a supraglottic airway can be used in a setting with a low endotracheal intubation success rate or a low level of training for endotracheal intubation techniques, including OHCA (Grade B evidence).
2. Placement of an endotracheal tube can be used in adults in cardiac arrest settings with a high endotracheal intubation success rate or optimal level of training for the clinical providers, including OHCA (Grade B evidence).
3. If an advanced airway technique is used in in-hospital cardiac arrest (IHCA), then experienced providers can choose either a supraglottic airway device or endotracheal intubation (Grade B evidence).
4. Frequent training for providers who perform endotracheal intubation is recommended (Grade B evidence).
5. If advanced airway placement interrupts chest compressions, then advanced airway placement should be deferred until the patient fails to respond to resuscitation measures or ROSC is obtained (Grade C evidence).
6. Continuous waveform capnography is the recommended method to confirm and monitor advanced airway placement (Grade C evidence).

Many of the advanced airway recommendations are derived from studies in OHCA settings. Studies showed no difference in the neurological and survival outcomes between supraglottic airway devices and endotracheal tube placement [12, 13]. In a randomized controlled trial comparing supraglottic airway placement (SGA) versus endotracheal intubation (ETI) in an OHCA setting, there was no difference in outcomes [14]. A comparison between SGA and ETI and their impact on cost-effectiveness and quality of life showed no difference between the groups [15].

The timing of the use of an advanced airway can be correlated with favorable outcomes. The timing of advanced airway placement has been the focus of a recent observational study that showed early endotracheal intubation is associated with favorable neurological outcomes [16]. In a secondary analysis of the Pragmatic Airway Resuscitation Trial (PART), the investigators evaluated the impact of early advanced airway placement in four cohorts (<5 min, 5–10 min, 10–15 min, and 15–20 min). They found no association between advanced airway placement and survival to hospital discharge [17]. However, a delay in advanced airway placement, defined as advanced airway placement after 20 min of CPR, may result in poor neurological outcomes [17, 18]. However, another study evaluating early intubation in an in-hospital cardiac arrest setting was associated with decreased survival to discharge [19]. Because of conflicting data, it is best to follow the AHA recommendations that placement of an advanced airway device is recommended when feasible, and the decision should be based on the clinical situation.

27.3.3 Endotracheal Intubation

Endotracheal intubation (ETI) during CPR in OHCA provides airway protection from gastric contents, the ability to provide high positive pressure ventilation, allows the providers to focus on other resuscitation tasks, and allows providers to continue chest compressions while ventilating without interruptions. However, these benefits may not be achieved without risks. Aspiration may occur before and during advanced airway placement, and high positive airway pressure may impact cardiac output. In addition, many studies assessing the use of advanced airway devices did not show improved survival with endotracheal intubation compared to a supraglottic device [7].

ETI can be challenging during OHCA. These challenges include the required frequent training for providers and the limited experience of first responders, resulting in decreased intubation success rates. In addition, ETI may result in interruptions in chest compressions and possible distraction from high-quality CPR. Therefore, to achieve high intubation success rates, it should be performed by the most experienced providers, minimizing interruptions in chest compressions to 5-s pauses only if needed. However, it is suggested not to interrupt chest compressions during ETI, which can also impact the intubation success rate, and to use video laryngoscopy when feasible.

The use of video laryngoscopy (VL) has been associated with a higher first-attempt success rate when compared to direct laryngoscopy (DL). Two studies comparing the success rate of intubation using VL versus DL during CPR showed improved success rates with VL [20, 21]. These results were also confirmed in a recent systematic review, mainly when clinicians are less experienced [22]. There is also evidence that VL may result in fewer interruptions in chest compressions. Despite this evidence, the use of VL in the OHCA setting may be limited by the presence of blood, secretions, and gastric contents, which may limit the intubation success rate. [20, 23, 24] In addition, VL may not be readily available in the OHCA setting.

27.3.4 Supraglottic Airway Devices (SGA)

Supraglottic airway devices may be viable alternatives to ETI in situations where advanced airway management skills are lacking or where the rate of first-pass endotracheal intubation success is low [25]. Supraglottic airway devices have been reported to be used more commonly than endotracheal intubation in OHCA since the COVID-19 pandemic [26]. Per the AHA guidelines, an SGA device is recommended as an alternative to endotracheal intubation, and the choice could be based on the providers' experience and success rate with intubation [5, 6] (Fig. 27.1). There is no clear evidence that ETI is superior to SGA in terms of outcomes, including survival to discharge and neurological outcomes. However, two randomized controlled trials in OHCA comparing ETI to SGA during CPR showed better survival to discharge and better neurological outcomes when the airway was managed using SGA [12, 13]. There are limited studies in IHCA, so the current recommendations are extrapolated from OHCA studies.

There are advantages and disadvantages to using SGA when compared to endotracheal intubation. Advantages include a shorter preparation time, minimal interruption of chest compressions, faster, and easier insertion, and a higher placement success rate, even by less experienced providers. In addition, SGA placement is less complex than intubation, which allows providers to train and improve clinical skills in placing an SGA. Disadvantages include air leaks and malpositioning during transport. The one potential disadvantage of placing an SGA is the increased regurgitation and aspiration risk. This risk of regurgitation and aspiration is conflicting in the literature, which could be related to the likely incidence of vomiting and aspiration before or at the beginning of cardiac arrest [9–11].

27.3.5 Waveform Capnography

Waveform capnography is 100% specific for confirming endotracheal tube placement during CPR. The use of waveform capnography to assess the placement of other advanced airways, like SGA, has not been studied yet [5, 6]. In addition, the sensitivity of waveform capnography may decrease after prolonged resuscitation due to low cardiac output, even if the endotracheal tube is confirmed to be in the correct depth in the trachea. Continuous monitoring of waveform capnography is recommended during CPR and after ROSC to minimize the risk of misplacement or malpositioning of the endotracheal tube. In addition to its utility in confirming ETT placement, it is used to evaluate the quality of CPR, predict ROSC, and for prognostication purposes [27–29]. A sustained increase in $ETCO_2$ (>40 mmHg) is an indication of ROSC. Recent recommendations from the international consensus on CPR and emergency cardiovascular care science endorse waveform capnography to ensure adequate ventilation and as an indicator for ROSC [30].

27.3.6 Cricoid Pressure

There is no evidence that cricoid pressure will reduce the risk of aspiration in cardiac arrest patients. Cricoid pressure may prevent adequate ventilation and successful placement of an SGA or an ETT, in addition to the increased risk of airway trauma during intubation while using cricoid pressure. [31] The AHA guidelines recommend against the routine use of cricoid pressure during airway management in adult cardiac arrest [5, 6].

27.4 Alternative Methods for Oxygen Delivery During CPR

27.4.1 Passive Oxygenation

It is hypothesized that chest compressions generate air movement, with enough movement to allow oxygenation. Therefore, CPR without ventilation is known as compression-only CPR. Continuous oxygen delivery via passive oxygen insufflation can be achieved using an oropharyngeal airway and an oxygen mask. Passive oxygen insufflation will prevent interruptions to chest compressions and decrease the risk of hyperventilation that may result in gastric insufflation. Passive oxygenation will also prevent a further decrease in cardiac output from the high positive pressure ventilation. However, there are disadvantages to using this technique, including atelectasis, and the need for additional equipment like high-flow oxygen techniques may result in hypercapnia and acidosis. Hypercapnia and acidosis may exacerbate the hemodynamic status of an adult cardiac arrest patient. This approach had been described in the 2010 AHA guidelines. However, due to a lack of evidence on the impact of this approach on outcomes, the updated AHA guidelines since 2015 advise against the routine use of passive oxygenation during CPR [5, 6].

27.4.2 Oxylator

The oxylator is a patient-responsive emergency ventilation device that can be used automatically or manually. In an automatic mode, it can deliver a breath during the decompression phase of chest compressions at 100 breaths/min [32]. It can also deliver a constant flow rate at 30 L per minute during inspiration until a preliminary airway pressure is achieved (45 cm H_2O), at which point it switches to a passive exhalation phase. The advantages of this device include consistency in ventilation and oxygenation at a set pressure and avoiding hyperventilation or gastric insufflation. In addition, it allows the providers to focus on other resuscitation efforts.

27.4.3 Impedance Threshold Devices

An impedance threshold device (ITD) creates a negative intrathoracic pressure during CPR [33, 34]. This device is integrated into the breathing circuit, allowing air to exit during chest compression but preventing airflow into the chest during decompression. The negative intrathoracic pressure allows increased venous return, which can improve cardiac output. A large randomized controlled trial did not show the beneficial effects of ITD. However, an ad-hoc analysis showed improved outcomes when an ITD is combined with high-quality CPR [33]. In the ResQTrial, the addition of an ITD to standard CPR improved hospital discharge survival [5, 6, 34, 35]. It is recommended as a class II recommendation by the AHA to be used during CPR to improve venous return during chest compression.

27.4.4 Extracorporeal Life Support (ECLS)

Extracorporeal life support (ECLS) may improve survival and neurological outcomes in select groups of patients with cardiac arrest, however its routine use is not recommended due to the limited high-quality evidence and the need for specialized personnel and resources. The 2025 AHA guidelines now recommend ECLS as an option for potentially reversible etiologies such as anaphylaxis or asthma, hypothermia, or specific poisoning scenarios, as well as cardiac arrest after cardiac surgery, interventional cardiology procedures, or pulmonary embolism [36–38].

27.5 Airway Management After Return of Spontaneous Circulation (ROSC)

Care for adult cardiac arrest patients after ROSC includes identifying the cause of the cardiac arrest, managing multisystem organ failure, targeted temperature management, and neurological prognostication. The most recent AHA guidelines highlight continued oxygenation and ventilation to prevent secondary injury to different organs [5, 6]. It is recommended to continue to deliver oxygen at the highest concentration during CPR and after ROSC until the providers can obtain arterial oxyhemoglobin saturation and or partial pressure of oxygen. Hypoxia should be avoided after ROSC, and supplemental oxygen should be titrated to a goal of an oxygen saturation range of 92–98%. Goals for ventilation should be aimed at maintaining $PaCO_2$ in the normal range (35–45 mmHg), mainly in comatose patients. Hyperoxemia should also be avoided, as there are physiological and pre-clinical data that hyperoxemia may result in increased inflammation, which can exacerbate brain injury [5, 6].

27.6 Challenges of Airway Management During CPR

27.6.1 Airway Management During Resuscitation in the Prone Position

The prone positioning is commonly used in surgical procedures, as well as in intensive care units when caring for patients with acute respiratory distress syndrome. Cardiac arrest in the prone position poses challenges to providers as they may not be familiar with how to administer CPR in this position. Recent data and recommendations by the international consensus on CPR and ECC related to special situations recommend initiating CPR in prone positions when an advanced airway is in place [30, 39]. If the patient is in a prone position without an advanced airway, it is recommended to turn the patient supine to begin CPR and airway management.

27.6.2 Airway Management During CPR in a Trauma Patient

Airway management during CPR in a trauma patient should follow the current stepwise approach. The first responder should use the head tilt-chin lift maneuver to open the airway when cervical spine injury is not suspected. However, in cases of suspected cervical spine injury or instability, the healthcare provider should open the airway using only jaw thrust without head tilt. An airway adjunct insertion is allowed with jaw thrust when the jaw thrust alone cannot open the airway. Maintaining a patent airway and providing adequate ventilation are essential steps during CPR. If a jaw thrust and adjunct airway are ineffective in opening the airway, a head tilt-chin lift should be used in this situation, as the need to open the airway outweighs the risk of spinal cord injury in an adult cardiac arrest patient [5, 6]. The AHA recommends manual in-line stabilization during airway management in patients with a suspected cervical spine injury, which may be challenging during airway management during CPR. Currently, no specific airway management technique has been shown to be "safest" for patients with a cervical spine injury. [40] The overall goal in patients with suspected cervical spine injury is to minimize cervical spine movement during CPR and airway management. Most patients with suspected cervical spine injury will be placed in a hard collar. See the Airway Management during Trauma Chapter in this book for details.

27.6.3 *Infection Risk*

As the COVID-19 pandemic continued for over 3 years, data related to OHCA and IHCA outcomes were evaluated. However, the COVID-19 pandemic highlighted concerns related to the aerosolization of infectious viral particles during CPR and airway management in COVID-19 patients. Hence, the AHA published guidelines related to BLS and ACLS in adults, pediatric, and neonatal patients with suspected or confirmed COVID-19 infection and addressed infection risk in the recently published 2025 AHA guidelines [36, 41, 42]. The summary of their recommendations focused on strategies that minimize the risk of exposure of healthcare professionals to viral particles and could be used in other situations where the risk of droplet infection is high. These strategies include:

1. The use of a high-efficiency particulate air filter (HEPA filter).
2. Patients in cardiac arrest should be intubated with a cuffed tube at the earliest opportunity.
3. It is best to minimize intubation attempts by allowing the most experienced provider to intubate.
4. It is recommended to pause chest compressions during intubation.
5. The use of videolaryngoscopy is recommended.
6. If intubation is delayed, it is advised to use an SGA with a HEPA filter.
7. Use of PPE before CPR, defibrillation, and airway management.

27.6.4 *Airway Management After Drowning*

Drowning results in an initial respiratory arrest from submersion-related hypoxia but can progress to cardiac arrest. Since drowning primarily causes hypoxia, restoring breathing is as important as restoring circulation. Providing rescue breaths early, before cardiac arrest occurs, is associated with lower mortality [36]. If possible and not a risk to rescuer safety, providing in-water rescue breaths is reasonable, and is associated with higher survival rates. Chest compressions and defibrillation may be required if the drowning victim progresses to cardiac arrest or presents with an initial cardiac etiology. It is also recommended to initiate pre-hospital oxygen therapy using 100% inspired oxygen until oxygen saturation or partial pressure of oxygen can be measured [36].

27.7 Airway Management During Other Circumstances

27.7.1 Airway Management During Pediatric Resuscitation

Most pediatric cardiac arrests are caused by respiratory insult; as a result, airway management and adequate ventilation are essential for CPR in the pediatric population. The 2025 AHA guidelines recommend bag-mask ventilation (BMV) as a reasonable approach compared to an advanced airway technique in managing pediatric cardiac arrest in the OHCA setting [37, 38]. Advanced airway devices in children may improve ventilation, reduce the risk of aspiration, and allow minimal interruption in chest compression; however, advanced airway management requires specialized equipment and skilled providers. When provided by inexperienced providers, pre-hospital airway management in pediatric patients showed an intubation failure rate of more than 50% [43]. However, when anesthesia providers are involved, this has demonstrated improved mortality and neurological outcomes [44]. Recent studies showed that ETI and BMV achieve similar surgical and neurological outcomes rates in pediatric OHCA. Similarly, there was no difference in outcomes when SGA was compared to ETI.

Identification and treatment of the respiratory causes of cardiac arrest in children is of utmost importance since it is the common reason for cardiac arrest. Disordered control of breathing, upper airway obstruction, lower airway obstruction, and foreign body aspiration are among other reasons for respiratory arrest. Assisted ventilation, relieving foreign body obstruction, and administering naloxone can be essential strategies to treat and reverse the cause of cardiac arrest in this population. The recommended assisted ventilation rate is one breath every 2–3 s (20–30 breaths/min), which has been increased from 1 breath every 3–5 s in previous guidelines. In patients with suspected opioid overdose, it is recommended to start with airway management and assisted ventilation, assuming the infant or the child has a pulse.

When healthcare providers opt for intubation, it is recommended to use a cuffed endotracheal tube. Healthcare providers should choose the appropriate ETT size, position, and cuff inflation pressure (not to exceed 20–25 cm H_2O). In contrast to the recommendations for adults, cricoid pressure may be considered during bag-mask ventilation in children and infants to minimize gastric insufflation. However, the routine use of cricoid pressure is not recommended and should be discontinued if it interferes with ventilation or intubation [37, 38]. The AHA guidelines also recommend using atropine at a dose of 0.02 mg/kg as a premedication before emergently intubating infants and children when there is a high risk of bradycardia.

27.7.2 Airway Management During Neonatal Resuscitation

It is estimated that 20% of newborn infants need help with initial breathing efforts at birth, and nearly 1% need intensive resuscitation [45]. In addition, 5% of term infants will require positive pressure ventilation, 2% require intubation, 0.1% will receive chest compressions, and 0.05% will require chest compressions with epinephrine [45]. For the neonates who do not initiate breathing after stimulation, the following stepwise approach by the healthcare provider can be implemented:

1. Deliver adequate ventilation using a face mask.
2. Check for airway patency and apply positive pressure ventilation.
3. An advanced airway management strategy should be utilized, either the placement of SGA or ETT.
4. Monitor heart rate while supporting ventilation and oxygenation. If HR < 60/min, then start chest compressions.
5. Suctioning the airway is only used when the airway appears obstructed and when positive pressure ventilation is needed. Per the 2025 guidelines, routine airway suctioning is not recommended, as it may result in bradycardia, apnea, and iatrogenic infection [30, 45].

The 2025 AHA guidelines also endorse the following recommendations:

1. For newborns receiving positive pressure ventilation (PPV):
   (a) For newborns gasping or apneic within 60 s, or HR <100, PPV should be provided without delay (Grade B evidence).
   (b) Use peak inflation pressure to achieve a rise in heart rate (Grade C evidence).
   (c) Provide peak end-expiratory pressure (PEEP) (Grade C evidence).
   (d) Avoid excessive peak inflation pressures (less than 20–25 cm H_2O) (Grade C evidence).
   (e) Deliver PPV at a rate of 40–60 inflations per minute (Grade C evidence).
   (f) Avoid routine inflation of more than 5 s in preterm newborns (data is lacking for full-term and late preterm newborns) (Grade B evidence).
2. Use continuous positive airway pressure (CPAP) over intubation or intermittent positive pressure ventilation (Grade A evidence).
3. In term and late preterm newborns (35 weeks or more of gestation) receiving respiratory support at birth, the initial use of 21% oxygen is reasonable (Grade B evidence).
4. In preterm newborns (less than 35 weeks of gestation) receiving respiratory support at birth, it may be reasonable to begin with 21% to 30% oxygen with subsequent oxygen titration based on pulse oximetry (Grade C evidence).
5. In term and late preterm newborns (35 weeks or more of gestation) receiving respiratory support at birth, 100% oxygen should not be used because it is associated with excess mortality (Grade B evidence).
6. The compression-to-ventilation ratio in newborn resuscitation is 3:1 (Grade C evidence).

27.7.3 Airway Management During Cardiac Arrest in a Pregnant Patient

Maternal cardiac arrest may occur in 1 in 12,000 admissions for delivery in the United States. Successful maternal resuscitation is the key factor in ensuring the best outcomes for both mother and fetus. Common causes of maternal cardiac arrest are hemorrhage, heart failure, amniotic fluid embolism, sepsis, venous thromboembolism, and anesthesia complications [5, 6]. The increased maternal metabolism, increased oxygen consumption, and decreased functional reserve capacity caused by the gravid uterus result in hypoxia, which can result in fetal hypoxia and poor outcomes for the mother and the fetus. Multiple factors play a role in the planning for airway management in unstable pregnant patients or those who experience cardiac arrest. As a result, an advanced airway management strategy should be planned and performed early in cardiac arrest. Perimortem cesarean delivery is anticipated during cardiac arrest in pregnant patients; hence, being prepared with an early airway management strategy is essential in anticipation of cesarean delivery.

The airway management of a pregnant patient is anticipated to be difficult. The difficult airway is due to the distorted landmarks caused by edema, and the increased risk of airway bleeding related to high vascularity during pregnancy. The pregnant patient desaturates quickly due to decreased pulmonary reserve and increased oxygen consumption. It is highly recommended that the most experienced healthcare professional perform the intubation. Ventilation should be maintained using high PEEP and a plateau pressure < 30 cm H_2O. Oxygenation requirements are expected to be higher compared to a non-pregnant patient to avoid fetal hypoxemia. Ventilation goals should aim for a $PaCO_2$ of 30 mmHg to maintain the maternal-fetal CO_2 gradient [46].

27.8 Summary of the Evidence-Based Recommendations (See Tables 27.1 and 27.2)

The 2025 AHA guidelines emphasize adequate oxygenation and ventilation over the selection of any specific airway management technique during CPR. Either bag-mask ventilation (BMV) or an advanced airway strategy may be considered for adult cardiac arrest in any setting, with the choice guided by the provider's skill set and the clinical situation (COR 2b, LOE B-R). Rescue breathing should be delivered at a rate of one breath every 6 seconds (10 breaths/min) regardless of whether BMV or an advanced airway device is used, and a compression-to-ventilation ratio of 30:2 is maintained until an advanced airway is secured.

Table 27.2 Updated airway management during pediatric cardiac arrest per the American Heart Association Guidelines

Grade of evidence	Recommendations for Pediatric and Neonatal Cardiac Arrest Patients
C	Unless a cervical spine injury is suspected, use a head tilt-chin lift maneuver to open the airway
C	For the trauma patient with suspected cervical spinal injury, use a jaw thrust without head tilt to open the airway
C	For the trauma patient with suspected cervical spinal injury, if the jaw thrust does not open the airway, use a head tilt-chin lift maneuver
C	Bag-mask ventilation is reasonable compared with advanced airway interventions (SGA and ETI) in the management of children during cardiac arrest in the out-of-hospital setting
C	It may be reasonable for rescuers to wean oxygen to target an oxyhemoglobin saturation between 94% and 99% after obtaining ROSC
C	It may be reasonable for practitioners to target a partial pressure of carbon dioxide ($PaCo_2$) after ROSC that is appropriate to the specific patient's underlying condition, and limit exposure to severe hypercapnia or hypocapnia
B	For newborns gasping or apneic within 60 s, or HR <100, PPV should be provided without delay
C	For newborns, use peak inflation pressure to achieve a rise in heart rate
C	For newborns, provide peak end-expiratory pressure (PEEP)
C	For newborns, avoid excessive peak inflation pressures (less than 20–25 cm H_2O)
C	For newborns, deliver PPV at a rate of 40–60 inflations per minute
B	For newborns, avoid routine inflation of more than 5 s in preterm newborns
A	Use continuous positive airway pressure (CPAP) over intubation or intermittent positive pressure ventilation in newborns
C	The compression-to-ventilation ratio in newborn resuscitation is 3:1 in newborns
B	In term and late preterm newborns (35 weeks or more of gestation) receiving respiratory support at birth, the initial use of 21% oxygen is reasonable
C	In preterm newborns (less than 35 week of gestation) receiving respiratory support at birth, it may be reasonable to begin with 21–30% oxygen with subsequent oxygen titration based on pulse oximetry
B	In term and late preterm newborns (35 week or more of gestation) receiving respiratory support at birth, 100% oxygen should not be used because it is associated with excess mortality

Sources:

Joyner BL Jr, Dewan M, Bavare A, de Caen A, DiMaria K, Donofrio-Odmann J, et al. Part 6: Pediatric Basic Life Support: 2025 American Heart Association and American Academy of Pediatrics Guidelines for Cardiopulmonary Resuscitation and Emergency Cardiovascular Care. Circulation. 2025 Oct 21;152(16_suppl_2):S424-S447

Lasa JJ, Dhillon GS, Duff JP, Hayes J, Kamath-Rayne BD, Levy A, et al. Part 8: Pediatric Advanced Life Support: 2025 American Heart Association and American Academy of Pediatrics Guidelines for Cardiopulmonary Resuscitation and Emergency Cardiovascular Care. Circulation. 2025 Oct 21;152(16_suppl_2):S479-S537

Lee HC, Strand ML, Finan E, Illuzzi J, Kamath-Rayne BD, Kapadia V, et al. Part 5: Neonatal Resuscitation: 2025 American Heart Association and American Academy of Pediatrics Guidelines for Cardiopulmonary Resuscitation and Emergency Cardiovascular Care. Circulation. 2025 Oct 21;152(16_suppl_2):S385-S423

When an advanced airway is required in out-of-hospital cardiac arrest (OHCA), a supraglottic airway (SGA) is preferred in systems with low endotracheal intubation success rates or limited training opportunities (COR 2a, LOE B-R). In systems with high intubation success rates or optimal training, either an SGA or endotracheal tube (ETT) may be used (COR 2a, LOE B-R). For in-hospital cardiac arrest (IHCA), expert providers trained in advanced airway management may use either device (COR 2a, LOE B-NR). Continuous waveform capnography is recommended as the standard method for confirming and monitoring advanced airway placement throughout resuscitation (COR 1, LOE C-EO). Advanced airway placement should be deferred if it interrupts chest compressions, unless the patient fails to respond to resuscitation or ROSC is achieved (COR 2b, LOE C-LD).

Routine use of cricoid pressure during cardiac arrest is not recommended. In pediatric OHCA, BMV is preferred over advanced airway interventions (COR 2a, LOE C-LD), while either approach may be reasonable in pediatric IHCA (COR 2b, LOE C-LD). When an advanced airway is in place in children, a ventilation rate of 20–30 breaths/min (one breath every 2–3 s) is targeted, with hyperventilation actively avoided (COR 2b, LOE C-LD). In neonatal resuscitation, positive pressure ventilation should be initiated promptly for apneic or gasping newborns or those with a heart rate below 100 beats/min, with a compression-to-ventilation ratio of 3:1. The use of continuous positive airway pressure (CPAP) is preferred over intubation in preterm infants when feasible (COR 1, LOE A). Initial inspired oxygen concentration should be 21% for term and late-preterm newborns, with titration guided by pulse oximetry.

In special circumstances, airway management principles remain consistent with the general approach. In prone-position cardiac arrest with an advanced airway already in place, prone CPR may be initiated without repositioning. In pregnant patients, early advanced airway placement is prioritized given rapid oxygen desaturation and anticipated airway difficulty. In drowning, early rescue breathing is critical and is associated with improved survival. In all high-infection-risk environments, providers should use appropriate personal protective equipment, video laryngoscopy, and cuffed ETTs with HEPA filters to minimize aerosolization risk.

27.9 Conclusion

Airway management during cardiopulmonary resuscitation has been the focus of recent American Heart Association guidelines updates. Recent updates focus on the quality and adequacy of ventilation and oxygenation over the choice of airway management technique. The choice of bag-mask ventilation versus an advanced airway device should be based on the skills of the provider and the success rate of advanced airway device placement. The choice of supraglottic airway placement versus endotracheal intubation should be based on the provider's experience and the patient's situation. No individual airway management technique is superior to the others in achieving improved survival and neurological outcomes (See the clinical scenario Table 27.3).

Table 27.3 Clinical scenario

A 150 kg trauma patient of unknown age presented to the emergency department after a motor vehicle accident. The patient presented with labored breathing at 30 breaths per minute, a heart rate of 120/min, and blood pressure 74/43 mmHg. Shortly after arrival in the emergency department, the patient became unresponsive with no palpable pulse. Chest compressions started and the presenting rhythm was pulseless ventricular tachycardia. The emergency department physician started preparing for advanced airway management as chest compression started.
Q. How could this patient be managed according to the updated guidelines?
A. Adult cardiac arrest patients presenting with shockable rhythm can have the advanced airway management delayed up to two cycles of CPR. It is a priority to deliver defibrillation to this patient before proceeding with an advanced airway. The healthcare provider could continue with bag mask ventilation while continuing CPR.
Q. The patient started vomiting during CPR. What is the most appropriate advanced airway management technique for this patient?
A. Advanced airway management technique can be decided based on the setting (IHCA in this situation) and the clinical experience of the healthcare provider. In this setting, a 150 kg trauma patient poses challenges to intubation. If a supraglottic airway management is easier to place and ensure adequate ventilation, it will not prevent the regurgitation and aspiration that already occurred in this patient. However, if the healthcare provider has the appropriate equipment and is able to proceed with videolaryngoscopy without the barriers of vomiting and blood in a trauma patient, they should proceed based on their clinical expertise.

References

1. Virani SS, Alonso A, Aparicio HJ, Benjamin EJ, Bittencourt MS, Callaway CW, et al. Heart disease and stroke Statistics-2021 update: a report from the American Heart Association. Circulation. 2021;143(8):e254–743.
2. Virani SS, Alonso A, Benjamin EJ, Bittencourt MS, Callaway CW, Carson AP, et al. Heart disease and stroke statistics—2020 update: a report from the American Heart Association. Circulation. 2020;141(9):e139–596.
3. Walker RG, White LJ, Whitmore GN, Esibov A, Levy MK, Cover GC, et al. Evaluation of physiologic alterations during prehospital paramedic-performed rapid sequence intubation. Prehosp Emerg Care. 2018;22(3):300–11.
4. Davis DP, Bosson N, Guyette FX, Wolfe A, Bobrow BJ, Olvera D, et al. Optimizing physiology during prehospital airway management: an NAEMSP position statement and resource document. Prehosp Emerg Care. 2022;26(sup1):72–9.
5. Kleinman ME, Buick JE, Huber N, Idris AH, Levy M, Morgan SG, et al. Part 7: Adult basic life support: 2025 American Heart Association Guidelines for Cardiopulmonary Resuscitation and Emergency Cardiovascular Care. Circulation. 2025;152(16_Suppl_2):S448–S478.6.
6. Wigginton JG, Agarwal S, Bartos JA, et al. Part 9: Adult advanced life support: 2025 American Heart Association guidelines for cardiopulmonary resuscitation and emergency cardiovascular care. Circulation. 2025;152(16_Suppl_2):S538–77. https://doi.org/10.1161/CIR.0000000000001376.
7. van Schuppen H, Boomars R, Kooij FO, den Tex P, Koster RW, Hollmann MW. Optimizing airway management and ventilation during prehospital advanced life support in out-of-hospital cardiac arrest: a narrative review. Best Pract Res Clin Anaesthesiol. 2021;35(1):67–82.
8. Gerber L, Botha M, Laher AE. Modified two-rescuer CPR with a two-handed mask-face seal technique is superior to conventional two-rescuer CPR with a one-handed mask-face seal technique. J Emerg Med. 2021 Sep;61(3):252–8.

9. Lupton JR, Schmicker RH, Stephens S, Carlson JN, Callaway C, Herren H, et al. Outcomes with the use of bag–valve–mask ventilation during out-of-hospital cardiac arrest in the pragmatic airway resuscitation trial. Acad Emerg Med. 2020;27(5):366–74.
10. Baekgaard JS, Triba MN, Brandeis M, Steinmetz J, Cohen Y, Gorlicki J, et al. Early-onset pneumonia following bag-mask ventilation versus endotracheal intubation during cardiopulmonary resuscitation: a substudy of the CAAM trial. Resuscitation. 2020;154:12–8.
11. Jabre P, Penaloza A, Pinero D, Duchateau FX, Borron SW, Javaudin F, et al. Effect of bag-mask ventilation vs endotracheal intubation during cardiopulmonary resuscitation on neurological outcome after out-of-hospital cardiorespiratory arrest: a randomized clinical trial. JAMA. 2018;319(8):779–87.
12. Benger JR, Kirby K, Black S, Brett SJ, Clout M, Lazaroo MJ, et al. Effect of a strategy of a Supraglottic airway device vs tracheal intubation during out-of-hospital cardiac arrest on functional outcome: the AIRWAYS-2 randomized clinical trial. JAMA. 2018;320(8):779–91.
13. Wang HE, Schmicker RH, Daya MR, Stephens SW, Idris AH, Carlson JN, et al. Effect of a strategy of initial laryngeal tube insertion vs endotracheal intubation on 72-hour survival in adults with out-of-hospital cardiac arrest: a randomized clinical trial. JAMA. 2018;320(8):769–78.
14. Benger JR, Lazaroo MJ, Clout M, Voss S, Black S, Brett SJ, et al. Randomized trial of the i-gel supraglottic airway device versus tracheal intubation during out of hospital cardiac arrest (AIRWAYS-2): patient outcomes at three and six months. Resuscitation. 2020 Dec 1;157:74–82.
15. Stokes EA, Lazaroo MJ, Clout M, Brett SJ, Black S, Kirby K, et al. Cost-effectiveness of the i-gel supraglottic airway device compared to tracheal intubation during out-of-hospital cardiac arrest: findings from the AIRWAYS-2 randomised controlled trial. Resuscitation. 2021;167:1–9.
16. Nakagawa K, Sagisaka R, Tanaka S, Takyu H, Tanaka H. Early endotracheal intubation improves neurological outcome following witnessed out-of-hospital cardiac arrest in Japan: a population-based observational study. Acute Med Surg. 2021;8(1):e650.
17. Fukuda T, Ohashi-Fukuda N, Inokuchi R, Kondo Y, Sekiguchi H, Taira T, et al. Association between time to advanced airway management and neurologically favourable survival during out-of-hospital cardiac arrest. Anaesth Crit Care Pain Med. 2021;40(4):100906.
18. Okubo M, Komukai S, Izawa J, Aufderheide TP, Benoit JL, Carlson JN, et al. Association of advanced airway insertion timing and outcomes after out-of-hospital cardiac arrest. Ann Emerg Med. 2022;79(2):118–31.
19. Andersen LW, Granfeldt A, Callaway CW, Bradley SM, Soar J, Nolan JP, et al. Association between tracheal intubation during adult in-hospital cardiac arrest and survival. JAMA. 2017;317(5):494–506.
20. Okamoto H, Goto T, Wong ZSY, Hagiwara Y, Watase H, Hasegawa K. Comparison of video laryngoscopy versus direct laryngoscopy for intubation in emergency department patients with cardiac arrest: a multicentre study. Resuscitation. 2019;136:70–7.
21. Min BC, Park JE, Lee GT, Kim TR, Yoon H, Cha WC, et al. C-MAC video laryngoscope versus conventional direct laryngoscopy for endotracheal intubation during cardiopulmonary resuscitation. Medicina (Mex). 2019 Jun;55(6):225.
22. Cox L, Tebbett A. Videolaryngoscopy versus direct laryngoscopy for endotracheal intubation of cardiac arrest patients in hospital: a systematic literature review. Resusc Plus. 2022;11:100297.
23. Park SO, Baek KJ, Hong DY, Kim SC, Lee KR. Feasibility of the video-laryngoscope (GlideScope®) for endotracheal intubation during uninterrupted chest compressions in actual advanced life support: a clinical observational study in an urban emergency department. Resuscitation. 2013;84(9):1233–7.
24. Tandon N, McCarthy M, Forehand B, Carlson JN. Comparison of intubation modalities in a simulated cardiac arrest with uninterrupted chest compressions. Emerg Med J. 2014;31(10):799–802.

25. Murphy TW, Cohen SA, Hwang CW, Avery KL, Balakrishnan MP, Balu R, et al. Cardiac arrest: an interdisciplinary scoping review of clinical literature from 2020. J Am Coll Emerg Physicians Open. 2022;3(4):e12773.
26. Lim ZJ, Ponnapa Reddy M, Afroz A, Billah B, Shekar K, Subramaniam A. Incidence and outcome of out-of-hospital cardiac arrests in the COVID-19 era: a systematic review and meta-analysis. Resuscitation. 2020;157:248–58.
27. Sandroni C, De Santis P, D'Arrigo S. Capnography during cardiac arrest. Resuscitation. 2018;132:73–7.
28. Crickmer M, Drennan IR, Turner L, Cheskes S. The association between end-tidal CO2 and return of spontaneous circulation after out-of-hospital cardiac arrest with pulseless electrical activity. Resuscitation. 2021;167:76–81.
29. Poppe M, Stratil P, Clodi C, Schriefl C, Nürnberger A, Magnet I, et al. Initial end-tidal carbon dioxide as a predictive factor for return of spontaneous circulation in nonshockable out-of-hospital cardiac arrest patients: a retrospective observational study. Eur J Anaesthesiol EJA. 2019;36(7):524.
30. Wyckoff MH, Singletary EM, Soar J, Olasveengen TM, Greif R, Liley HG, et al. International consensus on cardiopulmonary resuscitation and emergency cardiovascular care science with treatment recommendations: summary from the basic life support; advanced life support; neonatal life support; education, implementation, and teams; first aid task forces; and the COVID-19 working group. Resuscitation. 2021;169:229–311.
31. Asai T, Goy RWL, Liu EHC. Cricoid pressure prevents placement of the laryngeal tube and laryngeal tube-suction II. Br J Anaesth. 2007;99(2):282–5.
32. Schaller SJ, Altmann S, Unsworth A, Schneider G, Bogner-Flatz V, Paul T, et al. Continuous chest compressions with a simultaneous triggered ventilator in the Munich Emergency Medical Services: a case series. GMS Ger Med Sci. 2019;17:Doc06.
33. Yannopoulos D, Aufderheide TP, Abella BS, Duval S, Frascone RJ, Goodloe JM, et al. Quality of CPR: an important effect modifier in cardiac arrest clinical outcomes and intervention effectiveness trials. Resuscitation. 2015;94:106–13.
34. Frascone RJ, Wayne MA, Swor RA, Mahoney BD, Domeier RM, Olinger ML, et al. Treatment of non-traumatic out-of-hospital cardiac arrest with active compression decompression cardiopulmonary resuscitation plus an impedance threshold device. Resuscitation. 2013;84(9):1214–22.
35. Brooks SC, Anderson ML, Bruder E, Daya MR, Gaffney A, Otto CW, et al. Part 6: alternative techniques and ancillary devices for cardiopulmonary resuscitation: 2015 American Heart Association guidelines update for cardiopulmonary resuscitation and emergency cardiovascular care. Circulation. 2015;132(18 Suppl 2):S436–43.
36. Cao D, Arens AM, Chow SL, Easter SR, Hoffman RS, et al. Part 10: adult and pediatric special circumstances of resuscitation: 2025 American Heart Association guidelines for cardiopulmonary resuscitation and emergency cardiovascular care. Circulation. 2025;152(16_suppl_2):S578–672.
37. Joyner BL Jr, Dewan M, Bavare A, de Caen A, DiMaria K, Donofrio-Odmann J, et al. Part 6: pediatric basic life support: 2025 American Heart Association and American Academy of Pediatrics guidelines for cardiopulmonary resuscitation and emergency cardiovascular care. Circulation. 2025;152(16_suppl_2):S424–47.
38. Lasa JJ, Dhillon GS, Duff JP, Hayes J, Kamath-Rayne BD, Levy A, et al. Part 8: pediatric advanced life support: 2025 American Heart Association and American Academy of Pediatrics guidelines for cardiopulmonary resuscitation and emergency cardiovascular care. Circulation. 2025 Oct 21;152(16_suppl_2):S479–537.
39. Anez C, Becerra-Bolaños Á, Vives-Lopez A, Rodríguez-Pérez A. Cardiopulmonary resuscitation in the prone position in the operating room or in the intensive care unit: a systematic review. Anesth Analg. 2021;132(2):285–92.
40. Austin N, Krishnamoorthy V, Dagal A. Airway management in cervical spine injury. Int J Crit Illn Inj Sci. 2014;4(1):50.

41. Hsu A, Sasson C, Kudenchuk PJ, Atkins DL, Aziz K, Becker LB, et al. interim guidance to health care providers for basic and advanced cardiac life support in adults, children, and neonates with suspected or confirmed COVID-19. Circ Cardiovasc Qual Outcomes. 2021;14(10):e008396.
42. Atkins DL, Sasson C, Hsu A, Aziz K, Becker LB, Berg RA, et al. 2022 Interim guidance to health care providers for basic and advanced cardiac life support in adults, children, and neonates with suspected or confirmed COVID-19: from the emergency cardiovascular care committee and get with the guidelines-resuscitation adult and pediatric task forces of the American Heart Association in collaboration with the American Academy of Pediatrics, American Association for Respiratory Care, the Society of Critical Care Anesthesiologists, and American Society of Anesthesiologists. Circ Cardiovasc Qual Outcomes 2022 15(4):e008900.
43. Gausche M, Lewis RJ, Stratton SJ, Haynes BE, Gunter CS, Goodrich SM, et al. Effect of out-of-hospital pediatric endotracheal intubation on survival and neurological outcome. A controlled clinical trial. JAMA. 2000;283(6):783–90.
44. Pakkanen T, Nurmi J, Huhtala H, Silfvast T. Prehospital on-scene anaesthetist treating severe traumatic brain injury patients is associated with lower mortality and better neurological outcome. Scand J Trauma Resusc Emerg Med. 2019;27(1):9.
45. Lee HC, Strand ML, Finan E, Illuzzi J, Kamath-Rayne BD, Kapadia V, et al. Part 5: neonatal resuscitation: 2025 American Heart Association and American Academy of Pediatrics guidelines for cardiopulmonary resuscitation and emergency cardiovascular care. Circulation. 2025;152(16_Suppl_2):S385–423.
46. Hu KM, Hong AS. Resuscitating the crashing pregnant patient. Emerg Med Clin North Am. 2020;38(4):903–17.

Chapter 28
Documentation on Airway Management

Vassilis Athanassoglou and Rian Crandon

28.1 Introduction

Difficult airways present themselves in a variety of forms. As such, the management of each airway is dependent on the individual factors involved at that time. Each encounter brings with it a particular set of risks to the patient. For example, a difficult or failed airway is not the same as a difficult or failed intubation, and the same is true for a failed supraglottic airway and bag and mask ventilation. Documentation in these instances is crucial in mitigating future risk, as failure to effectively manage an airway not only has significant risks to the patient but also negative consequences to the airway practitioner. It is therefore vitally important to be able to not only describe and document the situation encountered, the attempts or procedures failed, and the method of successful management, but also for that information to be efficiently disseminated and accessible in the future.

The development of an effective and universally accepted airway documentation system is yet to be established, despite the global recognition of its need. As such, the method of documentation tends to be country, state, or even hospital dependent, bringing significant limitations in interpretation and access to important information that would otherwise help guide safe patient care. Critical care practitioners will likely all encounter a difficult airway at some stage in their career [1]. The definition of a difficult airway varies widely. Therefore, the reported incidence of such

V. Athanassoglou (✉)
Nuffield Department of Anaesthetics, Oxford University Hospitals, Oxford, UK
e-mail: Vassilis.Athanassoglou@ouh.nhs.uk

R. Crandon
Nuffield Department of Anaesthetics, Oxford University Hospitals, Oxford, UK

Vic Callanan Department of Anaesthetics, Townsville University Hospital, Douglas, QLD, Australia

M. Á. Gómez-Ríos, A. van Zundert (eds.), *Evidence-based Guide to Difficult Airway Management*, https://doi.org/10.1007/978-3-032-30769-9_28

an event varies depending on the definition used [2]. Difficult bag and mask ventilation is commonly reported from 0.9% to 5%, with impossible bag and mask ventilation between 0.07% and 1.4% [2–6]. Difficult supraglottic airway ventilation is quoted between 0.16% and 0.9% [7, 8] and difficult intubation is reported to be approximately 5.8% of the general population [2, 9–12]. Unanticipated difficult airway rates are reported between 1% and 3% of hospitalised patients [13–15].

With this in mind, it is the practitioner's responsibility to assess and plan patient management with a view to minimising the morbidity or even mortality from failed airway management. This inevitably involves a combination of clinical assessment of the patient, taking into account the well-documented risk factors and features associated with a difficult airway, as well as reviewing past documentation and anaesthetic history (this is covered in more detail in Chap. 5). The most accurate predictor of a difficult airway is previous difficult airway management [30, 43]. A recent publication by Sajayan et al., analysing the Difficult Airway Society (DAS) difficult airway database over a 5-year period, found that 58% of difficult airways were anticipated, and one in five patients had a history of previous or known difficult airway [30]. For this reason, access to clearly detailed documentation is essential in minimising patient risk. The consequences of failed airway management can be devastating for the patient and practitioner. One needs only to look at the well-publicised case of Elaine Bromiley seen in the United Kingdom in 2005. This case inspired the advancement of airway management algorithms and the widespread recognition of human factors influencing performance in crisis management. This chapter will endeavour to cover advances in documentation of the difficult airway and correlate current reporting systems and databases across the world.

28.2 Documentation of Airway Grade: Direct Laryngoscopy

Some of the difficulty in airway management documentation comes about from technological advances and uncertainty in describing practices. Cormack and Lehane defined laryngoscopy in terms of the best view of the glottis during conventional laryngoscopy and direct view (including the use of external laryngeal manipulation). This grading system is well known and established in airway management and documentation, with grades one through to four [16]. These grades were subsequently further modified, firstly by Yentis and Lee in 1998 and then by Cook in 2000, to divide grades 2 and 3 into "a" and "b" divisions (see Fig. 28.1). This is now known as the Modified Cormack and Lehane (CL) Classification [17, 18]. Although the CL classification was not intended to be used in this way, these grades correlate well with the likelihood of intubation failure, with grade 1 having less than 1% possibility of failure and grade 4 being very likely to fail intubation [17, 60]. Documentation in this way has been long established with clear interpretation (see Table 28.1 for the table of grades).

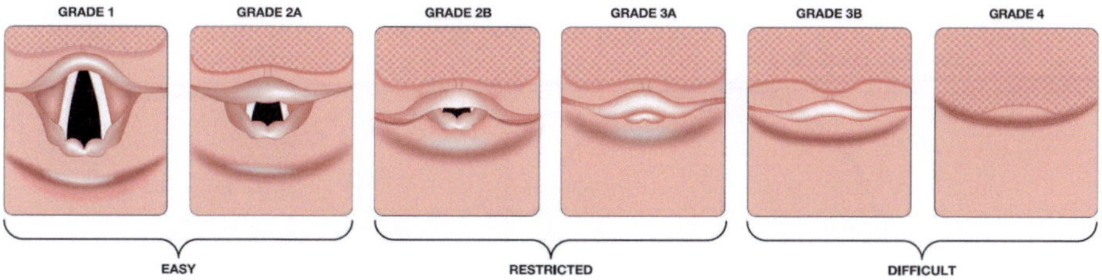

Fig. 28.1 Modified Cormack-Lehane view (author owned)

Table 28.1 Correlation between Cormack-Lehane view and intubation failure [17, 60].

Classification	Description	FREQ (%)	Possibility of intubation failure (%)
Grade 1	Full view of the glottis	68	<1
Grade 2a	Partial view of the glottis	24	4.3
Grade 2b	Only posterior portion of glottis or arytenoid cartilages	6.5	67.4
Grade 3a	Epiglottis **can** be lifted from the posterior pharyngeal wall	1.2	87.5
Grade 3b	Epiglottis **cannot** be lifted from the posterior pharyngeal wall	Very rare	Very likely
Grade 4	Neither glottis or epiglottis can be seen	Very rare	Very likely

Table adapted from Yentis et al. (1998), and ANZCA Airway Assessment (2016)

An alternative description to the modified Cormack-Lehane views was put forward by Levitan in 1998 [19, 20]. This system describes the laryngeal view in terms of the percentage of visible glottic opening (POGO). A score of 0% when none of the glottis is seen to 100% POGO score, which corresponds to visualisation of the entire glottic opening from the anterior commissure of the vocal cords to the inter-arytenoid notch between the posterior cartilages (see Fig. 28.2). The idea was that this system could be used in both direct and indirect laryngoscopy. In multiple studies from 1999 through to 2014 POGO has demonstrated improved inter-rater reliability compared to CL views [19, 20]. This feature is vitally important in documentation, as it means different operators are similarly describing the same conditions [19, 20]. Despite its advantages, the POGO system has not been widely adopted for direct laryngoscopy and has significant limitations when used alone for videolaryngoscopy. For example, a 100% view of the larynx with videolaryngoscopy does not translate to an easy intubation, and gives little information on the degree of difficulty and equipment required throughout the intubating process [26]. This poses a significant risk of misinterpretation and potentially false reassurance to an airway practitioner.

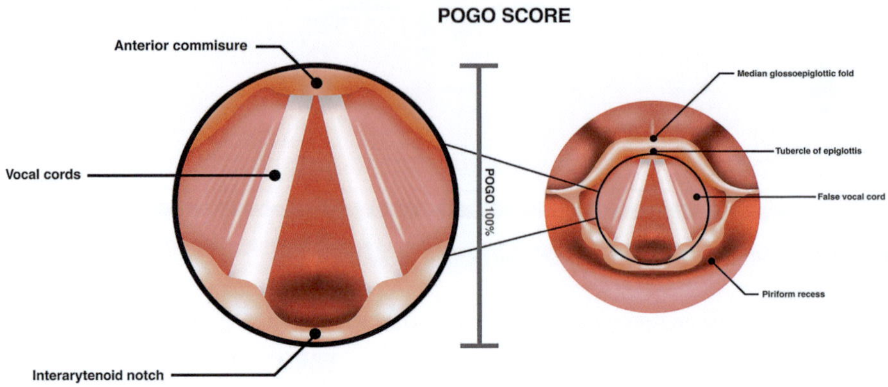

Fig. 28.2 Anatomy of the glottis in relation to POGO Score (author owned)

28.3 Documentation of Airway Grade: Videolaryngoscopy

The advancement of technology has led to improved patient safety in airway management. One such tool is the addition of videolaryngoscopy into the anaesthetic arsenal. Videolaryngoscopy is now widely available and in many parts of the world considered standard for every anaesthetic requiring intubation [21–24]. Furthermore, it is now recommended to be a routine part of airway management in the 2022 Universal Management of Airways Guidelines [27]. Despite the widespread use, however, there is a lack of clarity on how to clearly and accurately document airway difficulty when videolaryngoscopy is used. The issue is, videolaryngoscopy, unlike direct laryngoscopy, can create a situation where the view of the glottis is good, but intubation is difficult or impossible. Therefore, there is little value in describing the view of the glottis alone [26]. To date, a clear and robust classification and documentation tool for videolaryngoscopy is yet to be widely adopted into clinical practice [23–25]. Several systems have been proposed, including the Fremantle Videolaryngoscopy Score and, more recently, the Video Classification of Intubation (VCI) score [23, 29].

The Fremantle Videolaryngoscope Scoring system is a system proposed in 2012 by Swann and colleagues from Perth, Western Australia. It is a three-part system encompassing view, ease, and device (see Fig. 28.3). It was proposed as a simple, informative and reproducible score [25, 26, 28]. A score for the best laryngeal view obtained (with or without laryngeal manipulation) is described as full (F), partial (P), no view (N). A numerical score for the ease of use is described as 1 (easy, passed first time), 2 (modified, more than one attempt or required the use of an adjunct), 3 (unachievable). Lastly, the name of the specific device and blade is recorded [28]. The validity of the Fremantle Score for videolaryngoscopy was assessed in 2017 by O'Loughlin and colleagues, and demonstrated an accuracy of 73.9%, which was superior to CL views and comparable to POGO. Fremantle Score inter-rater reliability was also superior to the CL scoring system [26, 28]. Despite

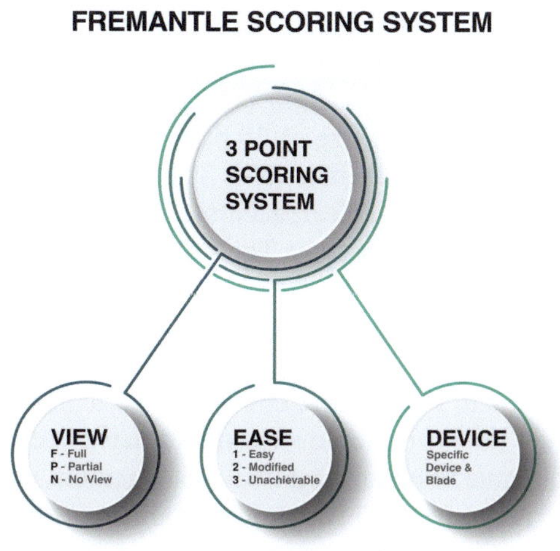

Fig. 28.3 The Fremantle scoring system (author owned)

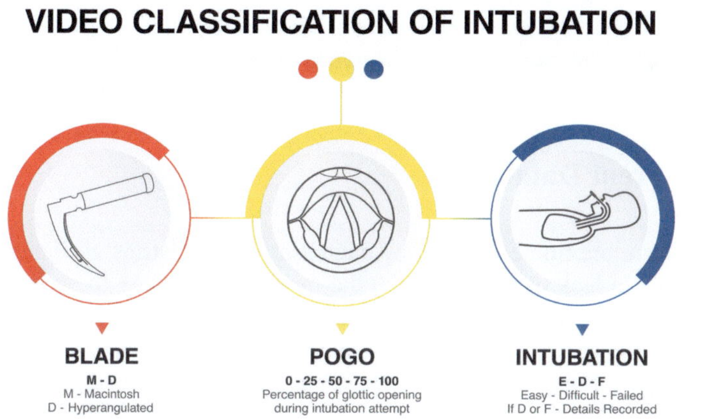

Fig. 28.4 VCI scoring system (author owned)

the potential noted in the Fremantle Score, its use in worldwide clinical practice remains limited.

The Video Classification of Intubation (VCI) score was developed in 2021 and, similar to the Fremantle Score, incorporates three components (see Fig. 28.4) [26, 28, 29]. Firstly, the type and shape of the videolaryngoscope blade used, Macintosh (M) or hyperangulated (D). Next, the percentage of glottic opening (POGO) is recorded as 0, 25, 50, 75, or 100%, but specifically at the moment of tracheal intubation. Lastly, the ease of tracheal intubation is described as easy (E), difficult (D), or failed (F). An easy intubation is one requiring no modifications, a difficult intubation requires modification of the tracheal tube, and a failed intubation is an unsuccessful attempt despite the use of extra equipment and modifications [29]. These three components are combined to provide a final score or description. In the instance of a failed intubation, it is recommended that a further and more detailed description be provided in the patient's notes. The VCI score has been validated in a small pilot study in manikins using a range of videolaryngoscope devices. Reproducibility in adult human subjects was also assessed over a 3-month period, where a sample size of 35 patients demonstrated 97.1% congruency in VCI scores from 58 anaesthetists [29]. The VCI score has shown promising results thus far, demonstrating a clear, accurate, easily interpreted, and reproducible scoring system for videolaryngoscopy. The VCI potentially has some advantages over the Fremantle Score. Firstly, the VCI doesn't require a device name and has been shown to be consistent among a range of videolaryngoscope devices. Secondly, the VCI incorporates POGO into the score, which provides a quantitative description of the view obtained. This feature could be used to assess disease progression and show a trend over time if multiple anaesthetics have occurred. This information would be highly valuable in planning airway management in patients with known pathology.

Although VCI has shown promising results, a larger cohort, multi-centre study is required to further assess its use, and will require comparison with other scoring systems such as the Fremantle Score. The incorporation of the VCI score into widespread clinical practice, however, is a valid option that could help to improve documentation, communication, and subsequently improve patient safety.

28.4 Current Databases

Currently, there are numerous airway databases and registries available across the world. Despite a lack of consensus on the most efficient way to establish, format, and run such a database, there seems to be a trend towards establishing national and international integration [31]. This, although difficult to achieve, has obvious benefits towards achieving the common goal of improving patient safety and furthering epidemiological and etiologic research. With these goals in mind, difficult airway databases can be divided into 3 broad types: (1) patient protective; (2) epidemiological and etiologic databases; and (3) combined patient protective, epidemiological, and etiologic databases (see Fig. 28.5) [31]. The particular use and functionality of

Fig. 28.5 Types of airway databases (author owned)

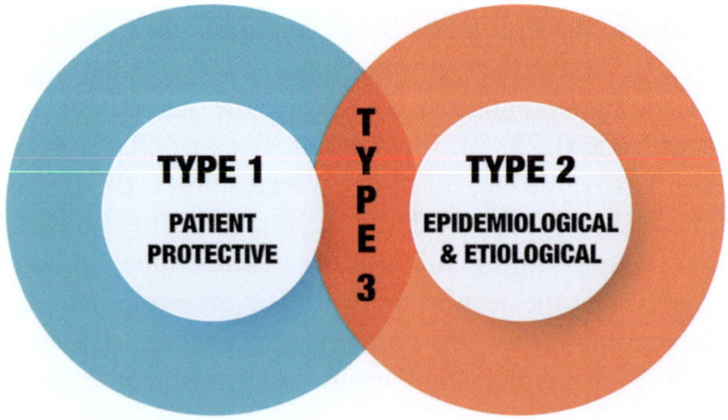

the database is determined by several factors, including the parameters recorded in the databank, the denominator of the total number of airway management occurrences (essential for assessment of incidence and prevalence), and the timeframe of data collection (prescribed or ongoing) [31]. We have reviewed the major difficult airway databases in use across the world and have grouped them according to the previously mentioned database taxonomy. We will discuss the main features and utility of each, although this is by no means an exhaustive list.

28.5 Type 1: Patient Protective Difficult Airway Database

A patient protective difficult airway database is established with the goal to protect individual patients during their hospital stay and provide information for future care [31]. In its basic form, anaesthetic departments and hospitals have been recording this information for local use for decades. Over time, this effort has grown to become a more formalised process with comprehensive records and incorporated alerts into patient records. These local alert systems have subsequently evolved into a general movement towards widespread, statewide, or even national integration systems providing up-to-date patient information. They do, however, lack the capacity for epidemiological and etiological research.

28.5.1 Queensland Difficult Airway Alert Project

Australia, like the rest of the world, has recognised the utility and need for a national integrated airway database; however, this has so far fallen short in its development. There have been multiple attempts over the years to develop such a system, however issues such as the strict privacy laws around the storage of medical information, the cost to run such a database, a differing in goals and agenda of lobbying groups (including consensus on the airway information collected), and the ability to make this information accessible across various health jurisdictions has to date made this unfeasible. Striving towards this goal regardless is an important step for both patient safety and advancement of airway research [43]. The Queensland Statewide Anaesthesia and Perioperative Care Clinical Network (SWAPNET) group has been working towards the development of a patient-protective statewide airway database, with a long-term view of expanding this to a national database [40]. With no easy solution to these difficulties in sight, the focus in Australia seems to have changed from developing a national database to developing consistency in reporting practices. This has led to the initiation of the Queensland Difficult Airway Alert Project.

The Queensland Difficult Airway Alert Project is endorsed by the Australian New Zealand College of Anaesthetists (ANZCA) and the Australian Society of Anaesthetists as the standard of care for how and when reporting of a difficult airway should occur and an alert be generated. It is essentially a project established to standardise the recording of difficult airways in Queensland, following a number of airway-related events in both public and private facilities. It incorporates the standardisation of the definition of difficult airway, development of a website, information and guidance on when an airway alert should be generated, standardisation of a difficult airways alert form and guidance on how it can be disseminated. A significant amount of work has gone into adjusting and standardising the language used in the systematised nomenclature of medicine clinical terms (SNOMED). This has allowed the incorporation of the difficult airway alert into the electronic patient record as of 2019. This ensures a generated airway alert will be flagged on the electronic patient record when an encounter for that patient is created, in any public facility statewide. Furthermore, SWAPNET is engaged in ongoing consultation with the Australian Digital Health Agency, with a plan to incorporate the airway alert into the national "My Health Record" system [40].

This is undoubtedly a positive step in patient safety; however, significant limitations remain. Firstly, the nature of public and private institutions in Australia limits accessibility. Not only are the public and private sectors not linked from a patient information point of view, but they also differ in the systems utilised to store patient records. So, a patient who has had an alert generated in a public hospital will not have that information available in any private setting. Secondly, there are differences between states and the information systems are again not connected. An individual who has had an anaesthetic in one state will not have that information available to anaesthetists who may be treating them in the future in another state. So, dissemination of information will remain a major issue until a national database can be created.

28.5.2 Veterans Affairs Healthcare System

In 2002, the Department of Veterans Affairs (VA) in the United States (US), launched the Department of Veterans Affairs Emergency Airway Management Initiative following the finding that 11,000 times per year within the US VA Hospitals, an emergency airway management event occurs outside of the operating theatre [39]. A survey was sent to all 163 VA Hospitals, receiving an 83% response rate. Respondents estimated that 12.3% of intubations in the VA Hospitals were unusually difficult to accomplish, and 6.5% of total intubations resulted in inadvertent oesophageal intubation. This equated to nearly four cases per day that were difficult and 2 cases per day that resulted in oesophageal intubation. After reviewing these results, the VA embarked on a national initiative to improve the standard of care with regard to airway management.

This initiative was then followed up in 2012 with the creation of the Out of Operating Room Airway Management Directive (VHA Directive 2012–032). This directive encompassed a comprehensive set of airway management standards and included guidelines stating that all VA hospitals must have a plan for the management of a known or emergent difficult airway, and a process for the dissemination of this information to patients involved. These guidelines were generalised, and the implementation of these guidelines was left to the individual VA hospital. The directive has since been updated in 2018 (VHA Directive 1157(1)) and now includes an updated Difficult Airway Algorithm and Rescue Cricothyrotomy (DAARC) plan, mandatory credentialing for those involved in airway management, and standardised documentation of those patients with difficult airways using the National Difficult Airway Template in the Computerised Patient Record System. This will subsequently appear in the patient's record and problem list for future rapid identification. The alert, once generated, will be visible in all VA hospitals due to the presence of a nationally integrated computerised Patient Record System.

28.6 Type 2: Epidemiological and Etiologic Difficult Airway Database

These databases are established for the purpose of furthering epidemiological and etiological research into difficult airways. It is a database for ongoing collection and anonymised data with a view to identifying the epidemiology of difficult airways and causative factors. It lacks real-time access for anaesthetists to search patients and obtain individualised difficult airway information.

28.6.1 National Audit Project 4 (NAP4)

The largest airway audit conducted, addressing major airway complications, the National Audit Project 4 (NAP4), was released in 2011. Data on adverse events were collected for a year between September 2008 and September 2009 [62]. NAP4 was a joint project between the Difficult Airway Society (DAS) and the Royal College of Anaesthetists. NAP4 was conducted to address poor understanding in the anaesthetic community of: (1) how frequently airway complications occur; (2) what is the nature of these complications; (3) how often do major complications lead to serious harm; and (4) whether these serious airway events are preventable. Data were collected prospectively on patients in whom airway management complications resulted in death, brain damage, emergency surgical airway/cricothyroidotomy, or unanticipated ICU admission [32–34]. Despite the prescribed timeframe of data collection being limited, the snapshot provided resulted in a large-scale re-examination of current practices in anaesthesia, emergency departments, and intensive care units across the UK and internationally [35]. The report led to over 160 recommendations designed to improve patient care [34, 35]. A follow-up survey conducted from 2013 to 2014, including 175 UK hospitals, demonstrated 95% anaesthetic, 80% of intensive care, and 59% of emergency department respondents reported changes to individual or institutional practice within a 2-year period after NAP 4 release [61]. Given that previous studies have reported an approximately 17-year time requirement for research to lead to significant changes in clinical practice, NAP 4 appears to have had a considerable impact on clinical practice in a short period of time [35, 36]. Over a decade has passed now since the release of NAP4, with the implementation of recommendations and changes in standard practice. Further evaluation assessing the ongoing impact on airway management and event rate would be an interesting follow-up audit.

28.6.2 Web-Based Anaesthetic Incident Reporting System (WebAIRS): —Australia and New Zealand

WebAIRS is an Internet-based voluntary de-identified anaesthetic incident recording system used by anaesthetists in Australia and New Zealand. It is owned and funded by three organisations: the Australian and New Zealand College of Anaesthetists (ANZCA), the Australian Society of Anaesthetists, and the New Zealand Society of Anaesthetists. The system has been in operation since 2009, allowing registered anaesthetists across Australia and New Zealand to report incidents via the webpage (www.anztadc.net). All anaesthesia-related incidents are recorded via a tick box and text format, allowing description of the incident and reflection on contributing and mitigating factors [55]. Airway management incidents are also included in this database. In 2020, a study was released analysing airway events in the first 4000 incidents reported in WebAIRS. The publication demonstrated risk factors including BMI over 30 $kg/m^{2,}$ undergoing emergency procedures, and human factors such as poor communication, lack of pre-operative assessment and planning [55]. An audit released in the same year, utilising a specifically designed WebAIRS portal, assessed airway incidents across 12 tertiary hospitals throughout Australia and New Zealand, collecting prospective data from April to October 2018. This audit further backed the previous findings and provided an up-to-date snapshot of airway events in typical Australian and New Zealand hospitals [56]. Following this, there has been an ongoing effort to improve the ease of access to medical information, preoperative assessments, preparation, and the execution of difficult airway management plans in Australia and New Zealand.

The database provides an easy and accessible means of incident reporting and the maintenance of anonymity. The primary limitation of this database is difficulty in accurately collecting a denominator, and the numerator data are submitted voluntarily, thereby prohibiting absolute risk calculations [55, 56]. The database also does not provide a means of accessing patient-specific difficult airway information.

28.6.3 Anaesthesia Quality Institute: Anaesthesia Incident Reporting System

The Anaesthesia Incident Reporting System (AIRS) is a database established in the United States by the Anaesthesia Quality Institute (AQI). It is a database that records all anaesthesia, pain management, and perioperative care-related incidents, including those related to airway management. AIRS is an online reporting tool allowing for either anonymous or confidential (sender information retained) reporting. The data collated are incorporated into the National Anaesthesia Clinical Outcomes Registry which includes more than 22 million cases [31]. The goal of AIRS is to collect and analyse anaesthesia-related incidents in order to improve the quality of anaesthetic care nationwide. The database provides a powerful source for airway research; however, it lacks the capacity for storage of individual patient information.

28.6.4 National Emergency Airway Registry and National Emergency Airway Registry for Children

The National Emergency Airway Registry (NEAR) was developed and coordinated by the Department of Emergency Medicine at Brigham and Women's Hospital in Boston, Massachusetts in 1998. It is a multi-centre observational intubation registry prospectively collecting emergency department intubation data from 26 locations. Data is entered via a web-based system through a standardised data collection form. Patients are deidentified and information is accessible to participating hospitals for analysis and publication purposes. The database is incapable of real-time access for information on individual patient airway management; however, it does collect information on all intubations, so it is one of the few databases capable of analysing incidence and prevalence of airway events [31]. Currently, the database has over 19,000 emergency department intubations and has produced several publications aiming to improve emergency department and prehospital airway management [49–54].

Following the development of NEAR, the NEAR for children, termed NEAR4KIDS, was developed. This is again a multi-centre prospective database focussed on paediatric airway management in paediatric intensive care units, with a primary goal of improving advanced airway management for critically ill children. The project has now grown to consist of 22 participating centres in North America [62].

28.6.5 American Society of Anaesthesiologists Closed Claims Project

The American Society of Anaesthesiologists (ASA) Closed Claims Project is an extremely well-known and established research database in operation [31]. The project was initially established due to rapidly escalating personal liability insurance premiums, with anaesthesiologists being considered "high" insurance risk [46]. Since its development in 1985, the group has analysed anaesthesia-related events resulting in completed legal claims in the United States [31, 44, 46]. It is a structured evaluation of adverse anaesthetic outcomes obtained from the closed claims files of 20 US insurance carriers [41]. Although the time from adverse event to mitigation of risk is long, the results obtained from the Closed Claims Project have had a profound positive impact on improving safe practice and understanding hazards in anaesthesia [31, 41, 45]. Data collection encompasses a wide range of anaesthetic events, with part of the data including difficult intubation. In 2019, a paper was released analysing 11,034 cases from 2000–2012 [42, 46]. Data included the type of surgery, details of anaesthetic care, patient demographics, outcomes, legal proceedings, and payments made [42]. 93 claims were found to have difficult intubation as the primary damaging event. Outcomes in these claims were poor with a high proportion of death claims relating to a difficult airway [42]. Despite such work, the value in this context is limited. This is due to the inherent bias where the data collected only includes those with negative outcomes (morbidity or mortality) as a result of failed or inadequate ventilation that resulted in legal contest [31]. The data utilised provides a quantitative appreciation for the severity and cost of claims for rare adverse respiratory events; however, it lacks inclusion of all airway events [46]. Absence of a denominator makes analysis of the incidence or prevalence of difficult airway and adverse respiratory events impossible. Furthermore, in most instances, the details provided in the case notes were inadequate to ascertain the primary cause of the event, leading to some ambiguity in the data [41, 31].

The limitations aside, the work done by the Closed Claims Project has certainly led to improvements in anaesthetic practice. This is seen as a general trend towards a reduction in the severity of injury in anaesthesia malpractice claims over the past 30 years, suggesting a significant improvement in anaesthesia safety [46].

28.7 Type 3: Combined Patient-Protective, Epidemiological, and Etiologic Difficult Airway Database

Combined databases are the most valuable, but labour-intensive and difficult to establish. They incorporate both the goals of improving patient safety by being an accessible database for anaesthetists and airway practitioners to access clinical information on their patients, but also provide a means of ongoing data collection for difficult airway research and analysis, leading to improvements in the field of difficult airway management.

28.7.1 DAS Airway Alert Card and Difficult Airway Database Project

The Difficult Airways Society (DAS) alert card and difficult airway database project was established as a pilot in 2016 and formalised in 2018. It is a streamlined national difficult airway reporting system aimed at improving recording and dissemination of difficult airway information to patients, GP's, and future airway practitioners

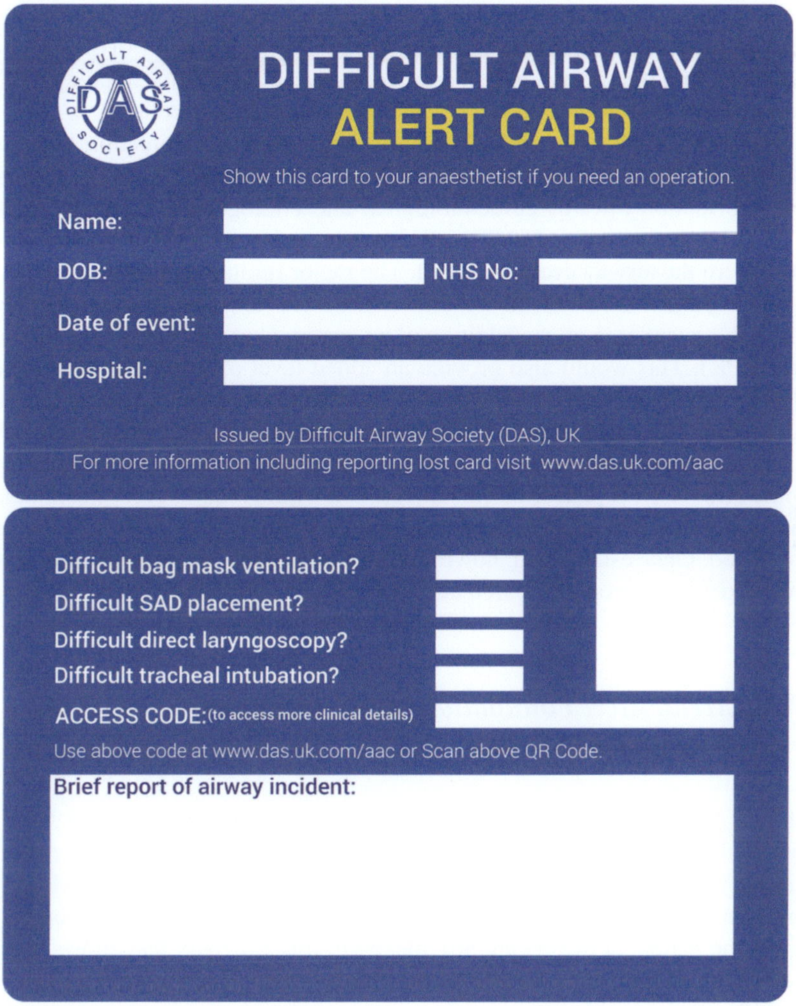
DIFFICULT AIRWAY SOCIETY
DAS
DIFFICULT AIRWAY
ALERT CARD
Show this card to your anaesthetist if you need an operation.
Name:
DOB:
NHS No:
Date of event:
Hospital:
Issued by Difficult Airway Society (DAS), UK
For more information including reporting lost card visit www.das.uk.com/aac
Difficult bag mask ventilation?
Difficult SAD placement?
Difficult direct laryngoscopy?
Difficult tracheal intubation?
ACCESS CODE:(to access more clinical details)
Use above code at www.das.uk.com/aac or Scan above QR Code.
Brief report of airway incident:

Fig. 28.6 Difficult Airway Alert Card. Reproduced from the Difficult Airway Society, DAS Airway Alert Card

alike. Patients involved in a difficult airway scenario are entered into a national database. The patient subsequently receives an "airway alert" card free of charge from DAS (see Fig. 28.6). This card can then be presented to the anaesthetist involved in any future anaesthetic. Each individual entered into the database receives an individual code that can be entered into the Internet accessible database, allowing the anaesthetist to access information pertaining to the patient's airway history. The patient information can also be searched using their NHS number (linked to the DAS code), which is also included in the registry. This is useful for circumstances where the patient has not brought the DAS alert card and code with them, but the anaesthetist is suspicious of a previous difficult airway event. The database is divided into two divisions, one containing patient identification that is stored by DAS offline, and the second, which is an anonymised version for ongoing data collection and research purposes.

This system, although in its infancy, is a step in the right direction towards the ideal database. It covers both improving patient safety and allows for the use of stored information towards epidemiological and etiological research. It is also a national database, meaning that this information can be accessed in any hospital, no matter where the airway event occurred. The major limitation, however, is the reliance on the patient to inform the anaesthetist of a previous airway event. This could be somewhat overcome by the addition of an airway alert into the electronic patient record (EPR). This would also provide an added level of safety for out-of-theatre locations such as the emergency department and the intensive care unit, flagging a difficult airway to practitioners as soon as a patient encounter is created. DAS is currently engaged in discussion with NHS Digital, with a view to incorporating this database into the EPR platform. This integration would require every hospital in the NHS to have a compatible electronic patient record in operation, which to date has not occurred. Once established, however, this system will prove a powerful tool for improved patient care and research alike.

28.7.2 MedicAlert Foundation: Difficult Airway/ Intubation Registry

The MedicAlert Foundation is a 501(c) nonprofit organisation started in 1956 by Dr. Marion Collins. MedicAlert innovated a national and international emergency medical identification emblem and 24-h emergency response system. The MedicAlert Foundation is a system patients join for an annual premium that needs to be covered by either the patient or healthcare provider [40]. It is a registry that allows updating of medical information and is easily accessible by medical professionals in an emergency [47]. Patients added to the registry are issued a MedicAlert bracelet or Smart ID (QR coded), identifying the individual as a member of the database. The database can then be accessed either via phone or by scanning the QR code present. The foundation was endorsed by the American Society of Anaesthesiologists in 1979, the World Federation of Societies of Anaesthesiologists in 1992, and the American Academy of Otolaryngology-Head and Neck Surgeons in 1993 [31]. In 1992, an Anaesthesia Advisory council consisting of anaesthetists, otolaryngologists and safety and risk management experts joined with MedicAlert Foundation to create the MedicAlert National Registry for Difficult Airway/Intubation, with a mission of (1) standardising documentation and dissemination of critical airway information, (2) establishing a database to store and transmit protected patient information (nationally and internationally), and (3) analyse the accumulated data to assess the effect of such a system on clinical outcomes and healthcare costs [31].

Between 1992 and 2014, there were nearly 12,000 enrolments in the difficult airway registry. In 2004, 113 patients who were mailed a post-operative difficult airway letter between 2000 and 2002 were surveyed. 41% of patients reported informing their primary care provider about the difficult airway. 92% of those who had undergone subsequent surgery reported informing their anaesthesiologist about their airway event. 23% had registered with MedicAlert Foundation. It therefore seems that the difficult airway alert letters have significant positive utility even if they did not lead to the patient obtaining an alert bracelet [48]. In a comprehensive preliminary survey of patient enrolments from 1992–2014, from all 50 states in the United States, approximately 12% of enrolments included "Dear Patient" letters from their health care providers. Review of these letters identified 3 categories of information. (1) generic difficult airway/intubation alert only, (2) generic difficult airway/intubation alert supplemented with database elements describing the nature of the event, (3) either category one or two with scanned original documents from the patient's medical record [31]. In response to this, in 2014, the Society for Airway Management MedicAlert Task Force updated the National Difficult Airway/Intubation registry form. Health care providers from any background or location can now access a web-based system and provide up-to-date documentation on airway factors, management, and outcomes [31]. The practitioner can either download the registry and complete it, giving a copy to the patient, or assist the patient in registering online. All information is stored securely and available for access by both the patient and practitioner.

This database is a well-designed tool for providing and disseminating airway management information. It has global, international access that is rapid and easily achievable. It is simple to update, keeping patient information current. The major limitations of MedicAlert include the cost of registration, which, although small, will limit patients from registering, and secondly, it requires the patient to actively register themselves and flag registration to their practitioner.

28.8 Clinical Practices

28.8.1 What Information to Include

In 2003, the American Society of Anaesthesiologists (ASA) published practice guidelines for the management of the difficult airway, which included the development of an airway management algorithm. A year later, in 2004, the Difficult Airway Society in the UK released their own version and guidelines, and in 2013, the Vortex approach was released in Australia [37]. Since this time, difficult airway management has evolved significantly, reflecting advances in knowledge and technology, and has subsequently led to multiple guideline updates, with the most recent being the DAS in 2015 and ASA in 2022 [38]. Irrespective of the society creating and releasing them, all guidelines present a common theme of attempting to standardise airway management, minimise task fixation, improve non-technical skills such as communication and recognition of the importance of human factors. Communication in difficult airway scenarios is certainly not limited to the event. Post-event documentation, dissemination of information, and communication with the patient and relevant healthcare professionals are just as important. Description and communication of the difficult airway event, both successful and unsuccessful strategies, provides valuable information for future airway practitioners to assess and plan safe and effective airway management. With the importance of this in mind, what exactly should be documented? Is there consensus, and is the description and language used important?

It is well documented that effective communication is a core non-technical skill that contributes to risk minimisation [57]. Standardised language and communication strategies, including terms or phrases with clear, mutually agreed meaning, termed "critical language" when employed in healthcare settings, reduce ambiguity, reduce errors, and facilitate a shared mental model [58]. This has been well established in relation to acute crisis management, but can easily be extrapolated to documentation post-event also. This mentality has led to a push by many groups to standardise difficult airway documentation, leading to practice guidelines and standardised forms being created from the ASA, ANZCA Airway Management Special Interest Group, and DAS, among others.

Although priorities and recommendations differ amongst groups, the recorded information is generally some combination of the following list:

1. Date of airway event.
2. Institution and location.
3. Practitioner identity and contact information.
4. Demographic information of the patient: airway examination, body mass index, co-morbidities.
5. Description of the difficulty encountered: including techniques attempted and success of each (bag and mask ventilation, supraglottic airways, intubation, and best view).
6. Recommendations and implications for future airway management.
7. Follow-up plan: patient discussion, dissemination of information, local alert, difficult airway database.

In the United States, the updated ASA difficult airway guidelines (2022) recommend the documentation of an encountered difficult airway, including the nature, reasons for difficulty, how intubation was achieved and the implications for patient care. This should be included in the patient's anaesthetic chart and medical record to guide and facilitate future care [38]. In Australia, the ANZCA Airway Management Special Interest Group has created a standardised Difficult Airway Alert form which includes a supporting document containing a glossary of terms (see Figs. 28.7 and 28.8 below). It defines terms such as difficult airway, grading of direct and videolaryngoscopy, and when to use a difficult airway alert. The alert form is a combination of a tick box and text that allows for a detailed description of the event. It includes information, including the date, nature of the surgery (emergency or elective), direct and videolaryngoscopy grade, and procedures attempted. This document also

Queensland Government

Difficult Airway Alert

Support document and glossary of terms

The *Difficult Airway Alert* form has been developed with the intention of being a concise and effective communication tool regarding a difficult airway event, in order to reduce the risk of future airway morbidity in at risk patients.

The need to balance level of detail with simplicity must be recognised. This form does not take the place of a detailed pre-anaesthetic airway assessment.

This support document is intended to complement the form and clarify potential areas of confusion.

Airway Management

Difficult airway	
The term "Difficult Airway" refers to the presence of any clinically significant threat to oxygenation and/or ventilation with difficulty in any of the key domains of airway management. That is, difficult or impossible bag-mask ventilation, supraglottic airway insertion, tracheal intubation or front of neck access[1,2].	
Bag mask ventilation (BMV)	
BMV can be graded objectively by its outcome on the capnograph[3]. Record the subjective feel of mask ventilation as Easy, Difficult or Impossible and grade the capnograph (A–D). Finally, document airway adjuncts and manoeuvres utilised to achieve the best capnograph, and whether or not muscle relaxant was used.	
Supraglottic airway (SGA) ventilation	
Consider describing difficulty with placing the device(s) as well as adequacy of ventilation.	
Easy	Placement of and adequate ventilation via SGA possible with first or second selected device
Difficult	SGA ventilation clinically inadequate* or unstable despite use of two or more different devices
Impossible	Unable to place or ventilate via SGA device
*Clinically adequate ventilation: greater than 7ml. kg-1 oropharyngeal leak pressure of greater than 20cm H_2O[1,4]	
Tracheal intubation	
Easy	Direct intubation achieved easily
Difficult	Intubation required multiple attempts or additional equipment
Impossible	Intubation failed
Neuromuscular blockade	
The use of neuromuscular blockade is an integral component of airway management. Document the elements of airway management for which muscle relaxant was used.	

Bag mask ventilation

Best capnograph achieved:

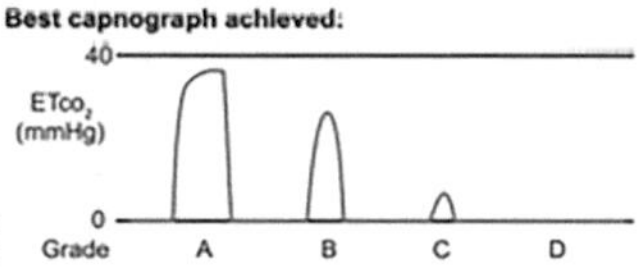

Image 1: Grading mask ventilation best capnograph
(Adapted from Lim & Nielsen. Br J Anaesth. 2016;117(6):828-9)

Grade A: plateau present
Grade B: no plateau, $ETco_2$ ≥10mmHg
Grade C: no plateau, $ETco_2$ <10mmHg
Grade D: no $ETco_2$

How this was achieved:
1 hand for mask
2 hands for mask
Oropharyngeal airway
Nasopharyngeal airway
Neuromuscular blocker

SW885

Department of Health — Difficult Airway Alert Support document v2.00 06/2021 Page 1 of 2

Fig. 28.7 QLD health glossary of terms, Australia

includes a specification of a follow-up plan: whether the patient has been alerted and a letter of the incident provided, a copy of the letter has been sent to the patient's General Practitioner, inclusion in the patient notes and electronic record, and inclusion in the anaesthetic department or relevant database.

Direct laryngoscopy

Grades 1 to 4 refer to the view as described by Cormack & Lehane[5]. Where possible, please also refer to modified categorisation as described by Cook[6].

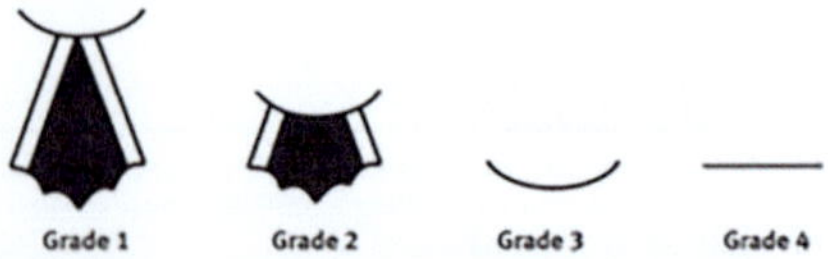

Image 2: Cormack and Lehane views (Clinical Excellence Division, Queensland Health 2018[7])

Modified C&L grade	Description	Direct laryngoscopy was
1	Most of cords visible	Easy
2a	Posterior part of cords visible	Easy
2b	Arytenoids only visible	Restricted
3a	Epiglottis visible and liftable	Restricted
3b	Epiglottis visible and adherent	Difficult
4	No laryngeal structures visualised	Difficult

Adapted from Cook. Anaesthesia. 1999; 54(5):496–7.

Videolaryngoscopy

The percentage of glottic opening (POGO) score represents the portion of the glottis visualised, having a linear span from the anterior commissure to the Interarytenoid notch[8].

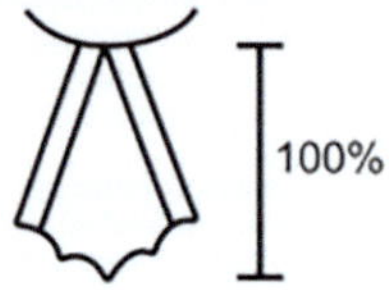

Image 3: POGO score 100% (Levitan et al. Anaesthesia. 1999; 54(10)1009–10)

Can I record my airway assessment?

Patient features contributing to difficulty (e.g. syndromes/ anatomical abnormalities) should be recorded in the free-text section addressing whether or not airway difficulty was predicted. A dedicated area to record airway assessment has not been included as this should be apparent when conducting a pre-operative airway assessment. Any conditions that are reversible or not obvious should be documented.

When should I use a Difficult Airway Alert?

Reason to report should include any clinically significant threat to the maintenance of oxygenation and/or ventilation. Consider the following suggested indications for providing an Alert.

Suggested indications for providing a Difficult Airway Alert

- Difficult or impossible **direct laryngoscopy:**
  - C&L 4
  - C&L 3 with difficulty passing ETT
- Difficult or impossible **videolaryngoscopy:**
  - POGO 0% or difficulty passing ETT
- Impossible **bag-mask ventilation**
- Impossible **supraglottic airway device** placement
- Any airway difficulty requiring awakening the patient and subsequent awake intubation
- Any 'cannot intubate, cannot oxygenate' events with or without emergency front of neck access
- Any permanent space-occupying lesions or barriers with the potential risk of airway obstruction[9]
- Patients where an awake intubation technique was required as the primary airway management plan

References:

1. Bradley P, et al. Airway Assessment. ANZCA, 2016. www.anzca.edu.au/getattachment/effa2b5d-46cf-46db-95ef-5e65ecb88c26/PU-Airway-Assessment-20160916v1
2. Baker P, et al. How do anaesthetists in New Zealand disseminate critical airway information? Anaesth Intensive Care 2013; 41:334–41
3. Lim, K & Nielsen, J. Objective description of mask ventilation. Br J Anaesth 2016;117(6):828–9
4. Kumar, CM et al. Time to consider supraglottic airway device oropharyngeal leak pressure measurement more objectively. Acta Anaesthesiol Scand 2021;65:142-5
5. Cormack R & Lehane J. Difficult tracheal intubation in obstetrics. Anaesthesia. 1984; 39(11):1105–11
6. Cook T. A grading system for direct laryngoscopy. Anaesthesia. 1999; 54(5):496–7
7. Clinical Excellence Division, Queensland Health 2018
8. Levitan R et al. A grading system for direct laryngoscopy. Anaesthesia. 1999; 54(10):1009–10
9. Shaeuble J & Ganter M. Clarifying the indications for difficult airway alert forms. Anaesthesia. 2015; 70(4):505–6

Acknowledgement:

The SWAPNet Steering Committee would like to acknowledge the Royal Brisbane and Women's Hospital Anaesthetic Department for providing the original draft of the DAA form and the commitment and significant efforts of the DAA and DAA Review Working Group members including Drs Elizabeth McLellan and Jane Elms (Co-Chairs), Linda Beckmann, Alexander Cottle, Christopher Stonell, Nicole Fairweather, James Hosking, Stacey Swinkels and Christina Hansson (The Viewer), Jenny Cooper (Digital) and Karen Hamilton (SWAPNet Coordinator). The SWAPNet Steering Committee would also like to thank anaesthetists from across the public and private sectors for their input and Drs Pierre Bradley and Kar-Soon Lim for their expertise and advice.

Department of Health Difficult Airway Alert Support document v2.00 06/2021 Page 2 of 2

Fig. 28.8 QLD health difficult airway alert form, Australia

28.9 Hospital Documentation

28.9.1 The Anaesthetic Record and Patient Chart

The primary goal of difficult airway documentation is to provide relevant information for future airway practitioners to make a safe and educated airway plan, minimising patient risk. This means the presence of a difficult airway should be clearly and accurately depicted in both the patient's anaesthetic record and as a separate entry in the patient's hospital chart. In modern days, this would include the electronic patient record (EPR) in many facilities. One of the main strengths of the electronic patient record is the ability to produce a separate "airway alert," which can be either highlighted on the EPR main page or may be included in the patient's "problems list," depending on the type of software utilised. This provides an added margin of safety, highlighting the patient's difficult airway history without having to sift through individual patient notes. One difficulty in written documentation in the anaesthetic chart and patient record lies in access. The hard copy patient record, in many instances, is kept offsite in a storage facility and may not be easily accessible to the airway practitioner at the time of need. This is somewhat overcome by the use of an EPR; however, may still be limited to an individual location, meaning the alert generated may be a local alert only. Some centres, such as those in Queensland, Australia, have set up a statewide integrated EPR system. Any alert or addition to the patient record, including the anaesthetic chart, is included in the EPR and accessible by any other public hospital in the state. A similar process is currently being established in the NHS and is also seen in the Veterans Affairs Hospitals in the United States [31].

28.10 Dissemination of Information

28.10.1 Patient Consultation

Patient consultation and open disclosure of an anaesthetic incident are considered the standard of care in most countries. Patients need to be consulted, the situation explained, and future implications detailed. This is vital as in many situations the patient is an essential link in informing the future anaesthetist of a difficult airway history. Patient explanation and discussion should include both written and oral communication. Factors such as post-operative pain, medications and analgesia, anxiety, disrupted sleep, and understanding of medical terminology all limit the ability of a patient to take in and remember information communicated by the anaesthetist [31]. For this reason, timing for delivery of information is important and should not take place in the post-operative care/recovery unit, but rather at a later date when anaesthetic medications are not impairing cognition. In a study conducted in 2004, 50% of patients did not remember having a post-operative consultation with their anaesthetist regarding a difficult airway event [31, 48]. It was found, however, that the addition of a "difficult airway letter" sent to the patient's home proved a significant benefit. In this study, 92% of patients who had undergone further surgery post a difficult airway event had informed their anaesthetist of a difficult airway history, 41% had informed their GP, and 23% had registered with MedicAlert following receipt of their difficult airway letter [48]. As such, it is imperative that the limitations of verbal communication be recognised, the timing of communication be planned accordingly, and verbal dissemination of information should not be used interchangeably with written information, but rather in addition to provide the best model of patient education.

28.10.2 Physician and Patient Letters

Informing a GP of their patient's difficult airway encounter and the information surrounding it is vital. This information can then be added to the patient's GP file and included with any surgical referral in the future. Both the ANZCA Airway Management SIG and the updated 2015 DAS Difficult Airway Algorithm include this step as part of the post-operative care recommendations. In 2013, a study analysing difficult airway communications between anaesthetists and GPs found that communication was poor but could likely be improved by utilising standardised, simplified difficult airway letters [59]. Figure 28.9 below is an example of a customisable template created by DAS and available for use.

Difficult Airway Society

DAS Difficult Airway Database
C/o Department of Anaesthetics
Good Hope Hospital
Rectory Road, Sutton Coldfield
B75 7RR

To

Reference:

Dear Mr/Ms

We have received information from your Anaesthetist that there was a difficulty in managing your airway during your anaesthetic. Your Anaesthetist has requested that we issue you the enclosed 'Airway Alert Card'. We understand that you have given written consent for sharing your details with us for this purpose and for using your anonymous clinical details for research purposes. If that is not the case, please contact us urgently.

This card has valuable and potentially lifesaving information, should you have another operation or procedure under anaesthesia or sedation in the future. This information will also be useful, if you ever need support with your breathing due to any reason like an accident, choking, severe asthma etc., Please retain this card safely and show it to healthcare professionals treating you in the future.

In addition to the information printed on this card, detailed information on what happened during your anaesthetic is also held in a secure national database. This can be accessed by doctors using a code printed on the card (same as the Reference above). More information about this card (e.g., lost card) and national database are available on our website www.das.uk.com/aac

If you no longer want to keep your information on our database, please let us know and we will remove all your details with immediate effect. We might get in touch with you occasionally to gather information that will help us to improve this service. If you do not want to be contacted, please let us know at the earliest convenience.

This card is provided by DAS free of cost to you as part of our charitable activities. However, if you need a replacement card, that might be chargeable.

Yours sincerely

Alert card and Difficult Airway Database Team Difficult Airway Society-UK

DAS reserve the right to modify or discontinue this project at our discretion.
V2 AS 03/2020

Fig. 28.9 Example of a patient letter. (Reproduced from the Difficult Airway Society, DAS Airway Alert Card and Difficult Airway Database)

28.11 Recommendations for the Future

Although the utility of an integrated national and international database is well documented, to this day, such a database does not exist. This is likely due to a number of factors, including privacy laws which differ between countries, lack of funding to establish and maintain such a project long term, differences in agenda between participating and campaigning groups, and differences in hospital and healthcare facilities' patient record systems. Despite these hardships, an integrated, widely accessible, and difficult airway database allowing real-time access is undoubtedly the most efficient and effective way to improve future patient safety following a difficult airway event. The ability to access this information empowers airway practitioners, allowing for assessment and planning of airway management both in and out of the operating theatre. The DAS Difficult Airway Database, when widely instituted, will likely be a powerful tool and hopefully lead to other countries throughout the world adopting similar systems. It is the only system present, on a large scale, that addresses both patient safety and research capabilities.

In addition to the use of registries, standardisation of information to be documented allows for universal understanding of terminology. Much the same as Cormack-Lehane's direct views are universally recognised, there is a need for standardisation of documentation of videolaryngoscopy. The Fremantle Scoring System and the Video classification of Intubation are two systems showing promise. The VCI has some potential benefits over the Fremantle Score as it is not device dependent and includes a POGO score providing a quantitative description that can be compared over time. Regardless, more large-scale studies looking at inter-rater reliability are warranted to better assess their utility.

Standardised Difficult Airway Alert forms have appeared in many centres in recent years and are providing a tool for a comprehensive description of airway events. These, in many institutions, include a glossary of terminology and guidance on who and when an alert form should be generated. Many also provide recommendations for follow-up care, including patient consultation, notification of the patient's primary care physician, inclusion into relevant difficult airway databases, and inclusion into the electronic patient record. The post-event procedure should include both verbal and written communication with an explanation of future implications to the patient. The primary goal of such processes is to minimise negative outcomes to both patient and practitioner, which, although rare, when occur, can be catastrophic.

Ultimately, safe and effective management relies on four key points:

1. Standardisation of terminology and difficult airway databases.
2. Maximisation of database access and, in particular, real-time accessibility of patient information.

3. Standardisation and improvement of information dissemination post-event.
4. Ongoing education for:
   - Patient implications.
   - Practitioner familiarisation with processes and practices post-event.
   - Critical language and communication.
   - Primary care providers' understanding of terminology and implications of a difficult airway event on future care.

References

1. Hagberg CA. Chapter 54. In: Benumof and Hagberg's airway management. 3rd ed. Philadelphia: Elsevier; 2012.
2. Rose DK, Cohen MM. The incidence of airway problems depends on the definition used. Can J Anaesth. 1996;43(1):30–4. https://doi.org/10.1007/BF03015954.
3. Langeron O, Masso E, Huraux C, Guggiari M, Bianchi A, Coriat P, Riou B. Prediction of difficult mask ventilation. Anesthesiology. 2000;92(5):1229–36. https://doi.org/10.1097/00000542-200005000-00009. PMID: 10781266
4. Kheterpal S, Han R, Tremper KK, et al. Incidence and predictors of difficult and impossible mask ventilation. Anesthesiology. 2006;105(5):885–91. https://doi.org/10.1097/00000542-200611000-00007.
5. Kheterpal S, Martin L, Shanks AM, Tremper KK. Prediction and outcomes of impossible mask ventilation: a review of 50,000 anesthetics. Anesthesiology. 2009;110:891–7. https://doi.org/10.1097/ALN.0b013e31819b5b87.
6. Kheterpal S, Healy D, Aziz MF, Shanks AM, Freundlich RE, Linton F, Martin LD, Linton J, Epps JL, Fernandez-Bustamante A, Jameson LC, Tremper T, Tremper KK. Incidence, predictors, and outcome of difficult mask ventilation combined with difficult laryngoscopy: a report from the multicenter perioperative outcomes group. Anesthesiology. 2013;119:1360–9. https://doi.org/10.1097/ALN.0000435832.39353.20.
7. Verghese C, Brimacombe JR. Survey of laryngeal mask airway usage in 11,910 patients: safety and efficacy for conventional and nonconventional usage. Anesth Analg. 1996;82(1):129–33. https://doi.org/10.1097/00000539-199601000-00023.
8. Di Filippo A, Adembri C, Paparella L, et al. Risk factors for difficult Laryngeal Mask Airway LMA-Supreme™ (LMAS) placement in adults: a multicentric prospective observational study in an Italian population. Minerva Anestesiol. 2021;87(5):533–40. https://doi.org/10.23736/S0375-9393.20.15001-6.
9. Asai T, Koga K, Vaughan RS. Respiratory complications associated with tracheal intubation and extubation. Br J Anaesth. 1998;80(6):767–75. https://doi.org/10.1093/bja/80.6.767.
10. Rose DK, Cohen MM. The airway: problems and predictions in 18,500 patients. Can J Anaesth. 1994;41(5 Pt 1):372–83. https://doi.org/10.1007/BF03009858.
11. Shiga T, Wajima Z, Inoue T, Sakamoto A. Predicting difficult intubation in apparently normal patients: a meta-analysis of bedside screening test performance. Anesthesiology. 2005;103(2):429–37. https://doi.org/10.1097/00000542-200508000-00027.
12. Faramarzi E, Soleimanpour H, Khan ZH, Mahmoodpoor A, Sanaie S. Upper lip bite test for prediction of difficult airway: a systematic review. Pak J Med Sci. 2018;34(4):1019–23. https://doi.org/10.12669/pjms.344.15364.
13. American Society of Anesthesiologists Task Force on Guidelines for Management of the Difficult Airway. Practice Guidelines for management of the difficult airway. Anesthesiology. 1993;78:597–602.

14. Caplan RA, Posner K, Ward RJ, et al. Adverse respiratory events in anesthesia: a closed claims analysis. Anesthesiology. 1990;72:828.
15. Rose DK, Cohen MM. The airway problem and predictors in 18,500 patients. Can J Anaesth. 1989;41:372.
16. Cormack RS, Lehane J. Difficult tracheal intubation in obstetrics. Anaesthesia. 1984;39(11):1105–11.
17. Yentis SM, Lee DJ. Evaluation of an improved scoring system for the grading of direct laryngoscopy. Anaesthesia. 1998;53(11):1041–4. https://doi.org/10.1046/j.1365-2044.1998.00605.x.
18. Cook TM. A new practical classification of laryngeal view. Anaesthesia. 2000;55(3):274–9. https://doi.org/10.1046/j.1365-2044.2000.01270.x.
19. Levitan RM, et al. Assessment of airway visualisation: validation of the percentage of glottic opening (POGO) scale. Acad Emerg Med. 1998;5(9):919–23.
20. Ochroch EA, et al. Assessment of laryngeal view: percentage of glottic opening score vs Cormack and Lehane grading. Can J Anaesth. 1999;46(10):987–90.
21. Cook TM, Kelly FE. A national survey of videolaryngoscopy in the United Kingdom. Br J Anaesth. 2017;118(4):593–600. https://doi.org/10.1093/bja/aex052.
22. Lewis SR, Butler AR, Parker J, Cook TM, Smith AF. Videolaryngoscopy versus direct laryngoscopy for adult patients requiring tracheal intubation. Cochrane Database Syst Rev. 2016;11(11):CD011136. Published 2016 Nov 15. https://doi.org/10.1002/14651858.CD011136.pub2.
23. Chaggar RS, Shah SV, Berry M, Saini R, Soni S, Vaughan D. The Video Classification of Intubation (VCI) score: a new description tool for tracheal intubation using videolaryngoscopy: a pilot study. Eur J Anaesthesiol. 2021;38(3):324–6. https://doi.org/10.1097/EJA.0000000000001374.
24. Arulkumaran N, Lowe J, Ions R, Mendoza M, Bennett V, Dunser MW. Videolaryngoscopy versus direct laryngoscopy for emergency orotracheal intubation outside the operating room: a systematic review and meta-analysis. Br J Anaesth. 2018;120(4):712–24. https://doi.org/10.1016/j.bja.2017.12.041.
25. Bradley WP, Bain C, Mehra R, Symons J. Scoring systems for videolaryngoscopes. Anaesth Intensive Care. 2013;41(1):122.
26. O'Loughlin EJ, Swann AD, English JD, Ramadas R. Accuracy, intra- and inter-rater reliability of three scoring systems for the glottic view at videolaryngoscopy. Anaesthesia. 2017;72(7):835–9. https://doi.org/10.1111/anae.13837.
27. Chrimes N, Higgs A, Hagberg CA, Baker PA, Cooper RM, Greif R, Kovacs G, Law JA, Marshall SD, Myatra SN, O'Sullivan EP, Rosenblatt WH, Ross CH, Sakles JC, Sorbello M, Cook TM. Preventing unrecognised oesophageal intubation: a consensus guideline from the Project for Universal Management of Airways and international airway societies*. Anaesthesia. 2022; https://doi.org/10.1111/anae.15817.
28. Swann AD, English JD, O'Loughlin EJ. The development and preliminary evaluation of a proposed new scoring system for videolaryngoscopy. Anaesth Intensive Care. 2012;40(4):697–701. https://doi.org/10.1177/0310057X1204000417.
29. Chaggar RS, Shah SV, Berry M, Saini R, Soni S, Vaughan D. The Video Classification of Intubation (VCI) score: a new description tool for tracheal intubation using videolaryngoscopy: A pilot study. Eur J Anaesthesiol. 2021;38(3):324–6. https://doi.org/10.1097/EJA.0000000000001374. PMID: 33538438
30. Sajayan A, Nair A, McNarry AF, Mir F, Ahmad I, El-Boghdadly K. Analysis of a national difficult airway database. Anaesthesia. 2022;77(10):1081–8. https://doi.org/10.1111/anae.15820.
31. Feinleib J, Foley L, Mark L. What we should all know about our patient's airway. Difficult airway communications, database registries and reporting registries. Anesthiol Clin. 2015;33(2):397–413.
32. Cook TM, Woodall N, Frerk C. Major complications of airway management in the UK: results of the 4th National Audit Project of the Royal College of Anaesthetists and the Difficult Airway Society. Part 1 Anaesthesia. Br J Anaesth. 2011;106:617–31.

33. Cook TM, Woodall N, Harper J, Benger J. Major complications of airway management in the UK: results of the 4th National Audit Project of the Royal College of Anaesthetists' and the Difficult Airway Society. Part 2 Intensive Care and Emergency Department. Br J Anaesth. 2011;106:632–42.
34. Fourth National Audit Project of the Royal College of Anaesthetists and Difficult Airway Society. Major Complications of Airway management in the United Kingdom. In: Cook TM, Woodall N, Frerk C, editors. Report and findings. London: Royal College of Anaesthetists; 2011. Available from http://www.rcoa.ac.uk/document-store/nap4-full-report. Accessed 1 July 2016.
35. Woodall N, Frerk C, Cook TM. Can we make airway management (even) safer? Lessons from National audit. Anaesthesia. 2011;66(Suppl 2):27–33.
36. Balas EA, Boren SA. Managing clinical knowledge for health care improvement. In: Bemmel J, McCray AT, editors. Yearbook of medical informatics 2000. patient centred systems. Stuffgart: Schattauer Verlagsgesellschaft mbH; 2000. p. 65–70.
37. Chrimes N. The Vortex: a universal 'high-acuity implementation tool' for emergency airway management. Br J Anaesth. 2016;117(Suppl 1):i20–7. https://doi.org/10.1093/bja/aew175. Epub 2016 Jul 20. PMID: 27440673
38. Apfelbaum JL, Hagberg CA, Connis RT, Abdelmalak BB, Agarkar M, Dutton RP, Fiadjoe JE, Robert Greif P, Klock A, Mercier D, Myatra SN, O'Sullivan EP, Rosenblatt WH, Sorbello M, Tung A. American Society of Anesthesiologists practice guidelines for management of the difficult airway. Anesthesiology. 2022;2022(136):31–81. https://doi.org/10.1097/ALN.0000000000004002.
39. Stalhandske EJ, Bishop MJ, Bagian JP. Department of veterans affairs emergency airway management initiative. In: Henriksen K, Battles JB, Keyes MA, et al., editors. Advances in patient safety: new directions and alternative approaches, vol. 1: Assessment. Rockville: Agency for Healthcare Research and Quality; 2008. Available from: https://www.ncbi.nlm.nih.gov/books/NBK43632/.
40. Van Zundert AA, Endlich Y, Beckmann LA, et al. 2021 Update on airway management from the Anaesthesia Continuing Education Airway Management Special Interest Group. Anaesth Intensive Care. 2021;49(4):257–67. https://doi.org/10.1177/0310057X20984784.
41. Caplan RA, Posner KL, Ward RJ, Cheney FW. Adverse respiratory events in anesthesia: a closed claims analysis. Anesthesiology. 1990;72:828–33. https://doi.org/10.1097/00000542-199005000-00010.
42. Joffe AM, Aziz MF, Posner KL, Duggan LV, Mincer SL, Domino KB. Management of difficult tracheal intubation: a closed claims analysis. Anesthesiology. 2019;131:818–29. https://doi.org/10.1097/ALN.0000000000002815.
43. Lundstrøm LH, Møller AM, Rosenstock C, Astrup G, Gätke MR, Wetterslev J. A documented previous difficult tracheal intubation as a prognostic test for a subsequent difficult tracheal intubation in adults. Anaesthesia. 2009;64:1081–8. https://doi.org/10.1111/j.1365-2044.2009.06057.x.
44. Metzner J, Posner KL, Lam MS, et al. closed claims analysis. Best Pract Res Clin Anaesthesiol. 2011;25(2):263–76.
45. Kent CD, Metzner JI, Domino KB. Anesthesia hazards: lessons from the anesthesia closed claims project. Int Anesthesiol Clin. 2020;58(1):7–12. https://doi.org/10.1097/AIA.0000000000000256. PMID: 31800409
46. Lee LA, Domino KB. The Closed Claims Project. Has it influenced anesthetic practice and outcome? Anesthesiol Clin North Am. 2002;20(3):485–501. https://doi.org/10.1016/s0889-8537(02)00006-8. PMID: 12298302
47. Wharry S. MedicAlert Foundation turns 35, issues warning to MDs about lookalike bracelets. CMAJ. 1996;154(6):919–20. PMID: 8634974; PMCID: PMC1487804
48. Trentman TL, Frasco PE, Milde LN. Utility of letters sent to patients after difficult airway management. J Clin Anesth. 2004;16(4):257–61. https://doi.org/10.1016/j.jclinane.2003.08.011. PMID: 15261315

49. Brown CA 3rd, Bair AE, Pallin DJ, Walls RM, NEAR III Investigators. Techniques, success, and adverse events of emergency department adult intubations. Ann Emerg Med. 2015;65(4):363–370.e1. https://doi.org/10.1016/j.annemergmed.2014.10.036. Epub 2014 Dec 20. Erratum in: Ann Emerg Med. 2017 May;69(5):540. PMID: 25533140
50. Brown CA 3rd, Cox K, Hurwitz S, Walls RM. 4,871 Emergency airway encounters by air medical providers: a report of the air transport emergency airway management (NEAR VI: "A-TEAM") project. West J Emerg Med. 2014;15(2):188–93. https://doi.org/10.5811/westjem.2013.11.18549. PMID: 24672610; PMCID: PMC3966436
51. Tollefsen WW, Brown CA 3rd, Cox KL, Walls RM. Two hundred sixty pediatric emergency airway encounters by air transport personnel: a report of the air transport emergency airway management (NEAR VI: "A-TEAM") project. Pediatr Emerg Care. 2013;29(9):963–8. https://doi.org/10.1097/PEC.0b013e3182a219ea. PMID: 23974713
52. Brown CA 3rd, Bair AE, Pallin DJ, Laurin EG, Walls RM. National Emergency Airway Registry (NEAR) Investigators. Improved glottic exposure with the Video Macintosh Laryngoscope in adult emergency department tracheal intubations. Ann Emerg Med. 2010;56(2):83–8. https://doi.org/10.1016/j.annemergmed.2010.01.033. Epub 2010 Mar 3. PMID: 20202720
53. Sagarin MJ, Barton ED, Chng YM, Walls RM, National Emergency Airway Registry Investigators. Airway management by US and Canadian emergency medicine residents: a multicenter analysis of more than 6,000 endotracheal intubation attempts. Ann Emerg Med. 2005;46(4):328–36. https://doi.org/10.1016/j.annemergmed.2005.01.009. PMID: 16187466
54. Sagarin MJ, Chiang V, Sakles JC, Barton ED, Wolfe RE, Vissers RJ, Walls RM, National Emergency Airway Registry (NEAR) Investigators. Rapid sequence intubation for pediatric emergency airway management. Pediatr Emerg Care. 2002;18(6):417–23. https://doi.org/10.1097/00006565-200212000-00004. PMID: 12488834
55. Endlich Y, Lee J, Culwick MD. Difficult and failed intubation in the first 4000 incidents reported on webAIRS. Anaesth Intensive Care. 2020;48(6):477–87. https://doi.org/10.1177/0310057X20957657.
56. Endlich Y, Beckmann LA, Choi S-W, Culwick MD. A prospective six-month audit of airway incidents during anaesthesia in twelve tertiary level hospitals across Australia and New Zealand. Anaesth Intensive Care. 2020;48(5):389–98. https://doi.org/10.1177/0310057X20945325.
57. Heitmiller E, Martinez E, Pronovost PJ. Identifying and learning from mistakes. Anesthesiology. 2007;106:654–6. https://doi.org/10.1097/01.anes.0000264753.39511.4c.
58. Chrimes N, Cook TM. Critical airways, critical language. Br J Anaesth. 2017;118:649–54. https://doi.org/10.1093/bja/aex075.
59. Wilkes M, Beattie C, Gardner C, McNarry AF. Difficult airway communication between anaesthetists and general practitioners. Scott Med J. 2013;58(1):2–6. https://doi.org/10.1177/0036933012474554. PMID: 23596019
60. Bradley P, Chapman G, Crooke B, Greenland K. ANZCA Airway Assessment. 2016. https://www.anzca.edu.au/resources/incident-reporting-docs/airway-docs/pu-airway-assessment-20160916v1
61. Cook TM, Woodall N, Frerk C. A national survey of the impact of NAP4 on airway management practice in United Kingdom hospitals: closing the safety gap in anaesthesia, intensive care and the emergency department. Br J Anaesth. 2016;117(2):182–90. https://doi.org/10.1093/bja/aew177. PMID: 27440629
62. Cook TM. Strategies for the prevention of airway complications – a narrative review. Anaesthesia. 2018;73:93–111. https://doi.org/10.1111/anae.14123.

Chapter 29
Airway Management in the Context of the Wider Healthcare Organisational Framework

Jaideep J. Pandit

Highlights

1. **Systemic Scheduling Mitigates Stress:** Poorly planned and overbooked operating lists create severe time pressures compromising team performance during an airway crisis; using proactive planning frameworks like probabilistic list scheduling manages this.
2. **Pre-Assessment:** Identifies the difficult airway, helping secure specialized helping secure specialized equipment in advance and preparing patients for advanced procedures like awake fiberoptic intubation.
3. **Human factors:** understanding and overcoming cognitive biases in airway management such as anchoring bias, task focus and groupthink, using team training and crisis management simulations.
4. **Standardizing Video-Laryngoscopy:** Utilize videolaryngoscopy as the default standard.
5. **Evidence-Based, Clinician-Led Technology Selection:** Transitioning from small, binary product clinical trials to large-scale, post-marketing observational studies (under the ADEPT-2 strategy) ensures hospitals stock a diverse, clinician-selected range of niche airway devices organized in difficult airway carts.

J. J. Pandit (✉)
Nuffield Department of Anaesthetics, Oxford University Hospitals, Oxford, UK

Nuffield Department of Clinical Neuroscience, University of Oxford, Oxford, UK
e-mail: jaideep.pandit@sjc.ox.ac.uk

M. Á. Gómez-Ríos, A. van Zundert (eds.), *Evidence-based Guide to Difficult Airway Management*, https://doi.org/10.1007/978-3-032-30769-9_29

29.1 Introduction

This chapter discusses the broader context in which airway management occurs. We discuss three aspects: (1) the organisation of operating lists, (2) human factors and teamwork, (3) technology availability.

29.2 Organisation of Operating Lists

Airway management does not take place in a vacuum, but, notwithstanding emergency interventions in the emergency department or the ward, most often in the context of a surgical operating list. The planning of such lists is therefore crucial to creating a supportive environment for managing difficult airway patients. This has been especially highlighted by issues pertaining to out-of-operating-theatre difficult airway management [1–3], and management of the airway during the COVID-19 pandemic [4].

Recent research has focused on optimal planning of operating lists and the increasing appreciation that poorly planned, especially overbooked lists, create pressures on anaesthetists facing the challenge of a difficult airway [5]. Overbooking or inadequate patient preparation due to suboptimal pre-assessment can create both time pressures through list overrunning and pressures through additional, unanticipated medical problems. A stressed team may underperform during an airway management crisis [6].

Planning is facilitated through several steps (grade of evidence D). In advance of the day of surgery, managers should review lists using a 6-4-2 system (where the numbers refer to the weeks in advance that each list is reviewed) [7]. Aspects of the list reviewed include whether: the correct staff by grade and number are available; the correct equipment is available; additional support, such as postoperative critical care beds, is booked; and if the number of cases scheduled is appropriate for the time scheduled.

This last factor is aided by quantitative, probabilistic scheduling. The principle of this is to employ the mean of the known or estimated duration of the planned operation (including anaesthesia time) plus the standard deviation (SD) [8]. For a series of cases, these means and SDs are combined to generate a probability that the list will finish on time or over-run. This method is shown to be more effective than simply using the means of operation times [9], but does require teams and managers to think in terms of probability and not certainties. The data for operation times can be obtained from operating room computer logs or can be estimated with broadly similar results, but individual patient factors must be taken into account in these estimates. This is important in patients known to present difficulties in airway management, where additional time needs to be added to the estimate if advanced management techniques are to be employed. For lists where this is commonplace or routine, such as head and neck surgery, these timings should be automatically factored.

In addition to the scheduling of patients into lists, the time allocated for the list itself should be optimised, and there are processes described for achieving this. For example, a list that habitually overruns due to demands should be allocated more time to reduce overruns. All this will reduce the stress of the day [10].

While start times are important, as delayed starts can lead to delayed finishes and contribute to staff exhaustion and stress [11], start times in themselves do not necessarily contribute to inefficiency [12]. Instead, the factors causing late starts should be considered. These can include suboptimal patient preparation or the need to await key information, such as bed state. Where these are the norm, the start time should be adjusted rather than aspire in vain to meet an arbitrary start time that is never achievable [13].

Pre-assessment to optimise the medical condition of patients is always essential [14], and in the realm of airway management, this should include prediction of the difficult airway (grade of evidence A) [15]. It is now well established that clinical assessment correctly identifies almost all patients who are difficult (it may overestimate the numbers, but rarely do the tests miss a difficult airway) [16]. This presents an opportunity to schedule additional equipment (e.g. for advanced airway management techniques) and to discuss plans with the patient in advance to prepare them for interventions such as awake fibreoptic intubation [17].

29.3 Human Factors and Teamwork

Human factors is the recognition that innate cognitive biases influence performance, and mitigate these through systems design (grade of evidence D). This is especially the case in airway management [18]. Recency bias occurs when a recent encounter with a similar pathology (e.g. bronchospasm) leads the practitioner to mistakenly believe it is the same diagnosis again (in fact, a blocked tracheal tube). Anchoring bias is where the first diagnosis is rigidly held to, despite mounting evidence to the contrary, or where that later evidence is misinterpreted to fit the erroneous belief. Groupthink is where the whole team thinks in a certain way, and there are no challenges (e.g. for someone to question if the tracheal tube is correctly sited). Task focus is the inappropriate fixation on a particular goal (tracheal intubation) without considering alternatives (supraglottic airway) [19]. It is beyond the scope of this chapter to discuss how these can be engineered out of the system, but team training in crisis management is one important way to help overcome these [20].

Other aspects of teamwork and communication are relevant [21]. Before the start of the list, the team should identify and declare, including the surgical team, any patients with difficult airways so that all are aware that this may take more time and that surgeons may be called for assistance (e.g. front of neck access). Before a patient is sent for, the anaesthesia team should rehearse and play out the steps to be employed for induction and airway management: this should include a check that all equipment, including backup, is available. Anaesthetists in neighbouring rooms should also be alerted (and ideally the system should provide a spare 'n + 1' anaesthetist for each theatre suite). It is now recommended that, after induction of anaesthesia, each step of intubation is verbalised so that the assistant and team know what the anaesthetist is seeing, doing, and thinking. This is particularly the case with confirmation of end-tidal CO2 as evidence of correct tracheal placement [22–25]. Video-laryngoscopy (VL) with screen technology means that assistants can see the same view as the anaesthetist, and VL should now be standard as a replacement for direct Macintosh laryngoscopy [25].

Patients who are difficult to intubate are also difficult to extubate, and the same procedures are needed at the end of surgery. The number of staff available and their positioning around the patient's bed are also important, and specific recommendations have been made [26].

29.4 Technology Availability

There are several pertinent questions. Which devices/technology should be available? Who and how decides which to obtain? How is the technology best stored or made available? What training is necessary?

Hitherto, the research emphasis was probably on ascertaining the 'best' device, such as the supraglottic airway (SGA) and this approach was underlined by clinical trial designs that sought to compare one device vs another for one or more apparently relevant end-points (grade of evidence A). Although the trials were generally small in size (<100 patients), at least they generated some objective evidence of efficacy [27]. The evidence became important as many SGAs were introduced to the market, often without any clinical trial evidence. The increasing concern became that hospitals would purchase only the cheapest devices, with no regard for clinical efficacy. As a result, at least in the UK, the Difficult Airway Society developed its 'Airway Device Evaluation Project Team' (ADEPT) guidance to address this [28]. The principle was to establish a clinical standard that no device should be purchased unless it had at least one relevant published trial, which could be a set of observational studies. The peer-reviewed nature of the publication would increase the evidence base to a much higher level than existing, albeit lower than ideal. The strategy was coupled with a proposal that the industry would fund the recommended trials and that this funding would be structured in a way that strengthened academic departments; academic anaesthesia was internationally appreciated to be in some crisis. However, organisational inertia, the reluctance of industry to buy in, and an ever-dwindling anaesthesia research base meant the first 'ADEPT trial' was published only recently [29].

It is now better appreciated that the question is not a binary one, but rather that each airway device has its niche in the complex set of interventions needed to maintain oxygenation. Comparative clinical trials are not the best way to ascertain this, and as a consequence, an updated ADEPT-2 strategy has been proposed [30]. This has an emphasis on larger-scale observational studies, particularly at the post-marketing stage in device history, which are easier to perform (ethical permissions are generally not needed), inexpensive (the industry typically provides the devices for trials), and, given their size, more effective in establishing complication rates [31]. ADEPT-2 also emphasises the need for evidence-driven decision-making, where clinicians, rather than non-clinical managers, lead purchasing decisions.

This updated approach leads logically to the need to stock a range of devices—whether these are SGAs or VLs, etc.—and not just one class or type. Because each has its niche, different devices will likely be needed in different situations or challenges.

In terms of storage, the 'difficult airway cart' has become standard, although exact layouts are best determined by local needs, and also by some consideration of human factors elements discussed above (grade of evidence D) [32]. For example, which devices should be placed in the top vs. the bottom drawers, and in what combination within a drawer? In general, a logical system for drawers is to map onto the escalating interventions that may be necessary, from SGAs through to complex laryngoscopy (e.g. polio or straight blades) through to front-of-neck access. The number of carts in a theatre suite should also be considered based on likely need, with audits of frequency of use guiding such decisions. For some equipment, such as HFNO, there should likely be one device needed in each anaesthesia room/operating theatre [33].

29.5 Conclusions

The safe conduct of airway management requires a supportive planning structure within the overall hospital management. Advanced and careful planning of lists, in all their aspects, and the acquisition of appropriate equipment in quantities and range as dictated by evidence and clinician choice are important. Support for regular training, not just in the technical use of devices, but also in teamwork, communication, and crisis management is essential. Finally, there is a responsibility for the speciality and clinicians to conduct and publish trials on devices to generate the evidence on which decisions can be made.

Recommendations Table for Healthcare and Airway

Recommendation	Grade of evidence
Planning operating lists using data	D
Predicting the difficult airway	A
Consideration of human factors in the planning of the list	D
Selecting appropriate airway equipment according to the evidence base	A
Storage of equipment in specifically arranged airway carts	D

References

1. Brindley PG, Beed M, Law JA, Hung O, Levitan R, Murphy MF, Duggan LV. Airway management outside the operating room: how to better prepare. Can J Anaesth. 2017;64(5):530–9. English. https://doi.org/10.1007/s12630-017-0834-z.
2. Asai T. Airway management inside and outside operating rooms-circumstances are quite different. Br J Anaesth. 2018 Feb;120(2):207–9. https://doi.org/10.1016/j.bja.2017.10.010.
3. Karamchandani K, Wheelwright J, Yang AL, Westphal ND, Khanna AK, Myatra SN. Emergency airway management outside the operating room: current evidence and management strategies. Anesth Analg. 2021;133(3):648–62. https://doi.org/10.1213/ANE.0000000000005644.
4. Wei H, Jiang B, Behringer EC, Hofmeyr R, Myatra SN, Wong DT, Sullivan EPO, Hagberg CA, McGuire B, Baker PA, Li J, Pylypenko M, Ma W, Zuo M, Senturk NM, Klein U. Controversies in airway management of COVID-19 patients: updated information and international expert consensus recommendations. Br J Anaesth. 2021;126(2):361–6. https://doi.org/10.1016/j.bja.2020.10.029.
5. Pandit JJ, Westbury S, Pandit M. The concept of surgical operating list 'efficiency': a formula to describe the term. Anaesthesia. 2007 Sep;62(9):895–903. https://doi.org/10.1111/j.1365-2044.2007.05174.x.
6. Groombridge CJ, Kim Y, Maini A, Smit V, Fitzgerald MC. Stress and decision-making in resuscitation: A systematic review. Resuscitation. 2019 Nov;144:115–22. https://doi.org/10.1016/j.resuscitation.2019.09.023.
7. Barbagallo S, Corradi L, de Ville de Goyet J, Iannucci M, Porro I, Rosso N, Tanfani E, Testi A. Optimization and planning of operating theatre activities: an original definition of pathways and process modeling. BMC Med Inform Decis Mak. 2015;15:38. https://doi.org/10.1186/s12911-015-0161-7.
8. Pandit JJ, Tavare A. Using mean duration and variation of procedure times to plan a list of surgical operations to fit into the scheduled list time. Eur J Anaesthesiol. 2011 Jul;28(7):493–501. https://doi.org/10.1097/EJA.0b013e3283446b9c.
9. Pandit JJ. Rational planning of operating lists: a prospective comparison of 'booking to the mean' vs. 'probabilistic case scheduling' in urology. Anaesthesia. 2020;75(5):642–7. https://doi.org/10.1111/anae.14958.
10. Pandit JJ, Dexter F. Lack of sensitivity of staffing for 8-hour sessions to standard deviation in daily actual hours of operating room time used for surgeons with long queues. Anesth Analg. 2009 Jun;108(6):1910–5. https://doi.org/10.1213/ane.0b013e31819fe7a4.
11. Wong J, Khu KJ, Kaderali Z, Bernstein M. Delays in the operating room: signs of an imperfect system. Can J Surg. 2010;53(3):189–95.
12. Pandit JJ, Abbott T, Pandit M, Kapila A, Abraham R. Is 'starting on time' useful (or useless) as a surrogate measure for 'surgical theatre efficiency'? Anaesthesia. 2012;67(8):823–32. https://doi.org/10.1111/j.1365-2044.2012.07160.x.
13. Wachtel RE, Dexter F. Reducing tardiness from scheduled start times by making adjustments to the operating room schedule. Anesth Analg. 2009;108(6):1902–9. https://doi.org/10.1213/ane.0b013e31819f9fd2.
14. Rai MR, Pandit JJ. Day of surgery cancellations after nurse-led pre-assessment in an elective surgical Centre: the first 2 years. Anaesthesia. 2003;58(7):692–9. https://doi.org/10.1046/j.1365-2044.2003.03189_3.x.
15. Meachin JA. Airway management: from pre-assessment to intubation. A student ODP's perspective. J Perioper Pract. 2011 Sep;21(9):309–12. https://doi.org/10.1177/175045891102100903.
16. Pandit JJ, Heidegger T. Putting the 'point' back into the ritual: a binary approach to difficult airway prediction. Anaesthesia. 2017;72(3):283–8. https://doi.org/10.1111/anae.13720.
17. Reed AF, Han DG. Preparation of the patient for awake intubation. Anesthesiol Clin North Am. 1991;9:69–81.

18. Cortese G, Sorbello M, Di Giacinto I, Cedrone M, Urdaneta F, Brazzi L. Human factors and airway management in COVID-19 patients: the perfect storm? J Clin Med. 2022;11(15):4271. https://doi.org/10.3390/jcm11154271.
19. Stiegler MP, Neelankavil JP, Canales C, Dhillon A. Cognitive errors detected in anaesthesiology: a literature review and pilot study. Br J Anaesth. 2012;108(2):229–35. https://doi.org/10.1093/bja/aer387.
20. Gaba DM. Crisis resource management and teamwork training in anaesthesia. Br J Anaesth. 2010 Jul;105(1):3–6. https://doi.org/10.1093/bja/aeq124.
21. Gumbert SD. Communication of the difficult airway and dissemination of critical airway information. In: The difficult airway: a practical guide. New York/Oxford: Academic; 2013.; online edn. https://doi.org/10.1093/med/9780199794416.003.0018.
22. Pandit JJ, Young P, Davies M. Why does oesophageal intubation still go unrecognised? Lessons for prevention from the coroner's court. Anaesthesia. 2022 Feb;77(2):123–8. https://doi.org/10.1111/anae.15634.
23. Pandit JJ. 'No trace, wrong place' does not mean 'positive trace, right place'. Identifying and managing misplaced or displaced tracheal tubes in cardiopulmonary resuscitation. Anaesthesia. 2022 Jan;77(1):16–21. https://doi.org/10.1111/anae.15526.
24. Qureshi T, Hutton P, Pandit JJ. Sharpening PUMA's teeth: improving guidance for capnography to confirm tracheal intubation in cardiopulmonary resuscitation. Anaesthesia. 2023; https://doi.org/10.1111/anae.16002.
25. Chrimes N, Higgs A, Hagberg CA, et al. Preventing unrecognised oesophageal intubation: a consensus guideline from the project for universal management of airways and international airway societies. Anaesthesia. 2022;77:1395–415.
26. Difficult Airway Society Extubation Guidelines Group, Popat M, Mitchell V, Dravid R, Patel A, Swampillai C, Higgs A. Difficult airway society guidelines for the management of tracheal extubation. Anaesthesia. 2012;67(3):318–40. https://doi.org/10.1111/j.1365-2044.2012.07075.x.
27. Pandit JJ, MacLachlan K, Dravid RM, Popat MT. Comparison of times to achieve tracheal intubation with three techniques using the laryngeal or intubating laryngeal mask airway. Anaesthesia. 2002;57(2):128–32. https://doi.org/10.1046/j.0003-2409.2001.02401.x.
28. Pandit JJ, Popat MT, Cook TM, Wilkes AR, Groom P, Cooke H, Kapila A, O'Sullivan E. The difficult airway society 'ADEPT' guidance on selecting airway devices: the basis of a strategy for equipment evaluation. Anaesthesia. 2011;66(8):726–37. https://doi.org/10.1111/j.1365-2044.2011.06787.x.
29. Ní Eochagáin A, Athanassoglou V, Cumberworth A, Morris O, Corbett S, Jefferson H, O'Sullivan EP, Pandit JJ. Assessing a novel second generation laryngeal mask airway using the 'ADEPT' approach: results from the LMA® protector™ observational study. J Clin Monit Comput. 2023;37(2):517–24. https://doi.org/10.1007/s10877-022-00910-5.
30. Athanassoglou V, O'Sullivan EP, van Zundert A, Pandit JJ. New guidelines for research in airway device evaluation: time for an updated approach (ADEPT-2) to the difficult airway Society's 'ADEPT' strategy? J Clin Monit Comput. 2023;37(2):345–50. https://doi.org/10.1007/s10877-022-00911-4.
31. Pandit JJ. If it hasn't failed, does it work? On 'the worst we can expect' from observational trial results, with reference to airway management devices. Anaesthesia. 2012;67(6):578–83. https://doi.org/10.1111/j.1365-2044.2012.07155.x.
32. Bjurström MF, Bodelsson M, Sturesson LW. The difficult airway trolley: a narrative review and practical guide. Anesthesiol Res Pract. 2019;2019:6780254. https://doi.org/10.1155/2019/6780254.
33. Patel A, El-Boghdadly K. Facemask or high-flow nasal oxygenation: time to switch? Anaesthesia. 2022;77(1):7–11. https://doi.org/10.1111/anae.15593.

Chapter 30
Teaching and Training

Bastian Grande and Corinna von Deschwanden

30.1 Introduction

The procedure for an expected difficult airway can be planned and trained. That for an unexpected difficult airway cannot be predicted in time or sequence. Both entities deserve their place in training and education; they are a (life-) important part of clinical practice that must be mastered [1].

In the past, there has often been a great focus on technical means, for example, coniotomy, and less on the concrete application of the procedure defined in the algorithms or on teamwork.

Recently, systematic debriefing of challenging clinical situations has also come to the fore. This allows teams to learn together from each other based on specific situations they have experienced [2].

In what follows, we will have a look at these three essential elements of difficult airway training: (1) training formats, (2) training organization, (3) clinical debriefings, and (4) institutional strategies.

Throughout the chapter, a guideline is given on how organizations can provide structured training on difficult airways for their staff and how individual clinicians can be prepared for rare situations through regular training, act safely in a team, and

B. Grande (✉)
Institute of Anesthesiology and Perioperative Medicine, University Hospital Zurich, Zürich, Switzerland

Department of Health Sciences and Technology, ETH Zurich, Zürich, Switzerland
e-mail: Bastian.Grande@usz.ch

C. von Deschwanden
Institute of Anesthesiology and Perioperative Medicine, University Hospital Zurich, Zürich, Switzerland
e-mail: Corinna.VonDeschwanden@usz.ch

M. Á. Gómez-Ríos, A. van Zundert (eds.), *Evidence-based Guide to Difficult Airway Management*, https://doi.org/10.1007/978-3-032-30769-9_30

reflect on them afterwards. Another focus is the assessment of the training, which can establish a comparability with other and similar institutions.

Because there is no training that covers all needs at the same time, i.e., that works for large and small clinics, helps beginners and experts, and addresses both technical aspects and teamwork, difficult airway training has to be planned individually and adaptively. At the same time, the training of an algorithm always requires structural clarity and unambiguity. In this tension lies the implementation of a difficult airway training program.

Institutions are responsible for bringing together simulation techniques, learner engagement, and assessment of the learning strategy. This can only succeed with a strategy that includes all of the above: training format, organization, debriefing, and assessment.

30.1.1 Different Forms of Training

To train the skills described in airway management algorithms, different forms of training can be considered. In the following, the most successful ones are described: technical skills training, deliberate practice, full-scale simulator training, and so-called booster training. To be able to think about which training form to consider, it is worth looking at the training content. Several studies have shown which content can be trained in which form. For example, purely technical training in various tools for airway management always leads to a purely technical skill and not to mastering a complex clinical situation in the context of daily work [3]. At the same time, the training effort has to be compared to the expected learning experience. Thus, it could be shown that full-scale simulator training does not necessarily lead to an improvement in technical and behavioral skills compared to low-scale training [4]. Table 30.1 lists the different types of training with their respective advantages and disadvantages.

Which recommendation can be given for training the expected difficult airway, and especially the unexpectedly difficult airway? Unfortunately, no outcome-relevant studies are available comparing how much more efficiently such clinically challenging situations are resolved with one of the different training forms. Drawing on existing evidence in advanced cardiac life support training, a similarly acute situation that is rare and requires structure, recommendations for combined technical and behavioral training can be made at evidence level E [5].

The algorithm of the expected and unexpected difficult airway is clear on the one hand, but on the other hand, a deviation is often observed in clinical practice. Practicing purely technical skills cannot replace the interactions between the different team members. At the same time, those skills are a necessary condition to master difficult airway situations. In an interdisciplinary study with anesthesiologists and intensive care staff, Weiss et al. were able to show how a mixed form of technical and non-technical training can represent both conditions, addressing technical and

Table 30.1 Different simulation training types

Method	Description	Stock	Learning point	Plus	Delta
Task training	Training of different skills	Models, anatomically correct	Procedure and performance of the task	Low threshold practice and different skill grades possible	No complex task, no CRM training
Full scale simulation	Realistic physiological simulation in the context of the work environment	Full-scale mannequin and trained instructors, video recording	Complex processes and team learning	Effective team training method for training in context	Elaborate setting, high costs
Booster training	Short low-threshold refresher, self-guided	Same as task training, poss. e-learning	Task and process refresher, single or team-centered	High psychological safety	No feedback on performance, no corrections in task management
In situ simulation	Simulation in an environment in which employees work	Like full scale but with portable materials	Extremely effective for procedures and testing structural changes	The context of the environment is highlighted	Very high cost, risk of mixing with everyday clinical practice

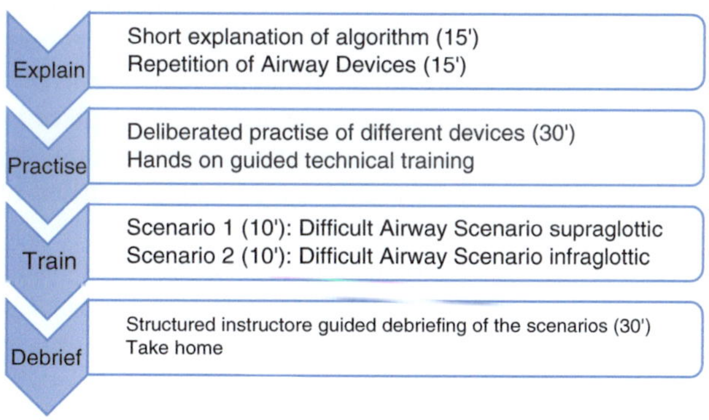

Fig. 30.1 Combined technical and behavioral airway management training

behavioral aspects [3]. Such combined training can first provide an overview of the different airway tools in the context of deliberate practice and then offer them in simple, low-scale scenarios that address the difficult airway (See Fig. 30.1) [6].

Similarly, low-threshold booster training is conceivable, where participants repeat what they have learned and deepen their knowledge and skills. Both forms are very straightforward to organize and make available to employees of clinical institutions [7, 8].

In summary, a mixture of different forms of training that addresses technical skills and behavior and is adapted to the circumstances of the clinical work of the employees is strongly recommended.

30.1.2 Training Organization

The goal of organized training in difficult airway management is to ensure that all clinicians who may be confronted with this task have the opportunity to practice the intended algorithm regularly. In addition, these individuals should be trained in the technical skills it requires and reflect simple team behaviors. This means that such training is always interprofessional and must be graduated on different skill levels.

The organization of such training regularly poses problems to institutions, mainly concerning the availability and working time of the staff. The organization has to be done individually, but the obstacles are usually the same and very solvable problems.

The availability of the employees and the working time allow only one solution: the training must take place during working hours and in situ, i.e., on site [9]. At the same time, it has proven useful to have these trainings accredited by the relevant professional association, so that the official character of a training is given and can serve as proof of participation for the employer [10].

There is always the possibility of a "self-guided-learning" versus an "instructor-guided-learning" in those trainings. In the former, the key is a clearly described learning path so that team members have clarity about learning content and objectives. In the second, the focus is on the training of the instructors and the role they take during the training. There is little evidence to support the benefits of one program or the other [11].

As necessary conditions, emphasis must be placed primarily on mastery of the technique, knowledge of the underlying algorithm, and essential aspects of team collaboration. All three points can be taught to different professions in a short time without losing the "red thread".

Mastering the use of different tools to secure the airway can be significantly improved by repetitive training. Biro et al. demonstrated in a prospective study how fast learning of common procedures (e.g., intubation with VAD, EGD, coniotomy) can be accomplished [12].

An algorithm underlying airway management can be theoretically practiced in the form of frontal teaching or digitally supported learning. Thus, the learner has theoretical knowledge, but not yet a handle on practical application. The comparison to learning a foreign language and the difficulties of applying it in everyday life in a foreign country is obvious. Therefore, based on existing evidence, it is not advisable to conduct theoretical tests of any kind. The learners or the instructors can do a repetition of the algorithm at the beginning of the training in a summarized form. Decisive importance is to be attached to the reflection of the application. Here, participants can learn from instructors, but instructors can also learn from participants who are confronted with respiratory problems in their everyday lives and help to improve both the training and the algorithm.

Lastly, teamwork cannot be captured in its complexity and depth in a short training. Emphasis should be placed on a few, but helpful, components such as role clarification, re-evaluation, and speaking up [6]. All other items found in the so-called crisis resource management (CRM) can, of course, also be practiced and alternately depending on the frequency of training [13, 14].

30.1.3 Clinical Debriefings

Management of a difficult airway does not occur in a social vacuum. Focusing on individual expertise in anesthesia is insufficient [15]. Operating room "tribes" influence management as do race and ethnicity. The operating room is an intense work environment where power imbalances, stereotypes, and unhealthy team dynamics interact to lead to poor communication, tension, and fatal patient outcomes [16]. The resulting challenges must be an integral part of the training in the management of difficult airways.

Increasing "collective competence" [15] to ensure sufficient difficult airway management includes, but is by no means limited to, the aforementioned forms of simulation-based training. In the clinical setting, briefings and debriefings represent the opportunity to collectively and continuously learn from defined performance episodes [17, 18]. Debriefings are structured meetings in which team members discuss, interpret, and learn from a specific event. They include both retrospective (e.g., "What did we do well and why?") and prospective considerations (e.g., "What can we improve? Why? How?"). Debriefings can follow a structure (Table 30.2) [sharing initial reactions, (c) collecting and analyzing perceptions, feedback, interactions, and (d) take-away messages [18].

Regular, brief debriefings are associated with improvements in team performance of greater than >20%, particularly in terms of clinical outcome and competence. When combined with briefings, debriefings improve team climate, coordination, and collaboration in the operating room.

At the same time, debriefings provide the space to establish a dialogue between and within the different professional groups. This possibility can lead to the fact that difficult airway management Training equally promotes the ability to reflect on these clinical situations. This so-called psychological safety also increases the ability to remain in exchange in real situations and not blindly rely on a single team leader.

30.1.4 Institutional Strategy

For institutions of any size, there is always the question of the return on training in rare situations compared to the cost. "If you think safety is expensive, try an accident." NASA's basic rule can be easily applied to critical medical situations. In BLS and ALS training, the premise has already become a reality—difficult airway

Table 30.2 Debriefing structure

Phase	Content	Example
Introduction	Setting the context for the debriefing and outlining the objectives	It is important to note that this debriefing is not about assigning blame or criticizing individuals, but rather about learning from our experiences and working together to improve. Are there any questions before we begin?
Reactions	Opportunity to share thoughts, feelings, and reactions, led by a facilitator, safe and non-judgmental	How do you feel after the scenario? What are your first thoughts or reactions?
Analysis, feedback	Provide a brief overview of the key events that took place during the event or activity being debriefed	What happened during the scenario? Who would like to start?
Interactions	Identify and discuss the positive aspects of the event, including any successes or achievements. Discuss any challenges or issues that arose during the event, and identify possible causes	What was your experience like? What did you learn? What was difficult? What was easy? What would you have done differently?
Take-away messages	Analyze the challenges and issues identified, and provide recommendations for addressing them in future events. Sum up the key points of the debriefing, and thank participants for their participation	Are there any final comments or questions before we conclude the debriefing? What do you take home? What are your key findings?

situations are no exception. The critical question is not whether training in difficult airway situations is conducted or not, but how it is conducted. This question can only be answered if the participants of the training evaluate the training and at the same time, a measurement of the participants' performance takes place. In this way, training can be continuously evaluated and, if necessary, measures can be introduced to bring about an improvement.

There are several validated questionnaires for the evaluation of training; meanwhile, the DASH® is the best-researched tool [19]. The participants should not be taken out of their psychological safety by individual performance observations during the training. It is much more worthwhile to keep the topic of difficult airway management in view institutionally via closed claims, CIRS, and individual reports. Such rapports can be completed after each use of difficult airway material and made available to staff. This step appears to be critical in learning from challenging situations, but should not lead to fear-based avoidance.

Overall, it is recommended not only to provide the strategy of the approach to the difficult airway in the form of algorithms but also to openly state the training strategy. The individual institutions are not only in charge of training, but they are also key to training competent teams.

References

1. Boulton AJ, Balla SR, Nowicka A, Loka TM, Mendonca C. Advanced airway training in the UK: a national survey of senior anesthetic trainees. J Anaesthesiol Clin Pharmacol. 2019;35(3):326–34.
2. Salas E, Rosen MA, King H. Managing teams managing crises: principles of teamwork to improve patient safety in the Emergency Room and beyond. Theor Issues Ergon Sci. 2007;8(5):381–94.
3. Grande B, Weiss M, Biro P, Grote G, Steiger P, Spahn D, et al. Ist Reden wichtig? Technisches versus kombiniert technisches/nicht-technisches Atemwegstraining in der Anästhesie und Intensivmedizin Is talking important? Technical versus combined technical/non-technical airway training in anaesthesia and intensive care medicine. Anästhesiol Intensivmed. 2015;01(56):5–12.
4. Lejus-Bourdeau C, Pousset F, Magne C, Bazin O, Grillot N, Pichenot V. Low-cost versus high-fidelity pediatric simulators for difficult airway management training: a randomized study in continuing medical education. Braz J Anesthesiol. 2021;
5. Kolbe M, Grande B. Team coordination during cardiopulmonary resuscitation. J Crit Care. 2013;28(4):522–3.
6. Grande B, Kolbe M, Biro P. Difficult airway management and training: simulation, communication, and feedback. Curr Opin Anaesthesiol. 2017;30(6):743–7.
7. Kerins J, McCully E, Stirling SA, Smith SE, Tiernan J, Tallentire VR. The impact of simulation-based mastery learning, booster session timing and clinical exposure on confidence in intercostal drain insertion: a survey of internal medicine trainees in Scotland. BMC Med Educ. 2022;22(1):621.
8. Sullivan A, Elshenawy S, Ades A, Sawyer T. Acquiring and Maintaining Technical Skills Using Simulation: Initial, Maintenance, Booster, and Refresher Training. Cureus. 2019;11(9):e5729.
9. Sabbagh AY, Alzaid HM, Almarshed AA, Azizalrahman AA, Elmasry S, Rosu CA, et al. A newly developed interprofessional in-situ simulation-based training for airway management of COVID-19 patients: identification of challenges and safety gaps, and assessment of the participants' reaction. J Clin Med Res. 2022;14(9):377–87.
10. Grande B, Zalunardo MP, Kolbe M. How to train thoracic anesthesia for residents and consultants? Curr Opin Anaesthesiol. 2022;35(1):69–74.
11. Sloth SB, Jensen RD, Seyer-Hansen M, Christensen MK, De Win G. Remote training in laparoscopy: a randomized trial comparing home-based self-regulated training to centralized instructor-regulated training. Surg Endosc. 2022;36(2):1444–55.
12. Biro P, Grande B, Kind SL, Spahn DR, Theusinger OM. Concluding results from the first phase of the Zurich unexpected difficult airway course based on exercise of technical skills. Anaesthesia. 2014;69(5):452–7.
13. Rall M, Dieckmann P. Safety culture and crisis resource management in airway management: general principles to enhance patient safety in critical airway situations. Best Pract Res Clin Anaesthesiol. 2005;19(4):539–57.
14. Gaba DM. Crisis resource management and teamwork training in anaesthesia. Br J Anaesth. 2010;105(1):3–6.
15. Lingard L. Paradoxical truths and persistent myths: reframing the team competence conversation. J Contin Educ Heal Prof. 2016;36(Suppl 1):S19–21.
16. Douglas RN, Stephens LS, Posner KL, Davies JM, Mincer SL, Burden AR, et al. Communication failures contributing to patient injury in anaesthesia malpractice claims☆. Br J Anaesth. 2021;127(3):470–8.
17. Kolbe M, Grande B, Spahn DR. Briefing and debriefing during simulation-based training and beyond: content, structure, attitude and setting. Best Pract Res Clin Anaesthesiol. 2015;29(1):87–96.
18. Kolbe M, Schmutz S, Seelandt JC, Eppich WJ, Schmutz JB. Team debriefings in healthcare: aligning intention and impact. BMJ. 2021;374:n2042.
19. Brett-Fleegler M, Rudolph J, Eppich W, Monuteaux M, Fleegler E, Cheng A, et al. Debriefing assessment for simulation in healthcare: development and psychometric properties. Simul Healthc. 2012;7(5):288–94.

MIX
Papier aus verantwortungsvollen Quellen
Paper from responsible sources
FSC® C105338

If you have any concerns about our products,
you can contact us on
ProductSafety@springernature.com

In case Publisher is established outside the EU,
the EU authorized representative is:
Springer Nature Customer Service Center GmbH
Europaplatz 3, 69115 Heidelberg, Germany

Printed by Libri Plureos GmbH
in Hamburg, Germany